ENVIRONMENTAL TOXICOLOGY:
Organic Pollutants

ELLIS HORWOOD BOOKS IN WATER AND WASTEWATER TECHNOLOGY

This collection of authoritative works reflects the awareness of the importance to the world of water, wastewater treatment, and closely related subjects. The titles are written and edited by experts from a wide range of countries closely concerned with research and development, monitoring and improving water quality and supplies, and treatment and disposal of wastewater.

Titles published in collaboration with the WATER RESEARCH CENTRE, UK

AQUALINE THESAURUS 2
Editor: G. BOTHAMLEY, Water Research Centre
BIOLOGICAL FLUIDISED BED TREATMENT OF WATER AND WASTEWATER
Editors: P. F. COOPER, Water Research Centre, and B. ATKINSON, University of Manchester Institute of Science and Technology
ENVIRONMENTAL TOXICOLOGY: Organic Pollutants
J. K. FAWELL and S. HUNT, Water Research Centre
ENVIRONMENTAL PROTECTION: Standards, Compliance and Costs
Editor: T. J. LACK, Water Research Centre
WATER RESEARCH TOPICS
Editor: I. M. LAMONT, Water Research Centre
SMALL WATER POLLUTION CONTROL WORKS: Design and Practice
E. H. NICOLL, Scottish Development Department, Edinburgh
RIVER POLLUTION CONTROL
Editor: M. J. STIFF, Water Research Centre

Other books in Water and Wastewater

WATER POLLUTION BIOLOGY
P. ABEL, Sunderland Polytechnic
ALKALINITY–pH CHANGES WITH TEMPERATURE FOR WATERS IN INDUSTRIAL SYSTEMS
A. G. D. EMERSON, Independent Consulting Technologist
CHEMICAL PROCESSES IN WASTE WATER TREATMENT
W. J. EILBECK, University College of North Wales, and
G. MATTOCK, Waste Water Treatment and Resource Recovery Consultant
BIOLOGICAL TREATMENT OF SEWAGE BY THE ACTIVATED SLUDGE PROCESS
K. HÄNEL, Research Leader of Purification of Sewage Team, Leipzig, East Germany
ANALYSIS OF SURFACE WATERS
H. HELLMANN, Federal German Institute of Hydrology, Koblenz
WATER-ABSTRACTION, STORAGE, TREATMENT, DISTRIBUTION
J. JEFFERY, General Manager, North Surrey Water Company
POLLUTION CONTROL AND CONSERVATION
Editor: M. KOVACS, Hungarian Academy of Sciences
NATURAL WATER SAMPLING
J. KRAJCA, Research Insitute of Geological Engineering, Brno, Czechoslovakia
GROUND RESOURCES AND YIELDS
H. KRIZ, Institute of Geography of the Czechoslovak Academy of Sciences, Czechoslovakia
PREVENTION OF CORROSION AND SCALING IN WATER SUPPLY SYSTEMS
L. LEGRAND, Former Head of the Water Dept. of City of Paris, and P. LEROY, Chemical Engineer of City of Paris, Chief of Corrosion Lab.
HANDBOOK OF WATER PURIFICATION Second Edition
W. LORCH, The Lorch Foundation
WATER MANAGEMENT IN INDUSTRY AND COMMERCE
P. MILLINGTON, Consulting Engineer, Staffordshire
BIOLOGY OF SEWAGE TREATMENT AND WATER POLLUTION CONTROL
K. MUDRACK, University of Hanover, FRG, and S. KUNST, Institute for Sanitary Engineering, Hanover, FRG
IMPROVING WATER QUALITY
M. RAPINAT, Compagnie Générale des Eaux, France
DRINKING WATER MATERIALS: Field Observations and Methods of Investigation
D. SCHOENEN and H. F. SCHÖLER, Hygiene-Institut der Universität, Bonn, FRG
HANDBOOK OF LIMNOLOGY
J. SCHWOERBEL, University of Freiburg, West Germany
BIOTECHNOLOGY OF WASTE TREATMENT AND EXPLOITATION
Editors: J. M. SIDWICK and R. S. HOLDOM, Watson Hawksley, Buckinghamshire
INTERACTION OF MICRO-ORGANISMS AND CHEMICAL POLLUTION OF WATER
D. TOTH and D. TOMASOVICOVA, Institute of Experimental Biology & Ecology, Bratislava
BIOLOGICAL TREATMENT OF WASTEWATER, 2nd Edition
M. WINKLER, University of Surrey

ELLIS HORWOOD BOOKS IN AQUACULTURE AND FISHERIES SUPPORT

Series Editor: Dr L. M. LAIRD, University of Aberdeen

BACTERIAL FISH PATHOGENS: Disease in Farmed and Wild Fish
B. AUSTIN and D. AUSTIN, Heriot-Watt University
MICROBIAL BIOTECHNOLOGY: Freshwater and Marine Environments
B. AUSTIN and D. AUSTIN, Heriot-Watt University
MICROBIOLOGICAL METHODS FOR FISH AND SHELLFISH
B. AUSTIN and D. AUSTIN, Heriot-Watt University
AQUACULTURE, Volumes I & II
G. BARNABÉ, Université des Sciences et Techniques du Languedoc
AUTOMATED BIOMONITORING
D. GRUBER and J. DIAMOND, Biological Monitoring Inc., Virginia, USA
SALMON AND TROUT FARMING
L. M. LAIRD and T. NEEDHAM, University of Aberdeen
MARINE FISH FARMING: Warm Water Marine Culture
J. F. MUIR, University of Stirling

ENVIRONMENTAL TOXICOLOGY: Organic Pollutants

J. K. FAWELL, B.Sc.
Head of Environmental Toxicology
and
S. HUNT, B.Sc.
Head of Mutagenicity
both of Water Research Centre, Medmenham, Bucks

ELLIS HORWOOD LIMITED
Publishers · Chichester

Halsted Press: a division of
JOHN WILEY & SONS
New York · Chichester · Brisbane · Toronto

First published in 1988 by
ELLIS HORWOOD LIMITED
Market Cross House, Cooper Street,
Chichester, West Sussex, PO19 1EB, England
The publisher's colophon is reproduced from James Gillison's drawing of the ancient Market Cross, Chichester.

Distributors:
Australia and New Zealand:
JACARANDA WILEY LIMITED
GPO Box 859, Brisbane, Queensland 4001, Australia
Canada:
JOHN WILEY & SONS CANADA LIMITED
22 Worcester Road, Rexdale, Ontario, Canada
Europe and Africa:
JOHN WILEY & SONS LIMITED
Baffins Lane, Chichester, West Sussex, England
North and South America and the rest of the world:
Halsted Press: a division of
JOHN WILEY & SONS
605 Third Avenue, New York, NY 10158, USA
South-East Asia
JOHN WILEY & SONS (SEA) PTE LIMITED
37 Jalan Pemimpin # 05–04
Block B, Union Industrial Building, Singapore 2057
Indian Subcontinent
WILEY EASTERN LIMITED
4835/24 Ansari Road
Daryaganj, New Delhi 110002, India

British Library Cataloguing in Publication Data
Environmental toxicology.
1. Drinking water. Organic pollutants
I. Fawell, J. K. (John Kirtley), *1945–*
II. Hunt, S. (Stephen), *1961–*
628.1'68

Library of Congress Card No. 88–12960

ISBN 0–7458–0194–3 (Ellis Horwood Limited)
ISBN 0–470–21157–1 (Halsted Press)

Typeset in Times by Ellis Horwood Limited
Printed in Great Britain by Hartnolls, Bodmin

Table of contents

Introduction

Drinking water usually contains a complex mixture of organic chemicals of a remarkably diverse range of chemical type. The substances are of natural and anthropogenic origin, although often a distinction between the two is difficult to make. Anthropogenic substances can be introduced into raw waters by industrial and domestic effluents, surface drainage, spillage etc and by less obvious routes such as synthesis during disinfection.

In the early 1970s, traces of chlorinated compounds were detected in drinking water. This discovery, along with the increasing tendency to draw supplies from water sources known to include effluent from industrial and domestic sewage works, and aided by the advent of advanced analytical techniques, which enabled the measurement of minute traces of organic compounds in water, was the stimulus for a large international programme of research into micro-contaminants in drinking water. The driving force behind this development was mainly concern over potential health risks, such as carcinogenicity, that may be associated with long-term exposure to small amounts of organic chemicals.

As part of the programme to study micro-contaminants in water, in the UK, the Water Research Centre carried out analysis of a range of raw and treated drinking waters using gas chromatography–mass spectrometry (GC–MS). In an initial study, a small number of raw and treated waters were taken from waterworks treating lowland river water which contained relatively high levels of wastewater. This was followed by a survey of 14 treated drinking waters derived from surface water, of a wide range in quality, and groundwater (Fielding *et al* 1981).

Several hundred compounds were identified, the majority of which were present in very low concentrations ($<1\ \mu g/l$) and most of which were identified in only a small proportion of the samples examined. These were grouped into classes and sub-classes (Table 1) in order to aid toxicological assessment. Subsequently a number of additional compounds were identified in a later, unpublished survey of treated waters.

Since a substantial number of compounds had been identified in drinking water the next stage was to assess whether the presence of these compounds constituted any hazard to the health of consumers. In order to facilitate this, critical reviews of the toxicology of individual and groups of compounds were prepared using data gathered primarily from published sources. This volume comprises the great majority of those reviews.

Although the reviews were written for the purpose outlined above it was considered that the collection of such a large body of information would be of value to others interested in the health aspects of organic contaminants in the environment.

The reviews were prepared between 1983 and 1987 and although it is recognised that some compounds reviewed are under continuing investigation the data included in this book represent a substantial proportion of the published literature on the toxicology of each compound. It is therefore intended that it should be used as a reference source by anyone interested in the toxicology of these compounds, many of which will be found not just as water pollutants but as common environmental pollutants.

It must be stated that the prime interest was long-term exposure to low levels of contaminants so, although acute toxicity was considered, greater emphasis was given to chronic toxicity and carcinogenicity where data were available. The extent of the discussion largely reflects the perceived importance, at the time, of each one as a drinking water contaminant in combination with the amount of information available.

Table 1. Classes of compounds identified in treated waters

A – Hydrocarbons
- A1. Hydrocarbons – saturated/unsaturated aliphatic
- A2. Hydrocarbons – alicyclic
- A3. Hydrocarbons – aromatic
- A4. Hydrocarbons – polynuclear aromatic

B – Halogenated compounds
- B1. Halogenated aliphatics
- B2. Halogenated aromatics
- B3. Halogenated ethers
- B4. Miscellaneous halogenated compounds

C – Carboxylic acids and esters
- C1. Acids
- C2. Esters of carboxylic acids

D – Oxygenated compounds
- D1. Ketones
- D2. Aldehydes
- D3. Ethers
- D4. Miscellaneous oxygenated compounds

REFERENCE

FIELDING M, GIBSON T M, JAMES H A, MCLOUGHLIN K, and STEEL C P (1981) Organic micropollutants in drinking water, Technical Report TR159 Water Research Centre, Marlow.

Acknowledgements

We wish to acknowledge the substantial contribution of the following in the preparation of these reviews: Mr C Barnett, Miss H Brand, Miss C Chrzanowska, Mr K Owen, Miss P Tilling, Mr T Robertson and Mr R Weaver.

We would like to thank Dr J W Ridgway for his criticism and Mrs P Dixon and Miss B Harris for preparing the manuscript.

Since some of the information in this monograph was collected and prepared as part of DoE funded work we wish to thank the department.

1

Chloroform

1. INTRODUCTION

Chloroform is a colourless volatile liquid at room temperature, with a sweet taste and a characteristic odour. It is relatively soluble in water compared to other haloalkanes, but also has a high lipid solubility.

Chloroform is still used as an industrial solvent and chemical intermediate.

CAS Reg No:	67-66-3
Molecular weight:	199.390
Boiling point:	61.2°C
Odour threshold in water at 60°C:	1.2 mg/l (Alexander *et al* 1982)
Taste threshold in water at 40°C	12 mg/l (Alexander *et al* 1982)

2. EXPOSURE

2.1 Air

Contamination from industrial sources makes chloroform a common air pollutant (Yung *et al* 1975). Mean concentrations for atmospheric chloroform range from 0.045 $\mu g/m^3$ to 5 $\mu g/m^3$ (Lillian *et al* 1975, Singh *et al* 1977, Grimsrud and Rasmussen 1975, Russell and Sandoff 1977). Chloroform has also been detected as a photochemical product in simulated ambient air containing trichloroethylene, and it is suggested that a portion of the atmospheric chloroform may result from photochemical reactions of trichloroethylene in air (Appleby *et al* 1976).

2.2 Food

Chloroform has been detected in dairy products, meat, oils and fats, beverages, fruits and vegetables up to a maximum level of 30 mg/kg (McConnell 1975, Pearson and McConnell 1975). In 1976 chloroform was banned as an additive in drug and cosmetic products in the United States, and its sale and use in the cosmetic and pharmaceutical industry in the United Kingdom has been restricted since 1986 (US Food and Drug Administration 1976, Statutory Instruments 1984).

2.3 Water

Chloroform was detected in all 14 drinking water samples in a WRc survey (Water Research Centre 1981). It is formed during the chlorination of water and sewage (Rook 1974, Symons *et al* 1975) via the haloform reaction (US Environmental Protection Agency 1980, Yung *et al* 1975), (NIOSH 1977, Bellar *et al* 1974, Symons *et al* 1975). Kroneld (1986) determined the monthly concentrations of chloroform in tap water over one year in Finland. The lowest concentration occurred in January, when chloroform concentration was 11.7 μg/l, and peaked in November, when the concentration reached 106.2 μg/l. The variation in concentration was probably due to seasonal temperatures influencing the rate of the haloform reaction, as there was a gradual rise in chloroform concentration as the year progressed. Water is possibly now the major source of environmental exposure to chloroform.

3. TOXICOKINETICS

Chloroform is rapidly and extensively absorbed through the lungs and from the gastrointestinal tract. Significant absorption through the skin has also been shown with liquid contact or submersion (Torkelson *et al* 1976).

Tsurata (1975, 1977) studied the percutaneous absorption of liquid chloroform applied to a shaved area of mouse abdominal skin. Absorption increased linearly with time over the 15-minute exposure period, and was directly related to water solubility. The absorption rate for chloroform was 329 nmol/min/cm^2 skin. This result was extrapolated to calculate the amount that would be absorbed into the human body as the result of 1-minute immersion of both hands (total area 800 cm^2) into liquid chloroform. The estimated amount absorbed, 29.7 mg/min, suggested that skin absorption from liquid contact could be a significant route of entry into the body for chloroform under these circumstances. However, the significance of these findings to skin absorption of chloroform from dilute aqueous solutions is not clear.

The rate of gastrointestinal absorption of chloroform after oral ingestion has not been specifically studied. However, absorption does occur readily with chloroform, due to its neutral and lipophilic properties (Sato and Nakajima 1979). Brown *et al* (1974a,b) concluded that [^{14}C]chloroform in olive oil given orally to mice, rats and monkeys at a dose of 60 mg/kg was totally absorbed, by virtue of a 93–98% recovery of radioactivity in exhaled air, urine and carcass. Absorption was rapid, with peak blood levels at one hour after administration in mice and monkeys.

After absorption, chloroform is distributed throughout the body, the concentration varying with the duration of the exposure and dose. Accumulation of chloroform occurs in tissues with a high fat content.

Kroneld (1986) carried out a 12-month study into the plasma chloroform concentration of patients with various diseases and healthy individuals drinking chlorinated tap water. Controls were healthy individuals drinking non-chlorinated well water. Only about 4% of the 200 healthy individuals had plasma concentrations of 20–25 nmol/l and 20–50 nmol/l for blood cell samples during the whole study period. Of the 210 patients, about 3% had plasma concentrations of 20–25 nmol/l and 20–55 nmol/l for blood cell samples. The control individuals, as well as their drinking water, showed no trace of chloroform. It would appear from this study that chronic ingestion of chloroform at levels from 11.7 μg/l (January) to 106.2 μg/l (November) resulted in very little change in the chloroform plasma concentration in patients and healthy individuals drinking chlorinated tap water.

Taylor *et al* (1974) have studied the distribution of chloroform in CF/LP, CBA and C57 Black mice. One group of male mice and one of female mice were dosed with 60 mg/kg (500 μCi/kg) [^{14}C]chloroform. At 3, 5, 7, and 24 hours post-treatment a single animal from each group was killed, and whole-body autoradiographs prepared. The results showed that male mice, irrespective of strain, accumulated most radioactivity in the liver and kidney, and by 3 hours there was a clear difference between the radioactive content of the renal cortex and medulla. High levels of radioactivity also appeared in the intestine, connective tissue and bladder, with smaller amounts in the salivary glands and brown fat. In the females, greater amounts of radioactivity appeared in the liver, intestine and bladder. Much less radioactivity was found in the kidney, and there was little difference between medulla and cortex. A similar distribution pattern was observed 5 and 7 hours after treatment. Twenty-four hours after dosing, radioactivity was reduced, but the distribution remained the same.

In additional studies on the kidney, male and female mice of each strain were dosed with 30 mg/kg (250 μCi/kg) [^{14}C]chloroform, and killed 5 hours after treatment (Taylor *et al* 1974). There was a highly significant difference between the activity present in the kidneys of males and females of each strain. The male CBA mice showing significantly higher amounts than either the CF/LP or C57 Black strains. For all three strains, livers of females contained more radioactivity than those of males, but differences in the amount of radioactivity between females of the same strain were not significant. There were no significant differences between the amount of radioactivity in brown fat or blood between sexes or strains.

A number of studies have suggested that the main pathway for chloroform metabolism is its oxidation to phosgene by an oxygen-dependent mixed function oxidase system (Sipes *et al* 1977, Pohl *et al* 1980a, b, Ilett *et al* 1973, Mansuy *et al* 1977). The initial step in this pathway involves the oxidation of the aliphatic carbon (C–H) to trichloromethanol by a phenobarbital-inducible cytochrome P-450 (Sipes *et al* 1977, Ilett *et al* 1973, Pohl *et al* 1980b). It is assumed that the highly unstable trichloromethanol spontaneously dehydrochlorinates to produce the highly reactive phosgene, which has been shown to be formed by rat liver microsomes *in vitro*. The electrophilic phosgene may then react with water to produce carbon monoxide, with macromolecules to form covalently bound products (Pohl *et al* 1977), or undergo condensation reactions with glutathione and possibly cysteine.

Pohl and Krishna (1978) have found that the metabolism of chloroform to phosgene by rat liver microsomes is oxygen and NADPH dependent. Carbon monoxide and SKF 525-A, known inhibitors of cytochrome P450, also inhibit chloroform metabolism, further supporting a role for cytochrome P450 in chloroform metabolism.

Additional evidence for oxidative dechlorination has been produced by Pohl *et al* (1980a), who measured the covalent binding of ^{14}C- and ^{3}H-labelled chloroform to

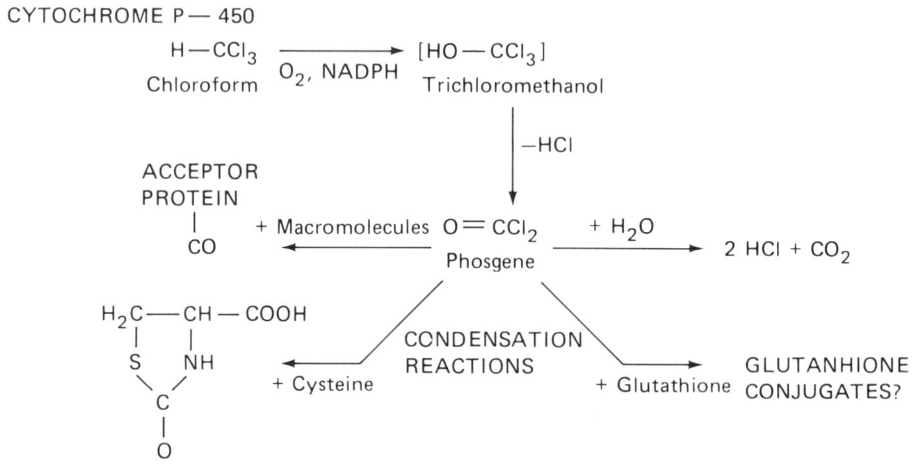

Fig. 1 — Major oxidative pathways of chloroform metabolism. Under normal oxygen conditions the major pathway is by oxidative dechlorination to trichloromethanol, but under hypoxic conditions the minor reductive pathway may become more prevalent, resulting in higher than normal production of the dichlormethyl radical.

cellular macromolecules. The results of this study showed that the majority of the label bound to cellular protein was from the ^{14}C-labelled chloroform. This study therefore suggests that reductive dechlorination is not the major pathway for chloroform metabolism under aerobic conditions. The finding that deuterated chloroform was metabolised more slowly than normal chloroform (Pohl and Krishna 1978, Pohl *et al* 1979) infers that cleavage of the C–H bond of chloroform is the rate-determining step in this enzymic pathway.

In the presence of cysteine and an [^{180}]oxygen atmosphere, [^{18}O]-oxygen was incorporated into the 2-oxo position of 2-oxothiazolidine-4-carboxylic acid due to a condensation reaction between phosgene and cysteine. This has been cited as further evidence for the production of phosgene by an oxidative dechlorination mechanism (Pohl *et al* 1977). Pretreatment of rats with cysteine tends to protect against the hepatotoxicity of chloroform. This may be an important *in vivo* protection mechanism, and may account for the depletion of cellular glutathione levels noted by many research groups.

Under anaerobic conditions about 30% of aerobic chloroform metabolism still occurs (Pohl *et al* 1980a), suggesting the presence of an alternative, reductive pathway. Tomasi *et al* (1985) have shown that several trihalomethanes, including chloroform, undergo reductive metabolism in isolated rat hepatocytes, incubated under nitrogen, giving rise to free radical intermediates.

The reductive metabolism of chloroform is also stimulated by pretreatment of rats with phenobarbital and reduced by cytochrome P-450 inhibitors. This would suggest that the cytochrome P-450 system is the site for both the oxidative and reductive pathways. Therefore, it would seem reasonable to suggest a dual activation pathway for chloroform; the major oxidative pathway relevant under normal oxygen conditions, and the minor reductive pathway occurring under relative hypoxia resulting, for example, from perturbation in the liver blood flow.

Taylor *et al* (1974) studied the cellular distribution of chloroform metabolites in the kidneys of male and female CF/LP mice. The mice were dosed with 60 mg/kg (500 μCi/kg) [^{14}C]chloroform, and killed 5 hours post-treatment. The kidneys were then homogenised, and the amount of radioactivity present in the fractions determined. This study showed that the quantities of radioactivity in the tissue fractions from the male kidneys are greater than the corresponding fractions for the females except in the nucleic acid fraction, where the amounts are approximately the same. Both the acid-soluble and lipid-soluble extracts from male kidneys contained about 2.5–3 times the radioactivity present in the female fractions, whereas the radioactivity in the protein residues from male kidneys was six times greater than from the females.

Pulmonary excretion of chloroform was investigated by Fry *et al* (1972) in male and female volunteers given 0.1–1.0 g [^{14}C]chloroform in olive oil in a gelatin capsule. Chloroform was determined in expired air by gas–liquid chromatography. Following a peak blood concentration of 0.5 mg/l for 500 mg dose 1 hour after oral dosage, absorption and distribution, the blood chloroform concentration declined exponentially with three components:

(1) A very rapid disappearance with half-life of 14 minutes, possibly due to the kinetics of organs with high blood flow and high diffusion rate constant.
(2) A slower disappearance with half-life of 90 minutes corresponding to the kinetics of muscle and skin.
(3) A very slow disappearance with very long half-life from adipose tissue. This half-life was not determined, but chloroform was detected in the blood and expired air 24 hours after administration.

Chloroform is not excreted unchanged in significant amounts from the body by any route other than the lungs. Brown *et al* (1974b) identified chloroform at high concentration in the bile of squirrel monkeys after oral [^{14}C]chloroform administration, and suggested a significant entero-hepatic recirculation in this species. For monkeys they found only 2% of dose in combined urine and faeces collected for 48 hours, and only 8% and 3% for rats and mice respectively.

4. HEALTH EFFECTS

4.1 Acute and subacute toxicity

Chloroform is of low acute toxicity in rodents, though males are slightly more sensitive than females. In young adult Sprague–Dawley rats the oral LD50s were 908 mg/kg in males and 1117 mg/kg in females (Chu *et al* 1980). In older adult males of the same strain the oral LD50 was 1188 mg/kg (Kimura *et al* 1971). In male ICR mice the oral LD50 was found to be 1120 mg/kg and in females 1400 mg/kg (Bowman *et al* 1978).

Vessell *et al* (1976) showed that C57BL/6J mice were four times more resistant to the acute toxic effects of chloroform than DBA/2J mice, while F1 hybrids showed intermediate susceptibility.

Torkelson *et al* (1976) found that one or two applications of chloroform on the skin of rabbits resulted in hyperaemia and moderate necrosis. When liquid was instilled into the eyes of rabbits some corneal injury was evident in addition to conjunctivitis.

Chloroform has been associated with the induction of hepatic enzymes in rats. Ornithine decarboxylase (ODC) induction has been suggested as a marker for liver and kidney regenerative hyperplasia. Savage *et al* (1982) studied the effect of chloroform on this enzyme in both liver and kidney. Fisher albino rats were dosed by intraperitoneal injection with 750 mg/kg chloroform, and sacrificed 18 hours post-treatment. Chloroform produced a 43.5 fold enhancement of hepatic ODC. Repeated administration of 500 mg/kg chloroform to male rats for 7 days resulted in a smaller induction of hepatic ODC than a single dose. They concluded that hepatic regenerative hyperplasia induced by chloroform in rats appeared to be associated with the induction of ODC, while this was not the case in the kidney. Similar results have been obtained by Pereira *et al* (1984).

A more comprehensive study on the effect of chloroform on hepatic enzymes has been carried out by Groger and Grey (1979). Eighteen groups of Wistar rats, 6 males and 6 females per group, were orally intubated with solutions of chloroform in groundnut oil to give dose levels of 0, 0.5, 1.0, 5.0, 25.0 and 50.0 mg/kg. One of the three groups at each dose level was killed after 1 dose, 5 doses and 10 doses. The rats treated 5 and 10 times received the dose once daily. A range of cellular enzymes from the cytosol, mitochondria, lysosomes and peroxisomes, and soluble phase were assayed. Most of the enzymes were induced by chloroform after the initial dose, but were either reduced or returned to near normal activity after repeated doses.

Yannai (1983) investigated the adrenocortical response to a single dose of chloroform in young male albino rats. The rats were dosed with 1.5 mg/kg chloroform in corn oil, while the controls received corn oil only. The rats were sacrificed over a 20-day period, and the adrenal glands removed. Samples of blood were also taken from the sacrificed animals for plasma corticosterone determination. Adrenal hypertrophy occurred 24 hours after treatment, and persisted for at least 12 days after treatment. A decrease in cholesterol content of the adrenal was taken as an indirect sign of increased adrenal activity, cholesterol being the precursor of the corticosteroids. The cholesterol content began to decrease 2 hours after chloroform administration, although this fall was not significant. However, 24 hours after treatment, cholesterol content was significantly increased and remained so until 12 days post-treatment. High plasma corticosterone levels were evident 15 minutes after treatment in both the treated and control animals. It is suggested that this was due to stress caused by administration by gavage. After 3 hours, the control plasma corticosterone levels returned to near normal levels, while in the treated animals the level remained high, peaking 24 hours after treatment. The author suggested that the hypersecretion of corticosterone results in increased demand for cholesterol, which would explain the increase in adrenal cholesterol content observed from days 3 to 16 post-treatment.

4.2 Chronic toxicity

Most data on the chronic toxicity of chloroform are derived from carcinogenicity studies (section 4.4).

Inhalation studies of rats, rabbits and guinea-pigs exposed to 25, 35, or 50 ppm for 7 hours/day 5 days/week for 6 months showed higher mortality, organ weight differences and histopathological changes in the liver and kidney when compared to controls. The changes in liver pathology appeared to be reversible at the lowest exposure (Torkelson *et al* 1976).

Guinea-pigs and rats were dosed orally with 0.4 mg/kg, 35 mg/kg or 125 mg/kg for 5 months. No adverse effects were seen in the animals dosed with 0.4 mg/kg. At the higher doses there were changes in haematology in the guinea pigs, and an impaired ability to develop new conditioned reflexes in the rat (Miklashevski *et al* 1966).

4.2.1 Nephrotoxicity

Chloroform has been found to cause nephrotoxicity in the mouse, rat and rabbit.

Smith *et al* (1984) showed that, in mice, males are more susceptible to chloroform-induced nephrotoxicity than females. Castration of male mice eliminated this susceptibility and reduced renal mixed function oxidase activity to that observed in female mice. Incubation of liver slices, isolated from rats treated with chloroform, in a carbon monoxide:oxygen atmosphere showed a reduction in chloroform toxicity, suggesting that microsomal metabolism potentiates the toxicity of chloroform in the mouse.

Smith *et al* (1985) investigated the renal toxicity of chloroform using adult male Fischer 344 and Sprague–Dawley rats. The results from this study suggest that rat kidney metabolises and responds differently qualitively and quantitatively from the mouse or rabbit kidney. In the rat renal cortical tissue, chloroform was metabolised to carbon dioxide and a reactive metabolite capable of binding to macromolecules. In addition, an atmosphere of carbon monoxide:oxygen, which inhibits cytochrome P-450, did not alter chloroform toxicity, whereas carbon monoxide did reduce toxicity in the mouse (Smith and Hook 1983). This suggests that intrarenal bioactivation of chloroform by cytochrome P-450 may not play a major role in chloroform nephrotoxicity in the rat.

Taylor *et al* (1974) studied the changes in chloroform distribution caused by hormone treatment in male and female CF/LP mice. Three males were injected daily with 1 mg/kg stilboestrol, and 3 females with 50 mg/kg testosterone for 14 days. Five CF/LP mice were castrated and allowed to recover. Two of these mice were then injected daily for 1 week with 4 mg/kg stilboestrol and one with testosterone. The other two mice received no further treatment. All the mice were then dosed with 60 mg/kg (500 μCi/kg) [^{14}C]chloroform and killed 5 hours after dosing. After testosterone administration to female mice, more radioactivity appeared in the renal cortex of these mice than in female controls. Stilboestrol appeared to have little effect upon the amount of radioactivity in the renal cortex of males. In comparison to the male control, less radioactivity appeared in the renal cortex after castration. However, castration and stilboestrol did not reduce the amount further, but testosterone administration to castrated mice restored the normal distribution.

4.3 Genotoxicity

In vitro studies using Ames *Salmonella typhimurium* strains, with and without S-9 or equivalent fractions for metabolic activation, have on the whole produced negative results (Rosenthal 1987).

Van Abbe *et al* (1982) tested chloroform in *Salmonella typhimurium* strains TA1535, TA100, TA1537, TA1538 and TA98. At a concentration of 10 mg/plate chloroform was toxic to all strains of *Salmonella*. Below this concentration there was no significant increase in revertant colonies in any of the strains.

Negative results for genotoxicity have also been obtained in *E. coli* strain K-12, and Chinese hamster lung fibroblast cells (V-79) exposed for 24 hours to 1–2.5% vapours of chloroform and then assayed for 8-azaguanine resistance (Sturrock 1977). Chinese hamster ovary cells in culture, with and without incorporation of S-9 rat liver fractions for metabolic activation, exposed to 0.7% chloroform vapour did not show an increase in sister chromatid exchange frequency (White *et al* 1979).

The morphology of mouse sperm following exposure to chloroform has been examined by Land *et al* (1979). Groups of four (C57B1/C3H) F1 mice were exposed by inhalation to 0.04 or 0.08% chloroform 4 hours/day for 5 days. Twenty-eight days after the first day of exposure, the mice were sacrificed and the sperm examined. A statisically significant increase in morphological abnormalities was found in the sperm of the chloroform-treated animals compared to the controls.

4.4 Carcinogenicity

The carcinogenicity of chloroform has been well studied in both mice and rats.

In a study by the National Cancer Institute (1976), groups of 50 male and 50 female B6C3F1 mice were exposed to chloroform by gavage in corn oil at two dose levels 5 days/week for 78 weeks. A matched control group of 20 animals per sex and pooled control groups of 77 males and 80 females were included in the study. Initially, the males were given 100 or 299 mg/kg, while females received 200 or 400 mg/kg beginning at 5 weeks of age. After 18 weeks, however, these doses were increased to 150 and 300 mg/kg for males and 250 and 500 mg/kg for females. All groups of chloroform-treated mice showed highly significant dose-dependent increases in hepatocellular carcinomas. Metastases were found in the lungs of some animals. Nodular hyperplasia was commonly found in the livers of low-dose males that did not develop hepatocellular carcinoma. Groups of 50 male and 50 female Osborne–Mendel rats were also studied. Males received dose levels of 90 or 180 mg/kg chloroform in corn oil by gavage 5 days/week from 7 weeks to 78 weeks of age. Females initially received 125 or 250 mg/kg, but after 22 weeks these doses were reduced to 90 and 180 mg/kg, yielding mean levels of 100 and 200 mg/kg. This study was terminated at 111 weeks. Survival time and weight gain were reduced in all treated groups when compared to controls. In male rats, a highly significant dose-dependent increased incidence of kidney epithelial tumours was found. No kidney tumours occurred in control or treated females. There have been many criticisms of this study, mainly due to the methods employed, including the absence of an untreated control group, a numerical imbalance between matched control groups, inadequate characterisation of the vehicle, for example, antioxidant content, and treatment on 5 days per week only.

Roe *et al* (1979) studied the long-term effect of chloroform administration in four strains of mice; C57BL, CBA, CF/1 and ICI. In three experiments, chloroform was administered to mice by gavage in a toothpaste base or arachis oil, in doses up to 60 mg/kg/day for 80 weeks. Control groups were left untreated or given vehicle only. Survival rates among the treated groups were generally greater than in the controls.

In the case of males in three of the strains, treatment had no effect on the incidence of tumours. In the males of the ICI strain at 60 mg/kg/day, administration of chloroform in a toothpaste base caused an increase in the incidence of epithelial tumours of the kidney. A higher incidence of tumours resulted when the ICI males received chloroform dissolved in arachis oil. In two of the three experiments kidney tumours were also seen in vehicle control ICI males as well as in the treated animals.

Palmer *et al* (1979) studied the long-term effect of chloroform administration in Sprague–Dawley rats. Fifty male and 50 female rats were dosed with 60 mg/kg/day chloroform in toothpaste base for 6 days/week for 80 weeks. The chloroform-treated rats of both sexes had a higher survival rate than the controls, although both groups showed a high degree of non-neoplastic respiratory and renal disease. Female rats showed a decreased plasma cholinesterase activity. There was no significant increase in tumour incidence in either sex when compared to the controls.

Heywood *et al* (1979) dosed beagle dogs with 15 or 30 mg/kg/day chloroform in a toothpaste base for 6 days/week for $7\frac{1}{2}$ years. Control animals received toothpaste without chloroform, while another group of 16 male and 16 female dogs received a non-chloroform toothpaste. The only significant toxic response was an increase in some serum enzyme levels, reaching a peak in the sixth year of the study. There was no treatment-related increase in the number of neoplasms observed.

Jorgenson *et al* (1985) carried out studies on the carcinogenicity of chloroform administered in drinking water to Osborne–Mendel rats and female B6C3F1 mice. Chloroform caused a dose-related increase in renal tubular adenomas and adenocarcinomas in male rats. A dose corresponding to a time-weighted average of 160 mg/kg/day for 104 weeks caused a 14% incidence of renal tubular adenomas and adenocarcinomas against 1% in the control group. These results are comparable to the results observed earlier by the National Cancer Institute (NCI 1976). A time-weighted average dose of 263 mg/kg chloroform in drinking water for 104 weeks administered to female B6C3F1 mice resulted in a 5% combined incidence of hepatocellular adenomas and carcinomas compared to a 6% incidence in control groups.

Tumasonis *et al* (1985) studied the effects of chloroform in male and female Wistar rats. Chloroform was administered to weanling rats in drinking water at 2.9 g/l for 72 weeks, after which point the dose was reduced to 1.45 g/l, due to increased water consumption by the animals. All surviving animals were necropsied after 185 weeks. Body weights for all treated animals were reduced for the duration of the experiment compared to the controls. The incidence of neoplastic nodules and a tumour the author classified as adenofibrosis in the liver was significantly increased in both males and females above the 0% incidence in controls. No significant increase in any other tumours was found.

Bull *et al* (1985) investigated the extent to which the vehicle was responsible for the different results in the studies by NCI and EPA by examining the effects of chloroform administered by gavage using corn oil versus a 2% Emulphor suspension as the vehicle. Chloroform was administered to male and female B6C3F1 mice at doses of 60, 130, and 270 mg/kg/day for 90 days. The liver of mice administered chloroform in corn oil displayed a significant degree of diffuse parenchymal degeneration (5/10 males and 1/10 females) and mild to moderate cirrhosis (5/10 males and 9/10 females). Pathological lesions were not observed in the animals receiving corn oil without chloroform or in the mice receiving 2% Emulphor containing chloroform. The data indicate that administration of chloroform in corn oil by gavage results in an enhanced hepatotoxic effect than when administered in an aqueous suspension. This would appear to explain the increased incidence of hepatocellular carcinoma observed in the 1976 NCI study, using corn oil as vehicle, compared to the incidence in the study using drinking water as the vehicle (Jorgenson *et al* 1985).

4.5 Reproductive toxicity

Schwetz *et al* (1974) exposed pregnant Sprague–Dawley rats 7 hours/day to either 0, 30, 100 or 300 ppm chloroform vapour on days 6–15 of gestation. Significant embryotoxicity and foetotoxicity, including reduced foetal size and weight, were observed in the 300 ppm dosage group, but not at the lower doses. Evidence of retarded foetal development as well as true terata were observed in the chloroform-exposed animals. Higher incidences of delayed sternebrae ossification and missing ribs, as well as subcutaneous oedema, were observed more often in the exposed animals than in controls. Acaudia and imperforate anus were each noted in three of 13 litters of the 100 ppm dosage group.

In a study by Murray *et al* (1979), pregnant CF-1 mice were exposed to 0 or 100 ppm chloroform for 7 hours/day from days 6 to 15, 1 to 7 or 8 to 15 of gestation. The ability of the females to maintain pregnancy was reduced in the dams exposed from days 1 to 7 or 6 to 15, but not significantly affected in females exposed from days 8 to 15. This suggests that the effect of chloroform on pregnancy occurred either prior to implantation or during the early stages of implantation. A significant increase in the incidence of cleft palate was observed among offspring of mice exposed to 100 ppm chloroform from days 8 to 15 of gestation. This was seen in foetuses with retarded growth, suggesting a secondary rather than primary effect.

5. DISCUSSION

Chloroform is a widely used industrial chemical. It is found in food, especially those with high lipid content, some pharmaceutical products and in water as a byproduct of chlorination. Chloroform has been banned as an additive in cosmetic and pharmaceutical products in the US since 1976, and new British legislation has restricted its sale and use in the British cosmetic and pharmaceutical industry. In some circumstances chlorinated drinking water may be the major source of exposure to chloroform.

Chloroform is readily absorbed from the lungs and gastrointestinal tract. Metabolism appears to be by the microsomal mixed function oxidase system. Much of the chloroform is excreted unchanged or metabolised to carbon dioxide, although covalent binding to cellular macromolecules and condensation reactions with glutathione and cysteine have been shown to occur *in vitro*.

The major effect of chloroform by acute inhalation exposure is on the central nervous system, causing anaesthesia. It produces both liver and kidney toxicity on high-dose acute exposure or chronic exposure to lower levels.

Studies on the mutagenic effects of chloroform in *Salmonella typhimurium* proved negative in all strains tested. These results have been supported by the results of other *in vitro* assays using Chinese hamster cells and *E. coli* strains.

In carcinogenicity studies, chloroform has been shown to produce liver and kidney tumours. The significance of the liver tumours is unclear, since this effect has not been confirmed, and in studies where they have been observed this may be due to increased hepatotoxicity caused by using corn oil as a vehicle. There is mounting evidence that chloroform possesses an epigenetic mechanism of carcinogenicity.

In inhalation studies, chloroform has been shown to be embryotoxic and possibly teratogenic in Sprague–Dawley rats and CF-1 mice, but only at high doses.

From the information available it appears that the toxicity and carcinogenicity of chloroform is species-, strain-, sex- and age-dependent in experimental animals. The concentrations of chloroform encountered in drinking water seem unlikely to produce hepatotoxicity or nephrotoxicity. A risk extrapolation on carcinogenicity using the NCI rat study data was used by WHO (1984) to set a guideline for chloroform in drinking water of 30 μg/l. This was based on an increased risk of 1 extra cancer in 100 000 of population with an exposure of 70 years. However, if chloroform has a truly epigenetic mechanism of carcinogenesis, as indicated by the inability to demonstrate genotoxicity , this model may substantially overestimate the risk to consumers from chloroform in drinking water.

REFERENCES

ALEXANDER H C, McCARTY W M, BARTLETT E A and SYVERUD A N (1982) Aqueous odour and taste threshold values of industrial chemicals. *Journal of the American Water Works Association* **74,** 595-599.

APPLEBY A, KAZAZIS J, LILLIAN D and SINGH H B (1976) Atmospheric formation of chloroform from trichloroethylene. *Journal of Environmental Science and Health* **A11,** 711-715.

BELLAR T A, LICHTENBURG J J and KRONER R C (1974) Occurrence of organohalides in chlorinated drinking water. *Journal of the American Water Works Association* **66,** 703-706.

BOWMAN F J, BORZELLECA J F and MUNSON A E (1978) The toxicity of some halomethanes in mice. *Toxicology and Applied Pharmacology* **44,** 213-215.

BROWN B R, SIPES I G and SAGALYN A M (1974a) Mechanism of acute hepatic toxicity: chloroform, halothane and glutathione. *Anesthesiology* **41,** 554-561.

BROWN D M, LANGLEY P F, SMITH D and TAYLOR D C (1974b) Metabolism of chloroform. 1. The metabolism of ^{14}C-chloroform by different species. *Xenobiotica* **4,** 151-163.

BULL R J, BROWN J, JORGENSON T A, MEIERHENRY E A, ROBINSON M and STOBER J A (1985) Enhancement of the hepatotoxicity of chloroform in female B6C3F1 mice by corn oil: implications for chloroform carcinogenesis. *Fundamental and Applied Toxicology* **5,** 760-769.

CHU I, SECOURS V, MARINO I and VILLENEUVE D C (1980) The acute toxicity of four trihalomethanes in male and female rats. *Toxicology and Applied Pharmacology* **52,** 351-353.

DAVIDSON I W F, SUMNER D D and PARKER J C (1982) Chloroform: a review of its metabolism, teratogenic, mutagenic and carcinogenic potential. *Drug and Chemical Toxicology* **5,** 1-87.

FRY J, TAYLOR T and HATHAWAY D F (1972) Pulmonary elimination of chloroform and its metabolites in man. *Archives of International Pharmacodynamics* **196,** 98-111.
GRIMSRUD E P and RASMUSSEN R A (1975) Survey and analysis of halocarbons in the atmosphere by gas chromatography–mass spectrometry. *Atmospheric Environment* **9,** 1014-1017.
GROGER W K L and GREY T F (1979) Effect of chloroform on the activities of liver enzymes in rats. *Toxicology* **14,** 23-38.
ILETT K F, REID W D, SIPES I G and KRISHNA G (1973) Chloroform toxicity in mice: correlation of renal and hepatic necrosis with covalent binding of metabolites to tissue macromolecules. *Experimental and Molecular Pathology* **19,** 215-229.
INTERNATIONAL AGENCY FOR RESEARCH ON CANCER (1979) Some halogenated hydrocarbons: chloroform. Volume 20, 401-427, Lyons.
JORGENSON T A, MEIERHENRY E F, RUSHBROOK C J, BULL R J, ROBINSON M and WHITMIRE C E (1985) Carcinogenicity of chloroform in drinking water to male Osborne–Mendel rats and female B6C3F1 mice. *Fundamental and Applied Toxicology* **5,** 760-769.
KIMURA E T, EBERT D M and DODGE P W (1971) Acute toxicity and limits of solvent residue for sixteen organic solvents. *Toxicology and Applied Pharmacology* **19,** 699.
KRONELD R (1986) Chloroform in tap water and human blood. *Bulletin of Environmental Contamination and Toxicology* **36,** 477-483.
LAND P C, OWEN E L and LINDE H W (1979) Mouse sperm morphology following exposure to anesthetics during early spermatogenesis. *Anesthesiology* **51,** 259.
LILLIAN D, SINGH H B, APPLEBY A, LOBBAN L, ARNTS R, GUMPERT R, HAGUE R, TOOMEY J, KAZAZIS J, ANTELL M, HANSEN D and SCOTT B (1975) Atmospheric fates of halogenated compounds. *Environmental Science and Technology* **9,** 1042-1048.
MANSUY D, BEAUNE P, CRESTEIL T, LANGE M and LEROUX J (1977) Evidence for phosgene formation during liver microsomal oxidation of chloroform. *Biochemical and Biophysical Research Communications* **79,** 513-517.
McCONNELL G (1975) Chlorinated hydrocarbons and the environment. *Endeavour* **34**(121), 13-18.
MIKLASHEVSKI V E, TUBARINOJA U N, RAKMANINA N L and YAGOVLEVA G P (1966) Toxicity of chloroform administered orally. *Gigiena i Sanitariia* **31,** 320-325.
MURRAY F G, SCHWETZ B A, McBRIDE M G and STAPLES R E (1979) Toxicity of inhaled chloroform in pregnant mice and their offspring. *Toxicology and Applied Pharmacology* **50,** 515.
NATIONAL CANCER INSTITUTE (1976) Report on the carcinogenesis bioassay of chloroform. National Technical Information Service PB-264018, Springfield, Virginia.
NIOSH (1977) National occupational hazard survey, Vol 3, Survey analysis and supplemental tables, USDHEW, Cincinnati 2864.
OETTEL H (1936) Wirkung auf die unverletzte menschliche haut. Schilderung der

einzelnen substangruppen aliphatische kohlen wasserstaffe. *Archiv fur Experimentelle Pathologie und Pharmacologie* **183,** 649-696.
PALMER A K, STREET A E, ROE F J C, WORDEN A N and VAN ABBE N J (1979) Safety evaluation of toothpaste containing chloroform. 2. Long-term studies in rats. *Journal of Environmental Pathology and Toxicology* **2**, 821-833.
PEARSON C R and McCONNELL G (1975) Chlorinated C1 and C2 hydrocarbons in the marine environment. *Proceedings of the Royal Society of London B* **189,** 305-332.
PEREIRA M A, SAVAGE R E Jr and GUION C W (1984) Effect of chloroform on hepatic and renal DNA synthesis and ornithine decarboxylase activity in mice and rats. *Toxicology Letters* **21,** 357-364.
POHL L R and KRISHNA G (1978) Deuterium isotope effect in bioactivation and hepatoxicity of chloroform. *Life Sciences* **23,** 1067-1072.
POHL L R, BHOOSHAN B, WHITAKER N F and KRISHNA G (1977) Phosgene: a metabolite of chloroform. *Biochemical and Biophysical Research Communications* **79,** 684-691.
POHL L R, GEORGE J W, MARTIN J L and KRISHNA G (1979) Deuterium isotope effect in *in vivo* bioactivation of chloroform to phosgene. *Biochemical Pharmacology* **28,** 561-563.
POHL L R, MARTIN J L and GEORGE J W (1980a) Mechanism of metabolic activation of chloroform by rat liver microsomes. *Biochemical Pharmacology* **29,** 3271-3276.
POHL L R, MARTIN J L, TABURET A M and GEORGE J W (1980b) Oxidative bioactivation of haloforms into hepatotoxins. In: *Microsomes, drug oxidations and chemical carcinogenesis,* edited by M J Coon, A H Conney, R W Estabrook, H V Gelboin, J R Gillette and P J O'Brien, pp. 881-884. Academic Press, New York.
ROE F J C, PALMER A K, WORDEN A N and VAN ABBE N J (1979) Safety evaluation of toothpaste containing chloroform. 1. Long-term studies in mice. *Journal of Environmental Pathology and Toxicology* **2,** 821-833.
ROOK J J (1974) Formation of haloforms during chlorination of natural waters. *Journal of Water Treatment and Examination* **23,** 234-243.
ROSENTHAL R L (1987) A review of the mutagenicity of chloroform. *Environmental and Molecular Mutagenesis* **10,** 211-226.
RUSSELL J W and SANDOFF L A (1977) The sampling and determination of halocarbons in ambient air using concentration on porous polymer. *Journal of Chromatography* **134,** 375-384.
SATO A and NAKAJIMA T (1979) A structure relationship of some chlorinated hydrocarbons. *Archives of Environmental Health* **34,** 69-75.
SAVAGE R E, WESTRICH C, GUION C and PEREIRA M A (1982) Chloroform induction of ornithine decarboxylase activity in rats. *Environmental Health Perspectives* **16,** 157-162.
SCHWETZ B A, LEONG B K J and GEHRING P J (1974) Embryo- and foetotoxicity of inhaled chloroform in rats. *Toxicology and Applied Pharmacology* **28,** 442-451.
SINGH H B, SALAS L J and CAVANAGH L A (1977) Distribution, sources and sinks of atmospheric halogenated compounds. *Journal of the Air Pollution*

Control Association **27,** 332-336.

SIPES I G, KRISHNA G and GILETTE J R (1977) Bioactivation of carbon tetrachloride, chloroform and bromotrichloromethane: role of cytochrome P-450. *Life Sciences* **20,** 1541-1548.

SMITH J H and HOOK J B (1983) Mechanism of chloroform nephrotoxicity. *Toxicology and Applied Pharmacology* **70,** 467-480.

SMITH J H, MAITA K, SLEIGHT S D and HOOK J B (1984) Effect of sex hormone status on chloroform nephrotoxicity and renal mixed function oxidases in mice. *Toxicology* **30,** 305-316.

SMITH J H, HEWITT W R and HOOK J B (1985) Role of bioactivation in chloroform induced nephrotoxicity in rats. *Toxicology and Applied Pharmacology* **79,** 166-174.

STURROCK J (1977) Lack of mutagenic effect of halthane or chloroform on cultured cells using the azaguanine test system. *British Journal of Anaesthesia* **49,** 207-210.

SYMONS J M (1975) National Organics Reconnaissance Survey for halogenated organics. *Journal of the American Water Works Association* **67,** 634-647.

SYMONS J M, BELLAR T A, CARSWELL J K, DeMARCO J, KROPP K L, ROBECK G G, SEEGER D R, SLOCUM C J, SMITH B L and STEVENS A A (1975) National reconnaissance survey for halogenated organics. *Journal of the American Water Works Association* **67,** 634-647.

TAYLOR D C, BROWN D M, KEEBLE R and LANGLEY P F (1974) Metabolism of chloroform. 2. A sex difference in the metabolism of ^{14}C-chloroform in mice. *Xenobiotica* **4,** 165-174.

TOMASI A, ALBANO E, BIASI F, SLATER T R, VANNINI V and DIANZANI M U (1985) Activation of chloroform and related trihalomethanes to free radical intermediates in isolated hepatocytes and in the rat in vivo as detected by the ESR–spin trapping technique. *Chemicobiological interactions* **55,** 303-316.

TORKELSON T R, OYEN F and ROWE V K (1976) The toxicity of chloroform as determined by single and repeated exposure of laboratory animals. *American Industrial Hygiene Association Journal* **37,** 697-705.

TSURATA H (1975) Percutaneous absorption of organic solvents. 1. Comparative study of the *in vivo* percutaneous absorption of chlorinated solvents in mice. *Industrial Health* **13,** 227-236.

TSURATA H (1977) Percutaneous absorption of organic solvents. 2. A method for measuring the penetration rate of chlorinated solvents through excised ratskin. *Industrial Health* **15,** 131-139.

TUMASONIS C F, MCMARTIN D N, BUSH B (1985) Lifetime toxicity of chloroform and bromodichloromethane when administered over a lifetime to rats. *Ecotoxicology and Environmental Safety* **9,** 233-240.

US ENVIRONMENTAL PROTECTION AGENCY (1980) Ambient water quality criteria for chloroform. EPA 440/5-80-033, October 1980, C-35-C40.

US FOOD AND DRUG ADMINISTRATION (1976) Chloroform as an ingredient of human drug and cosmetic production. *Federal Register* **41,** 26842-26845.

US OCCUPATIONAL SAFETY and HEALTH ADMINISTRATION (1978) Air contaminents. US Code Federal Regulations Title 29, part 1910.1000 637.

VAN ABBE N J, HEYWOOD R, SORTWELL R J, NOEL P R B, STREET A E,

PRENTICE D E, ROE F J C, WADSWORTH P F and WORDEN A N (1979) Safety evaluation of toothpaste containing chloroform. 3. Long term study in beagle dogs. *Journal of Environmental Pathology and Toxicology* **2,** 835-851.

VAN ABBE N J, GREEN T J, JONES E, RICHOLD M and ROE F J C (1982) Bacterial mutagenicity studies on chloroform in vitro. *Food and Chemical Toxicology* **20,** 557-561.

VESSELL E S, LANG M C, WHITE W J, PASSANANTI G T, HILL R N, CLEMENS T L, LIU DK and JOHNSON D W (1976) Environmental and genetic factors affecting the response of laboratory animals to drugs. *Federation of American Society for Experimental Biology Proceedings* **35,** 1125-1132.

WATER RESEARCH CENTRE (1981) Organic micropollutants in drinking water. Technical Report TR 159. Water Research Centre, Marlow.

WEISBURGER E K (1977) Carcinogenicity studies on halogenated hydrocarbons. *Environmental Health Perspectives* **21,** 7-16.

WHITE A E, TAKEHISON S, EGER E I, WOLFF S and STEVENS W C (1979) Sister chromatid exchanges induced by inhaled anaesthetics. *Anesthesiology* **50,** 426-430.

YANNAI S (1983) Adrenocortical response to single and repeated doses of chloroform in rats. *Archives of Toxicology* **54,** 145-156.

YUNG Y L, McELROY M B and WOFSY S C (1975) Atmospheric halocarbons: a discussion with emphasis on chloroform. *Geophysical Research Letters* **2,** 397-399.

2

The trihalomethanes

1. INTRODUCTION

Trihalomethanes (THMs) are found in all chlorinated drinking waters. They are formed as a result of the reaction between chlorine and organic precursors, typically naturally occurring substances like humic acids. Many of the trihalomethanes have no industrial use, and are known to man only as a result of these reactions during drinking water disinfection. One, however, tribromomethane (bromoform), is used industrially as a gauge fluid, as a heavy liquid in solids separation, and as a chemical intermediate.

The most frequently identified compound, trichloromethane (chloroform), is the subject of Chapter 1.

2. EXPOSURE

2.1 Air

Little information is available on the level of these compounds in the atmosphere. Minimal quantities may be inhaled from the atmosphere above swimming pools (Lahl *et al* 1981), while some could also be taken in as a result of the reactions of chlorine released from sterilising tablets.

2.2 Food

There is little information on the occurrence of these compounds in food, although minimal contamination is likely in foods where water is used during production.

2.3 Water

In addition to chloroform, seven trihalomethanes were identified in UK drinking water in the WRc survey (Fielding *et al* 1981). Of these, the most frequently detected were:

Bromodichloromethane	14/14 samples

Tribromomethane	14/14 samples
Chlorodibromomethane	14/14 samples

The other four halomethanes identified were:

Bromochloroiodomethane	8/14 samples
Dichloroiodomethane	7/14 samples
Dibromoiodomethane	2/14 samples
Chlorodiiodomethane	1/14 samples

Studies have shown that trihalomethanes result primarily from reactions between chlorine and naturally occurring organic matter in water, such as humic acids (Rook 1974, 1976). Chlorine can oxidise bromide and iodide present in water to their respective hypo-acids, which in turn can react with humic acids to produce brominated and iodinated trihalomethanes. The quantities of trihalomethanes found in drinking water are very variable, and concentrations up to 40 μg/l of each of the three non-iodinated trihalomethanes may be detected on occasion (Symons *et al* 1975, Kasso and Wells 1981, Pinchin 1986). The iodinated compounds occur at much lower concentrations.

3. TOXICOKINETICS

The metabolism of bromodichloromethane, chlorodibromomethane and tribromomethane has been studied in male Sprague–Dawley rats and male B6C3F1 mice (Mink *et al* 1986). Each compound was dissolved in corn oil, and administered by intragastric intubation at doses of 100 mg/kg (rats) and 150 mg/kg (mice). Although all three compounds behaved similarly in this study, there was a significant difference in the way in which the trihalomethanes were metabolised by rats and mice. Eight hours following dosing in rats, most was eliminated unchanged in the expired air. Much smaller concentrations were metabolised and excreted in the urine or in the expired air as carbon dioxide. However, 8 hours following dosing in mice, most was metabolised to carbon dioxide and eliminated in the expired air. The portion of the dose remaining in the tissues of both rats and mice was generally less than 10%. The half-lives reported for these compounds in rats were 0.8 hours for tribromomethane, 1.2 hours for chlorodibromomethane, and 1.5 hours for bromodichloromethane. In mice, the half-lives were 8 hours for tribromomethane and 2.5 hours for both chlorodibromomethane and bromodichloromethane.

Intraperitoneal injection of 253 mg/kg of tribromomethane in male Sprague–Dawley rats resulted in elevation of blood carbon monoxide levels (Anders *et al* 1978). Formation of carbon monoxide from trihalomethanes was demonstrated *in vitro* using rat liver microsomes. The rate of production was dependent on the halogen substitution, that is, in the order $CHI_3>CHBr_3>CHBr_2Cl>CHBrCl_2>CHCl_3$ (Ahmed *et al* 1977). There is also evidence from *in vitro* studies (Tomasi *et al* 1985) that trihalomethanes may to some extent be metabolised to free radical intermediates. The production of free radical intermediates was again in the order $CHI_3>CHBr_3>CHBrCl_2>CHCl_3$.

There appear to be no data available on the metabolism of these trihalomethanes in man.

4. HEALTH EFFECTS

4.1 Acute and subacute toxicity

The following oral LD50 data in rats and mice have been published. The major pathological changes occurred in the liver and kidney (Bowman *et al* 1978, Chu *et al* 1980, 1982a).

		Oral LD50 (mg/kg) (95% confidence limits)	
		Sprague-Dawley rats	ICR Swiss mice
Bromodichloromethane	male	916 (779–1083)	450 (326–621)
	female	969 (764–1198)	900 (811–999)
Chlorodibromomethane	male	1186 (997–1421)	800 (667–960)
	female	848 (576–1090)	1200 (945–1524)
Tribromomethane	male	1388 (1167–1693)	1400 (1205–1595)
	female	1147 (890–1524)	1550 (1165–2062)

The effects of trihalomethanes on the liver and kidney in male Sprague–Dawley rats were studied following acute oral exposure (Hewitt *et al* 1983). Chlorodibromomethane and bromodichloromethane did not produce liver injury until near-lethal doses were administered. Compared to chloroform, both were weak hepatotoxins. However, pretreatment of rats with acetone markedly potentiated the hepatotoxic effects of bromodichloromethane and chlorodibromomethane. Neither compound produced appreciable kidney injury. Agarwal and Mehendale (1983) found no evidence of hepatotoxicity in male Sprague–Dawley rats given single doses of 72–867 mg/kg of tribromomethane by intraperitoneal injection. Animals given 578 and 867 mg/kg were in deep sedation and prostration for up to 8 hours.

Changes in hepatic lipid metabolism in rats were demonstrated shortly after administration of an oral dose of 215 mg/kg of bromodichloromethane (Koyama and Nakazawa 1985). However, studies in rat liver slices showed that effects on lipid metabolism were more pronounced with tribromomethane and chlorodibromomethane than bromodichloromethane and chloroform (Koyama and Nakazawa 1986). Rats given a single oral dose of 1000 mg/kg of tribromomethane and killed 18 hours after treatment exhibited lowered hepatic cytochrome P-450 and ALA-dehydratase, but increased hepatic porphyrins and glutathione (Moody and Smuckler 1986).

In a 14-day study (Munson *et al* 1982), groups of 6–12 male and female CD-1 mice were given oral doses of 0, 50, 125 and 250 mg/kg body weight/day of either bromodichloromethane, chlorodibromomethane or tribromomethane. The solutions for gavage were prepared in 10% Emulphor in deionized water. Although there were no deaths in any group, a wide range of effects was noted in the high-dose groups. These included depression of body weight gain, elevated liver weight/body weight ratio, lowered spleen weight/body weight ratio, changes in haematology, changes in clinical chemistry indicative of liver damage, and some evidence of depression of both humoral and cell-mediated immunity. Some of these changes were also evident at 125 mg/kg, but there were almost no effects at 50 mg/kg. All three compounds gave similar results in this study.

In another study (Condie *et al* 1983), no effects on body weight were found in CD-1 mice given oral doses of bromodichloromethane (37, 74 and 148 mg/kg/day), chlorodibromomethane (37, 74 and 147 mg/kg/day) and tribromomethane (72, 145 and 289 mg/kg/day), dissolved in corn oil, for 14 days. Elevated serum alanine aminotransferase activity, indicative of liver damage, was found at the high dose levels with all three compounds. Although clinical chemistry measurements of renal function (blood urea nitrogen, creatinine) revealed little evidence of toxicity, uptake of *p*-aminohippurate into renal cortical slices was inhibited at the high dose levels of all three compounds, and also at the mid-dose level with bromodichloromethane. Histopathological changes were evident in the liver and kidney at the high dose levels. Milder changes were found at the mid-dose levels, but only very slight effects were noted at the low dose levels.

No effects on body weight, histopathology of a wide range of organs, serum biochemical parameters or hepatic microsomal enzyme activities were observed in groups of 10 male Sprague–Dawley rats given drinking water containing 0, 5, 50 or 500 mg/l bromodichloromethane, chlorodibromomethane or tribromomethane for 28 days. Slight increases in relative kidney weights were found in the groups exposed to 500 mg/l of tribromomethane and 5 and 500 mg/l of bromodichloromethane (Chu *et al* 1982a).

4.2 Chronic toxicity

In recent studies on chlorodibromomethane (United States National Toxicology Program 1985, Dunnick *et al* 1985), groups of 10 male and 10 female F-344 rats and B6C3F1 mice were given oral doses of 0, 15, 30, 60, 125 or 250 mg/kg body weight/day in corn oil on 5 days/week for 13 weeks. Of the rats, 9/10 males and 9/10 females given 250 mg/kg died before the end of the study. Histopathological changes were found in the liver, kidney and salivary glands of these animals, but not in those given 125 mg/kg. Although there were no deaths of mice which were treatment-related, histopathological changes in the liver and kidney were evident in the high-dose males.

Chu *et al* (1982b) studied the reversibility of toxicological changes produced by trihalomethanes in Sprague–Dawley rats. Groups of 20 male and 20 female animals were given drinking water containing 0, 50, 500 and 2500 mg/l bromodichloromethane, chlorodibromomethane or tribromomethane for 90 days. Ten rats from each group were killed at this time. The remaining animals received ordinary tap water for a further 90 days before they were sacrificed. At the end of the 90-day treatment period, depression of body weight gain was observed in rats exposed to 2500 mg/l of bromodichloromethane. Mild histological changes were found in the livers and thyroids of rats in most treatment groups, though their severity reflected the dose. Serum lactate dehydrogenase activity was depressed in male and female rats exposed to 2500 mg/l of tribromomethane. Most of these changes were not found in the animals given a 90-day recovery period.

In a lifetime study of bromodichloromethane in Wistar rats (Tumasonis *et al* 1985), females developed an increased incidence of neoplastic nodules and lesions described as hepatic adenofibrosis. Full details of this study are described in Section 4.4.

Slight effect on behaviour was reported in a 90-day study in which male ICR mice were given oral doses of either 1.2 or 11.6 mg/kg/day of bromodichloromethane, 1 or 10 mg/kg/day of chlorodibromomethane or 0.9 or 9.2 mg/kg/day of tribromomethane dissolved in 1 : 8 Emulphor : water. However, for bromodichloromethane and tribromomethane, exposure to 100 and 400 mg/kg/day for 60 days affected operant behaviour. For chlorodibromomethane, effects on operant behaviour were observed only at 400 mg/kg/day. In each case, effects were noted early in the treatment period, and tolerance soon developed (Balster and Borzelleca 1982).

Rats exposed by inhalation to tribromomethane at up to 0.25 mg/l for 4 hours/day over 2 months induced disorders of prothrombin synthesis, liver glycogenesis and renal filtration capacity at doses above 0.05 mg/l (Dykan 1962).

4.3 Genotoxicity

Simmon (1977) found that bromodichloromethane, chlorodibromomethane and tribromomethane were mutagenic to *Salmonella typhimurium* TA100 only when the assays were carried out in a desiccator. Other Ames studies on bromodichloromethane and tribromomethane in which the assays were not carried out in an enclosed system have shown very little evidence of mutagenic activity (Haworth *et al* 1983, Mortelmans *et al* 1986).

Morimoto and Koizumi (1983) have shown that bromodichloromethane, chlorodibromomethane and tribromomethane induce sister chromatid exchanges in human lymphocytes *in vitro* and in mouse bone marrow cells *in vivo*. Of the three compounds, tribromomethane was the most potent *in vitro*, but the three compounds were not markedly different in their ability to induce sister chromatid exchanges *in vivo*.

In *Drosophila* studies, tribromomethane gave some evidence for induction of sex-linked recessive lethal mutations following feeding, but not after intraperitoneal injection. It gave negative results in the reciprocal translocation test (Woodruff *et al* 1985).

Only a very low level of DNA binding was found in the livers of Sprague–Dawley rats given a single intragastric dose of 380 mg/kg body weight of radiolabelled tribromomethane (Pereira *et al* 1982).

No dominant lethal effects were reported in a study of chlorodibromomethane in ICR Swiss mice (Borzelleca *et al* 1980).

There appears to be no information available as to the mutagenicity of the iodinated compounds.

4.4 Carcinogenicity

In the US National Toxicology Program study on chlorodibromomethane (United States National Toxicology Program 1985, Dunnick *et al* 1985), groups of 50 male and 50 female F-344 rats were given oral doses of 0, 40 or 80 mg/kg body weight/day in corn oil on 5 days/week for 104 weeks. There were no significant differences in survival between groups, but there was a slight depression in body weight gain in high-dose males. Comparison of tumour incidences between treated and control animals did not reveal any evidence of carcinogenic activity for chlorodibromomethane. In the mouse study, groups of 50 male and 50 female animals of the B6C3F1 strain were given oral doses of 0, 50 or 100 mg/kg body weight/day in corn oil on 5 days/week for 105 weeks. However, an overdose of chemical was given to the low-dose animals at week 58, which resulted in the death of 35 males but no females. The low-dose male group was therefore considered inadequate for analysis of tumour data. Evaluation of tumour data from female mice revealed a significant increase in hepatocellular adenomas (vehicle control 2/50, low-dose 4/49, high-dose 11/50) and also for hepatocellular adenomas and carcinomas when the numbers are combined (vehicle control 6/50, low-dose 10/49, high-dose 19/50). The incidence of hepatocellular carcinomas was significantly increased in high-dose male mice (vehicle control 10/50, high-dose 19/50) but the combined incidence of hepatocellular adenomas and carcinomas was similar to that of control (vehicle control 23/50, high-dose 27/50).

US National Toxicology Program studies on bromodichloromethane showed clear evidence of carcinogenicity in rats and mice with increases in kidney tubular adenomas and adenocarcinomas in rats and male mice, tumours of the large intestine in rats and liver tumours in female mice (Dunnick *et al.* 1987). Studies on tribromomethane are still in progress.

The effects of bromodichloromethane administered in drinking water have been examined in a lifetime study in rats (Tumasonis *et al* 1985). Groups of 58 male and 58 female Wistar rats received drinking water containing 2.4 g/l bromodichloromethane until 72 weeks, at which point the concentration was halved due to increasing water consumption by the experimental rats. The controls comprised 22 male and 22 female animals. During the experiment, both treated male and female animals exhibited depression of body weight gain. At autopsy, sections of livers from all rats and sections from other organs with grossly observable lesions were examined histologically. In females, there was a significant increase in the incidence of hepatic neoplastic nodules (control 0/18, treated 17/53), and also a number of lesions described as adenofibrosis (control 0/18, treated 12/53). There was no evidence of carcinogenicity in males.

Theiss *et al* (1977) tested bromodichloromethane and tribromomethane in a short-term assay in strain A mice. Male animals were dosed by intraperitoneal injection, thrice weekly, for up to 8 weeks. The dose levels employed were 20, 40 and 100 mg/kg for bromodichloromethane and 4, 48 and 100 mg/kg for tribromomethane. Twenty animals were used at each dose level, including vehicle control (tricaprylin) and positive control (urethan). Mice were sacrificed 24 weeks after the first injection, and the frequency of lung tumours in each group was compared with that of the vehicle-treated controls. A slight increase in the frequency of lung tumours was found with tribromomethane at 48 mg/kg. However, there is considerable doubt as to the significance of this finding, since there was no dose response, only the middle dose gave an increase in tumours, and several other compounds produced significantly fewer tumours than the vehicle controls. In addition, the response compared to that of urethan, the positive control, was marginal.

Tribromomethane gave no evidence for carcinogenic initiating activity in a study in rats. A group of 12 male Sprague–Dawley rats were given single oral doses of 200 mg/kg body weight of tribromomethane in tricaprylin. Three days later the animals began receiving drinking water containing 200 mg/l of a promoter, phenobarbital. Exposure to phenobarbital was terminated after 47 days. The animals were then left for 6 days before being killed, and the livers examined for gamma-glutamyl transpeptidase-positive foci, an increase in which is thought to be indicative of carcinogenicity. Tribromomethane did not increase the incidence of gamma-glutamyl transpeptidase-positive foci, but the positive control, diethylnitrosamine, gave a clear response (Pereira et al 1982).

4.5 Reproductive toxicity

Groups of up to 15 pregnant Sprague–Dawley rats were dosed by gavage with 50, 100 or 200 mg/kg body weight/day of tribromomethane, bromodichloromethane or chlorodibromomethane in corn oil on days 6–15 of gestation. Controls received vehicle alone. Bromodichloromethane and tribromomethane gave some evidence of embryotoxicity at the highest dose levels, but no evidence of teratogenicity. Chlorodibromomethane gave no evidence of either embryotoxicity or teratogenicity. At the top dose, exposure to bromodichloromethane and chlorodibromomethane did result in depression of maternal body weight gain. The dams given bromodichloromethane also exhibited increased liver weight to body weight ratios at all dose levels, and increased relative kidney weight to body weight ratios and brain weight to body weight ratios at the highest dose levels, but there appeared to be no pathological changes in these organs (Ruddick *et al* 1983).

In an abstract of multigeneration and teratogenicity studies, Borzelleca *et al* (1980) reported dose-dependent effects on survival and weight gain of pups and viability and lactation indices, but no evidence of teratogenicity in ICR mice exposed to 0, 0.1, 1 or 4 mg/l of chlorodibromomethane in drinking water (Emulphor : water 1 : 1000).

5. DISCUSSION

Trihalomethanes are widespread in treated water and occur as a result of the reaction between chlorine and naturally occurring organic matter.

Information on the metabolism and toxicology of these compounds is restricted to bromodichloromethane, chlorodibromomethane and tribromomethane.

The limited information available on toxicokinetics suggests that the trihalomethanes are handled differently in rats and mice. There appear to be no data available in man.

These trihalomethanes are of low acute oral toxicity in rats and mice. In subacute and chronic studies the main target organ is the liver, though the kidney is sometimes affected. All three compounds were mutagenic in the Ames assay when tested in an enclosed system. There is also some evidence for genotoxicity from *in vivo* experiments. In the National Toxicology Program study, chlorodibromomethane was classified as carcinogenic in the mouse but not in the rat. In another study, very high concentrations of bromodichloromethane in drinking water resulted in an increased incidence of hepatic neoplastic nodules in rats. There was no evidence that these compounds were teratogenic in rats and mice.

Although much more information on the toxicity of the trihalomethanes has become available in the last five years, data on carcinogenicity is still lacking. More attention must also be given to the metabolism of these compounds in different species, and its influence on toxicity and carcinogenicity.

REFERENCES

AGARWAL A K and MEHENDALE H M (1983) Absence of potentiation of bromoform hepatotoxicity and lethality by chlordecone. *Toxicology Letters* **15**, 251-257.

AHMED A E, KUBIC V L and ANDERS M W (1977) Metabolism of haloforms to carbon monoxide: 1. *In vitro* studies. *Drug Metabolism and Disposition* **5**, 198-204.

ANDERS M W, STEVENS J L, SPRAGUE R W, SHAATH Z and AHMED A E (1978) Metabolism of haloforms to carbon monoxide. 2. *In vivo* studies. *Drug Metabolism and Disposition* **6**, 556-560.

BALSTER R L and BORZELLECA J F (1982) Behavioral toxicity of trihalomethane contaminants of drinking water in mice. Environmental Health Perspectives **46**,127-136.

BORZELLECA J F, SKALSKY H L and RIDDLE B L (1980) Effects of dibromochloromethane and trichloromethane in drinking water on reproduction and development in mice. *Federation Proceedings* **39**, 999.

BOWMAN F J, BORZELLECA J F and MUNSON A E (1978) The toxicity of some halomethanes in mice. *Toxicology and Applied Pharmacology* **44**, 213-215.

CHU I, SECOURS V, MARINO I and VILLENEUVE D C (1980) The acute toxicity of four trihalomethanes in male and female rats. *Toxicology and Applied Pharmacology* **52**, 351-353.

CHU I, VILLENEUVE D C, SECOURS V E, BECKING G C and VALLI V E (1982a) Toxicity of trihalomethanes: 1. The acute and subacute toxicity of chloroform, bromodichloromethane, chlorodibromomethane and bromoform in rats. *Journal of Environmental Science and Health B* **17**, 205-224.

CHU I, VILLENEUVE D C, SECOURS V E, BECKING G C and VALLI V E (1982b) Trihalomethanes: 2. Reversibility of toxicological changes produced by chloroform, bromodichloromethane, chlorodibromomethane and bromoform in rats. *Journal of Environmental Science and Health B* **17**, 225-240.

CONDIE L W, SMALLWOOD C L and LAURIE R D (1983) Comparative renal and hepatotoxicity of halomethanes: bromodichloromethane, bromoform, chloroform, dibromochloromethane and methylene chloride. *Drug and Chemical Toxicology* **6**, 563-578.

DUNNICK J K, HASEMAN J K, LILJA H S and WYAND S (1985) Toxicity and carcinogenicity of chlorodibromomethane in Fischer 344/N rats and B6C3F1 mice. *Fundamental and Applied Toxicology* **5**, 1128-1136.

DUNNICK J K, EUSTIS S L and LILJA H S (1987) Bromodichloromethane, a trihalomethane that produces neoplasms in rodents. Cancer Research **47**, 5189–5193.

DYKAN V A (1962) *Chemical Abstracts* **60,** 8541d.

FIELDING M, GIBSON T M, JAMES H A, McLOUGHLIN K and STEELE C P (1981) Organic micropollutants in drinking water. WRc Technical Report TR159.

HAWORTH S, LAWLOR T, MORTELMANS K, SPECK W and ZEIGER E(1983) Salmonella mutagenicity test results for 250 chemicals. *Environmental Mutagenesis* **5**, Supplement 1, 3-142.

HEWITT W R, BROWN E M and PLAA G L (1983) Acetone-induced potentiation of trihalomethane toxicity in male rats. *Toxicology Letters* **16**, 285-296.

KASSO W B and WELLS M R (1981) A survey of trihalomethanes in the drinking water system of Murfreesboro, Tennessee. *Bulletin of Environmental Contamination and Toxicology* **27**, 295-302.

KOYAMA Y and NAKAZAWA Y (1985) Acute effect of bromodichloromethane on lipid metabolism in rat liver microsomes. *Toxicology Letters* **29**, 123-130.

KOYAMA Y and NAKAZAWA Y (1986) Comparison of the effect of trihalomethanes on lipid metabolism in rat liver slice. *Toxicology Letters* **31**, 37-44.

LAHL U, BATJER K, DUSZELN J v, GABEL B, STACHEL B and THIEMANN W (1981) Distribution and balance of volatile halogenated hydrocarbons in the water and air of covered swimming pools using chlorine for water disinfection. *Water Research* **15**, 803-814.

MINK F L, BROWN T J and RICKABAUGH J (1986) Absorption, distribution, and excretion of 94C-trihalomethanes in mice and rats. *Bulletin of Environmental Contamination and Toxicology* **37**, 752-758.

MOODY D E and SMUCKLER E A (1986) Disturbances in hepatic heme metabolism in rats administered alkyl halides. *Toxicology Letters* **32**, 209-214.

MORIMOTO K and KOIZUMI A (1983) Trihalomethanes induce sister chromatid exchanges in human lymphocytes *in vitro* and mouse bone marrow cells *in vivo*. *Environmental Research* **32**, 72-79.

MORTELMANS K, HAWORTH S, LAWLOR T, SPECK W, TAINER B and ZEIGER E (1986) Salmonella mutagenicity test results: 2. Results from the testing of 270 chemicals. *Environmental Mutagenesis* **8**, Supplement 7, 1-119.

MUNSON A E, SAIN L E, SANDERS V M, KAUFFMANN B M, WHITE K L Jr, PAGE D G, BARNES D W and BORZELLECA J F (1982) Toxicology of organic drinking water contaminants: trichloromethane, bromodichloromethane, dibromochloromethane and tribromomethane. *Environmental Health Perspectives* **46**, 117-126.

PEREIRA M A, LIN L-H C, LIPPITT J M and HERREN S L (1982) Trihalomethanes as initiators and promoters of carcinogenesis. *Environmental Health Perspectives* **46**, 151-156.

PINCHIN M J (1986) A study of the trace organic profiles of raw and potable water systems. *Journal of the Institution of Water Engineers and Scientists* **40**, 81-99.

ROOK J J (1974) Formation of haloforms during chlorination of natural waters. *Water Treatment and Examination* **23**, 234-243.

ROOK J J (1976) Haloforms in drinking water. *Journal of the American Water Works Association* **68**, 168-172.

RUDDICK J A, VILLENEUVE D C, CHU I and VALLI V E (1983) A teratological assessment of four trihalomethanes in the rat. *Journal of Environ-*

mental Science and Health B **18**, 333-349.
SIMMON V F (1977) Mutagenic activity of chemicals identified in drinking water. In: *Progress in Genetic Toxicology*, edited by D Scott, B A Bridges and F H Sobels. Elsevier/North-Holland Biomedical Press, pp. 249-258.
SYMONS J M *et al* (1975) National organics reconnaissance survey for halogenatedorganics. *Journal of the American Waterworks Association* **67**, 634-647.
THEISS J C, STONER G D, SHIMKIN M B and WEISBURGER E K (1977) Test for carcinogenicity of organic contaminants of United States drinking waters by pulmonary tumor response in strain A mice. *Cancer Research* **37**, 2717-2720.
TOMASI A, ALBANO E, BIASI F, SLATER T F, VANNINI V and DIANZANI M U (1985) Activation of chloroform and related trihalomethanes to free radical intermediates in isolated hepatocytes and in the rat *in vivo* as detected by the ESR-spin trapping technique. *Chemicobiological Interactions* **55**, 303-316.
TUMASONIS C F, McMARTIN D N and BUSH B (1985) Lifetime toxicity of chloroform and bromodichloromethane when administered over a lifetime in rats. *Ecotoxicology and Environmental Safety* **9**, 233-240.
UNITED STATES NATIONAL TOXICOLOGY PROGRAM (1985) Toxicology and carcinogenesis studies of chlorodibromomethane in F344/N rats and B6C3F1 mice. US National Toxicology Program, Technical Report Series No 282.
WOODRUFF R C, MASON J M, VALENCIA R and ZIMMERING S (1985) Chemical mutagenesis testing in *Drosophila*. V. Results of 53 coded compounds tested for the National Toxicology Program. *Environmental Mutagenesis* **7**, 677-702.

3

Trichloroethylene

1. INTRODUCTION

Trichloroethylene (trichloroethene, acetylene trichloride, ethylene trichloride, Tri, Trilene, TCE) is an important industrial solvent, used for degreasing metals and as a dry-cleaning agent. It has been used as an anaesthetic by inhalation, although this use is now infrequent. Commercial grades of trichloroethylene usually have a purity of greater than 98%; the stabilisers added include amines (0.001–0.01%) or combinations of epoxides and esters (0.2–2.0% total) (Health and Safety Executive 1985).

CAS Reg No:	79-01-6
Molecular weight:	131.38
Boiling point:	86.7 °C
Solubility:	1.0 g/l at 20 °C (Torkelson and Rowe 1982)
Odour threshold:	10 mg/l in water (Verschueren 1983)

2. EXPOSURE

Although trichloroethylene is not known to occur naturally, it is widely distributed in the environment, and has been detected in air, food and water.

2.1 Air

Trichloroethylene is a common contaminant of air, and has been detected at levels normally in the range 1–20 $\mu g/m^3$ (McConnell *et al* 1975, Fishbein 1976, Ziglio *et al* 1983, World Health Organization 1985). Analyses of concentrations of trichloroethylene in air in Western Europe during the period 1972–1976 indicated that levels were between 0.5 and 20 $\mu g/m^3$ (Correia *et al* 1977). However, concentrations up to 90 $\mu g/m^3$ have been reported in an urban area containing many dry-cleaning establishments (Ziglio *et al* 1983). Atmospheric contamination with trichloroethylene has been implicated as a possible factor in the depletion of the ozone layer (Lovelock 1974).

2.2 Food

Trichloroethylene is used as a solvent in food processing, and this may account for its occurrence in food. It has been detected at levels of 10 μg/kg in butter, 16 μg/kg in steak and 60 μg/kg in tea (McConnell *et al* 1975). Wallace *et al* (1984) found 920 μg/kg trichloroethylene in margarine, but concentrations in other foodstuffs were negligible. There have been proposals by the US Food and Drug Administration to discontinue the use of trichloroethylene in food processing (US Code of Federal Regulations 1976). At present, the level of trichloroethylene in coffee is limited to 10 mg/kg dry weight in decaffeinated instant coffee and 25 mg/kg in decaffeinated ground coffee (US Code of Federal Regulations 1976). Some manufacturers now use methylene chloride as an alternative for decaffeinating coffee (Waters *et al* 1977).

2.3 Water

Trichloroethylene was identified in 13 out of 14 drinking water samples examined in a WRc survey (Water Research Centre 1981). Concentrations between 0.02 and 5.4 μg/l have been detected in domestic drinking water supplies in the United States (Wallace *et al* 1984). In rainwater, trichloroethylene was detected at levels of up to 0.07 μg/l (Pearson and McConnell 1975, Andelman 1985a). This compound was found as a common contaminant in groundwater in Britain, the Netherlands, France, Italy and the United States of America (Correia *et al* 1977, Fielding *et al* 1981, Water Research Centre 1985, Zoeteman *et al* 1981, Ziglio *et al* 1983, Wang *et al* 1985). In general, levels are below 2 μg/l although, in cases of gross pollution, figures of approximately 1500 μg/l and 40 000 μg/l have been reported (Wang *et al* 1985, Andelman 1985a). Since trichloroethylene is virtually insoluble in water, and has a specific gravity heavier than water, any pollution of groundwater is likely to persist. There is no indication that trichloroethylene is produced from chlorination of natural waters (World Health Organization 1985).

Although ingestion is the main route of exposure for most waterborne chemicals, inhalation may also be important for compounds such as trichloroethylene which are particularly volatile. Andelman (1985a, 1985b) measured air concentrations of trichloroethylene in showers, using trichloroethylene-contaminated groundwater, and has shown that this can be a substantial source of exposure.

3. TOXICOKINETICS

3.1 Absorption

Trichloroethylene is absorbed into the body through the lungs, gastrointestinal tract and the skin.

Following oral administration of 5, 10 and 25 mg/kg to male Sprague–Dawley rats, trichloroethylene appeared rapidly in the blood, with concentrations peaking after 6–10 minutes (D'Souza *et al* 1985). This compound is easily absorbed across the gastrointestinal tract in man, and many cases of acute poisoning following oral ingestion have been reported (Waters *et al* 1977).

Concentrations of 0.5 ppm trichloroethylene were detected in the expired air of volunteers following the immersion of one thumb in the chemical for 30 minutes (Stewart and Dodd 1964). This indicates that trichloroethylene is absorbed through the skin in man, although the significance of this route of exposure for dilute aqueous solutions is still unclear.

3.2 Distribution

Trichloroethylene is distributed primarily to the adipose tissue, due to its high fat solubility.

In guinea pigs, trichloroethylene concentrations of 38 mg/kg fresh tissue were recorded in body fat and adrenal tissue following inhalation of 7 mg/l for 5 hours/day over a period of 23 days (Fabre and Truhaut 1952). Levels in the blood, lungs and liver were below 10 mg/kg fresh tissue.

Low concentrations of trichloroethylene were detected in human tissue, ranging from less than 1 μg/kg wet tissue in the brain and kidney, to 32 μg/kg in body fat (McConnell *et al* 1975).

Transplacental diffusion has been demonstrated in humans, and trichloroethylene was detected in foetal blood (Laham 1970).

3.3 Metabolism

This compound is readily metabolised by rodents, primates and man.

Metabolism of trichloroethylene has been extensively studied in both *in vivo* and *in vitro* systems (Ertle *et al* 1972, Henschler 1977, Uehleke *et al* 1977, Hathway 1980, Muller *et al* 1982, Dekant and Henschler 1983, Miller and Guengerich 1983, Costa and Ivanetich 1984, Rouisse and Chakrabarti 1986). In the liver, metabolic breakdown of trichloroethylene is thought to involve transformation by mixed function oxidase enzymes to a reactive epoxide. The instability of this epoxide has been attributed to its non-symmetrical arrangement of chlorine atoms (Henschler 1977). A rearrangement of the epoxide results in the formation of chloral. This may be either oxidised to trichloroacetic acid, or reduced to trichloroethanol. Trichloroethanol products may also be conjugated to form glucuronides. The identification of *N*-(hydroxyacetyl)-aminoethanol (HAAE) and oxalic acid in the urine of rats and mice 72 hours after a single oral dose of 200 mg/kg radiolabelled trichloroethylene indicates that dechlorination reactions may also occur in the breakdown of this compound (Dekant *et al* 1984). HAAE was also detected in the urine of two volunteers exposed to 200 ppm trichloroethylene for 6 hours. However, in man the principal metabolites following absorption of trichloroethylene appear to be trichloroacetic acid and trichloroethanol.

Recent studies suggest that trichloroethylene may also be metabolised to some extent in the kidney, to form a cysteine conjugate (Green and Odum 1985, Dekant *et al* 1986a, Elfarra *et al* 1986). The production of reactive intermediates during this process may explain the nephrotoxicity and nephrocarcinogenicity of trichloroethylene observed in rats.

Following a single oral dose of up to 2000 mg/kg radiolabelled trichloroethylene in corn oil, the breakdown of this compound into its major metabolites, trichloroacetic acid, trichloroethanol and chloral, became constant and independent of dose above 1000 mg/kg in male Osborne–Mendel and Wistar-derived rats, while it remained a linear process in male B6C3F1 and Swiss–Webster mice over the range of doses tested (Prout *et al* 1985). It appears that in rats metabolism is a dose-dependent and saturable process, whereas in mice it is independent of dose at doses up to 2000 mg/kg body weight (Stott *et al* 1982, Prout *et al* 1985, Dekant *et al* 1986b). Trichloroethylene metabolism also appears to be a dose-dependent process in man (Ikeda 1977).

A factor of clinical significance is that alcohol in the blood inhibits metabolism of this compound (Muller *et al* 1975). Factory workers exposed to trichloroethylene, who are prone to drinking, may suffer from 'Degreaser's flush'. Symptoms include drowsiness and reddening of the face and upper body.

3.4 Excretion

The major route of elimination is via the lungs. In female Wistar rats, 72 hours after a single oral dose of 200 mg/kg radiolabelled trichloroethylene in corn oil, 52% was recovered as unchanged trichloroethylene in the exhaled air and 2% as radiolabelled carbon dioxide (Dekant *et al* 1984). A further 41% of the radioactivity was eliminated in the urine. In contrast to this, female NMRI mice exhaled 11% of the recovered radioactivity as unchanged trichloroethylene, 6% as carbon dioxide and 76% as urinary metabolites.

Elimination of a dose of 50 mg/kg radiolabelled trichloroethylene, (vehicle unspecified), administered by intramuscular injection, was studied in three primate species: chimpanzees, baboons and rhesus monkeys (Muller *et al* 1982). The recovery of radioactivity in the urine ranged from 40 to 60% in chimpanzees, 11 to 28% in baboons and 7 to 40% in rhesus monkeys. Chimpanzees excreted only 2–5% of the total dose in the faeces, baboons excreted 25–34% and rhesus monkeys excreted 18–23% of the radioactivity by this route. It appears that biliary excretion occurs to a greater extent in baboons and rhesus monkeys than in chimpanzees.

Following metabolism of trichloroethylene, the elimination of various metabolites in the urine occurs at different rates. In volunteers exposed to 170 ppm trichloroethylene for 7 hours, trichloroethanol was excreted most rapidly shortly after exposure ceased, and trichloroacetic acid 42–69 hours later (Ogata *et al* 1971). The slower excretion rate of trichloroacetic acid compared to trichloroethanol may be due to its higher affinity for proteins.

4. HEALTH EFFECTS

The health effects associated with exposure to trichloroethylene have been well documented, due to concern over industrial exposure.

4.1 Acute and subacute toxicity

Trichloroethylene is of moderate to low acute toxicity via the oral route. The oral LD50 in female mice was 2443 mg/kg body weight, and in male mice it was 2402 mg/kg, when this compound was administered by gavage, in a 10% solution of Emulphor (Tucker *et al* 1982). The oral LD50 in the rat was 4920 mg/kg (Torkelson and Rowe 1982).

In Wistar rats, no deaths were observed following exposure to trichloroethylene, by inhalation, for 0.4 hours at 20 000 ppm, 0.6 hours at 12 000 ppm, 1.4 hours at

6400 ppm and 7.0 hours at 3000 ppm (Adams *et al* 1951). However, trichloroethylene exerted an anaesthetic effect, and animals exhibited depression of the CNS, in the form of stupor and a drunken gait.

Although trichloroethylene affects the CNS, no changes in levels of acid phosphatase, an enzyme marker for brain damage, were observed in the brains of rats, mice and gerbils exposed continuously to 150 ppm trichloroethylene vapour for 30 days (Kjellstrand *et al* 1982). Neither were there any changes in the levels of brain acetylcholinesterase, glutamine synthetase and glutamate dehydrogenase in NMRI mice exposed to 170 ppm trichloroethylene for 30 days, indicating no effect on nerve or glial cells (Kanje *et al* 1981). In contrast, butyrylcholinesterase, a marker for liver damage, increased twofold in male mice. Levels of this enzyme in the plasma of female mice were unaffected.

Mice appear to be more sensitive to the hepatotoxic effects of trichloroethylene than rats. Male B6C3F1 mice treated with 250, 500, 1200 or 2400 mg/kg trichloroethylene in corn oil, by gavage, 5 days/week for 3 weeks, showed a dose-related increase in liver weight, decrease in hepatic DNA per gram of tissue and development of pathological changes in the liver (swelling of centrilobular hepatocytes, giant cell inflammation and cell mineralisation) (Stott *et al* 1982). In contrast to this, there was an increase in liver weight, but no decrease in DNA per gram of hepatic tissue, or appearance of histopathological changes in male Osborne–Mendel rats exposed to up to 1100 mg/kg/day trichloroethylene in corn oil, under the same conditions. Mice appear to metabolise this compound to a greater extent than rats, and this may explain their increased susceptibility to hepatotoxic effects.

In a subacute inhalation study, NMRI mice, Sprague–Dawley rats and Mongolian gerbils exposed to 150 ppm trichloroethylene continuously for 30 days showed a statistically significant increase in relative liver weight in comparison with relative liver weight of control animals (relative organ weights were expressed in percentages of body weight) (Kjellstrand *et al* 1981). An increase of 75% in relative liver weight occurred in mice; the increase in liver weight in rats and gerbils was smaller but still significant. Relative kidney weights were increased in all three species, but they were only statistically significant in gerbils.

Relative kidney weight was unaffected, and no histopathology was observed in the renal tissue of male B6C3F1 mice exposed to 2400 mg/kg/day, or male Osborne–Mendel rats exposed to 1100 mg/kg/day trichloroethylene in corn oil, by gavage, 5 days/week for 3 weeks (Stott *et al* 1982).

There is evidence that short-term exposure of mice to trichloroethylene vapour can have immunosuppressive effects. A group of 275 female CD 1 mice were exposed to 50 ppm trichloroethylene vapour for 3 hours, while a group of 275 controls were exposed to filtered air only (Aranyi *et al* 1986). Both groups were then challenged with a streptococcal infection. There was a statistically significant increase in mortality in the trichloroethylene-exposed animals. Further evidence of immunological effects were obtained in a 14-day study of male CD-1 mice dosed by gavage with 24 mg/kg and 240 mg/kg trichloroethylene in 10% Emulphor (Sanders *et al* 1982). Cell-mediated immune reactions to red blood cells of sheep were significantly decreased at both dose levels. It appears that trichloroethylene inhibits T-lymphocytes of the immune system in mice. The white cell count in five cross-bred dogs exposed to 700 ppm trichloroethylene vapour for 1 hour dropped in comparison with the cell count in 15 control animals exposed to fresh air (Hobara *et al* 1984). However, recovery occurred shortly after the end of exposure, indicating that the effect was reversible.

Depression of the CNS is the primary effect of acute exposure to trichloroethylene in man. Inhalation of concentrations of 5000 ppm and 20 000 ppm have been used for light anaesthesia and deep anaesthesia respectively in medicine (World Health Organization 1985). Symptoms resulting from industrial exposure by inhalation include giddiness, mental confusion and impaired vision. Neurotoxic effects were still evident in a man 18 years after acute, industrial exposure to an unknown concentration of heated trichloroethylene vapour for a period of approximately 1½ hours (Feldman *et al* 1985). Nerve conductivity was impaired, there was loss of sensitivity in the facial region, eye reflexes were reduced, and short-term memory was affected. The lipid-soluble nature of trichloroethylene may explain its neurotoxicity; it is thought that this solvent alters the lipid composition of myelin, leading to nerve degeneration.

The visual motor performance of 8 male volunteers, exposed to 0, 100, 300 and 1000 ppm trichloroethylene vapour for 2 hours, was compared with their performance after zero exposure for 2 hours (Vernon and Ferguson 1969). At the highest dose trichloroethylene impaired performance in two out of six standard coordination tests carried out. No effects were seen below this level.

Cases of solvent abuse and glue sniffing have been reported, some of which have been fatal due to cardiac arrest (James 1963, Hayden *et al* 1976, Wells 1982).

4.2 Chronic toxicity

Male Swiss–Cox mice exposed to doses of 100–3200 mg/kg/day trichloroethylene in corn oil, by gavage, for 6 weeks, showed an increase in relative liver weight in all dose groups, with an increase of 75% compared to controls in the highest dose group (Buben and O'Flaherty 1985). Hepatic glucose-6-phosphatase activity was depressed at dose levels of 800 mg/kg/day and above, but the levels of liver triglycerides or serum glutamate–pyruvate transaminase were unaffected, even at the highest dose.

There was a depression in the growth rate of 11 male Wistar rats exposed by inhalation to 400 ppm trichloroethylene for up to 173 7-hour periods over 243 days, compared to the growth rate of 12 air-exposed controls (Adams *et al* 1951). Under the same conditions, 15 female rats exhibited normal development. In both sexes liver and kidney weights were significantly increased in exposed animals, but there was no effect on the weight of lung, heart or spleen tissue, compared with control animals. Similar effects were observed in guinea-pigs. In groups of 8 male and 8 female guinea-pigs exposed to 167 7-hour exposures of 400 ppm trichloroethylene over 235 days, males showed a depression in the growth rate, and there was a significant increase in liver weight in both sexes compared to air-exposed controls. Chlorinated hydrocarbons increase fat incorporation into the liver, and this may explain the occurrence of liver enlargement in these two species.

Male and female CD-1 mice received trichloroethylene at concentrations of 100, 1000, 2500 and 5000 mg/l in 1% Emulphor for 4 or 6 months (Tucker *et al* 1982). Fluid consumption in male and female mice treated with the highest dose of trichloroethylene was less than for mice consuming the vehicle in drinking water only. After 6 months exposure there was an increase in the relative liver weight of males given 1000, 2500 and 5000 mg/l trichloroethylene, and in females exposed to 5000 mg/l. Microsomal enzymes were measured over this period, but there were no consistent trends. Relative kidney weights were also increased in both sexes at the highest dose level after 6 months. Urinalysis indicated that protein and ketone levels were elevated in females treated with 5000 mg/l and in males treated with 2500 and 5000 mg/l.

Nephrosis was observed in 96/98 male F344/N rats, 97/97 female rats, 45/50 male B6C3F1 mice and 49/49 female mice exposed to 1000 mg/kg trichloroethylene (epichlorohydrin-free) administered in corn oil, by gavage, 5 days/week for 103 weeks (US NTP 1983). Pathological changes included the enlargement of tubular cells near the cortico-medullary junction of the kidney, which progressed to dilation of tubules in the sub-capsular cortex. There were no effects in the kidneys of any corn oil control rats or mice.

In female Mongolian gerbils exposed continuously to 50 and 150 ppm trichloroethylene vapour for 12 months, small changes in the lipid composition of the hippocampal and cerebral cortex regions of the brain were observed (Kyrklund *et al* 1983). There were no significant effects on the total protein content or the distribution of lipid classes, although the ratio of cholesterol to phospholipid decreased in the cortex of exposed animals.

The behaviour of male rats exposed by inhalation to 100–1000 ppm trichloroethylene for an unspecified period of hours, 5 days/week, for 5 weeks showed a decline in total activity of up to 24%, compared with the behaviour of unexposed controls (Silverman and Williams 1975). However, in an exploration–thirst behaviour test rats exposed to 100, 200 or 1000 ppm trichloroethylene found water sooner than control animals, without moving faster around the cage. This indicates a loss of inhibition in unfamiliar situations in rats, following exposure to trichloroethylene vapour.

The immunological effects of trichloroethylene were assessed in male and female CD-1 mice given drinking water containing 100, 1000, 2500 and 5000 mg/l trichloroethylene dissolved in 1% Emulphor for 4 or 6 months (Sanders *et al* 1982). Tests for humoral immunity, cell-mediated immunity, lymphocyte responsiveness, bone marrow function and macrophage function indicated that males were unaffected, while in females cell-mediated and bone marrow responses were inhibited at all dose levels after 4 months. Following 6 months exposure, bone marrow function was affected by all dose levels, but cell-mediated immunity was only reduced by the highest dose in female animals. Toxicity was more pronounced after 4 months than 6 months exposure.

Workers chronically exposed to trichloroethylene may suffer central nervous effects such as headaches, dizziness and impaired sensitivity to touch and pain. The trigeminal nerve appears to be particularly affected from long-term exposure (Mitchell and Parsons–Smith 1969, Barret *et al* 1982). Disturbance in heart muscle conduction was reported in dry-cleaning workers (Vyskocil 1953).

Where work involves frequent skin contact with trichloroethylene, this solvent causes defatting of tissues, so hands and skin become rough and chapped. Dermatitis and secondary infections may develop as a consequence (Torkelson and Rowe 1982).

4.3 Genotoxicity

There is conflicting evidence that trichloroethylene is mutagenic in *in vitro* systems. To some extent this has been due to differences in the purity and nature of additives present in the samples tested.

No mutagenic activity was observed in TA98 and TA100 strains of *Salmonella typhimurium* exposed to 10% Trilene, a commercial grade of trichloroethylene of unspecified purity, in air for 48 hours at 37 °C, in the presence of rat liver homogenate (Waskell 1978). Trichloroethylene (purity of 99.5%) was tested in an Ames plate incorporation assay (Bartsch *et al* 1979). A concentration of 8% trichloroethylene in air, incubated with strains TA1530 and TA100 for 2 hours at 37 °C in the presence of mouse liver S–9, showed no mutagenic activity. Under the same conditions, a concentration of 20% trichloroethylene was toxic to the bacteria. However, if plates were preincubated with liver S–9 for 4 hours at 37 °C, before exposure to 5% trichloroethylene for 2 hours, there was a two fold increase in the spontaneous mutation rate. Dose-dependent mutagenicity was reported in *Salmonella typhimurium* TA1535 and TA1538 exposed to 10, 100 and 1000 mg/ml trichloroethylene (unspecified purity) in the absence of metabolic activation, although no experimental details were given (Cerna and Kypenova 1977).

In the absence of metabolic activation, 3 mM trichloroethylene did not induce gene mutations in *Escherichia coli* K-12 (Greim *et al* 1975). In the presence of mouse liver S-9 there was a doubling of the percentage of the spontaneous mutation rate in one of four gene mutation systems.

A small increase in point mutations and gene conversions were observed in *Saccharomyces cerevisiae* D7 after exposure to 40 mM trichloroethylene (unspecified purity) in the presence of mouse liver S-9 (Bronzetti *et al* 1978). No mutagenic activity was observed in the absence of metabolic activation. A twofold increase in gene conversions was also reported in the same strain of *Saccharomyces cerevisiae* exposed to 15 mM trichloroethylene (unspecified purity) (Callen *et al* 1980). Pure (99% purity) and technical grade trichloroethylene, at concentrations of up to 25 mM, did not induce forward mutations in the yeast *Schizosaccharomyces pombe*, either in the presence or absence of metabolic activation (Rossi *et al* 1983). However, positive results were obtained with 6.4 mM epichlorohydrin and 6.4 mM epoxybutane, two stabilisers contained in the technical grade sample. These contaminants were not mutagenic in two *in vivo* host-mediated assays.

Trichloroethylene (free of epoxide stabilisers) was tested for its ability to induce gene mutations and chromosome damage in a haploid and diploid strain of the fungus *Aspergillus nidulans* (Crebelli *et al* 1985). In the haploid strain, there was no induction of gene mutations (methionine suppressors) when the fully grown fungus was exposed to 20 000 ppm trichloroethylene, but a weak response was reported when growing colonies of the fungus were exposed to 5000 ppm of the compound. Exposure to 17 500 ppm trichloroethylene for 24 hours caused a statistically significant disruption to mitotic segregation in growing colonies of the diploid strain of *Aspergillus*.

Exposure of 50 male NMRI mice to concentrations of up to 450 ppm trichloroethylene (99.5% purity) for 24 hours did not produce mutations in the dominant lethal assay (Slacik–Erben *et al* 1980).

There were no interactions *in vitro* between radiolabelled trichloroethylene (99% purity) and DNA from calf thymus in the absence of metabolic activation (Bergman 1983). However, a significant increase in the covalent binding of radiolabelled trichloroethylene to DNA, compared to control values, was observed in the presence of mouse liver S–9 from phenobarbital-pretreated mice. *In vivo*, radioactivity was detected in the DNA of all tissues examined following intraperitoneal administration of 33.6 mg/kg radiolabelled trichloroethylene in peanut oil twice daily for 5 days to 10 male NMRI mice. Radioactivity was found in the brain, kidney, testis, lung, pancreas, liver and spleen, with the highest concentrations in the spleen.

The induction of single strand breaks in the DNA of liver, kidney and lung tissue was investigated in male NMRI mice, 1 hour or 24 hours after intraperitoneal injection of 4–10 mmol/kg trichloroethylene (99.5% purity), dissolved in Tween-80 (Walles 1986). Control animals received the vehicle, Tween-80, only. There was a dose-dependent increase in single strand breaks in liver and kidney DNA, compared with control values, 1 hour after administration of trichloroethylene. However, 24 hours after administration, the incidence of single strand breaks in these tissues returned to normal. No effect was observed in lung DNA.

Unscheduled DNA synthesis was induced in human lymphocytes by concentrations of 2.5, 5 and 10.5 μl/ml trichloroethylene (97–99% purity) dissolved in 0.5% dimethyl sulphoxide, during a 4-hour incubation period, both with or without S–9 mix (Perocco and Prodi 1981). Chromosome aberrations were observed in the lymphocytes of 9 out of 28 workers exposed to trichloroethylene for an unspecified period of time (Konietzko *et al* 1978).

The mutagenic activity of trichloroethylene metabolites has also been investigated. The cysteine conjugate, *S*-1,2-dichlorovinylcysteine, was mutagenic in the Ames test to *Salmonella typhimurium* TA100, TA2638 and TA98, in the absence of metabolic activation (Dekant *et al* 1986c).

The data available at present are inconsistent and inadequate to evaluate the genotoxic potential of trichloroethylene.

4.4 Carcinogenicity

In the National Cancer Institute study (1976) groups of 50 male B6C3F1 mice were given doses of 1200 or 2400 mg/kg body weight and females were given 900 or 1800 mg/kg body weight of trichloroethylene (99% purity, 0.19% epoxybutane stabiliser) in corn oil, by gavage, 5 days/week for 78 weeks. Twenty animals of each sex and species were given the vehicle alone, as controls. A significant increase in hepatocelluar carcinomas was found in treated mice of both sexes compared with control animals. There was also a slightly increased incidence of lung tumours in both sexes. No evidence of liver tumours was observed in groups of 50 Osborne–Mendel rats of both sexes given doses of 500 or 1000 mg/kg body weight of trichloroethylene (99% purity, 0.19% epoxybutane) in corn oil, by gavage, 5 days/week for 78 weeks.

Recent evidence from long-term gavage studies suggests that concentrations of 250 mg/kg body weight trichloroethylene produce a low incidence of renal adenocarcinomas in male rats. This type of tumour occurs very rarely in untreated control animals (WHO 1985, Dekant *et al* 1986a).

The carcinogenicity of trichloroethylene, with or without two epoxide stabilisers, epichlorohydrin (0.8% w/w) and epoxybutane (0.8% w/w) was investigated in Swiss mice, a strain with a low frequency of spontaneous liver tumours (Henschler *et al* 1984). Males were dosed with 2.4 g/kg and females were dosed with 1.8 g/kg trichloroethylene in corn oil, or trichloroethylene with epichlorohydrin and/or epoxybutane, by gavage, 5 days/week, for 18 months. Gross and microscopic examination of liver, stomach, spleen, kidney, adrenal, lung and heart tissue indicated a statistically significant increase in the incidence of forestomach tumours in mice treated with trichloroethylene plus epichlorohydrin, and mice treated with trichloroethylene plus epichlorohydrin and epoxybutane. No effect was observed in mice treated with pure, epoxybutane-stabilised and amine stabilised trichloroethylene.

In female ICR mice, exposed by inhalation to 0, 50, 150 or 450 ppm trichloroethylene (99% purity) 7 hours/day, 5 days/week for 104 weeks, there was a statistically significant increase in the incidence of lung adenocarcinomas in the two highest dose groups compared to controls (Fukuda *et al* 1983). There was no change in the incidence of tumours in groups of 50 female Sprague–Dawley rats, exposed by inhalation to 0, 50, 150 and 450 ppm trichloroethylene under the same conditions.

The carcinogenicity of amine-stabilised trichloroethylene was examined in NMRI mice, Wistar rats and Syrian hamsters (Henschler *et al* 1980). Exposure was by inhalation, at concentrations of 0, 100 and 500 ppm for 6 hours/day, 5 days/week over 18 months. Groups of 30 animals of each sex were used for each dose level. There was no increase in tumours of the spleen, liver, kidneys, lungs or heart of any species. In female mice, there was significant increase in the incidence of malignant lymphomas. However, the biological importance of this finding is unclear since there is a high spontaneous incidence of this type of tumour in NMRI mice.

No skin tumours were observed in female ICR Swiss mice following skin application of 25 mg/ml trichloroethylene oxide (10% dichloroacetyl chloride impurity) in acetone, three times per week, or subcutaneous injection of 2 mg/ml trichloroethylene oxide in tricaprylin once a week, for an unspecified period of time (Van Duuren *et al* 1983).

In a cell transformation assay, 250 μg/ml trichloroethylene was weakly positive after 72 hours, using BALB/c–3T3 cell line (Tu *et al* 1985).

At present, epidemiological studies are inadequate to evaluate the risk of cancer in man from exposure to trichloroethylene. Limitations include uncertain estimation of the degree and duration of exposure to the chemical, simultaneous exposure to other potentially carcinogenic chemicals, small cohort size, and a follow-up period which may be shorter than the latency period for a cancer to develop. The risk of death from cancer due to exposure to dry-cleaning fluids, including trichloroethylene, was investigated from the mortality figures of 330 dry-cleaning and laundry workers recorded between 1957 and 1977 (Blair *et al* 1979). The frequency of deaths from cancer was compared with the predicted frequency of deaths from cancer in the normal population. There was an increased occurrence of lung cancer, cervical cancer and leukaemia in the exposed group, although the difference was not significant. Lung cancer is often associated with low socio-economic status, and it is likely that this was a major contributing factor to the increased frequency observed. The results were also unclear because tetrachloroethylene, carbon tetrachloride and petroleum solvents were also present in the dry-cleaning fluids. In Finland, no significant difference was observed in either total mortality or cancer mortality between a cohort of 1148 men and 969 women, occupationally exposed to trichloroethylene between 1963 and 1976, and the national average mortality figures (Tola *et al* 1980). However, the period of exposure to trichloroethylene was not specified. In a retrospective study, comparing two information sources, the Cancer Registry of liver cancer and a list of past employees at Imperial Chemical Industries, Runcorn, there was only one probable match, and one possible match between the occurrence of liver cancer and occupational exposure. However, on further investigation these two possibilities proved to be negative since the subjects diagnosed with liver cancer had never worked on the Runcorn site (Paddle 1983).

4.5 Reproductive toxicity

Female Swiss–Webster mice were exposed, by inhalation, to 300 ppm trichloroethylene (99% purity), 7 hours/day, on days 6–15 of gestation (Schwetz *et al* 1975). There was no effect on litter size, foetal resorptions, or incidence of gross external, soft tissue or skeletal abnormalities in foetuses from 12 treated females compared with those from 30 control females exposed to filtered air. No embryotoxic or teratogenic effects were observed in the litters of 12 Sprague–Dawley rats exposed to the same conditions, but there was a significant decrease in maternal weight following exposure.

Female Long–Evans rats exposed, by inhalation, to 1800 ppm trichloroethylene 6 hours/day, 5 days/week for 2 weeks before mating and/or 6 hours/day, 7 days/week from day 1 to 20 during gestation showed no signs of toxicity or change in weight gain compared to females exposed to filtered air (Dorfmueller *et al* 1979). Litter size, number of resorptions and sex ratios were unaffected by treatment. Two minor abnormalities were observed in the litters of females exposed during pregnancy alone. These were incomplete ossification of the sternum and displacement of the right ovary. However, it is unlikely that these represent malformations, but indicate delayed skeletal development and variations in soft tissue development. Displacement of the ovary tissue appears to be a strain-specific effect in Long–Evans rats. No behavioural effects were observed in offspring at 10, 20 and 100 days of age, following maternal exposure.

The development of the CNS in the offspring of female rats exposed to 312, 625 or 1250 mg/l trichloroethylene in drinking water throughout gestation until 21 days post-partum was examined by locomotor and behavioural tests (Taylor *et al* 1985). Exploratory behaviour was higher in 60-day-old offspring from all the treatment groups than offspring from the control group. Locomotor activity (running wheel) was also significantly increased in the highest dose group.

The distribution and retention of trichloroethylene and its metabolites in maternal and foetal tissues was studied in C57BL mice following inhalation of radiolabelled trichloroethylene for 10 minutes on days 11, 14 or 17 of gestation (Ghantous *et al* 1986). The distribution of radioactivity in maternal tissues indicated high uptake in the liver, kidneys, bronchi and nasal mucosa. Foetal uptake of radioactivity appeared to be evenly distributed throughout the tissues. There was high retention of the metabolite, trichloroacetic acid, in the amniotic fluid, which was greatest 4 hours after exposure. Additional evidence indicated that some of the trichloroacetic acid present was formed by metabolism of trichloroethylene within the placental tissue itself.

Fertility of female Long–Evans rats was not affected following exposure to 10, 100 or 1000 mg/kg/day trichloroethylene in corn oil, by gavage, for 2 weeks before mating, during mating, and up to day 21 of gestation (Manson *et al* 1984). A significant depression in weight gain in females of the highest dose group indicated maternal toxicity, and neonatal survival was also significantly low in this group. Retention of trichloroethylene was high in the ovaries, adrenals and fat tissues at the end of the pre-mating exposure period.

There was no effect on sperm count, sperm motility, sperm morphology or plasma testosterone levels in male Long–Evans rats exposed to 10, 100 or 1000 mg/kg trichloroethylene in corn oil, by gavage, 5 days/week for 6 weeks (Zenick *et al* 1984). Copulatory behaviour was disrupted in the highest dose group, but returned to normal 4 weeks post-exposure. This reproductive impairment may have been a consequence of the effects of trichloroethylene on the CNS.

In male mice, following administration by intratesticular injection of 100 and 1000 mg/kg trichloroethylene, in an unspecified vehicle, there was a decrease in DNA synthesis in the testes (Borzelleca and Carchman 1982). However, the reproductive significance of this is not known.

5. DISCUSSION

Trichloroethylene is a common contaminant in water, and has been identified in 13 out of 14 drinking water samples in a WRc survey (Water Research Centre 1981). Exposure to high concentrations from polluted groundwater sources may be important under certain circumstances.

Absorption from the gastrointestinal tract is rapid and distribution is primarily to the adipose tissue. This compound is readily metabolised to trichloroacetic acid, trichloroethanol and trichloroethanol glucuronides, which are excreted in the urine. However, the major route of elimination is unchanged in the expired air.

The toxicology of trichloroethylene has been well studied and it appears to be of low acute and chronic toxicity. The principal target organs are the CNS and liver, although recent evidence suggests that trichloroethylene may be nephrotoxic in rodents following long-term exposure.

There is conflicting evidence that trichloroethylene is mutagenic. Both positive and negative results were reported in the Ames test with and without metabolic activation. Trichloroethylene does not appear to be mutagenic in yeast in the absence of metabolic activation, but the position is unclear in the presence of S-9. Under certain conditions of growth, trichloroethylene disrupts mitotic segregation in the fungus *Aspergillus nidulans*. Unscheduled DNA synthesis and chromosome aberrations were reported in human lymphocytes following exposure to this compound. The metabolite *S*-1,2-dichlorovinylcysteine was mutagenic in the Ames test without metabolic activation. The differences in mutagenicity observed in these studies may be partly explained by the purity and nature of the additives present in the samples tested. Both epichlorohydrin and epoxybutane, two stabilisers found in technical grade trichloroethylene, were mutagenic *in vitro*. At present, there are inadequate data to evaluate the mutagenic potential of this chemical.

In 1976 the National Cancer Institute study found an increase in liver tumours in C6B3F1 mice following chronic oral [illegible] trichloroethylene. An increase in forestomach tumours in Swiss mice and lung tumours in NMRI mice from oral and inhalation exposure have also been reported. The carcinogenic potential of trichloroethylene appears to be affected by the presence of stabilisers. There was no evidence of hepatocarcinogenicity in Osborne–Mendel rats. However, a number of renal adenocarcinomas have been recently reported in rats following long-term oral administration, which are rare in untreated controls. Epidemiology studies are insufficient to assess whether trichloroethylene causes cancer in man.

Trichloroethylene appears to be of low reproductive toxicity. There were no significant effects on fertility, teratogenicity or neonatal development in rodents. Delayed ossification of the sternum and displacement of the right ovary were observed in the offspring of treated Long–Evans rats, but these do not represent important embryotoxic effects.

Based on data from the mouse carcinogenicity study (National Cancer Institute 1976), the World Health Organization derived a tentative guideline level of 30 μg/l for trichloroethylene in drinking water (WHO 1984). However, the guideline value was calculated using a low-dose extrapolation model based on a genotoxic mechanism of action, but there is evidence that this is not the case with trichloroethylene. Elcombe (1985) has proposed that induction of peroxisome proliferation (an epigenetic mechanism) by the metabolite trichloroacetic acid is important in the carcinogenicity of trichloroethylene in mouse liver. However, there appear to be species differences between mice and man, both in the ability to metabolise trichloroethylene to trichloroacetic acid, and susceptibility to peroxisome proliferation in general. Both of these factors would tend to diminish the carcinogenic potential of trichloroethylene in man. In conclusion, it is probable that a practical threshold of effect exists for the carcinogenicity of trichloroethylene, and the application of low-dose extrapolation models of carcinogenesis would be inappropriate.

REFERENCES

ADAMS E M, SPENCER H C, ROWE V K, McCOLLISTER D D and IRISH D D (1951) Vapour toxicity of trichloroethylene determined by experiments on laboratory animals. *Archives of Industrial Hygiene and Occupational Medicine* **4**, 469-481.

ANDELMAN J B (1985a) Human exposures to volatile halogenated organic chemicals in indoor and outdoor air. *Environmental Health Perspectives* **62**, 313-318.

ANDELMAN J B (1985b) Inhalation exposure in the home to volatile organic contaminants of drinking water. *Science of the Total Environment* **47**, 443-460.

ARANYI C, O'SHEA W J, GRAHAM J A and MILLER F J (1986) The effects of inhalation of organic chemical air contaminants on murine lung host defences. *Fundamental and Applied Toxicology* **6**, 713-720.

BARRET L, ARSAC P, VINCENT M, FAURE J, GARREL S and REYMOND F (1982) Evoked trigeminal nerve potential in chronic trichloroethylene intoxication. *Journal of Toxicology–Clinical Toxicology* **19**, 419-423.

BARTSCH H, MALAVEILLE C, BA[illegible]N A and PLANCHE G (1979) Mutagenic and alkylating metabolite[illegible]lenes, chlorobutadienes and dichlorobutenes produced by rodent or human liver tissues. *Archives of Toxicology* **41**, 249-277.

BERGMAN K (1983) Interactions of trichloroethylene with DNA *in vitro* and with RNA and DNA of various mouse tissues *in vivo. Archives of Toxicology* **54**, 181-193.

BLAIR A, DECOUFLE P and GRAUMAN D (1979) Causes of death among laundry and dry cleaning workers. *American Journal of Public Health* **69**, 508-511.

BORZELLECA J F and CARCHMAN R A (1982) Effects of selected organic drinking water contaminants on male reproduction. United States Environmental Protection Agency EPA-600/S1-82-009.

BRONZETTI G, ZEIGER E and FREZZA D (1978) Genetic activity of trichloroethylene. *Journal of Environmental Pathology and Toxicology* **1**, 411-418.

BUBEN J A and O'FLAHERTY E J (1985) Delineation of the role of metabolism in the hepatotoxicity of trichloroethylene and perchloroethylene: A dose-effect study. *Toxicology and Applied Pharmacology* **78**, 105-122.

CALLEN D F, WOLF C R and PHILPOT R M (1980) Cytochrome P-450 mediated genetic activity and cytotoxicity of seven halogenated aliphatic hydrocarbons in *Saccharomyces cerevisiae. Mutation Research* **77**, 55-63.

CERNA M and KYPENOVA H (1977) Mutagenic activity of chloroethylenes analysed by screening system tests. *Mutation Research* **46**, 214-215.

CORREIA Y, MARTENS G J, VAN MENSCH F H and WHIM B P (1977) The occurrence of trichloroethylene, tetrachloroethylene and 1,1,1-trichloroethane in Western Europe in air and water. *Atmospheric Environment* **11**, 1113-1116.

COSTA A K and IVANETICH K M (1984) Chlorinated ethylenes: their metabolism and effect on DNA repair in rat hepatocytes. *Carcinogenesis* **5**, 1629-1636.

CREBELLI R, CONTI G, CONTI L and CARERE A (1985) Mutagenicity of trichloroethylene, trichloroethanol and chloral hydrate in *Aspergillus nidulans. Mutation Research* **155**, 105-111.

DEKANT W and HENSCHLER D (1983) New pathways of trichloroethylene metabolism. *Toxicology Letters* **18**, supplement 1, 121.

DEKANT W, METZLER M and HENSCHLER D (1984) Novel metabolites of trichloroethylene through dechlorination reactions in rats, mice and humans. *Biochemical Pharmacology* **33**, 2021-2027.

DEKANT W, METZLER M and HENSCHLER D (1986a) Identification of *S*-1,2-dichlorovinyl-*N*-acetyl-cysteine as a urinary metabolite of trichloroethylene: a possible explanation for its nephrocarcinogenicity in male rats. *Biochemical Pharmacology* **35**, 2455-2458.

DEKANT W, SCHULZ A, METZLER M and HENSCHLER D (1986b) Absorption, elimination and metabolism of trichloroethylene: a quantitative comparison between rats and mice. *Xenobiotica* **16**, 143-152.

DEKANT W, VAMVAKAS S, BERTHOLD K, SCHMIDT S, WILD D and HENSCHLER D (1986c) Bacterial beta-lyase mediated cleavage and mutagenicity of cysteine conjugates derived from the nephrocarcinogenic alkenes trichloroethylene, tetrachloroethylene and hexachlorobutadiene. *Chemicobiological Interactions* **60**, 31-45.

DORFMUELLER M A, HENNE S P, YORK R G, BORNSCHEIN R L and

MANSON J M (1979) Evaluation of teratogenicity and behavioural toxicity with inhalation exposure of maternal rats to trichloroethylene. *Toxicology* **14**, 153-166.

D'SOUZA R W, BRUCKNER J V and FELDMAN S (1985) Oral and intravenous trichloroethylene pharmacokinetics in the rat. *Journal of Toxicology and Environmental Health* **15**, 587-601.

ELCOMBE C R (1985) Species differences in carcinogenicity and peroxisome proliferation due to trichloroethylene: A biochemical human hazard assessment. *Archives of Toxicology*, Supplement 8, 6-17.

ELFARRA A A, JAKOBSON I and ANDERS M W (1986) Mechanisms of *S*-(1,2-dichlorovinyl)glutathione-induced nephrotoxicity. *Biochemical Pharmacology* **35**, 283-288.

ERTLE T, HENSCHLER D, MULLER G and SPASSOWSKI M (1972) Metabolism of trichloroethylene in man. *Archives of Toxicology* **29**, 171-188.

FABRE R and TRUHAUT R (1952) Toxicology of trichloroethylene. 2. Results of experimental animal studies. *British Journal of Industrial Medicine* **9**, 39-43.

FELDMAN R G, WHITE R F, CURRIE F N, TRAVERS P H and LESSELL S (1985) Long-term follow-up after single toxic exposure to trichloroethylene. *American Journal of Industrial Medicine* **8**, 119-126.

FIELDING M, GIBSON T M and JAMES H A (1981) Levels of trichloroethylene, tetrachloroethylene and *p*-dichlorobenzene in groundwaters. *Environmental Technology Letters* **2**, 545-550.

FISHBEIN L (1976) Industrial mutagens and potential mutagens. 1. Halogenated aliphatic derivatives. *Mutation Research* **32**, 267-279.

FUKUDA K, TAKEMOTO K and TSURUTA H (1983) Inhalation carcinogenicity of trichloroethylene in mice and rats. *Industrial Health* **21**, 243-254.

GHANTOUS H, DANIELSSON B R G, DENCKER L, GORCZAK J and VESTERBERG O (1986) Trichloroacetic acid accumulates in murine amniotic fluid after tri- and tetrachloroethylene inhalation. *Acta Pharmacologica et Toxicologica* **58**, 105-114.

GREEN T and ODUM J (1985) Structure/activity studies of the nephrotoxic and mutagenic action of cysteine conjugates of chloro- and fluoroalkenes. *Chemico-biological Interactions* **54**, 15-31.

GREIM H, BONSE G, RADWAN Z, REICHERT D and HENSCHLER D (1975) Mutagenicity *in vitro* and potential carcinogenicity of chlorinated ethylenes as a function of metabolic oxirane formation. *Biochemical Pharmacology* **24**, 2013-2017.

HATHWAY D E (1980) Consideration of the evidence for mechanisms of 1,1,2-trichloroethylene metabolism, including new identification of its dichloroacetic acid and trichloroacetic acid metabolites in mice. *Cancer Letters* **8**, 263-269.

HAYDEN J W, COMSTOCK E G and COMSTOCK B S (1976) The chemical toxicology of solvent abuse. *Clinical Toxicology* **9**, 169-184.

HEALTH AND SAFETY EXECUTIVE (1985) Trichloroethylene: Health and safety precautions. HSE Guidance Note, Environmental Hygiene Series 5, 1-7 HMSO.

HENSCHLER D (1977) Metabolism and mutagenicity of halogenated olefins – a comparison of structure and function. *Environmental Health Perspectives* **21**,

61-64.

HENSCHLER D, ROMEN W, ELSASSER H M, REICHERT D, EDER E and RADWAN Z (1980) Carcinogenicity study of trichloroethylene by long-term inhalation in three animal species. *Archives of Toxicology* **43**, 237-248.

HENSCHLER D, ELSASSER H, ROMEN W and EDER E (1984) Carcinogenicity study of trichloroethylene, with and without epoxide stabilisers, in mice. *Journal of Cancer Research and Clinical Oncology* **107**, 149-156.

HOBARA T, KOBAYASHI H, HIGASHIHARA E, KAWAMOTO T and SAKAI T (1984) Acute effects of 1,1,1-trichloroethane, trichloroethylene and toluene on the haematologic parameters in dogs. *Archives of Environmental Contamination and Toxicology* **13**, 589-593.

IKEDA M (1977) Metabolism of trichloroethylene and tetrachloroethylene in human subjects. *Environmental Health Perspectives* **21**, 239-245.

JAMES W R L (1963) Fatal addiction to trichloroethylene. *British Journal of Industrial Medicine* **20**, 47-49.

KANJE M, KJELLSTRAND P, FEX K and WALLDORF A (1981) Neurotransmitter metabolising enzymes and plasma butyrylcholinesterase in mice exposed to trichloroethylene. *Acta Pharmacologica et Toxicologica* **49**, 205-209.

KJELLESTRAND P, KANJE M, MANSSON L, BJERKEMO M, MORTENSEN I, LANKE J and HOLMQUIST B (1981) Trichloroethylene: effects on body and organ weights in mice, rats and gerbils. *Toxicology* **21**, 105-115.

KJELLESTRAND P, EDSTROM A, BJERKEMO M and HOLMQUIST B (1982) Effects of trichloroethylene inhalation on acid phosphatase in rodent brain. *Toxicology Letters* **10**, 1-5.

KONIETZKO H, HABERLANDT W, HEILBRONNER H, REILL G and WEICHARDT H (1978) Chromosome studies on trichloroethylene workers. *Archives of Toxicology* **40**, 201-206.

KYRKLUND T, ALLING C, HAGLID K and KJELLSTRAND P (1983) Chronic exposure to trichloroethylene: lipid and acyl group composition in gerbil cerebral cortex and hippocampus. *Neurotoxicology* **4**(4), 35-42.

LAHAM S (1970) Studies on placental transfer: trichloroethylene. *Industrial Medicine and Surgery* **39**, 46-49.

LOVELOCK J E (1974) Atmospheric halocarbons and stratospheric ozone. *Nature* **252**, 274-278.

MANSON J M, MURPHY M, RICHDALE N and SMITH M K (1984) Effects of oral exposure to trichloroethylene on female reproductive function. *Toxicology* **32**, 229-242.

McCONNELL G, FERGUSON D M and PEARSON C R (1975) Chlorinated hydrocarbons and the environment. *Endeavour* **34**, 13-18.

MILLER R E and GUENGERICH F P (1983) Metabolism of trichloroethylene in isolated hepatocytes, microsomes and reconstituted enzyme systems containing cytochrome P-450. *Cancer Research* **43**, 1145-1152.

MITCHELL A B S and PARSONS-SMITH B G (1969) Trichloroethylene neuropathy. *British Medical Journal* **1**, 422-423.

MULLER G, SPASSOVSKI M and HENSCHLER D (1975) Metabolism of trichloroethylene in man. 3. Interaction of trichloroethylene and ethanol. *Archives of Toxicology* **33**, 173-189.

MULLER W F, COULSTON F and KORTE F (1982) Comparative metabolism of [^{14}C]trichloroethylene in chimpanzees, baboons and rhesus monkeys. *Chemosphere* **11**, 215-218.

NATIONAL CANCER INSTITUTE (1976) Carcinogenesis bioassay of trichloroethylene. Carcinogenesis Technical Report Series Number 2, DHEW Publication No (NIH) 76-802.

OGATA M, TAKATSUKA Y and TOMOKUNI K (1971) Excretion of organic chlorine compounds in the urine of persons exposed to vapours of trichloroethylene and tetrachloroethylene. *British Journal of Industrial Medicine* **28**, 386-391.

PADDLE G M (1983) Incidence of liver cancer and trichloroethylene manufacture: joint study by industry and a cancer registry. *British Medical Journal* **286**, 846.

PEARSON C R and McCONNELL G (1975) Chlorinated C and C hydrocarbons in the marine environment. *Proceedings of the Royal Society London Series B,* **189**, 305-332.

PEROCCO P and PRODI G (1981) DNA damage by haloalkanes in human lymphocytes cultured *in vitro*. *Cancer Letters* **13**, 213-218.

PROUT M S, PROVAN W M and GREEN T (1985) Species differences in response to trichloroethylene. 1. Pharmacokinetics in rats and mice. *Toxicology and Applied Pharmacology* **79**, 389-400.

ROSSI A M, MIGLIORE L, BARALE R and LOPRIENO N (1983) *In vivo* and *in vitro* mutagenicity studies of a possible carcinogen, trichloroethylene, and its two stabilisers, epichlorohydrin and 1,2-epoxybutane. *Teratogenesis, Carcinogenesis and Mutagenesis* **3**, 75-87.

ROUISSE L and CHAKRABARTI S K (1986) Dose-dependent metabolism of trichloroethylene and its relevance to hepatotoxicity in rats. *Environmental Research* **40**, 450-458.

SANDERS V M, TUCKER A N, WHITE K L, KAUFFMANN B M, HALLETT P, CARCHMAN R A, BORZELLECA J F and MUNSON A E (1982) Humoral and cell-mediated immune status in mice exposed to trichloroethylene in the drinking water. *Toxicology and Applied Pharmacology* **62**, 358-368.

SCHWETZ B A, LEONG B K J and GEHRING P J (1975) The effect of maternally inhaled trichloroethylene, perchloroethylene, methyl chloroform and methylene chloride on embryonal and fetal development in mice and rats. *Toxicology and Applied Pharmacology* **32**, 84-96.

SILVERMAN A P and WILLIAMS H (1975) Behaviour of rats exposed to trichloroethylene vapour. *British Journal of Industrial Medicine* **32**, 308-315.

SLACIK-ERBEN R, ROLL R, FRANKE G and UEHLEKE H (1980) Trichloroethylene vapours do not produce dominant lethal mutations in male mice. *Archives of Toxicology* **45**, 37-44.

STEWART R D and DODD H C (1964) Absorption of carbon tetrachloride, trichloroethylene, tetrachloroethylene, methylene chloride and 1,1,1-trichloroethane through the human skin. *American Industrial Hygiene Association Journal* **25**, 439-446.

STOTT W T, QUAST J F and WATANABE P G (1982) The pharmacokinetics and macromolecular interactions of trichlorethylene in mice and rats. *Toxicology and Applied Pharmacology* **62**, 137-151.

TAYLOR D H, LAGORY K E, ZACCARO D J, PFOHL R J and LAURIE R D (1985) Effect of trichloroethylene on the exploratory and locomotor activity of rats exposed during development. *Science of the Total Environment* **47**, 415-420.

TOLA S, VILHUNEN R, JARVINEN E and KORKALA M L (1980) A cohort study on workers exposed to trichloroethylene. *Journal of Occupational Medicine* **22**, 737-740.

TORKELSON T R and ROWE V K (1982) Halogenated aliphatic hydrocarbons containing chlorine, bromine and iodine. In *Patty's Industrial Hygiene and Toxicology* Volume 2B, edited by G D Clayton and F E Clayton, 3553-3560, Chapter 48. J Wiley and Sons.

TU A S, MURRAY T A, HATCH K M, SIVAK A and MILMAN H A (1985) *In vitro* transformation of BALB/c–3T3 cells by chlorinated ethanes and ethylenes. *Cancer Letters* **28**, 85-92.

TUCKER A N, SANDERS V M, BARNES D W, BRADSHAW T J, WHITE K L, SAIN L E, BORZELLECA J F and MUNSON A E (1982) Toxicology of trichloroethylene in the mouse. *Toxicology and Applied Pharmacology* **62**, 351-357.

UEHLEKE H, TABARELLI-POPLAWSKI S, BONSE G and HENSCHLER D (1977) Spectral evidence for 2,2,3-trichloro-oxirane formation during microsomal trichloroethylene oxidation. *Archives of Toxicology* **37**, 95-105.

US CODE OF FEDERAL REGULATIONS (1976) Code of Federal Regulations 21 CFR 8: 305.

US NTP (1983) Technical report on the carcinogenesis studies of trichloroethylene (without epichlorohydrin) in F344/n rats and BCF mice. Research Triangle Park, NC, National Toxicology Program, NIH Publication No 83-1979, NTP TR 243.

VAN DUUREN B L, KLINE S A, MELCHIONNE S and SEIDMAN I (1983) Chemical structure and carcinogenicity relationships of some chloroalkene oxides and their parent olefins. *Cancer Research* **43**, 159-162.

VERNON R J and FERGUSON R K (1969) Effects of trichloroethylene on visual-motor performance. *Archives of Environmental Health* **18**, 894-900.

VERSCHUEREN K (1983) *Handbook of environmental data on organic chemicals*, second edition. Van Nostrand Reinhold Company.

VYSKOCIL J (1953) Effect of trichloroethylene on the central nervous system. *Lekarske Listy* **8**, 269-273.

WALLACE L A, PELLIZZARI E, HARTWELL T, ROSENZWEIG M, ERICKSON M, SPARACINO C and ZELON H (1984) Personal exposure to volatile organic compounds. 1. Direct measurements in breathing-zone air, drinking water, food and exhaled breath. *Environmental Research* **35**, 293-319.

WALLES S A S (1986) Induction of single-strand breaks in DNA of mice by trichloroethylene and tetrachloroethylene. *Toxicology Letters* **31**, 31-35.

WANG T C, LENAHAN R, KANIK M and J TENEYCK J (1985) The removal of trichloroethylene contaminated groundwater at Vero Beach, Florida. *Archives of Environmental Contamination and Toxicology* **14**, 719-723.

WASKELL L (1978) A study of the mutagenicity of anaesthetics and their metabolites. *Mutation Research* **57**, 141-153.

WATER RESEARCH CENTRE (1981) Organic micropollutants in drinking water. WRc Technical Report TR 159.

WATER RESEARCH CENTRE (1985) Trace organics in British aquifers – a baseline survey. WRc Technical Report TR 223.

WATERS E M, GERSTNER H B and HUFF J E (1977) Trichloroethylene. 1. An Overview. *Journal of Toxicology and Environmental Health* **2**, 671-707.

WELLS J C D (1982) Abuse of trichloroethylene by oral self-administration. *Anaesthesia* **37**, 440-441.

WORLD HEALTH ORGANIZATION (1984) Guidelines for drinking-water quality. 1. Recommendations. World Health Organization, Geneva, p 66.

WORLD HEALTH ORGANIZATION (1985) Trichloroethylene. Environmental Health Criteria, EHC 50, World Health Organization, Geneva.

ZENICK H, BLACKBURN K, HOPE E, RICHDALE N and SMITH M K (1984) Effects of trichloroethylene exposure on male reproductive function in rats. *Toxicology* **31**, 237-250.

ZIGLIO G, FARA G M, BELTRAMELLI G and PREGLIASCO F (1983) Human environmental exposure to trichloro- and tetrachloroethylene from water and air in Milan, Italy. *Archives of Environmental Contamination and Toxicology* **12**, 57-64.

ZOETEMAN B C J, De GREEF E and BRINKMAN J J (1981) Persistency of organic contaminants in groundwater, lessons from soil pollution incidents in the Netherlands. *Science of the Total Environment* **21**, 187-202.

4

Tetrachloroethylene

1. INTRODUCTION

Tetrachloroethylene (perchloroethylene, PER, ethylene tetrachloride) is used as a solvent, principally in dry-cleaning and the manufacture of textiles, but it is also used as a constituent of rubber solutions, paint removers, printing inks and metal cleaning fluids.

CAS Reg No:	127-18-4
Molecular weight:	165.8
Boiling point:	121.4°C
Solubility:	150 mg/l at 25°C

2. EXPOSURE

Since tetrachloroethylene is not known to occur naturally (International Agency for Research on Cancer 1979) contamination from manufacturing processes accounts for its presence in the environment. It has been detected in air, food and water.

2.1 Air

World-wide production of tetrachloroethylene in 1973 was estimated to be just over one million tons (McConnell *et al* 1975), and it is likely that over 80% of this was lost to the atmosphere by evaporation during subsequent use. There have been a number of reports of the detection of tetrachloroethylene in air (McConnell *et al* 1975, Lillian *et al* 1975, Cox *et al* 1977, Singh *et al* 1977, Russell and Shadoff 1977, Ziglio *et al* 1983). In New York City, levels ranged between 0.1 and 8.7 $\mu g/m^3$ (Lillian *et al* 1975). Atmospheric measurements of tetrachloroethylene in urban Milan were reported between 9 and 15 $\mu g/m^3$, whereas concentrations in rural areas were much lower (Ziglio *et al* 1983). This solvent was detected at concentrations as high as 20–300 mg/m^3 near dry-cleaning firms (Engels *et al* 1975).

2.2 Food

Tetrachloroethylene is used to extract oil and fat from meat so contamination of food may result from this process (NATO/CCMS 1974). Levels of 1 μg/kg have been detected in beef, up to 2 μg/kg in fruit and vegetables, 3 μg/kg in tea and coffee, and ranging from 7 μg/kg in olive oil to 13 μg/kg in butter (McConnell *et al* 1975).

2.3 Water

Tetrachloroethylene was detected in 11 out of 14 drinking water samples examined in a WRc survey (Water Research Centre 1981). Concentrations varied from less than 1 μg/l to about 10 μg/l in some groundwaters. There are many reports of contamination of water supplies by tetrachloroethylene, in both Europe and the United States of America (Trouwborst 1981, Kawamura and Kaplan 1983, Larson *et al* 1983, Ziglio *et al* 1983).

Tetrachloroethylene has been found in rainwater at 0.15 μg/l, groundwaters and rivers, and in tapwater at 45 μg/l (Giger and Molnar-Kubica 1978, Wakeham *et al* 1980, Grob and Grob 1974). Drinking water supplies in Milan contained levels between 4 and 20 μg/l (Ziglio *et al* 1983). Chlorination at sewage treatment plants can result in small quantities of tetrachloroethylene being present in water (Bellar *et al* 1974).

Although ingestion is the main route of exposure for most waterborne chemicals, inhalation may also be important for compounds such as tetrachloroethylene which are particularly volatile. Andelman (1985a,b) has measured air concentrations of trichloroethylene in showers using trichloroethylene-contaminated groundwater, and has shown that this can be a substantial source of exposure.

Leaching of tetrachloroethylene from vinyl-toluene-lined asbestos-cement pipes was reported in two American studies (Larson *et al* 1983, Demond 1985). Concentrations ranged from a few micrograms per litre to 3.5 mg/l tetrachloroethylene in the dead-end pipes of water distribution systems lined with vinyl-toluene.

3. TOXICOKINETICS

3.1 Absorption

Tetrachloroethylene is absorbed through the lungs, gastrointestinal tract and the skin (Steward and Dodd 1964).

Absorption from the gastrointestinal tract is poor, although some tetrachloroethylene can be detected in the exhaled air following gavage experiments in laboratory animals (Torkelson and Rowe 1982).

In both man and animals uptake of tetrachloroethylene through the skin is thought to be slow, and of less toxicological importance than for trichloroethylene (Steward and Dodd 1964).

3.2 Distribution

In rats and man, most of an inhaled dose of tetrachloroethylene is excreted unchanged in the exhaled air, and the remainder is distributed primarily to the adipose tissue.

Within 72 hours following oral administration of 1 mg/kg of radiolabelled tetrachloroethylene in corn oil to adult male Sprague–Dawley rats, 70% of the body burden of radioactivity was exhaled unchanged, 26% was metabolised and excreted, and 4% remained in the body (Pegg *et al* 1979). Following doses of 500 mg/kg radiolabelled tetrachloroethylene, 89% was exhaled, 9% was metabolised and excreted, and 2% remained in body tissues. Similar distribution patterns were observed following inhalation exposure to 10 or 600 ppm radiolabelled tetrachloroethylene for 6 hours.

Concentrations of tetrachloroethylene measured in different tissues in man varied from less than 1 μg/kg wet tissue in the brain to almost 30 μg/kg in the adipose layers (McConnell *et al* 1975).

3.3 Metabolism

Tetrachloroethylene is readily metabolised by rodents and man.

In the liver, metabolic breakdown of this compound is thought to involve oxidation by mixed function oxidase enzymes to an epoxide (Bonse *et al* 1975, Leibman and Ortiz 1977, Henschler 1977). The structural symmetry of this epoxide contrasts with the non-symmetrical arrangement of chlorine atoms in the trichloroethylene epoxide, and this may account for the different toxic properties of tetrachloroethylene and trichloroethylene. A chloride shift within the tetrachloroethylene epoxide results in the formation of an acyl chloride, trichloroacetyl chloride. The chloride is then hydrolysed to form trichloroacetic acid, the principal metabolite of tetrachloroethylene breakdown (Bonse *et al* 1975, Leibman and Ortiz 1977, Ziglio *et al* 1984). In mice, oxalic acid has been detected as a urinary metabolite, and this could originate from hydration of the tetrachloroethylene epoxide, followed by a dechlorination reaction (Yllner 1961).

A total of five metabolites were identified in unspecified biological fluids of humans, rats, mice and guinea-pigs (Reichert 1983). Quantitatively, the two most important compounds were trichloroacetic acid and oxalic acid; the identity of the three other compounds was not given.

Trichloroacetic acid was one of two trichloro compounds detected in the urine of male volunteers exposed by inhalation to 87 ppm of tetrachloroethylene for 3 hours (Ogata *et al* 1971). It could not be confirmed that the second compound was trichloroethanol.

There appears to be a species difference in the extent to which tetrachloroethylene is broken down (Schumann *et al* 1980). Male B6C3F1 mice metabolised 8.5 times more tetrachloroethylene per kilogram of body weight than male Sprague–Dawley rats following a 6-hour exposure, by inhalation, to 10 ppm of radiolabelled tetrachloroethylene.

However, in all species metabolism is dose-dependent, and saturable; above certain exposure an increase in tetrachloroethylene no longer leads to an increase in metabolites in the urine (Filser and Bolt 1979, Buben and O'Flaherty 1985).

In man, of the 2% inhaled tetrachloroethylene that is metabolised, most appears to be converted to trichloroacetic acid.

3.4 Excretion

The major route of elimination is via the exhaled air. In rats, 72 hours after oral administration of 1–500 mg/kg radiolabelled tetrachloroethylene, 70–89% of the unchanged compound was exhaled, together with 0.5–2.5% of radiolabelled carbon dioxide. Between 4.6 and 17.0% of the total radioactivity was measured in the urine, and 4.0–6.0% in the faeces (Pegg *et al* 1979). Yllner (1961) obtained similar results in mice. Following inhalation of tetrachloroethylene for 2 hours 70% of the radioactivity was found in the expired air, 20% was in the urine, and trace amounts in the faeces.

The distribution of tetrachloroethylene in human volunteers, exposed by inhalation to 50 ppm tetrachloroethylene for 8 hours, (Ohtsuki *et al* 1983) was found to be as follows: 38% exhaled unchanged; 2% metabolised, and excreted in the urine; 60% remained in the body tissues.

Urinalysis was carried out on male volunteers exposed to 87 ppm tetrachloroethylene for 3 hours, and samples were collected up to 100 hours after the start of the experiment (Ogata *et al* 1971). Trichloroacetic acid was identified, plus another chlorinated hydrocarbon, possibly trichloroethanol. The excretion rate of trichloroacetic acid initially rose to almost 0.2 mg/hour, then returned to a rate of about 0.05 mg/hour 64 hours later. The maximum rate of excretion of trichloroacetic acid after exposure to tetrachloroethylene is faster than that following exposure to trichloroethylene.

Results from a range of studies indicate that exhalation is the major route of elimination for tetrachloroethylene.

4. HEALTH EFFECTS

4.1 Acute and subacute toxicity

Tetrachloroethylene is of moderate to low acute toxicity via the oral route. The oral LD50 using corn oil as the vehicle of administration was 8.85 g/kg in the mouse, and 2.60 g/kg in the rat (Torkelson and Rowe 1982). When administered in drinking solutions the oral LD50 value of tetrachloroethylene in Charles River rats was 3.84 g/kg for males, and 3.00 g/kg in females (Hayes *et al* 1986).

Rats exposed to very high concentrations of tetrachloroethylene exhibited CNS depression. Unconsciousness did not occur at a level of 2000 ppm, but was observed after several hours at 3000 ppm, and within a few minutes at 6000 ppm (Rowe *et al* 1952).

Acute cardiotoxic properties of tetrachloroethylene have been studied in laboratory animals. The mean threshold dose that disturbed the rhythm and contractility of heart tissue following intravenous injection was 6.5 mg/kg in the rabbit, 24.0 mg/kg in the cat, and 6.5 mg/kg in the dog (Kobayashi *et al* 1981).

In 140 female CD-1 mice exposed to 50 ppm tetrachloroethylene vapour for 3 hours there was an increase in mortality compared with 140 controls, exposed to filtered air for 3 hours, following an experimental challenge to a streptococcal infection, *Streptococcus zooepidemicus* (Aranyi *et al* 1986). This indicates that acute exposure to tetrachloroethylene may alter the immune defence system, and increase susceptibility to respiratory infections in the mouse.

The major effect of acute tetrachloroethylene exposure in man is CNS depression, ranging from lightheadedness and loss of muscular coordination at low concentrations, to unconsciousness and respiratory paralysis at high concentrations (Steward 1969).

Burning and lacrimation of the eyes may be caused at levels above 200 ppm, due to membrane irritation. Ingestion may result in bleeding, diarrhoea and bloody stools also as a result of irritation to the gastrointestinal membranes (Torkelson and Rowe 1982).

Since tetrachloroethylene removes the natural oils from the skin, prolonged cutaneous exposure causes chapping, and often dermatitis.

Single doses of tetrachloroethylene for antihelminth purposes have been prescribed at levels of 0.1 ml/kg up to a maximum of 5 ml for adults, which can be repeated after 4–7 days. A dose of 500 mg/kg was reported not to be lethal in humans (Torkelson and Rowe 1982).

4.2 Chronic toxicity

Chronic exposure to tetrachloroethylene most readily affects the CNS and liver.

In a subchronic study tetrachloroethylene was administered in the drinking water of male and female Charles River rats at doses of 14, 400 and 1400 mg/kg body weight for 90 consecutive days (Hayes *et al* 1986). In order to make tetrachloroethylene soluble in drinking water, it was homogenised in 4% Emulphor, a polyethylated vegetable oil, for several hours. Animals in the three test groups received tetrachloroethylene dissolved in 4% Emulphor, administered in the drinking water. There were two control groups. Negative control animals received deionised water and vehicle controls received 4% Emulphor solution. Animals in each group (20 males and 20 females per group) were dosed by gavage. At the end of the 90-day exposure period females receiving 400 or 1400 mg/kg and males receiving 1400 mg/kg tetrachloroethylene had lower body weights than controls. Liver and kidney to body weight ratios for all animals in the highest dose group were higher than ratios for control animals. There were no deaths, and there were no significant changes in haematology, or urinalyses in any group. 5′-Nucleotidase enzyme levels were raised in males at 400 and 1400 mg/kg, and in females at the highest dose, which may be indicative of liver damage. Other serum chemistry parameters were unaffected.

In a chronic inhalation study, rats exposed to 400 ppm for 7 hours/day over a period of 183 days did not exhibit any ill-effects (Rowe *et al* 1952). Rabbits, guinea-pigs and monkeys were also exposed to repeated doses of tetrachloroethylene over different periods of time (13–179 exposures in 18–250 days). No adverse effects were observed at 100 ppm exposure, except in female guinea-pigs, which showed an increase in liver weight. Hepatic effects included an increase in liver weight, fatty degeneration, and a drop in hepatic ATP levels. A loss of coordination and balance plus CNS depression were observed at 255 ppm in rabbits, and at 1600 ppm in rats.

Biochemical changes in the CNS following chronic exposure to tetrachloroethylene have been investigated (Kyrklund *et al* 1984, Rosengren *et al* 1986). Male Mongolian gerbils were exposed by inhalation to a low dose (below the anaesthetic level) of 120 ppm tetrachloroethylene over a period of 12 months, with only short interruptions for cleaning the inhalation chambers (Kyrklund *et al* 1984). At the end of exposure the brains were taken for biochemical examination. Results indicated that the fatty acid composition of the membranes in the cerebral cortex and hippocampus had altered.

The hepatotoxicity of tetrachloroethylene was studied in a sub-chronic, inhalation experiment in female mice (Kylin *et al* 1965). Mice were exposed to 200 ppm tetrachloroethylene, 4 hours/day, 6 days/week for 1, 2, 4 and 8 weeks. There were no signs of cell death or increase in fibrous tissue (cirrhosis) in the liver, but fatty degeneration did occur, which became more severe with longer exposure. No adverse effects on the kidney were observed.

It appears that tetrachloroethylene only exerts a weak toxic effect on the kidneys at high doses. Sublethal oral doses of tetrachloroethylene in mice caused swelling, and some cell degeneration in kidney tubules (Klaassen and Plaa 1966).

Most of the information on the chronic effects of tetrachloroethylene in humans is from occupational data on dry-cleaners. The common symptoms of toxicity are dizziness, sleepiness, and irritation to the eyes, nose and throat (National Institute for Occupational Safety and Health 1976). Russian authors have reported other neurophysiological effects following occupational exposure, such as a reduced ability to perceive colour (Alieva *et al* 1985).

Neurological, physiological and behavioural tests were carried out on ten male and nine female volunteers exposed for 1, 3 or 7.5 hours/day, 5 days/week (for an unspecified period of time) to 20, 100 or 150 ppm tetrachloroethylene (Hake and Stewart 1977). No effects were observed at exposure levels of 20 ppm. Males showed a decrease in coordination skills at 100 and 150 ppm.

Behavioural, renal, hepatic and pulmonary tests were carried out on two groups of subjects: those occupationally exposed to tetrachloroethylene and a control group (Lauwerys *et al* 1983). The exposed group consisted of 26 subjects (24 female and 2 male) working in dry-cleaning establishments and occupationally exposed to 21 ppm tetrachloroethylene (time-weighted average exposure) over a period of 6 years; the control group was composed of 33 subjects (31 female and 2 male) working in a chocolate factory and who had never been occupationally exposed to organic solvents. No differences were found between the two groups.

Chronically exposed individuals may develop a tolerance to the solvent. Single and repeated experimental exposures to 100 ppm tetrachloroethylene vapour were carried out in subjects for either a single 7-hour period, or 7 hours/day for 5 days (Steward *et al* 1970). Subjects repeatedly exposed had fewer subjective and objective complaints (headaches, speech difficulty, dizziness, nose and throat irritation) than those who were exposed for only a single, 7-hour period.

4.3 Genotoxicity

At concentrations of 4 mM tetrachloroethylene was not mutagenic in the Ames test to *Salmonella typhimurium* TA 100, either in the presence or absence of mouse liver S-9 (Bartsch *et al* 1979). A concentration of 5 mM was toxic to the bacteria.

There is one report of a mutagenic effect in a host-mediated assay, using female ICR mice and *Salmonella typhimurium* TA1950, TA1951 and TA1952 (Cerna and Kypenova 1977).

At a concentration of 20 mM, tetrachloroethylene had no mutagenic effect in *Escherichia coli* K12, with or without metabolic activation (Greim *et al* 1975).

A dose of up to 85 mM tetrachloroethylene was tested in *Saccharomyces cerevisiae* D7 for three types of genotoxic effect, mitotic gene conversion, mitotic crossing over and reverse mutation. No mutagenicity was observed during a 2-hour incubation period (Bronzetti *et al* 1983). However, Callan *et al* (1980) using the same strain of yeast and comparable concentrations of tetrachloroethylene did report mutagenic activity in a 1-hour incubation test. No activity was reported during 4-hour incubation periods.

Tetrachloroethylene did not induce chromosomal aberrations in the bone marrow cells of mice or rats after single, repeated or long-term exposure to the compound *in vivo* (Cerna and Kypernova 1977).

4.4 Carcinogenicity

In the National Cancer Institute study (1977) groups of 48 B6C3F1 mice and Osborne–Mendel rats of both sexes were given doses of 500 or 1000 mg/kg body weight of tetrachloroethylene in corn oil by gavage, 5 days/week for 78 weeks. A significant increase in hepatocellular carcinomas was found in treated male and female B6C3F1 mice at both low and high dose levels. No other organs or tissues appeared to be affected.

In contrast there was no evidence of an increase in liver tumours in Osborne–Mendel rats treated with the same dose levels of tetrachloroethylene administered in corn oil. However, the survival rate was poor (Weisburger 1977).

In an inhalation study by Rampy *et al* (1977) there was no significantly increased incidence of any type of tumour in either male or female Sprague–Dawley rats exposed to 315 ppm or 602 ppm tetrachloroethylene for 6 hours/day, 5 days/week for 12 months. Observations were carried out over the animals' lifetime. However, inhalation of tetrachloroethylene for two years at 200 or 400 ppm in rats and 100 or 200 ppm in mice resulted in an increased incidence of leukaemia in rats and liver tumours in mice (USNTP 1986).

Tetrachloroethylene had no effect in two mouse skin-painting studies (Van Duuren *et al* 1979). Doses of 18 and 54 mg in acetone were applied to the shaved dorsal surface of male and female mice three times per week for 440–594 days. Also, a single application of 163 mg tetrachloroethylene was followed by thrice weekly applications of a promoter for 428–576 days. Control groups included one for promoter, one for acetone and one for no treatment.

A dose of 7.5 mg tetrachloroethylene epoxide in acetone applied three times weekly to the dorsal skin of female ICR/Ha Swiss mice for their lifespan resulted in three mice with benign skin tumours, and one with a squamous carcinoma out of 60 animals (Van Duuren *et al* 1983). No skin tumours were observed in the control group of 100 animals treated with acetone.

In an *in vitro* test, 16.08 mg/ml tetrachloroethylene induced cell transformation in the Fischer rat embryo (F1706) tissue culture system following a 48-hour incubation period (Price *et al* 1978). However, Tu *et al* (1985) reported that tetrachloroethylene at concentrations of up to 250 μg/ml gave negative results in an *in vitro* transformation assay using BALB/c–3T3 cells.

Evidence that tetrachloroethylene causes cancer in humans is unclear.

Blair *et al* (1979) investigated a group of 330 dry-cleaning and laundry workers who had been exposed to tetrachloroethylene for periods of up to 20 years. The frequency of specific causes of deaths for this group was compared with that for the general population, and the frequency of deaths from cancer was higher than the predicted frequency for the normal population (87 recorded; 68 expected), although the difference was only small. Lung, cervical and skin cancer were mainly responsible for the increased mortality rate, but there was also a slightly elevated occurrence of leukaemia and liver cancer. Although tetrachloroethylene was the main constituent of the cleaning fluid, other solvents such as carbon tetrachloride and trichloroethylene were also present, so any effects cannot be attributed to tetrachloroethylene alone. Also, a high incidence of lung cancer is associated with low socio-economic class. Since laundry workers tend to belong to this social group this could have been an important contributing factor to the elevated mortality rate from cancer, rather than the single effect of exposure to tetrachloroethylene.

Another study (Pesticide and Toxic Chemical News 1985) reported an unspecified excess of bladder and kidney cancers among 1690 dry-cleaning workers exposed to tetrachloroethylene. However, since exposure cannot be attributed to this solvent alone, due to the presence of other solvent compounds, the significance of the results is unclear.

4.5 Reproductive toxicity

The reproductive toxicity of tetrachloroethylene in rats and mice was investigated by Schwetz *et al* (1975). Seventeen Sprague–Dawley rats were exposed by inhalation to 300 ppm (2000 mg/m^3) tetrachloroethylene for 7 hours daily on days 6–15 of gestation. Maternal body weight dropped slightly, and there was a small but significant increase in the number of resorptions. No other abnormalities were observed in rats, but all 17 litters of mice exposed to the same conditions showed delayed ossification of skull bones. There was also an increase in the incidence of subcutaneous oedema. These findings are not considered to be gross disruptions of foetal development, and tetrachloroethylene did not cause any major teratogenic effects. However, the experiments were only conducted at one dose level.

A series of behavioural, neurochemical and neuropathological tests were carried out on the offspring of 15 Sprague–Dawley rats exposed by inhalation to 900 ppm tetrachloroethylene for 7 hours daily during days 7–13 of gestation (Nelson *et al* 1980). Mothers exposed to tetrachloroethylene gained less weight than the control animals. Behavioural tests to measure CNS function at different stages of development were carried out on the offspring before weaning. Pups from mothers exposed to tetrachloroethylene during gestation performed poorly in neuromuscular tests, but only on certain days of testing. Also, neurochemical analysis of brain tissue indicated a significant reduction in acetylcholine and dopamine levels in these offspring. No behavioural effects were observed in similar tests carried out on the offspring of rats exposed to 100 ppm tetrachloroethylene for 7 hours/day during days 14–20 of gestation.

Ghantous *et al* (1986) studied the distribution and retention of tetrachloroethylene and its metabolites in the maternal and foetal tissues of pregnant C57BL mice exposed by inhalation to ^{14}C-labelled tetrachloroethylene for 10 minutes. The distribution of radioactivity in maternal tissues indicated a high uptake in body fat, brain, liver, kidney and lung. [^{14}C]Tetrachloroethylene and its metabolites were found to be evenly distributed in foetal tissues. However, there was high retention of the metabolite, trichloroacetic acid, in the amniotic fluid. There was also evidence to suggest that some of the trichloroacetic acid was produced by metabolism of tetrachloroethylene within the placental tissue itself. This high level of trichloroacetic acid may contribute to long-term exposure of the foetus by absorption through its skin, or by swallowing the amniotic fluid. Any foeto-toxic effects cannot be attributed to tetrachloroethylene alone, but may also be caused by its metabolites.

From the evidence available it appears that mice are more susceptible than rats to embryo-toxic effects from tetrachloroethylene.

5. DISCUSSION

Tetrachloroethylene is a common environmental pollutant. It has been identified in groundwater, surface waters and treated drinking water, and these are likely to represent an important source of exposure. High concentrations of tetrachloroethylene vapour near dry-cleaning factories represent local sources of exposure from air.

Absorption of tetrachloroethylene from the gastrointestinal tract is poor; other routes of absorption include the lungs and skin. Tetrachloroethylene is distributed primarily to the adipose tissue. There appear to be species differences in the metabolism of this compound. In mice, oxalic acid and trichloroacetic acid are formed as metabolites, but in man only trichloroacetic acid has been identified as a metabolite. Excretion is primarily through exhalation of the unchanged compound.

Tetrachloroethylene is of relatively low acute toxicity in experimental animals. LD50 values in the rat indicate that tetrachloroethylene is slightly more toxic when administered in corn oil than in drinking water. The principal target organs for both acute and chronic toxicity are the CNS and liver.

Tetrachloroethylene does not appear to be mutagenic in the Ames test, with or without metabolic activation, but there is one report of mutagenic activity in a host-mediated assay. Evidence for mutagenicity in the yeast *Saccharomyces cerevisiae* D7 is equivocal, and no chromosomal aberrations were induced in rats or mice following acute or chronic exposure to the compound *in vivo.*

Although the National Cancer Institute study (1977) reported an increase in liver tumours in B6C3F1 mice following long-term exposure to tetrachloroethylene, there was no evidence of carcinogenicity in Osborne–Mendel rats, in inhalation studies in Sprague–Dawley rats or in mouse skin-painting assays. In view of the concern over the significance of liver tumours in the mouse, and the increasing evidence that the use of corn oil as a vehicle may not represent exposure via drinking water, care needs to be taken in the interpretation of the NCI study. A study of the carcinogenic potential of tetrachloroethylene administered in drinking water compared with corn oil as a solvent is essential. Epidemiological studies on dry-cleaning and laundry workers are insufficient to assess whether tetrachloroethylene causes cancer in man. Considering the lack of mutagenic activity together with negative findings in carcinogenicity studies, the evidence that tetrachloroethylene may cause cancer in man through ingestion in drinking water is limited.

Tetrachloroethylene does not appear to be teratogenic in rats, but delayed ossification of skull bones indicated foeto-toxic effects in the offspring of mice exposed to 300 ppm during days 6–15 of gestation.

The World Health Organization (WHO 1984) set a tentative guideline value of 10 μg/l for tetrachloroethylene in drinking water. This was based on data from the mouse carcinogenicity study (NCI 1977), using corn oil as the solvent. However, it is possible that the use of corn oil as a vehicle may overestimate the toxicity that might be expected following exposure through water.

REFERENCES

ALIEVA Z A, SULTANOV M Y and MIRZOEV T A (1985) Reduced acuity of color perception resulting from exposure to styrene and tetrachloroethylene vapours. *Gigiena Truda i Professional'nykh Zabolevanii* **2**, 11–13.

ANDELMAN J B (1985a) Human exposures to volatile halogenated organic chemicals in indoor and outdoor air. *Environmental Health Perspectives* **62**, 313–318.

ANDELMAN J B (1985b) Inhalation exposure in the home to volatile organic contaminants of drinking water. *Science of the Total Environment* **47**, 443–460.

ARANYI C, O'SHEA W J, GRAHAM J A and MILLER F J (1986) The effects of inhalation of organic chemical air contaminants on murine lung host defences. *Fundamental and Applied Toxicology* **6**, 713–720.

BARTSCH H, MALAVEILLE C, BARBIN A and PLANCHE G (1979) Mutagenic and alkylating metabolites of halo-ethylenes, chlorobutadienes and dichlorobutenes produced by rodent or human liver. Evidence for oxirane formation by P450-linked microsomal mono-oxygenases. *Archives of Toxicology* **41**, 249–277.

BELLAR T A, LECHTENBERG J J and KRONER R C (1974) The occurrence of organohalides in chlorinated drinking waters. *Journal of the American Water Works Association* **66**, 703–706.

BLAIR A, DECOUFLE P and GRAUMAN D (1979) Causes of death among laundry and dry cleaning workers. *American Journal of Public Health* **69**, 508–511.

BONSE G, URBAN T, REICHERT D and HENSCHLER D (1975) Chemical reactivity, metabolic oxirane formation and biological reactivity of chlorinated ethylenes in the isolated, perfused rat liver preparation. *Biochemical Pharmacology* **24**, 1829–1934.

BRONZETTI G, BAUER C, CORSI C, DEL CARRATORE R, GALLI A, NIERI R and PAOLINI M (1983) Genetic and biochemical studies on perchloroethylene *in vitro* and *in vivo*. *Mutation Research* **116**, 323–331.

BUBEN J A and O'FLAHERTY (1985) Delineation of the role of metabolism in the hepatotoxicity of trichloroethylene and perchloroethylene: A dose–effect study. *Toxicology and Applied Pharmacology* **78**, 105–122.

CALLAN D F, WOLF C R and PHILPOT R M (1980) Cytochrome P–450 mediated genetic activity and cytotoxicity of seven halogenated aliphatic hydrocarbons in *Saccharomyces cerevisiae*. *Mutation Research* **77**, 55–63.

CERNA M and KYPERNOVA H (1977) Mutagenic activity of chloroethylenes analysed by screening system tests. *Mutation Research* **46**, 214–215.

COX R A, DERWENT R G, EGGLETON A E J and LOVELOCK J E (1977) Photochemical oxidaton of halocarbons in the troposphere. *Atmospheric Environment* **10**, 305–308.

DEMOND A H (1985) Leaching of tetrachloroethylene from vinyl-lined pipe. *Journal of Environmental Engineering* **111**, 1–9.

ENGELS L H, SCHNETZ A and WOLF D (1975) Perchloroethylene in dry cleaning, pollutant situation and technical prophylaxis. *Staub Reinhalt Luft* **3**, 412–415.

FILSER U G and BOLT H M (1979) Pharmacokinetics of halogenated ethylenes in rats. *Archives of Toxicology* **42**, 123–136.

GHANTOUS H, DANIELSSON B R G, DENCKER L, GORCZAK J and VESTERBERG O (1986) Trichloroacetic acid accumulates in murine amniotic fluid after Tri- and Tetrachloroethylene inhalation. *Acta Pharmacologica et Toxicologica* **58**, 105–114.

GIGER W and MOLNAR-KUBICA E (1978) Tetrachloroethylene in contaminated ground and drinking waters. *Bulletin of Environmental Contamination and Toxicology* **19**, 475–480.

GREIM H, BONSE G, RADWAN Z, REICHERT D and HENSCHLER D (1975) Mutagenicity *in vitro* and potential carcinogenicity of chlorinated ethylenes as a function of metabolic oxirane formation. *Biochemical Pharmacology* **24**, 2013–2017.

GROB K and GROB G J (1974) Organic substances in drinking water and their precursor Part 2. Applications in the area of Zurich. *Journal of Chromatography* **90**, 303-313.

HAKE C L and STEWART R D (1977) Human exposure to tetrachloroethylene: Inhalation and skin contact. *Environmental Health Perspectives* **21**, 231–238.

HAYES J R, CONDIE L W and BORZELLECA J F (1986) The subchronic toxicity of tetrachloroethylene (perchloroethylene) administered in the drinking water of rats. *Fundamental and Applied Toxicology* **7**, 119–125.

HENSCHLER D (1977) Metabolism and mutagenicity of halogenated olefins — a comparison of structure and function. *Environmental Health Perspectives* **21**, 61–64.

INTERNATIONAL AGENCY FOR RESEARCH ON CANCER (1979) Some halogenated hydrocarbons. In *Monographs on the evaluations of carcinogenic risk of chemicals to man,* Vol 20. Lyons, International Agency for Research on Cancer, pp. 491–514.

KAWAMURA K and KAPLAN I R (1983) Organic compounds in the rain-water of Los Angeles. *Environmental Science and Technology* **17**, 497–501.

KLAASSEN C D and PLAA G L (1966) Relative effects of various chlorinated hydrocarbons on liver and kidney function in mice. *Toxicology and Applied Pharmacology* **9**, 139–151.

KOBAYASHI S, HUTCHEON D and REGAN J (1981) Acute cardiotoxic properties of tetrachloroethylene. *Federation Proceedings* **40**, 698.

KYLIN B, SUMEGI I and YLLNER S (1965) Hepatotoxicity of inhaled trichloroethylene and tetrachloroethylene. Longterm exposure. *Acta Pharmacologica et Toxicologica* **22**, 379–385.

KYRKLUND T, ALLING C, KJELLSTRAND P and HAGLID K (1984) Chronic effects of perchloroethylene on the composition of lipid and acyl groups in cerebral cortex and hippocampus of the gerbil. *Toxicology Letters* **22**, 343–349.

LARSON C D, LOVE O T and REYNOLDS G (1983) Tetrachloroethylene leached from lined asbestos-cement pipe into drinking water. *Journal of the American Water Works Association* **75**, 184–188.

LAUWERYS R, HERBRAND J, BUCHET J P, BERNARD A and GAUSSIN J (1983) Health surveillance of workers exposed to tetrachloroethylene in dry-cleaning shops. *International Archives of Occupational and Environmental Health* **52**, 69–77.

LEIBMAN K C and ORTIZ E (1977) Metabolism of halogenated ethylenes. *Environmental Health Perspectives* **21**, 91–97.

LILLIAN D, SINGH H B, APPLEBY A, LOBBAN L, ARNTS R, GUMPERT R, HAGUE R, TOOMEY J, KAZAZIS J, ANTELL M, HANSEN D and SCOTT B (1975) Atmospheric fates of halogenated compounds. *Journal of the Air Pollution Control Association* **26**, 141–143.

McCONNELL G, FERGUSON D M and PEARSON C R (1975) Chlorinated hydrocarbons and the environment. *Endeavour* **34**(121), 13–18.

NATIONAL CANCER INSTITUTE (1977) Bioassay of tetrachloroethylene for possible carcinogenicity, DHEW Publication No (NIH) 77–813, Bethesda, MD.

NATIONAL INSTITUTE FOR OCCUPATIONAL SAFETY AND HEALTH (1976) Criteria for a recommended standard occupational exposure to tetrachloroethylene. DHEW Publication No (NIOSH), 76–185.

NATO/CCMS (1974) Draft of the Joint Committee on the medical aspects of water quality, for NATO/CCMS Health Effects group, 8 June 1974, DHSS, Friars House, 157–168 Blackfriars Road, London SE1.

NELSON B K, TAYLOR B J, SETZER J V and HORNUNG R W (1980) Behavioural teratology of perchloroethylene in rats. *Journal of Environmental Pathology and Toxicology* **3**, 233–250.

OGATA M, TAKATSUKA Y and TOMOKUNI K (1971) Excretion of organic chlorine compounds in the urine of persons exposed to vapours of trichloroethylene and tetrachloroethylene. *British Journal of Industrial Medicine* **28**, 386–391.

OHTSUKI T, SATO K, KOIZUMI A, KUMAI M and IKEDA M (1983) Limited capacity of humans to metabolise tetrachloroethylene. *International Archives of Occupational and Environmental Health* **51**, 381–390.

PEGG D G, ZEMPEL J A, BRAUN W H and WATANABE P G (1979) Disposition of tetrachloro(^{14}C)ethylene following oral and inhalation exposure in rats. *Toxicology and Applied Pharmacology* **51**, 465–474.

PESTICIDE AND CHEMICAL NEWS (1985) Urinary tract cancers noted for dry cleaning workers; results confounded. *Pesticide and Chemical News* **13**, 39, 7.

PRICE P J, HASSETT C M and MANSFIELD J I (1978) Transforming activities of trichloroethylene and proposed industrial alternatives. *In Vitro* **14**, 290–293.

RAMPY L W, QUAST J F, LEONG B K L and GEHRING P J (1977) Results of long-term inhalation toxicity studies on rats of 1,1,1,-trichloroethane and perchloroethylene formulations. International Congress of Toxicology, Toronto, Canada, p 27.

REICHERT D (1983) Biological actions and interactions of tetrachloroethylene. *Mutation Research* **123**, 411–429.

ROSENGREN L E, KJELLSTRAND P and HAGLID K G (1986) Tetrachloroethylene: Levels of DNA and S-100 in the gerbil CNS after chronic exposure.

Neurobehavioural Toxicology and Teratology **8**, 201–206.

ROWE V K, McCOLLISTER D D, SPENCER H C, ADAMS E M and IRISH D D(1952) Vapor toxicity of tetrachloroethylene for laboratory animals and human subjects. *Archives of Industrial Hygiene and Occupational Medicine* **5**, 566–579.

RUSSELL J W and SHADOFF L A (1977) The sampling and determination of halocarbons in ambient air using concentration on porous polymer. *Journal of Chromatography* **134**, 375–384.

SCHUMANN A M, QUAST J F and WATANABE P G (1980) The pharmacokinetics and macromolecular interactions of perchloroethylene in mice and rats as related to oncogenicity. *Toxicology and Applied Pharmacology* **55**, 207–219.

SCHWETZ B A, LEONG B K J and GEHRING P J (1975) The effect of maternally inhaled trichloroethylene, perchloroethylene, methyl chloroform and methylene chloride on embryonal and fetal development in mice and rats. *Toxicology and Applied Pharmacology* **32**, 84–96.

SINGH H B, SALAS L J and CAVANAGH L A (1977) Distribution, sources and sinks of atmospheric halogenated compounds. *Journal of the Air Pollution Control Association* **27**, 332–336.

STEWARD R (1969) Acute tetrachloroethylene intoxication. *Journal of the American Medical Association* **208**, 1490–1492.

STEWARD R D, BARETTA E D, DODD H C and TORKELSON T R (1970) Experimental human exposure to tetrachloroethylene. *Archives of Environmental Health* **20**, 224–229.

STEWARD R D and DODD H C (1964) Absorption of carbon tetrachloride, trichloroethylene, tetrachloroethylene, methylene chloride and 1,1,1-trichloroethane through the human skin. *American Industrial Hygiene Association Journal* **25**, 439–446.

TORKELSON T R and ROWE V K (1982) Halogenated aliphatic hydrocarbons containing chlorine, bromine and iodine. In: *Patty's Industrial Hygiene and Toxicity,* Volume 2B, edited by G D Clayton and F E Clayton, pp. 3553–3560, Chapter 48. J Wiley and Sons.

TROUWBORST T (1981) Groundwater pollution by volatile halogenated hydrocarbons; sources of pollution and methods to estimate their relevance. *Science of the Total Environment* **21**, 41–46.

TU A S, MURRAY T A, HATCH K M, SIVAK A and MILMAN H A (1985) *In vitro* transformation of BALB/c–3T3 cells by chlorinated ethanes and ethylenes. *Cancer Letters* **28**, 85–92.

UNITED STATES NATIONAL TOXICOLOGY PROGRAM (1986) Toxicology and carcinogenesis of tetrachloroethylene in F344/N rats and B6C3F1 mice. NTP TR 311 Research Triangle Park N.C.

VAN DUUREN B L, GOLDSCHMIDT B M, LOEWENGART G, SMITH A C, MELCHIONNE S, SEIDMAN I and ROTH D (1979) Carcinogenicity of halogenated olefinic andaliphatic hydrocarbons in mice. *Journal of the National Cancer Institute* **63**, 1433–1439.

VAN DUUREN B L, KLINE S A, MELCHIONNE S and SEIDMAN I (1983) Chemical structure and carcinogenicity relationships of some chloroalkene oxides andtheir parent olefins. *Cancer Research* **43**,, 159–162.

WAKEHAM S G, DAVIS A C, WITT R T, TRIPP B W and FREW N M (1980)

Tetrachloroethylene contamination of drinking water by vinyl-coated asbestos-cement pipe. *Bulletin of Environmental Contamination and Toxicology* **25**, 639–645.

WATER RESEARCH CENTRE (1981) Organic micropollutants in drinking water. WRc Technical Report TR 159.

WEISBURGER E K (1977) Carcinogenicity studies on halogenated hydrocarbons. *Environmental Health Perspectives* **21**, 7–16.

WORLD HEALTH ORGANIZATION (1984) Guidelines for drinking-water quality, Volume 1 – Recommendations, Geneva, World Health Organization.

YLLNER S (1961) Urinary metabolites of ^{14}C-tetrachloroethylene in mice. *Nature* **191**, 820.

ZIGLIO G, FARA G M, BELTRAMELLI G and PREGLIASCO F (1983) Human environmental exposure to trichloro- and tetrachloroethylene from water and air in Milan, Italy. *Archives of Environmental Contamination and Toxicology* **12**, 57–64.

ZIGLIO G, BELTRAMELLI G and PREGLIASCO F (1984) A procedure for determining plasmatic trichloroacetic acid in human subjects exposed to chlorinated solvents at environmental levels. *Archives of Environmental Contamination and Toxicology* **13**, 129–134.

5

The aromatic hydrocarbons

1. INTRODUCTION

The structures of several of the aromatic hydrocarbons reviewed are shown in Figure 1. These compounds are used in industry in very large quantities.

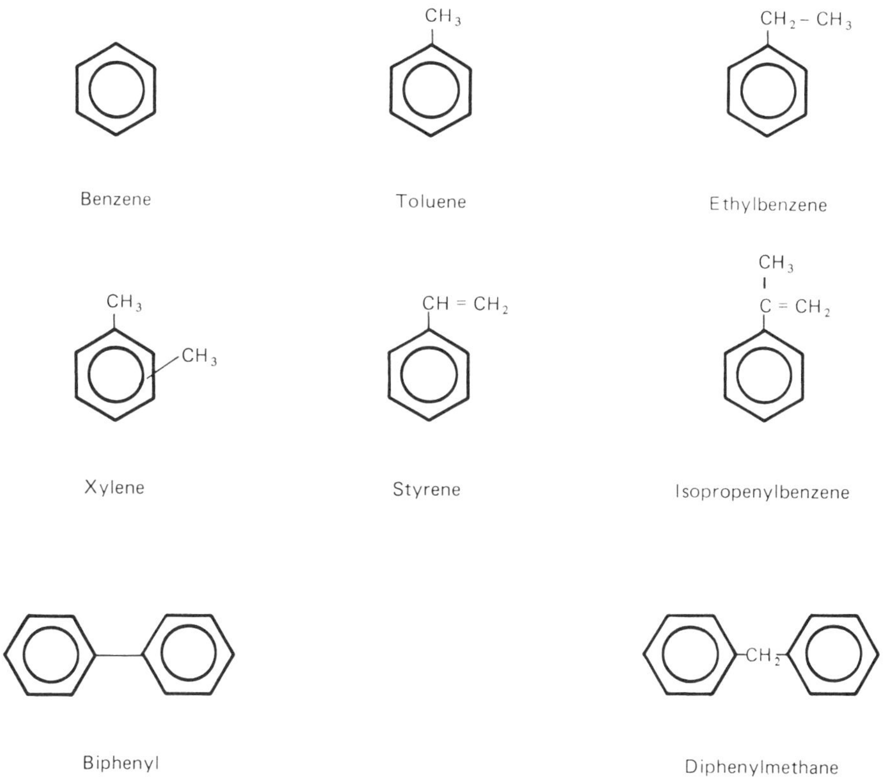

Fig. 1 — Structures of some of the aromatic hydrocarbons identified in drinking water.

The most important sources of environmental exposure are air and food. Water is only a minor source, except where specific pollution incidents have occurred. In the WRc survey, benzene, toluene and xylene were the most frequently detected compounds, occurring in 13/14, 14/14 and 14/14 samples respectively.

Toxicological information on the aromatic hydrocarbons varies markedly. Benzene, toluene, styrene and biphenyl are the most comprehensively studied, but there is relatively little or no information available on the other compounds.

2. BENZENE

2.1 Introduction

Benzene has been the most extensively studied of all the aromatic hydrocarbons, and the literature has been reviewed by several groups (Health and Welfare Canada 1979, Van Raalte and Grasso 1982, National Academy of Sciences 1977, 1980, Leong 1977, Sandmeyer 1978, United States Environmental Protection Agency 1980). Benzene is principally produced by fractional distillation of crude oil, catalytic dehydrogenation, and solvent extraction. Estimated annual world-wide production is over 15 million tonnes. Benzene is used as a solvent and a fuel additive, but primarily as a raw material in the manufacture of ethylbenzene, styrene, cyclohexane, nylon, dyes, pesticides, resins and detergents.

CAS Reg No:	71-43-2
Molecular weight:	78.1
Boiling point:	80.1°C
Solubility:	1780 mg/l at 20°C (Verschueren 1977)
Evaporative half-life in water of depth 1 m:	4.81 hours at 25°C (Mackay and Leinonen 1975)
Threshold odour concentration in water:	2–31 mg/l (Zoeteman *et al* 1974).

2.2 Exposure

2.2.1 Air

The major source of atmospheric benzene is vehicle exhausts (Pilar and Graydon 1973). Most data suggest that average benzene levels are in the low ppb range, although much higher levels have been reported in the vicinity of benzene-associated industries (Mara and Lee 1978) and in the ambient air of petrol stations (National Academy of Sciences 1977). An analysis of atmospheric benzene in the UK (Thorburn and Colenutt 1979) has reported higher levels than those found elsewhere. In a relatively rural area a level of 61 ppb was found, while near the M1 at Luton benzene was measured at 155 ppb.

2.2.2 Food

Benzene is found in many foodstuffs and beverages at significant levels, and the NCI have estimated that an individual could ingest as much as 250 μg/day of benzene from this source (National Cancer Institute 1977).

2.2.3 Water

Exposure data for water are rather limited, though both American and Canadian studies have suggested average drinking water concentrations in the nanogram per litre range (Health and Welfare Canada 1979, Van Raalte and Grasso 1982). The US EPA study reported the highest level of benzene found in a finished water as 10 μg/l. The survey by the WRc identified benzene in 13 out of 14 treated water samples examined (Water Research Centre 1981).

2.2.4 Relative exposure

In an assessment of the relative exposure of an individual to benzene by the US EPA, water was suggested to contribute 1.4%, food 17.7% and ambient air 80.9% to an overall daily intake of 1.1 mg of benzene (Van Raalte and Grasso 1982). This calculation was based on perhaps a rather low ambient air benzene level of 1 ppb, a rather high water level of 10 μg/l and an intake from food of 250 μg/day. The Canadians, however, have calculated an average yearly intake of 125 mg of benzene, of which 91 mg is derived from food, 33 mg from air, 0.007 mg from water and 1 mg from other sources (Health and Welfare Canada 1979). The more realistic assumptions included in this calculation are a drinking water concentration of 10 ng/l, an intake from food of 250 μg/day, and an ambient air level of 2.5 ppb, of which 50% is retained by the body.

These estimates indicate that exposure to waterborne benzene at current levels is almost insignificant in comparison to exposure from other sources.

2.3 Toxicokinetics

2.3.1 Absorption

No information appears to be available with regard to the gastrointestinal absorption of benzene, though a value of around 40–50% has been reported in several studies for respiratory absorption in humans (Srbova *et al* 1950, Hunter 1966, Hunter and Blair 1972). Percutaneous absorption has been demonstrated to occur slowly in man and rhesus monkey (Hanke *et al* 1961, Maibach and Anjo 1981).

2.3.2 Distribution

Autoradiographic and pharmacokinetic studies have shown that benzene has an affinity for nervous and adipose tissue, with high levels also found in the bone marrow, liver, spleen and blood (Bergman 1979, Rickert *et al* 1979, Rusch *et al* 1977).

2.3.3 Metabolism

Benzene is metabolised primarily in the liver to phenol, catechol, quinol and hydroxyquinol, and subsequently to conjugates of ester sulphates and glucuronides. In bone marrow, phenol appears to be the major metabolite shortly after exposure, though catechol and hydroquinone predominate subsequently (Rickert *et al* 1979). It is thought that secondary metabolites of the latter two compounds are probably responsible for the toxic effects of benzene in the bone marrow (Ikeda *et al* 1972, Drew and Fouts 1974, Greenlee *et al* 1981).

2.3.4 Excretion

The elimination of benzene by the lungs has been reported to be around 12% of the retained dose in humans but up to 70% in experimental animals (Hunter 1966, Parke and Williams 1953). Excretion in the urine as free or conjugated phenols accounts for 50–87% of retained benzene in humans, but only 23% is eliminated in this way by rodents (Hunter 1966, Cornish and Ryan 1965).

2.4 Health effects

2.4.1 Acute and subacute toxicity

Severe human exposure to benzene can cause convulsions, coma, paralysis and death from respiratory or cardiac failure. At sublethal doses, CNS excitation followed by depression, giddiness, headaches, nausea and unconsciousness is often found. Pathological effects include petechial haemorrhages of several tissues, cerebral oedema, hypo- and hyperplasia of the bone marrow, and congestion of the kidney (Gerarde 1960, Winek and Collom 1971).

Benzene has a low oral LD50 in the rat of 5.6 g/kg, though younger animals show a slightly increased susceptibility (Leong 1977, Wolf *et al* 1956, Kimura *et al* 1971). The inhalatory narcotic threshold of benzene in experimental animals has been estimated to be 4000 ppm, whilst concentrations above 10 000 ppm tend to be lethal (Gerarde 1960). Sudden deaths due to ventricular fibrillation have also been reported in laboratory animals (Nahum and Hoff 1934).

2.4.2 Chronic toxicity

The most commonly observed effects of chronic benzene toxicity in experimental studies are associated with the depression of bone marrow function, and normally take the form of pancytopenia, a reduction in the numbers of many kinds of blood cells. Much recent work has been involved in the study of these effects and the ultimate reactive species responsible.

Male C57BL/6 mice exposed intermittently by inhalation to 4000 ppm benzene for 6 weeks developed leukopenia without altering bone marrow cellularity, though at lower exposure levels decreased peripheral cell counts and decreased marrow cellularity were noted (Gill *et al* 1980). In another report, AKR/J mice exposed to 100 ppm of benzene in air for their lifetime exhibited excess bone marrow hypoplasia, anaemia and lymphocytopenia, while C57BL/6J mice also exposed by inhalation to 300 ppm of benzene for their lifetime developed anaemia, lymphocytopenia, neutrophilia and bone marrow hyperplasia (Snyder *et al* 1980). CD-1 mice exposed to benzene for 5 days showed reductions in marrow lymphocytes, splenic lymphocytes and marrow granulocytes at most exposure levels, though granulocytopenia and lymphocytopenia were only observed at doses above 103 ppm. Further animals exposed to 9.6 ppm for 50 days (equivalent to 5 days at 103 ppm) exhibited elevated spleen weight and cellularity. Lymphocytopenia and anaemia were evident in animals inhaling 302 ppm of benzene for 26 weeks (Green *et al* 1981).

Repeated, subcutaneous administration of 0.25 or 0.5 ml/kg/day of benzene to rabbits produced an 80% reduction in total numbers of lymphocytes after 10 days. The decrease was reported to be primarily due to a large reduction in B-cells (Irons and Moore 1980). Four groups of domestic pigs exposed by inhalation to 0, 20, 100 and 500 ppm of benzene for 3 weeks exhibited significant depressions of white cell counts, total lymphocytes and E-rosette-forming lymphocytes (T-cells) at the highest dose level (Johnston *et al* 1972). A significant decrease in the numbers of white cells and the proportion of T-cells, but not total lymphocytes, was found at the 100 ppm level.

Several other recent studies in experimental animals have provided further information, including a possible potentiation of benzene haematotoxicity by ethanol (Harigaya *et al* 1981, Tunek *et al* 1981, Longacre *et al* 1981, Wierda *et al* 1981, Snyder *et al* 1981).

Epidemiological studies have also often reported associations between benzene exposure and haematological abnormalities. A study of 217 workers exposed occupationally to between 30 and 210 ppm benzene in air for up to 17 years found abnormalities in 51% of subjects, including a 9.7% incidence of leukopenia and a 1.84% incidence of thrombocytopenia (Aksoy *et al* 1971). Chronic effects on the immune system have been suggested in workers exposed to benzene, toluene and xylene, where decreased levels of IgG and IgA, and increased levels of IgM were noted (Lange *et al* 1973). Additionally, suppressed complement activity has been observed in workers exposed to benzene, an effect also seen in rabbits after chronic benzene dosing (Smolik *et al* 1973, D'Angelo and Forcardi 1963, Raddi *et al* 1964). Many other reports on the epidemiology of benzene are available in the literature, but these have been comprehensively reviewed (Health and Welfare Canada 1979, Van Raalte and Grasso 1982, National Academy of Sciences 1977, 1980, Leong 1977, Sandmeyer 1978, United States Environmental Protection Agency 1980).

Neurological abnormalities were reported in four out of six pancytopenic individuals exposed to benzene, but the significance of this single report is unclear (Baslo and Aksoy 1982).

The mechanism of action of benzene on the bone marrow is an area of much research attention. The most plausible hypothesis has been forwarded by Greenlee *et al* (1981) who, based on both their own data and other published information (Irons and Neptun 1980, Tunek *et al* 1980), proposed that autoxidation of the benzene metabolites hydroquinone and 1,2,4-benzenetriol results in the production of reactive species such as semiquinones and oxygen radicals, which bind to critical cellular macromolecules. However, a great deal more work is needed before the toxic mechanism of benzene is fully understood.

2.4.3 Genotoxicity

Although there is strong evidence for benzene-related genetic damage in mammalian systems, mutagenicity of benzene has yet to be demonstrated in bacterial assays (Forni 1978, Dean 1978).

Lyon (1976) reported negative findings for benzene mutagenicity in a host-mediated assay and in bacterial plate assays with *Salmonella typhimurium* TA98 and TA100, but found chromosomal aberrations in bone marrow cells of rats given 0.5 ml/kg of benzene by intraperitoneal injection. This compound has given positive results in one forward gene mutation assay: resistance to 6-thioguanine at the HGPRT locus in a metabolically competent human lymphoblastoid cell line (Crespi and Penman 1984). Significant dose-related increases in micronucleated polychromatic erythrocytes have been reported in both rats and mice (Lyon 1976, Hite *et al* 1980, Siou *et al* 1981), though Siou *et al* (1981) were unable to report similar clastogenic effects in Chinese hamsters. Chromosomal aberrations have been induced in both rat and rabbit bone marrow cells *in vivo* and also in human leukocytes and Hela cells *in vitro* (Kissling and Speck 1971, Philip and Jensen 1970, Dobrokhotov 1972, Lyapkalo 1973, Koizumi *et al* 1974, Morimoto 1976). An increased incidence of sister chromatid exchanges has been observed in the peripheral blood lymphocytes of DBA mice exposed by inhalation to 10, 100 or 1000 ppm for 6 hours (Erexson *et al* 1984). Benzene or phenol were not found to induce the frequency of sister chromatid exchanges in cultured human lymphocytes, though catechol and hydroquinol were potent in this respect (Morimoto and Wolff 1980). In a more recent study of cultured human lymphocytes in which a rat liver microsomal preparation was incorporated as a metabolising system, benzene was found to induce sister chromatid exchanges (Morimoto 1983).

Many cytogenetic studies of human populations exposed to benzene have also indicated the genotoxic potential of this compound. Two studies (Vigliani and Forni 1969, Picciano 1979) have shown significantly increased incidences of peripheral lymphocyte chromosomal aberrations in exposed workers. Changes in chromosomal structure, including heteroploidy and aneuploidy, have been associated with benzene-induced blood dyscrasias (Pollini and Colombi 1964, Pollini *et al* 1964, Tough and Court-Brown 1965, Forni and Moreo 1967, 1969). In an investigation of 25 subjects with a clinical history of benzene haemopathies, chromosomal aberrations were still evident several years after exposure (Forni *et al* 1971). A two- to threefold increase in chromosomal aberrations has also been observed in a group of 52 workers exposed to benzene for varying durations (Kilian and Daniel 1978). No significant increase in sister chromatid exchange frequency was found in a study of 22 workers exposed to 0.2–12.4 ppm of benzene in air for an average of 11 years (Sarto *et al* 1984).

Despite the clear association between benzene and chromosomal damage in mammalian systems, the interpretation of studies is difficult due to the lack of *in vivo* dose–response data and also the lack of information at lower levels of exposure.

2.4.4 Carcinogenicity

With the exception of leukaemias, the only other tumours which have been associated with exposure to benzene are zymbal gland carcinomas and mammary carcinomas reported in a single study by Maltoni and Scarnato (1979). In this study, Sprague–Dawley rats dosed orally with 250 mg/kg of benzene for 52 weeks developed 4/33 leukaemias in males, 8/32 zymbal gland carcinomas and 7/32 mammary carcinomas in females. Control values were 3/30 mammary carcinomas, 1/30 leukaemias and 0/30 zymbal gland carcinomas in females, and 0/30 for both leukaemias and zymbal gland carcinomas in males. It was also noted that the latency period for mammary tumours was reduced from 110 weeks to 88 weeks.

Gavage studies of benzene in corn oil at doses of 0–200 mg/kg in male rats and 0–100 mg/kg in female rats and male and female mice gave rise to an increase in tumours at multiple sites (US National Toxicology Program 1986).

The evidence for the leukaemogenicity of benzene is derived largely from epidemiological studies, most attempts at inducing leukaemias in experimental animals having proved unsuccessful, although some evidence was found of leukaemias in mice exposed for 16 weeks to 300 ppm of benzene 6 hours/day, 5 days/week and then held for lifetime observations (Cronkite *et al* 1984). Aksoy *et al* (1974) calculated a leukaemia risk of 13 per 100 000 among 28 500 shoe workers exposed to a maximum of 210–650 ppm of benzene for 1–15 years. The risk of 6 per 100 000 for the general population is significantly lower.' In another study, a twentyfold increased risk of leukaemia has been calculated for workers exposed to benzene in northern Italy (Vigliani and Saita 1964). Infante *et al* (1977) found a fivefold increased risk of leukaemia in 748 workers exposed to benzene in the rubber industry, and deaths due to lymphatic and haemopoietic cancers have been reported to be 31% higher than expected for 5000 male workers exposed to benzene and other industrial solvents in tyre manufacturing plants (United States Environmental Protection Agency 1977). A study of survivors of the two atomic bombings of Japan found a doubled risk for leukaemia in subjects also occupationally exposed to benzene (Ishimaru *et al* 1971). Although Thorpe (1974) was unable to find a significantly increased incidence of leukaemia in 38 000 petroleum workers, the methodology of the study has been criticised (Brown 1975). Conversely, Vianna and Polan (1979) did report a significant excess of lymphomas in workers using benzene and/or coal tar fractions, but again the methodology is in some doubt (Enterline 1979).

Wong (1987) presented data from cohorts of workers from a number of chemical plants which further support the leukaemogenic potential of benzene in man. Rinsky *et al* (1987) calculated that protection from benzene-induced leukaemia would increase exponentially with any reduction in the permissible exposure limit.

In a short review of the role of benzene in carcinogenesis, Boyland (1981) argues convincingly that the results of both the epidemiological and experimental studies outlined above support the view that benzene acts as a tumour promoter. Recent evidence also suggests that for tumour promoters there may well be threshold levels below which no effect occurs. If this is the case, it is likely that exposure to very low levels of benzene would not constitute a cancer risk.

2.4.5 Reproductive toxicity

Transplacental transfer of benzene is a poorly studied subject, though one report has found similar levels of benzene in both maternal and cord-blood under low-level exposure conditions (Dowty *et al* 1976).

Indications of embryotoxicity were observed in CF-1 mice and New Zealand white rabbits exposed by inhalation to 500 ppm of benzene, 7 hours/day, from days 6 to 15 (mice) and 6 to 18 (rabbits) of gestation. No teratogenic effects, however, were observed in either species (Murray *et al* 1979). Similarly, no teratogenicity was observed in a study of CFY rats exposed to 313 ppm of benzene from days 9 to 14 of gestation, though decreased mean foetal weight was reported (Hudak and Ungvary 1978). Retardation of foetal development and a low incidence of skeletal and visceral abnormalities were reported in the offspring of Sprague–Dawley rats exposed by inhalation to 500 ppm of benzene on days 6 to 15 of gestation (Kuna and Kapp 1981). Some evidence for teratogenicity has been reported in CF-1 mice given 3 ml/kg of benzene by subcutaneous injection on the thirteenth day of gestation (Watanabe and Yoshida 1970). This study is difficult to interpret, however, due to the absence of control data. No teratogenic effects were seen in the susceptible chick embryo system (Roche and Hine 1968).

In general, the evidence would not indicate a teratogenic potential for benzene. Retardation of foetal development, the most common reproductive effect, is characterised by decreased foetal weight and ossification. This effect appears to occur only at doses which also cause a decrease in maternal weight gain. The retardation in foetal development may therefore be due to the toxicity of benzene in the mother.

2.5 Discussion

Assessments of relative exposure indicate that the contribution of waterborne benzene to overall exposure is almost insignificant in comparison to exposure from other sources.

Both epidemiological and animal studies have shown that pancytopenia is the most common effect of chronic exposure to benzene. This compound has been reported to cause chromosomal abnormalities *in vitro* and *in vivo* in mammals, but has not yet been shown to be mutagenic in bacterial assays. There is good evidence that benzene can cause leukaemia in man, and some indication that it does also in experimental animals. This carcinogenic action of benzene also appears to be consistent with that of tumour promotion. There is no evidence of any other benzene-related tumours, apart from zymbal gland carcinomas and mammary carcinomas reported in one rat study. Benzene can cause retardation of foetal development at high doses, but does not appear to be teratogenic.

As studies have shown that benzene is associated with leukaemia and that it can cause depression of bone marrow function at fairly low levels of exposure, benzene is of concern as an environmental pollutant. However, the contribution of benzene in drinking water to the estimated exposure from the whole environment is extremely small. It is also unlikely that these concentrations in themselves would give rise to concern.

References

AKSOY M, DINCOL K, AKGUN T, ERDEM S and DINCOL G (1971) Haematological effects of chronic benzene poisoning in 217 workers. *British Journal of Industrial Medicine* **28,** 296-302.

AKSOY M, ERDEM S and DINCOL G (1974) Leukemia in shoe workers exposed chronically to benzene. *Blood* **44,** 837-841.

BASLO A and AKSOY M (1982) Neurological abnormalities in chronic benzene poisoning. A study of six patients with aplastic anemia and two with preleukemia. *Environmental Research* **27,** 457-465.

BERGMAN K (1979) Whole body autoradiography and allied tracer techniques in distribution and elimination studies of some organic solvents. *Scandinavian Journal of Work Environment and Health* **5** Suppl 1.

BOYLAND E (1981) The role of benzene in carcinogenesis. IRCS, *Medical Science: Biochemistry* **9,** 560-561.

BROWN S M (1975) Leukemia and potential benzene exposure. *Journal of Occupational Medicine* **17,** 5.

CORNISH H H and RYAN R R (1965) Metabolism of benzene in nonfasted, fasted and arylhydroxylase inhibited rats. *Toxicology and Applied Pharmacology* **7,** 767.

CRESPI C L and PENMAN B W (1984) The mutagenicity of benzene in a metabolically competent human lymphoblastoid cell line. *Environmental Mutagenesis* **6,** 425.

CRONKITE E P, BULLIS J, INOUE T and DREW R T (1984) Benzene inhalation produces leukaemia in mice. *Toxicology and Applied Pharmacology* **75,** 358-361.

D'ANGELO V and FORCARDI L (1963) Immunisation processes in experimental benzene poisoning. I. Complementary potential in native serum. *Lavoro Umani* **17,** 326.

DEAN B J (1978) Genetic toxicology of benzene, toluene, xylenes and phenols. *Mutation Research* **47,** 75-97.

DOBROKHOTOV V B (1972) The mutagenic influence of benzene and toluene under experimental conditions. *Gigiena i Sanitariia* **37,** 36-39.

DOWTY B J, LASETER J L and STORER J (1976) The transplacental migration and accumulation in blood of volatile organic constituents. *Pediatric Research* **10,** 696-701.

DREW R T and FOUTS J R (1974) The lack of effects of pretreatment with phenobarbital and chlorpromazine in the acute toxicity of benzene in rats. *Toxicology and Applied Pharmacology* **27,** 183-193.

ENTERLINE P E (1979) Lymphomas and benzene. *Lancet* **2,** 1021.

EREXSON G L, WILMER J L, AUMAN C D and KLIGERMAN A D (1984) Induction chromatid exchanges and micronuclei in male DBA/2 mice after inhalation of benzene. *Environmental Mutagenesis* **6,** 408.

FORNI A (1978) Chromosome changes and benzene exposure. A review. *Reviews on Environmental Health* **III,** 5-17.

FORNI A and MOREO L (1967) Cytogenetic studies in a case of benzene leukaemia. *European Journal of Cancer* **3,** 251-255.

FORNI A and MOREO L (1969) Chromosome studies in a case of benzene induced erythroleukaemia. *European Journal of Cancer* **5,** 459-463.

FORNI A M, CAPPELLINI A, PACIFICO E and VIGLIANI E C (1971) Chromosome changes and their evolution in subjects with past exposure to benzene. *Archives of Environmental Health* **23,** 385-391.

GERARDE H W (1960) Toxicology and biochemistry of aromatic hydrocarbons. New York, Elsevier Monographs, Elsevier Publishing Co.

GILL D P, JENKINS V K, KEMPEN R R and ELLIS S (1980) The importance of pluripotential stem cells in benzene toxicity. *Toxicology* **16,** 163-171.

GREEN J D, SNYDER C A, LoBUE J, GOLDSTEIN B D and ALBERT R E (1981) Acute and chronic dose/response effect of benzene inhalation on the peripheral blood, bone marrow, and spleen cells of CD-1 male mice. *Toxicology and Applied Pharmacology* **59,** 204-214.

GREENLEE W F, SUN J D and BUS J S (1981) A proposed mechanism of benzene toxicity: Formation of reactive intermediates from polyphenol metabolites. *Toxicology and Applied Pharmacology* **59,** 187-195.

HANKE J (1961) The absorption of benzene through the skin in men. *Medycyna Pracy* **12,** 413-426.

HARIGAYA K, MILLER M E, CRONKITE E P and DREW R T (1981) The detection of *in vivo* hematotoxicity of benzene by *in vitro* liquid bone marrow cultures. *Toxicology and Applied Pharmacology* **60,** 346-353.

HEALTH AND WELFARE, CANADA (1979) Benzene. Human health implications of benzene at levels found in the Canadian environment and workplace, 79-EHD-40.

HITE M, PECHARO M, SMITH I and THORNTON S (1980) The effect of benzene in the micronucleus test. *Mutation Research* **77,** 149-155.

HUDAK A and UNGVARY G (1978) Embryotoxic effects of benzene and its methyl derivatives: toluene, xylene. *Toxicology* **11,** 55-63.

HUNTER C G (1966) Aromatic solvents. *Annals of Occupational Hygiene* **9,** 191-197.

HUNTER C G and BLAIR D (1972) Benzene: Pharmacokinetic studies in man. *Annals of Occupational Hygiene* **15,** 193.

IKEDA M, OHTSUJI H and IMAMURA I (1972) *In vivo* suppression of benzene and styrene oxidation by co-administered toluene in rats and effects of phenobarbital. *Xenobiotica* **2,** 101-110.

INFANTE P F, RINSKY R A, WAGONER J K and YOUNG R J (1977) Leukemia in benzene workers. *Lancet* **2,** 76-78.

IRONS R D and MOORE B J (1980) Effect of short-term benzene administration on circulating lymphocyte subpopulations in the rabbit: Evidence of a selective B-lymphocyte sensitivity. *Research Communications in Chemical Pathology and Pharmacology* **27,** 147-155.

IRONS R D and NEPTUN D A (1980) Effects of the principle hydroxy-metabolites of benzene on microtubule polymerization. *Archives of Toxicology* **45,** 297-305.

ISHIMARU T, OKADA H, TOMIYASU T, TSUCHIMOTO T, HOSHINO T and ICHIMARU M (1971) Occupational factors in the epidemiology of leukemia in Hiroshima and Nagasaki. *American Journal of Epidemiology* **93,** 157-165.

JOHNSTON R V, PINKERTON M N, MENSIK D C, SWAIM L D, LINSCOMBE V A, BENGE M C, BARNA-LLOYD G and KILIAN D J (1972) Hematologic and myologenous effects of inhaled benzene in the pig and the rat. *Journal of Toxicology and Environmental Health* **5,** 1025-1035.

KILIAN D J and DANIEL R C (1978) A cytogenetic study of workers exposed to benzene in the Texas division of Dow Chemical, USA. Freeport, TX, Dow Chemical.

KIMURA E T, EBERT D M and DODGE P W (1971) Acute toxicity and limits of solvent residue for sixteen organic solvents. *Toxicology and Applied Pharmacology* **19,** 699-704.

KISSLING M and SPECK B (1971) Chromosome aberrations in experimental benzene intoxication. *Helvetica Medica Acta* **36,** 59-66.

KOIZUMI A, DOBACHI Y, TACHIBANA Y, TSUDA K and KATSUNUMA H (1974) Cytokinetic and cytogenetic changes in cultured human leucocytes and Hela cells induced by benzene. *Industrial Health – Kawasaki* **12,** 23-29.

KUNA R A and KAPP R W (1981) The embryotoxic/teratogenic potential of benzene vapor in rats. *Toxicology and Applied Pharmacology* **57,** 1-7.

LANGE A, SMOLIK R, ZATONSKI W and GLAZMAN H (1973) Serum immunoglobulin levels in workers exposed to benzene, toluene, and xylene. *Internationale Archiv fur Arbeitsmedizin* **31,** 37-44.

LEONG B K J (1977) Experimental benzene intoxication. *Journal of Toxicology*

and Environmental Health Suppl 2, 45-61.
LONGACRE S L, KOCSIS J J and SNYDER R (1981) Influence of strain differences in mice on the metabolism and toxicity of benzene. *Toxicology and Applied Pharmacology* **60,** 398-409.
LYAPKALO A A (1973) Genetic activity of benzene and toluene. *Gigiena Truda i Professional'nye Zabolevaniia* **17,** 24.
LYON J P (1976) Mutagenicity studies with benzene. *Dissertation Abstracts International, Series B* **36,** 5537.
MACKAY D and LEINONEN P J (1975) Rates of evaporation of low-solubility contaminants from water bodies to atmosphere. *Environmental Science and Technology* **9,** 1178-1180.
MAIBACH H I and ANJO D M (1981) Percutaneous penetration of benzene and benzene contained in solvents used in the rubber industry. *Archives of Environmental Health* **36,** 156-160.
MALTONI C and SCARNATO C (1979) Long-term bioassays on Sprague–Dawley rats by oral administration. *Medicina del Lavoro* **70,** 352-357.
MARA S J and LEE S S (1978) Assessment of human exposures to atmospheric benzene. US EPA, EPA-450/3-78-031.
MORIMOTO K (1976) Analysis of combined effects of benzene with radiation on chromosomes in cultured human leukocytes. *Japanese Journal of Industrial Health* **18,** 23-24.
MORIMOTO K (1983) Induction of sister chromatid exchanges and cell division delays in human lymphocytes by microsomal activation of benzene. *Cancer Research* **43,** 1330-1334.
MORIMOTO K and WOLFF S (1980) Increase of sister chromatid exchanges and perturbations of cell division kinetics in human lymphocytes by benzene metabolites. *Cancer Research* **40,** 1189-1193.
MURRAY F J, JOHN J A, RAMPY L W, KUNA R A and SCHWETZ B A (1979) Embryotoxicity of inhaled benzene in mice and rabbits. *American Industrial Hygiene Association Journal* **40,** 993-998.
NAHUM L H and HOFF H E (1934) Mechanism of sudden death in experimental acute benzol poisoning. *Journal of Pharmacology and Experimental Therapeutics* **50,** 336.
NATIONAL ACADEMY OF SCIENCES (1977) Drinking water and health, vol 1. Washington DC, National Academy of Sciences.
NATIONAL ACADEMY OF SCIENCES (1980) Drinking water and health, vol 3. Washington DC, National Academy Press.
NATIONAL CANCER INSTITUTE (1977) Occurrence, metabolism, and toxicity including reported carcinogenicity of benzene. Washington DC, National Cancer Institute.
PARKE D V and WILLIAMS R T (1953) Studies in detoxification XLIX: Metabolism of benzene containing ^{14}C-benzene. *Biochemical Journal* **54,** 231-238.
PHILIP P and JENSEN M K (1970) Benzene induced chromosome abnormalities in rat bone marrow. *Acta Pathologica et Microbiologica Scandinavica* **78,** 489-490.
PICCIANO D (1979) Cytogenetic study of workers exposed to benzene. *Environmental Research* **19,** 33-38.

PILAR S and GRAYDON W F (1973) Benzene and toluene distribution in Toronto atmosphere. *Environmental Science and Technology* **7,** 628-631.

POLLINI G and COLOMBI R (1964) Lymphocyte chromosome damage in benzene blood dyscrasia. *Medicina del Lavoro* **55,** 641-654.

POLLINI G, STROSELLI E and COLOMBI R (1964) Relationship between chromosomal alterations and severity of benzene blood dyscrasia. *Medicina del Lavoro* **55,** 735-751.

RADDI R, D'ANGELO V and GIULIANI V (1964) Immunisation potential in experimental benzene poisoning. III. Variations in serum complementary power following active immunisation. *Lavoro Umani* **16,** 29.

RICKERT D E, BAKER T S, BUS J S, BARROW C S and IRONS R D (1979) Benzene disposition in the rat after exposure by inhalation. *Toxicology and Applied Pharmacology* **49,** 417-423.

RINSKY R A, SMITH A B, HORNUNG R, FILLOON T G, YOUNG R J, OKUN A H and LANDRIGAN P J (1987) Benzene and leukemia. An epidemiologic risk assessment. *The New England Journal of Medicine* **316,** 1044-1050.

ROCHE S M and HINE C H (1968) The teratogenicity of some industrial chemicals. *Toxicology and Applied Pharmacology* **12,** 327.

RUSCH G M, LEONG B K J and LASKIN S (1977) Benzene metabolism. *Journal of Toxicology and Environmental Health* Suppl 2, 23-36.

SANDMEYER E E (1978) Aromatic hydrocarbons. In: Clayton G D and Clayton F E (eds) *Patty's industrial hygiene and toxicology* vol 2B, 3rd revised edition. Wiley, pp 3260-3282.

SARTO F, COMINATO I, PINTON A M, BROVEDANI P G, MERLER E, PERUZZI M, BIANCHI V and LEVIS A G (1984) A cytogenetic study on workers exposed to low concentrations of benzene. *Carcinogenesis* **5,** 827-832.

SIOU G, CONAN L and EL HAITEM M (1981) Evaluation of the clastogenic action of benzene by oral administration with 2 cytogenetic techniques in mouse and Chinese hamster. *Mutation Research* **90,** 273-278.

SMOLIK R, GRZYBEK-HRYNCEWICZ K, LANGE A and ZATONSKI W (1973) Serum complement level in workers exposed to benzene, toluene and xylene. *Internationale Archiv fur Arbeitsmedizin* **31,** 243.

SNYDER C A, GOLDSTEIN B D, SELLAKUMAR A R, BROMBERG I, LASKIN S and ALBERT R E (1980) The inhalation toxicology of benzene: Incidence of hematopoietic neoplasms and hematotoxicity in AKR/J and C578L/6J mice. *Toxicology and Applied Pharmacology* **54,** 323-331.

SNYDER C A, BAARSON K A, GOLDSTEIN B D and ALBERT R E (1981) Ingestion of ethanol increases the hematotoxicity of inhaled benzene in C57BL mice. *Bulletin of Environmental Contamination and Toxicology* **27,** 175-180.

SRBOVA J, TEISINGER J and SKRAMOVSKY S (1950) Absorption and elimination of inhaled benzene in man. *AMA Archives of Industrial Hygiene and Occupational Medicine* **2,** 1-8.

THORBURN S and COLENUTT B A (1979) A gas chromatographic comparison of volatile organic compounds in urban and rural atmospheres. *International Journal of Environmental Studies* **13,** 265-271.

THORPE J J (1974) Epidemiological survey of leukemia in persons potentially

exposed to benzene. *Journal of Occupational Medicine* **16,** 375-382.
TOUGH I M and COURT-BROWN W M (1965) Chromosome aberrations and exposure to ambient benzene. *Lancet* **1,** 684.
TUNEK A, PLATT K L, PRZYBYLSKI M and OESCH F (1980) Multi-step metabolic activation of benzene. Effect of superoxide dismutase on covalent binding to microsomal macromolecules and identification of glutathione conjugates using high pressure liquid chromatography and field desorption mass spectrometry. *Chemicobiological Interactions* **33,** 1-17.
TUNEK A, OLOFSSON T and BERLIN M (1981) Toxic effects of benzene and benzene metabolites on granulopoietic stem cells and bone marrow cellularity in mice. *Toxicology and Applied Pharmacology* **59,** 149-156.
US ENVIRONMENTAL PROTECTION AGENCY (1977) Benzene health effects assessment. Washington DC, US EPA.
US ENVIRONMENTAL PROTECTION AGENCY (1980) Ambient water quality criteria for benzene. US EPA, EPA 440/5-80-018.
US NATIONAL TOXICOLOGY PROGRAM (1986) Toxicology and carcinogenesis studies of benzene in F344/N rats and B6C3F1 mice (gavage studies). National Toxicology Technical Report Series No 289, Research Triangle, NL.
VAN RAALTE H G S and GRASSO P (1982) Hematological, myelotoxic, clastogenic, carcinogenic, and leukemogenic effects of benzene. *Regulatory Toxicology and Pharmacology* **2,** 153-176.
VERSCHUEREN K (1977) *Handbook of environmental data on organic chemicals.* Van Nostrand Reinhold Company.
VIANNA N J and POLAN A (1979) Lymphomas and occupational benzene exposure. *Lancet* **1,** 1394-1395.
VIGLIANI E C and FORNI A (1969) Benzene, chromosome changes and leukemia. *Journal of Occupational Medicine* **11,** 148-149.
VIGLIANI E C and SAITA G (1964) Benzene and leukemia. *New England Journal of Medicine* **271,** 872-876.
WATANABE G I and YOSHIDA S (1970) The teratogenic effects of benzene in pregnant mice. *Acta Medica Biologica* **17,** 285-291.
WATER RESEARCH CENTRE (1981) Organic micropollutants in drinking water. WRc Technical Report TR 159.
WIERDA D, IRONS R D and GREENLEE W F (1981) Immunotoxicity in C57BL/6 mice exposed to benzene and Aroclor 1254. *Toxicology and Applied Pharmacology* **60,** 410-417.
WINEK C L and COLLOM W D (1971) Benzene and toluene fatalities. *Journal of Occupational Medicine* **13,** 259.
WOLF M A, ROWE V K, McCOLLISTER D D, HOLLINGSWORTH R L and OYEN F (1956) Toxicological studies of certain alkylated benzenes and benzene. *AMA Archives of Industrial Health* **14,** 387-398.
WONG O (1987) An industry wide mortality study of chemical workers occupationally exposed to benzene. 1. General results. *British Journal of Industrial Medicine* **44,** 365-381.
ZOETEMAN B C J, PIET G J, RUYGROK C T M and HEUVEL R V D (1974) Threshold odour concentrations in water of chemical substances. RID-MEDEDELING, 74-3.

3. TOLUENE

3.1 Introduction

Toluene (toluol, phenylmethane, methylbenzene, methacide) is a volatile and flammable aromatic hydrocarbon commercially produced by the petrochemicals industry. Most is converted to benzene but some is used directly in the manufacture of dyes, saccharin, perfumes, caprolactam, pharmaceuticals, detergents and TNT. It is also used as a gasoline additive and solvent.

CAS Reg No:	108-88-3
Molecular weight:	92.13
Boiling point:	110.6°C
Solubility:	515 mg/l at 20 °C (Verschueren 1977)
Evaporative half life in water of depth 1 m:	5.18 hours at 25°C (Mackay and Leinonen 1975)
Threshold odour concentration in water:	1 mg/l (Zoeteman *et al* 1984).

3.2 Exposure

3.2.1 Air

Atmospheric contamination by toluene has been linked with automobile exhaust emissions on several occasions (Pilar and Graydon 1973, Thorburn and Colenutt 1973, Grob and Grob 1971). One study of Toronto air samples reported a correlation between traffic density and atmospheric toluene (Pilar and Graydon 1973), while a British study found a rural toluene level of 29 ppb at Freshwater (IOW) and an urban toluene concentration of 72 ppb near the M1 at Luton (Thorburn and Colenutt 1973).

3.2.2 Food

Very little information is available with regard to the levels of toluene in foodstuffs, although it has been detected in fish (Ogata and Miyake 1973).

3.2.3 Water

Toluene has been identified in several surveys of raw and treated water in the US at average concentrations of less than 1 μg/l. The highest level recorded was 11 μg/l in New Orleans finished water (United States Environmental Protection Agency 1980). Toluene was found to be present in all 14 drinking water samples in the WRc survey. Levels in surface waters were generally less than 1 μg/l, but up to 5 μg/l was found in some groundwaters (Water Research Centre 1981).

3.3 Toxicokinetics

3.3.1 Absorption

The pulmonary retention of toluene, which is dependent on the atmospheric concentration, ventilation rate and body weight, was estimated to be about 50% of the inhaled dose in volunteers after 5 hours (Astrand *et al* 1972). Although gastrointestinal absorption is slower than respiratory absorption, it is likely that most of an oral dose of toluene would be retained (Pyykko *et al* 1977). Toluene can be absorbed through the skin, but the process is far slower than through either the lungs or the gastrointestinal tract (Dutkiewicz and Tyras 1968).

3.3.2 Distribution

Due to the high affinity of toluene for fat, its distribution is dependent primarily on the lipid content of individual tissues. Body fat provides a large reservoir for toluene, as illustrated in a mouse study in which tissue saturation was not reached after a 3-hour exposure to 4000 ppm of toluene vapour (Bruckner and Peterson 1976).

3.3.3 Metabolism

The metabolism of toluene by the liver has been well characterised. Toluene is metabolised rapidly through its methyl side-chain, via benzyl alcohol and benzaldehyde, to benzoic acid. Benzoic acid is conjugated with glycine, and excreted in the urine as hippuric acid. Some conjugation of side-chain metabolites with glutathione has been reported in rats (Van Doorn *et al* 1980). There is also evidence that a small amount of ring oxidation can occur during toluene metabolism. *Ortho-*, *meta-* and *para-*cresols have been detected in the urine of workers exposed to toluene (Woiwode *et al* 1979, Hasegawa *et al* 1983).

3.3.4 Excretion

The major mode of excretion for toluene is via the urine, largely as hippuric acid. However, variation of urinary hippuric acid concentrations due to dietary factors makes this parameter a poor index of exposure, especially at low levels (Woiwode *et al* 1979). Some unchanged toluene can be eliminated in the expired air.

3.4 Health effects

There are several comprehensive reviews of the health effects of toluene (United Stated Environmental Protection Agency 1980, Cohr and Stokholm 1979, Hayden *et al* 1977, National Academy of Sciences 1977, 1980, Benignus 1981, Sandmeyer 1981). Much of the information has arisen from occupational exposure and from the abuse of solvents and glues which contain toluene.

3.4.1 Acute and subacute toxicity

Acute exposure to toluene results in CNS depression and membrane irritation, though sudden deaths due to cardiac arrhythmias have been reported in some cases of toluene abuse. There is little evidence to indicate that toluene is acutely toxic to any organ system other than the CNS even at very high doses. The oral LD50 for rats is about 7.0 g/kg (Wolf *et al* 1956, Kimura *et al* 1971).

Two subacute studies in rats have noted slight increases in hepatic cytochrome P-450 levels (Elovaara *et al* 1979, Chand and Clausen 1982).

3.4.2 Chronic toxicity

Studies in experimental animals have on the whole failed to show significant organ damage, even after exposure to very high doses of toluene. Rodents exposed to 12 000 ppm of toluene vapour in 3-hour cycles, 5 times/week for 8 weeks, exhibited inebriation but no lung, liver or kidney damage (Bruckner and Peterson 1978). In another inhalation study where rats, guinea pigs, monkeys and dogs were exposed continuously (107 ppm for 90–127 days) or intermittently (1085 ppm, 8 hours/day, 5 days/week for 6 weeks) to toluene, no changes in body weight gain, haematological parameters or the morphology of several organ systems were reported in any species (Jenkins *et al* 1970). Both male and female rats exposed to 30, 100, 300, or 1000 ppm of toluene for 13 weeks also failed to show any significant effects, even at the highest dose level (Rhudy *et al* 1978). No changes in clinical chemistry, urinalysis, haematology, histopathology or ophthalmology were found in groups of 120 male and 120 female F-344 rats exposed by inhalation to 0, 30, 100 or 300 ppm, 6 hours/day, 5 days/week for up to 2 years (Gibson and Hardisty 1983). This very low toxicity of toluene has also been found in other studies (Wolf *et al* 1956, Carpenter *et al* 1976). Toxic effects, similar to those found with benzene, reported in early experiments on toluene are likely to be attributable to benzene contamination rather than to the toxicity of toluene itself.

Apart from several studies where visual signs of nervous distress were evident following exposure to high doses, relatively few studies have been carried out to assess the effects of toluene on the nervous system of experimental animals (Benignus 1981). However, changes in EEG patterns have been reported in rats and cats (Takeuchi and Hisanaga 1977, Suzuki and Kaziyama 1972).

Several studies of occupationally exposed subjects have suggested health effects of toluene, most of which are associated with the nervous system. Matsushita *et al* (1975) reported abnormal tendon reflexes, reduced grasping power and decreased finger agility in a group of 38 female shoemakers. In two studies of car painters, one found moderate impairment of concentration, emotional reactivity and hand agility, while the other was unable to find differences in EEGs or nerve conduction velocities. Average exposure levels were suggested to be about 30 ppm (Hanninen *et al* 1976, Seppalainen *et al* 1978). An early study found an increased incidence of hepatomegaly in painters exposed to solvent mixtures, of which toluene was the major component, at 100–1000 ppm (Greenburg *et al* 1942). Immunotoxicity has been associated with occupational exposure to toluene on some occasions, but in each case concurrent exposure to other solvents makes an evaluation very difficult (Capurro 1976, Lange *et al* 1973, Smolik *et al* 1973).

Studies of 'glue sniffers' have found results consistent with those from occupationally exposed subjects and from animal studies. There is very little evidence for haematological effects, although Press and Done (1967) documented eosinophilia in four out of 16 cases. There is also little evidence for liver and kidney toxicity. With regard to the effects of toluene on the CNS of 'glue sniffers', effects observed include cerebellar degeneration, encephalopathy, changes in personality, atrophy, slurred speech, clumsiness, memory and concentration disturbances (Grabski 1961, Knox and Nelson 1966, Satran and Dodson 1963, Boor and Hurtig 1977). Many accounts, however, have indicated that the adverse effects are reversible, provided that solvent abuse is ceased and that previous exposure had not been too severe. A report of toluene abuse, a study of six inmates in a Mexico prison, found blood toluene levels ranging from 9.8 to 31.2 mg/l in samples taken shortly after inhalation. The authors described the subjects to be 'in no distress, exhibiting only moderate signs of intoxication such as slurred speech, impaired ability to concentrate, and slow, unsteady movements' (Garriott *et al* 1981).

3.4.3 Genotoxicity

Toluene has given negative results in the Ames test with *Salmonella typhimurium* TA100, TA1535, TA1537, TA1538 and TA98, both in the presence and absence of rat liver S-9 or hamster liver S-9, at doses ranging from 10 to 2000 μg/plate (Bos *et al* 1981, Haworth *et al* 1983).

Bos *et al* (1981) reported that toluene was negative for unscheduled DNA synthesis in primary rat hepatocytes, but no experimental details were given.

In vivo clastogenic effects of toluene have been documented in the bone marrow of rats injected with 1 g/kg daily for 12 days (Lyapkalo 1973) and in another study where rats were exposed by inhalation to 112 ppm, 4 hours daily, for 4 months (Dobrokhotov and Enikeev 1977). In the latter study it was estimated that 0.8 g/kg/day of toluene induced the same frequency of chromosomal damage as 0.2 g/kg/day of benzene. Donner *et al* (1980) were unable to show an increased incidence of chromosomal aberrations in the bone marrow cells of Wistar rats exposed to 300 ppm, for 6 hours/day, 5 days/week, for 15 weeks. However, there was a significant increase in sister chromatid exchanges at 11 and 13 weeks, but not at 15 weeks. Toluene was not found to induce recessive lethal mutations in *Drosophila melanogaster* (Donner *et al* 1980).

Chromosomal studies of toluene-exposed workers have also produced equivocal results for clastogenic activity. Forni *et al* (1971) did not detect a significant increase in lymphocyte chromosomal aberrations in workers exposed to the compound for up to 15 years. Similarly, Donner *et al* (1980) found no increased incidence of lymphocyte chromosomal aberrations in a group of 32 rotogravure workers exposed to toluene. However, a study of workers in chemical laboratories and a rotoprinting factory did indicate a significantly increased frequency of abnormal lymphocytes and chromosome breaks (Funes-Cravioto *et al* 1977), while Bauchinger *et al* (1982) found an increased incidence of chromosome aberrations and sister chromatid exchanges in the lymphocytes of 20 male workers exposed solely to toluene for more than 16 years in a rotogravure plant.

Dean (1978) speculated that as toluene is highly lipophilic, high concentrations could alter the transport of other mutagenic compounds into the cell.

3.4.4 Carcinogenicity

In an inhalation study, groups of 120 male and 120 female F-344 rats were exposed to 0, 30, 100 or 300 ppm of toluene for 6 hours/day, 5 days/week for up to 2 years. No significant increase in tumour incidence was found (Gibson and Hardisty 1983).

Two skin painting studies in mice, one for lifetime and the other for one year, also found no evidence of carcinogenicity (Poel 1963, Doak *et al* 1976). Lijinsky and Garcia (1972) did report one skin papilloma and one skin carcinoma in a group of 30 mice receiving topically applied toluene (16–20 μl) twice weekly for 72 weeks.

Toluene has not been tested for carcinogenicity by the oral route.

3.4.5 Reproductive toxicity

Nawrot and Staples (1979) have provided some evidence for the teratogenicity of toluene. CD-1 mice were given 0.3, 0.5 or 1.0 ml/kg body weight of toluene by gavage on days 6–15 of gestation. Increased embryonic mortality was apparent at all doses, decreased foetal weight was noted at 0.5 and 1.0 ml/kg, and a significantly increased incidence of cleft palate was found at the highest dose. There was no evidence for maternal toxicity at any dose level. Embryotoxicity was observed in mice exposed by inhalation to 133 ppm on days 6–13 of gestation, and in rats exposed to 399 ppm, 8 hours/day on days 1–21 of gestation (Hudak and Ungvary 1978).

Mice were exposed to 0, 200 or 400 ppm toluene by inhalation on days 6–16 of gestation. There was a significant shift in the foetal rib profile at 400 ppm and an increase in dilated renal pelvis at 200 ppm. At 400 ppm neonatal weight was significantly increased at day 1 post partum (Courtney *et al* 1986).

3.5 Discussion

Toluene was identified in all 14 drinking water samples of the WRc survey. The contribution of waterborne toluene to overall exposure is unclear at present, due to the lack of information on levels in food. Toluene is metabolised rapidly by the liver, and eliminated, primarily in the urine, as hippuric acid.

There is little evidence to indicate that exposure to toluene results in toxicity to any particular tissue or organ, apart from the CNS. With early chronic toxicity studies, exposure to other compounds, notably benzene, probably led to misleading results. The evidence that toluene has clastogenic potential is equivocal. An inhalation study in rats and two skin painting studies in mice proved negative for carcinogenicity, but toluene has yet to be tested by the oral route. Toluene has been shown to be embryotoxic at high doses in rodents, and there is some evidence for teratogenicity.

The Cosmetic Ingredient Review Panel of the American College of Toxicology concluded that toluene was sage as a cosmetic ingredient for cosmetic use at the present practices of use and concentration (CIRP 1987).

Although there are some gaps in the information on the toxicology of toluene, notably long-term oral studies, the evidence indicates that this compound is of very low toxicity. This, together with the low concentrations present in drinking water, would suggest that toluene is unlikely to constitute a hazard to human health.

References

ASTRAND I, EHRNER-SAMUEL H, KILBOM A and OVRUM P (1972) Toluene exposure: I. Concentration in alveolar air and blood at rest and during exercise. *Scandinavian Journal of Work and Environmental Health* **9,** 119-130.

BAUCHINGER M, SCHMID E, DRESP J, KOLIN-GERRESHEIM J, HAUF R and SUHR E (1982) Chromosome changes in lymphocytes after occupational exposure to toluene. *Mutation Research* **102,** 439-445.

BENIGNUS V A (1981) Health effects of toluene: A review. *Neurotoxicology* **2,** 567-588.

BOOR J W and HURTIG H I (1977) Persistent cerebellar ataxia after exposure to toluene. *Annals of Neurology* **21,** 440.

BOS R P, BROUNS R M E, VAN DOORN R, THEUWS J L G and HENDERSON P Th (1981) Non-mutagenicity of toluene, *o-*, *m-* and *p*-xylene, *o*-methylbenzylalcohol and *o*-methylbenzylsulfate in the Ames assay. *Mutation Research* **88,** 273-279.

BRUCKNER J V and PETERSON R G (1976) Evaluation of toluene toxicity, utilizing the mouse as an animal model of human solvent abuse. *Pharmacology* **18,** 244.

BRUCKNER J V and PETERSON R G (1978) Effect of repeated exposure of mice and rats to concentrated toluene and acetone vapours. *Toxicology and Applied Pharmacology* **45,** 359.

CAPURRO P U (1976) Hydrocarbon exposure and cancer. *Lancet* **1,** 253-254.

CARPENTER C P, GEARY D L Jr, MYERS R C, NACHREINER D J, SULLIVAN L J and KING J M (1976) Petroleum hydrocarbon toxicity studies. XIII. Animal and human response to vapors of toluene concentrate. *Toxicology and Applied Pharmacology* **36,** 473-490.

CHAND P and CLAUSEN J (1982) Effects of toluene on cytochrome P-450 mixed function oxygenase and glutathione-*S*-transferase activities in rat brain and liver. *Bulletin of Environmental Contamination and Toxicology* **28,** 542-545.

COHR K H and STOKHOLM J (1979) Toluene: A toxicologic review. Scandinavian *Journal of Work Environment and Health* **5,** 71-90.

COSMETIC INGREDIENT REVIEW PANEL OF THE AMERICAN COLLEGE OF TOXICOLOGY (1987) Final report on the safety assessment of toluene. *Journal of the American College of Toxicology* **6,** 77-120.

COURTNEY K D, ANDREWS J E, SPRINGER J, MENACHE M, WILLIAMS T, DALLEY L and GRAHAM J A (1986) A perinatal study of toluene in CD-1 mice. *Fundamental and Applied Toxicology* **6,** 145-154.

DEAN B J (1978) Genetic toxicology of benzene, toluene, xylenes and phenol. *Mutation Research* **47,** 75-97.

DEAN B J (1985) Recent findings on the genetic toxicology of benzene, toluene, xylenes and phenols. *Mutation Research* **154,** 153-181.

DOAK S M A, SIMPSON B J E, HUNT P F and STEVENSON D E (1976) The carcinogenic response in mice to the topical application of propane sultone to the skin. *Toxicology* **6,** 139-154.

DOBROKHOTOV V B and ENIKEEV M I (1977) Mutagenic effect of benzene, toluene, and a mixture of these hydrocarbons in a chronic experiment. *Gigiena i Sanitariia* **1,** 32-34.

DONNER M, HUSGAFVEL-PURSIAINEN K, MAIKI-PAAKKANEN J, SORSA M and VAINIO H (1980) Genetic effects of *in vivo* exposure to toluene. *Abstracts of the Tenth Annual Meeting of EEMS, Athens, September 1980.*

DUTKIEWICZ T and TYRAS H (1968) The quantitative estimation of toluene skin absorption in man. *Internationale Archiv fur Gewerbepathologie und Gewerbehygiene* **24,** 253-257.

ELOVAARA E, SAVOLAINEN H, PFAFFLI P and VAINIO H (1979) Effects of subacute toluene inhalation on its metabolism and disposition in rat. *Archives of Toxicology* Suppl 2, 345-348.

FORNI A, PACIFICO E and LIMONTA A (1971) Chromosome studies in workers exposed to benzene or toluene or both. *Archives of Environmental Health* **22,** 373-378.

FUNES-CRAVIOTO F, ZAPATA-GAYON C, KOLMODIN-HEDMAN B, LAMBERT B, LINDSTEN J, NORBERG E, NORDENSKJOLD M, OLIN R and SWENSSON A (1977) Chromosome aberrations and sister-chromatid exchange in workers in chemical laboratories and a rotoprinting factory and in children of women laboratory workers. *Lancet* **2,** 322-325.

GARRIOTT J C, FOERSTER E, JUAREZ L, DE LA GARZA F, MENDIOLA I and CUROE J (1981) Measurement of toluene in blood and breath in cases of solvent abuse. *Clinical Toxicology* **18,** 471-479.

GIBSON J E and HARDISTY J F (1983) Chronic toxicity and oncogenicity bioassay of inhaled toluene in Fischer-344 rats. *Fundamental and Applied Toxicology* **3,** 315-319.

GRABSKI D A (1961) Toluene sniffing producing cerebellar degeneration. *American Journal of Psychiatry* **118,** 461.

GREENBURG L, MAYERS M R, HEIMANN H and MOSKOWITZ S (1942) The effects of exposure to toluene in industry. *Journal of the American Medical Association* **118,** 573-578.

GROB K and GROB G (1971) Gas–liquid chromatographic/mass spectrometric investigation of C_6-C_{20}-organic compounds in an urban atmosphere. *Journal of Chromatography* **62,** 1-13.

HANNINEN H, ESKELINEN L, HUSMAN K and NURMINEN M (1976) Behavioural effects of long-term exposure to a mixture of organic solvents. *Scandinavian Journal of Work Environment and Health* **2,** 240-255.

HASEGAWA K, SHIOJIMA S, KOIZUMI A and IKEDA M (1983) Hippuric acid and *o*-cresol in the urine of workers exposed to toluene. *International Archives of Occupational and Environmental Health* **52,** 197-208.

HAWORTH S, LAWLOR T, MORTELMANS K, SPECK W and ZEIGER E (1983) *Salmonella* mutagenicity test results for 250 chemicals. *Environmental Mutagenesis* **5** Suppl 1, 3-142.

HAYDEN J W, PETERSON R G and BRUCKNER J V (1977) Toxicology of toluene (methylbenzene): Review of current literature. *Clinical Toxicology* **11,** 549-559.

HUDAK A and UNGVARY G (1978) Embryotoxic effects of benzene and its methyl derivatives. *Toxicology* **11,** 55-63.

JENKINS L J Jr, JONES R A and SIEGEL J (1970) Long term inhalation screening studies of benzene, toluene, *o*-xylene, and cumene on experimental animals. *Toxicology and Applied Pharmacology* **16,** 818-823.

KIMURA E T, EBERT D M and DODGE P W (1971) Acute toxicity and limits of solvent residue for sixteen organic solvents. *Toxicology and Applied Pharmacology* **19,** 699-704.

KNOX J W and NELSON J R (1966) Permanent encephalopathy from toluene inhalation. *New England Journal of Medicine* **275,** 1494-1496.

LANGE A, SMOLIK R, ZATONSKI W and SZYMANSKA J (1973) Serum immunoglobulin levels in workers exposed to benzene, toluene and xylene. *Internationale Archiv fur Arbeitsmedizin* **31,** 37-44.

LIJINSKY W and GARCIA H (1972) Skin carcinogenesis tests of hydrogenated derivatives of anthracene and other polynuclear hydrocarbons. *Zeitschrift fur Krebsforschung und Klinische Onkologie* **77,** 226.

LYAPKALO A A (1973) Genetic activity of benzene and toluene. *Gigiena Truda Professional'nye Zabolevaniia* **17,** 24-28a.

MACKAY D and LEINONEN P J (1975) Rates of evaporation of low-solubility contaminants from water bodies to atmosphere. *Environmental Science and*

Technology **9,** 1178-1180.
MATSUSHITA T, ARIMATSU Y, UEDA A, SATOH K and NOMURA S (1975) Hematological and neuro-muscular response of workers exposed to low concentration of toluene vapor. *Industrial Health – Kawasaki* **13,** 115-121.
NATIONAL ACADEMY OF SCIENCES (1977) Drinking water and health, vol 1. Washington DC, US NAS.
NATIONAL ACADEMY OF SCIENCES (1980) Drinking water and health, vol 3. Washington DC, National Academy Press.
NAWROT P S and STAPLES R E (1979) Embryo-fetal toxicity and teratogenicity of benzene and toluene in the mouse. *Teratology* **19,** 41A.
OGATA M and MIYAKE Y (1973) Identification of substances in petroleum causing objectionable odor in fish. *Water Research* **7,** 4.2 1493-1504.
PILAR S and GRAYDON W F (1973) Benzene and toluene distribution in Toronto atmosphere. *Environmental Science and Technology* **7,** 628-631.
POEL W E (1963) Skin as a test site for the bioassay of carcinogens and carcinogen precursors. *National Cancer Institute Monographs* **10,** 611.
PRESS E and DONE A K (1967) Solvent sniffing. Physiological effects and community control measures for intoxication from the intentional inhalation of organic solvents. I and II. *Pediatrics* **39,** 451-460.
PYYKKO K, TAHTI H and VAPAATALO H (1977) Toluene concentrations in various tissues of rats after inhalation and oral administration. *Archives of Toxicology* **38,** 169-176.
RHUDY R L, LINDBERG D C, GOODE J W, SULLIVAN D J and GRALLA E J (1978) Ninety-day subacute inhalation study with toluene in albino rats. *Toxicology and Applied Pharmacology* **45**, 284-285.
SANDMEYER E E (1981) Aromatic hydrocarbons. In: Clayton G D and Clayton F E (eds) *Patty's industrial hygiene and toxicology,* vol 2B, 3rd Revised Edition. Wiley and Sons, pp 3283-3291.
SATRAN R and DODSON V N (1963) Toluene habituation. Report of a case. *New England Journal of Medicine* **268,** 719-721.
SEPPALAINEN A M, HUSMAN K and MARTENSON C (1978) Neurophysiological effects of long-term exposure to a mixture of organic solvents. *Scandinavian Journal of Work Environment and Health* **4,** 304-314.
SMOLIK R, GRZYBEKA-HRYNCEWICZ K, LANGE A and ZATONSKI W (1973) Serum complement level in workers exposed to benzene, toluene and xylene. *Internationale Archiv fur Arbeitsmedizin* **31,** 243.
SUZUKI Y and KAZIYAMA K (1972) Effects of a thinner preparation and its constituents on EEG of the cat. *Japanese Journal of Pharmacology* **22,** 68.
TAKEUCHI Y and HISANAGA N (1977) The neurotoxicity of toluene: EEG changes in rats exposed to various concentrations. *British Journal of Industrial Medicine* **34,** 314.
THORBURN S and COLENUTT B A (1973) A gas chromatographic comparison of volatile organic compounds in urban and rural atmospheres. *International Journal of Environmental Studies* **13,** 265-271.
US ENVIRONMENTAL PROTECTION AGENCY (1980) Ambient water quality criteria for toluene. Washington DC, US EPA, EPA 440/5-80-075.
VAN DOORN R, BOS R P, BROUNS R M E, LEIJDEKKERS C M and

HENDERSON P T (1980) Effect of toluene and xylenes on liver glutathione and their urinary excretion as mercapturic acids in the rat. *Archives of Toxicology* **43,** 293-304.

VERSCHUEREN K (1977) *Handbook of environmental data on organic chemicals.* Van Nostrand Reinhold Company.

WATER RESEARCH CENTRE (1981) Organic micropollutants in drinking water. WRc Technical Report TR 159.

WOIWODE W, WOOARZ R, DRYSCH K and WEICHARDT H (1979) Metabolism of toluene in man: Gas-chromatographic determination of *o-, m-* and *p*-cresol in urine. *Archives of Toxicology* **43,** 93-95.

WOLF M A, ROWE V K, McCOLLISTER D D, HOLLINGSWORTH R L and OYEN F (1956) Toxicological studies of certain alkylated benzenes and benzene. *AMA Archives of Industrial Health* **14,** 387-98.

ZOETEMAN B C J, PIET G J, RUYGROK C T M and HEUVEL R V D (1974) Threshold odour concentrations in water of chemical substances. RID-MEDEDELING, 74-3.

4. ETHYLBENZENE

4.1 Introduction

Ethylbenzene is commercially manufactured by the chemical industry as a byproduct of the refining of petroleum products. Ethylbenzene is used in the manufacture of acetophenone and styrene, as a constituent of asphalt, naphtha and gasoline, and as a general solvent.

A petition to remove this compound from the USA Clean Water Act list of toxic pollutants was submitted by the Dow Chemical Company in 1979 (United States Federal Register 1979), but this was rejected (United States Federal Register 1981).

CAS Reg No:	100-41-4
Molecular weight:	106.2
Boiling point:	136.2°C
Solubility:	152 mg/l at 20°C (Verschueren 1977)
Evaporative half-life in water:	No data available
Threshold odour concentration in water:	0.1 mg/l (Zoeteman *et al* 1974)

4.2 Exposure

4.2.1 Air

Two studies have reported higher levels of ethylbenzene in urban air compared to rural air. Thorburn and Colenutt (1979) detected an ethylbenzene concentration of 33.9 ppb near the M1 at Luton and a level of 11.3 ppb at Freshwater (IOW). Holzer et al (1977) found markedly higher levels of ethylbenzene in Tuscaloosa, USA urban air compared to air in a US National Forest.

4.2.2 Food

No data appear to be available with regard to ethylbenzene in food.

4.2.3 Water
In the WRC survey (Water Research Centre 1981), ethylbenzene was identified in 5/14 drinking water samples tested. This compound has been found at 11 μg/l in the Kanahawa river, USA (Dostal *et al* 1965).

4.3 Toxicokinetics
4.3.1 Absorption
The retention of inhaled ethylbenzene has been estimated to be 44% in rats (Chin *et al* 1980) and 64% in humans (Bardodej and Bardodejova 1970). Ethylbenzene is quite readily absorbed through the skin (Dutkiewicz and Tyras 1967). Although there are no specific data on gastrointestinal absorption, it appears likely that the majority of ingested ethylbenzene would be absorbed.

4.3.2 Distribution
Following inhalation of radiolabelled ethylbenzene by rats, small quantities were found in the lungs, gastrointestinal tract, liver and fatty tissues. However, almost 80% of the label remained in the rest of the carcass (Chin *et al* 1980).

4.3.3 Metabolism
In rabbits (Smith *et al* 1954, Elmasry *et al* 1956), about 35% of an oral dose of ethylbenzene (I) is converted to hippuric acid (XVII), 35% to methylphenyl carbinyl glucosiduronic acid (VII), 10–20% to phenaceturic acid (V) and about 2% to mandelic acid (XIV). Metabolism of ethylbenzene to phenaceturic acid (V) is thought to occur via 2-phenylethanol (II), phenylethanal (III) and phenylacetic acid (IV) intermediates. The precise metabolic pathway for biotransformation of ethylbenzene to hippuric acid is not clear (Kiese and Lenk 1974, Sullivan *et al* 1976, Ohtsuji and Ikeda 1971). A number of intermediates are thought to be involved and a number of different routes are possible (Figure 2).

Studies of human exposure to ethylbenzene have reported the occurrence of mandelic acid (XIV), 1-phenylethanol (VI), phenylglyoxylic acid (XV) and 2-ethylphenol (XVIII) in the urine (Bardodej and Bardodejova 1970, Leibman 1975, Angerer and Lehnert 1979).

4.3.4 Excretion
Following either an oral dose or inhalation of ethylbenzene, almost all of the dose is excreted as metabolites in the urine (Chin *et al* 1980, Smith *et al* 1954, Elmasry *et al* 1956).

4.4 Health effects
4.4.1 Acute and subacute toxicity
Ethylbenzene is primarily a membrane irritant which can cause erythema and blistering of the skin. Wolf *et al* (1956) reported moderate irritation and necrosis of rabbit skin after contact with ethylbenzene. Acute exposure of guinea pigs to ethylbenzene vapour has been reported to be fatal within a few minutes at 10 000

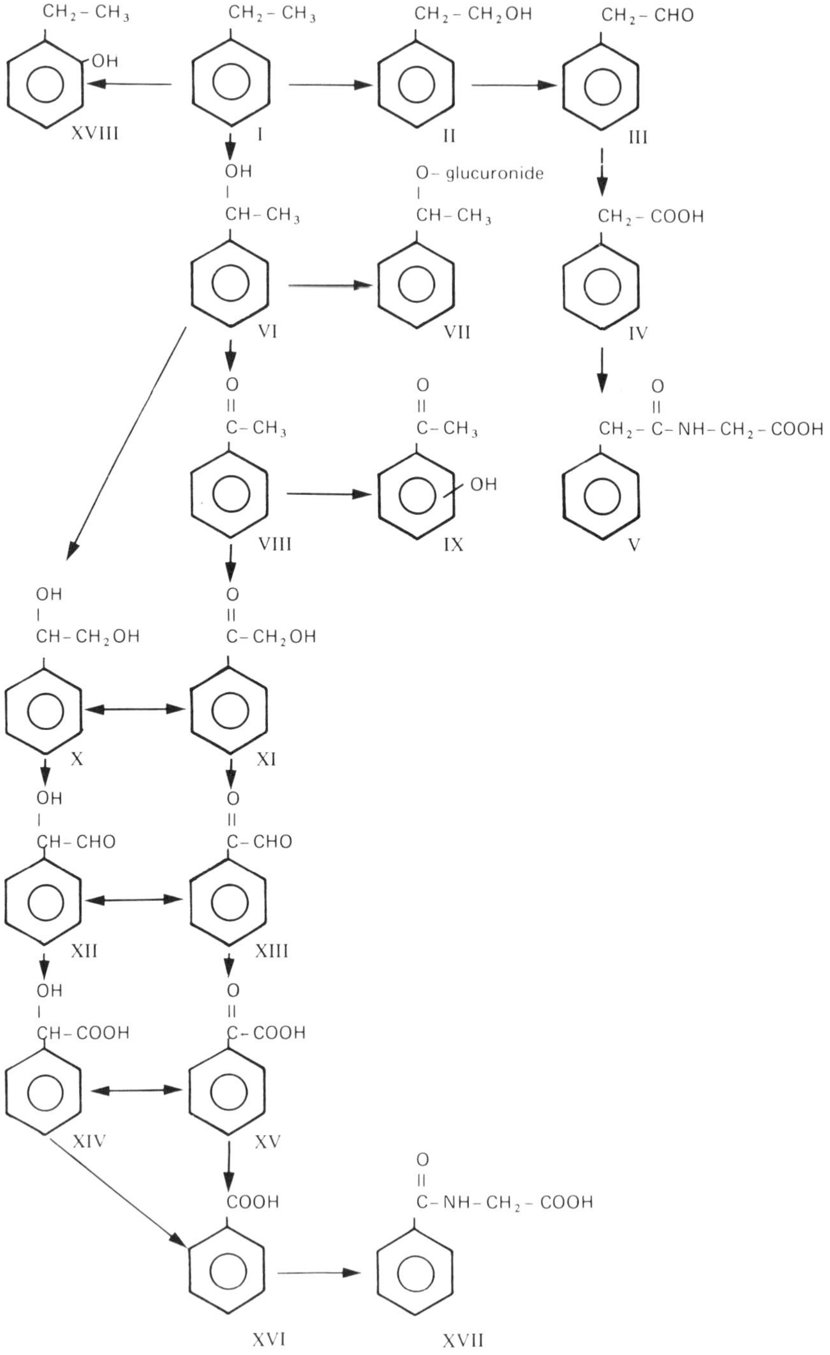

Fig. 2 — Biotransformation of ethylbenzene.

ppm, but caused no serious disturbance at 1000 ppm for several hours (Yant *et al* 1930). In man, an intolerable irritation of nose, eyes and throat is apparent after exposure for only a few seconds to 5000 ppm of ethylbenzene vapour. Quite severe membrane irritation and lacrimation followed by dizziness can be observed after a short time at 2000 ppm, but eye irritation was found to diminish after a few minutes at 1000 ppm (Yant *et al* 1930). The acute oral LD50 of ethylbenzene in rats is 3.5 g/kg (Wolf *et al* 1956).

In a subacute study (Gerarde 1956), 40 male Wistar rats were given daily subcutaneous injections of 1 ml/kg of ethylbenzene in olive oil, for 2 weeks. The animals exhibited CNS depression, but no significant changes were found in peripheral blood leukocyte counts, thymus and spleen weights, femoral marrow nucleated cell counts or femoral marrow nucleic acid. Andersson *et al* (1981) found pronounced changes in dopamine and noradrenaline levels in different areas of the hypothalamus and forebrain of rats exposed by inhalation to 2000 ppm of ethylbenzene, 6 hours/day, for 3 days. Although no behavioural effects were observed, it was suggested that the subtle changes in neurotransmitter levels may affect the secretion of hormones, such as prolactin. The mechanism of action of ethylbenzene on the nervous system is likely to be membrane-related.

Male rats exposed to ethylbenzene vapour at concentrations of 0, 50, 300 or 600 ppm for 6 hours/day, 5 days/week and killed after 2, 5, 9 or 16 weeks of exposure showed a variety of biochemical changes in liver and kidney particularly at the highest dose with the longest exposure period (Elovaara *et al* 1985).

4.4.2 Chronic toxicity

In an oral study (Wolf *et al* 1956), groups of 10 female rats were each given 13.6, 136, 408 or 680 mg/kg of ethylbenzene in olive oil, 5 days/week for 6 months. No effects of any type were observed in animals of the two lower dose groups, but slight effects on liver and kidney weights and on the histopathology of these two organs were noted in animals dosed with 408 or 680 mg/kg. A more detailed inhalation study (Wolf *et al* 1956) was performed on groups of 10–25 rats, 5–10 guinea pigs, 1–2 rabbits and 1–2 monkeys exposed to different vapour concentrations of ethylbenzene, 7 hours/day, 5 days/week for up to 6 months. Exposure to 400 ppm resulted in some effects on liver and kidney weights in rats, but no effects on any other species; while after exposure to 600 ppm, slight effects on testicular histopathology were observed in the rhesus monkey and rabbit, and liver weight changes were evident in the monkey, guinea-pig and rat. Only rats were exposed to 2200 ppm and were found to have a moderate growth depression and slight pathological changes in the liver and kidney.

4.4.3 Genotoxicity, carcinogenicity and reproductive toxicity

Ethylbenzene was not found to induce sister chromatid exchanges in human lymphocytes *in vitro* (Norppa and Vainio 1983), nor did it induce micronuclei in polychromatic erythrocytes of mice (Mohtashamipur *et al* 1985). It did not cause mutations in *Salmonella typhimurium* TA 1535, TA 1537, TA1538, TQ98, TA100, *E. coli* WP2, 2P2 uvrA or *S. cerivisiae* JD1 tested with or without metabolic activation. Ethylbenzene did not cause chromosome damage in rat liver cells (Dean *et al* 1985).

No studies have been found which relate to carcinogenic potential or reproductive effects apart from a gavage study in mice and rats with mixed xylenes and ethylbenzene which was negative (USNTP 1986).

4.5 Discussion

Ethylbenzene has been identified in air and water samples, but the lack of information on ethylbenzene in food, together with limited information on levels in air and water, provide insufficient data for an assessment of relative exposure. This compound would be expected to be readily absorbed in the gut, and rapidly metabolised by side-chain oxidation in the liver. Almost all of a dose of ethylbenzene would be excreted in the urine as metabolites.

From the limited information available it would appear that ethylbenzene has a low acute and chronic toxic potential in experimental animals. At high doses, ethylbenzene causes membrane irritation, CNS depression and pathological changes in the liver and kidney. No information on the genotoxicity, carcinogenicity, or reproductive toxicity of this compound appears to be available.

Although ethylbenzene does not appear to warrant concern as a micropollutant in drinking water, there are large areas of its toxicology in which information is completely lacking.

References

ANDERSSON K, FUXE K, NILSEN O G, TOFTGARD R, ENEROTH P and GUSTAFSSON J-K (1981) Production of discrete changes in dopamine and noradrenaline levels and turnover in various parts of the rat brain following exposure to xylene, *ortho-*, *meta-*, and *para*-xylene, and ethylbenzene. *Toxicology and Applied Pharmacology* **60,** 535-548.

ANGERER J and LEHNERT G (1979) Occupational chronic exposure to organic solvents. VIII. Phenolic compounds – metabolites of alkylbenzenes in man. Simultaneous exposure to ethylbenzene and xylenes. *International Archives of Occupational Environmental Health* **43,** 145-150.

BARDODEJ Z and BARDODEJOVA E (1970) Biotransformation of ethylbenzene, styrene and x-methyl-styrene in man. *American Industrial Hygiene Association Journal* **31,** 206-209.

CHIN B H, McKELVEY J A, TYLER T R, CALISTI L J, KOZBELT S J and SULLIVAN L J (1980) Absorption, distribution and excretion of ethylbenzene; ethylcyclohexane, and methylethylbenzene isomers in rats. *Bulletin of Environmental Contamination and Toxicology* **24,** 477-483.

DEAN B J, BROOKS T M, HODSON-WALKER G and HUTSON D H (1985) Genetic toxicology testing of 41 industrial chemicals. *Mutation Research* **153,** 57-77.

DOSTAL K A, PIERSON R C, HAGER D G and ROBECK G G (1965) Carbon bed design criteria study at nitro, Wva. *Journal of the American Water Works Association* **57,** 663-674.

DUTKIEWICZ T and TYRAS H (1967) A study of skin absorption of ethylbenzene in man. *British Journal of Industrial Medicine* **24,** 330-332.

ELMASRY A M, SMITH J N and WILLIAMS R T (1956) The metabolism of alkylbenzenes: *n*-propylbenzene and *n*-butylbenzene with further observations on ethylbenzene. *Biochemical Journal* **64,** 50-56.

ELOVAARA E, ENGSTROM K, NICKELS J, AITO A and VAINIO H (1985) Biochemical and morphological effects of long-term inhalation exposure of rats to ethylbenzene. *Xenobiotica* **15,** 299-308.

GERARDE H W (1956) Toxicological studies on hydrocarbons II. A comparative study of the effect of benzene and certain mono-*n*-alkylbenzenes on hemopoiesis and bone marrow metabolism in rats. *AMA Archives of Industrial Health* **13,** 468-474.

HOLZER G, SHANFIELD H, ZLATKIS A, BERTSCH W, JUAREZ P, MAYFIELD H and LIEBICH H M (1977) Collection and analysis of trace organic emissions from natural sources. *Journal of Chromatography* **142,** 755-764.

KIESE M and LENK W (1974) Hydroxyacetophenones: urinary metabolites of ethylbenzene and acetophenone in the rabbit. *Xenobiotica* **4,** 337-343.

LEIBMAN K C (1975) Metabolism and toxicity of styrene. *Environmental Health Perspectives* **11,** 115-119.

MOHTASHAMIPUR E, NORPATH K, WOELKE U and HUBER P (1985) Effects of ethylbenzene, toluene and xylene on the induction of micronuclei in bone marrow polychromatic erythrocytes of mice. *Archives of Toxicology* **58,** 106-109.

NORPPA H and VAINIO H (1983) Induction of sister-chromatid exchanges by styrene analogues in cultured human lymphocytes. *Mutation Research* **116,** 379-387.

OHTSUJI H and IKEDA M (1971) The metabolism of styrene in the rat and the stimulatory effect of phenobarbitol. *Toxicology and Applied Pharmacology* **18,** 321-328.

SMITH J N, SMITHIES R H and WILLIAMS R T (1954) The metabolism of alkylbenzenes. Stereochemical aspects of the biological hydroxylation of ethylbenzene to methylphenylcarbinol. *Biochemical Journal* **56,** 320-324.

SULLIVAN H R, MILLER W M and McMAHON R E (1976) Reaction pathways of *in vivo* stereoselective conversion of ethylbenzene to (−)-mandelic acid. *Xenobiotica* **6,** 49-54.

THORBURN S and COLENUTT B A (1979) A gas chromatographic comparison of volatile organic compounds in urban and rural atmospheres. *International Journal of Environmental Studies* **13,** 265-271.

UNITED STATES FEDERAL REGISTER (1979) 44, 64555-64557.

UNITED STATES FEDERAL REGISTER (1981) 46, 2267-2273.

UNITED STATES NATIONAL TOXICOLOGY PROGRAM (1986) Toxicology and carcinogenesis studies of xylenes (mixed) in F344/N rats and B6C3F1 mice. NTP TR 327, Research Triangle Park.

VERSCHUEREN K (1977) *Handbook of environmental data on organic chemicals.* Van Nostrand Reinhold Company.

WATER RESEARCH CENTRE (1981) Organic micropollutants in drinking water. WRc Technical Report TR 159.

WOLF M A, ROWE V K, McCOLLISTER D D, HOLLINGSWORTH R L and OYEN F (1956) Toxicological studies of certain alkylated benzenes and benzene. *AMA Archives of Industrial Health* **14,** 387-398.

YANT W P, SCHRENK H H, WAITE C P and PATTY F A (1930) Acute response of guinea pigs to vapors of some new commercial organic compounds. II. Ethylbenzene. *US Public Health Reports* **45,** 1241.

ZOETEMAN B C J, PIET G J, RUYGROK C T M and HEUVEL R V D (1974) Threshold odour concentrations in water of chemical substances. RID-MEDEDELING, 74-3.

5. XYLENE

5.1 Introduction

Xylene (dimethylbenzene) is produced by the chemical industry and from the distillation of petroleum, coal tar and coal gas. It is used as a solvent in resins, lacquers, enamels and rubber cements, in aviation fuel, and in the manufacture of polyester, pharmaceuticals, dyes, insecticides, asphalt and naphtha. The three isomeric forms of xylene (*ortho-, meta-* and *para-*) all possess similar physicochemical properties.

CAS Reg No (mixed):	1330-20-7
Molecular weight:	106.17
Boiling point:	138°C
Solubility:	180 mg/l at 20°C (Verschueren 1977)
Evaporative half-life in water of depth 1 m:	5.61 hours at 25°C (Mackay and Leinonen 1975)
Threshold odour concentration in water:	1–2 mg/l (Zoeteman *et al* 1974).

5.2 Exposure

5.2.1 Air

Thorburn and Colenutt (1979) detected a xylene concentration of around 16 ppb in the rural atmosphere of Freshwater (IOW) and a level of 49 ppb near the M1 at Luton. Data by Holzer *et al* (1977) also suggest higher levels of xylene in urban air compared to rural air in the US.

5.2.2 Food

No data appear to be available with regard to the presence of xylene in food.

5.2.3 Water

The xylenes were identified in all 14 treated water samples of the WRc survey (Water Research Centre 1981). A Japanese study detected xylene in both filtered river water and in tap water (Akiyama *et al* 1980). The US EPA have reported a xylene concentration of 4.1 μg/l in the treated water supply to New Orleans (United States Environmental Protection Agency 1975).

5.3 Toxicokinetics

5.3.1 Absorption

In man, about 60% of inhaled xylene is retained by the lungs (Sedivec and Flek 1976,

Astrand *et al* 1978). Percutaneous absorption also occurs readily (Engstrom *et al* 1977). Although there are no data on gastrointestinal absorption, xylene would be expected to be readily absorbed in view of its lipophilic nature.

5.3.2 Distribution

The distribution of xylene in the body is dependent on the fat content of individual tissues. The highest levels of xylene are found in lipid-rich tissues such as the adipose tissue, subcutaneous fat, adrenal glands, brain and liver.

5.3.3 Metabolism

The metabolic pathways differ for each xylene isomer. The *meta*- and *para*-isomers are 80–90% metabolised to the corresponding toluic acids and glycine conjugates (Williams 1959). Only 60% of *ortho*-xylene is transformed to *ortho*-toluic acid, and of this roughly half remains free, about half is conjugated with glucuronide, and only 0.3% is conjugated with glycine (Bray *et al* 1949, Ogata *et al* 1970). Aromatic ring oxidation to hydroxyxylenes (xylenols) has also been reported for each isomer, but this appears to be only a very minor route (Bakke and Scheline 1970). Methylbenzylmercapturic acids have also been identified as metabolites of xylenes, though only transformation of *ortho*-xylene in this manner appears to be of any quantitative significance (Van Doorn *et al* 1980).

5.3.4 Excretion

Xylene is excreted in the urine as methylhippuric acids, free toluic acids, toluoglucuronic acids, dimethylphenols and methylbenzylmercapturic acids. A small amount of unchanged xylene can be exhaled from the lungs (Sedivec and Flek 1976).

5.4 Health effects

Although the toxicology of xylene has not been comprehensively reviewed, there are several sources available which provide useful information (Gerarde 1960, Sandmeyer 1981, TSCA Interagency Committee 1977, Bruckner and Peterson 1977, National Academy of Sciences 1977, 1980).

5.4.1 Acute and subacute toxicity

Acute exposure to very high doses of xylene can cause erythema, dehydration, defatting and blistering of the skin, irritation of mucous membranes, peripheral vasodilation, giddiness, fatigue, 'drunkenness', narcosis and unconsciousness.

Studies on experimental animals have shown that xylene has a relatively low order of acute toxic potential. Mixed xylenes have an oral LD50 in the rat of 4.3 g/kg (Wolf *et al* 1956) and an inhalation LC50 in the rat of 6700 ppm (Carpenter *et al* 1975), while *para*-xylene has an inhalation LC50 in the same species of 4740 ppm (Harper *et al* 1974).

The most common effects of acute exposure to lower levels of xylene are CNS-related. Gamberale *et al* (1978) exposed 8 healthy men to 1300 mg/m^3 of xylene in inspired air for 70 minutes, 30 minutes of which was spent on a bicycle ergometer (100 W). The authors reported clear evidence of performance decrement in three out of a battery of behavioural tests. Changes in dopamine and noradrenaline levels in selected areas of the brain have been found in rats exposed by inhalation to 2000 ppm of xylene, 6 hours/day for 3 days (Andersson *et al* 1981).

Fabacher and Hodgson (1977) were unable to demonstrate enhanced hepatic microsomal *O*- or *N*-demethylase activity, or changes in the liver weight/body weight ratio of mice given daily intraperitoneal injections of 100 mg/kg of xylene for 3 days. In another study, increased serum ornithine-carbamyl transferase activity and higher levels of hepato-lipids were found in guinea-pigs following intraperitoneal injection of 1 g/kg of xylene in corn oil (Divincenzo and Krasavage 1974).

Combined administration of ethanol and xylene appears to result in additive effects on both the CNS and hepatic enzyme activities (Elovaara *et al* 1980, Savolainen 1980, Riihimaki *et al* 1982).

5.4.2 Chronic toxicity

Despite previous indications that xylene may possess the haematotoxic properties of benzene, the evidence from more recent studies would not support this. It is likely that contamination of xylene samples by benzene may have been responsible for the effects seen in earlier studies.

No significant changes in blood parameters were found in rats and rabbits exposed by inhalation to 690 ppm of mixed xylenes, 8 hours/day, 6 days/week for 130 days. Exposure of rabbits to 1150 ppm for 55 days in the same study was found to result in lowered numbers of erythrocytes and leukocytes, and an increase in platelet numbers (Fabre and Truhaut 1954). A long-term inhalation study of *ortho*-xylene in several species failed to show significant changes in body weight or haematological parameters after continuous exposure to 78 ppm of xylene vapour for 90 days, or after 30 repeated exposures to 780 ppm of xylene (Jenkins *et al* 1970). Similarly, no myelotoxic effects were observed in rabbits given 300 mg/kg/day of xylene by subcutaneous injection for 6 weeks or 700 mg/kg/day of xylene for 9 weeks (Speck and Moeschlin 1968).

Enhanced activities of hepatic microsomal 7-ethoxycoumarin *O*-deethylase, 2,5-diphenyloxazole hydroxylase and UDP-glucuronyltransferase have been reported in rats exposed by inhalation to 300 ppm of technical grade xylene, 6 hours/day, 5 days/week for 18 weeks. Histological examination did not reveal liver damage (Elovaara *et al* 1980).

5.4.3 Genotoxicity

All three isomers of xylene have given negative results for mutagenicity in the Ames test with *Salmonella typhimurium* TA98, TA100, TA1535, TA1537 and TA1538, both in the presence and absence of either rat liver or hamster liver S-9, and at doses ranging from 1.0 to 500 μg/plate (Bos *et al* 1981, Haworth *et al* 1983).

Xylenes have been shown not to be mutagenic in the *Salmonella*/microsome assay, bacterial DNA repair, not cause chromosome aberrations or sister chromatid exchanges in mammalian cells *in vitro*. Equivocal results were obtained in *Drosophila* germ cells but they did not cause chromosome aberrations in rat bone marrow *in vivo* (Dean 1978, 1985).

Dose levels of 0.0152–1.52 mg/ml of xylene were not found to increase chromosome aberrations or sister chromatid exchanges in human lymphocytes *in vitro*

(Gerner-Smidt and Friedrich 1978). Although no experimental data were given, Bos *et al* (1981) reported that *ortho-, meta-* and *para*-xylene had given negative results for unscheduled DNA synthesis in primary cultures of rat hepatocytes.

Mohtashamipur *et al* (1985) report that *ortho, meta-* and *para*-xylenes did not induce micronuclei in the bone marrow polychromatic erythrocytes of mice.

5.4.4 Carcinogenicity

Although no evidence for carcinogenicity was found in two 6-month skin painting experiments in mice (Kennaway 1924, Berenblum 1941), these studies were of insufficient duration, and therefore only very limited conclusions can be drawn. Long-term studies of mixed xylenes (60% *meta*, 14% *para* and 9% *ortho-* and 17% ethylbenzene) given by gavage at doses of 250 or 500 mg/kg to rats and 500 or 1000 mg/kg to mice, indicated no evidence of carcinogenicity (US National Toxicology Program 1986).

5.4.5 Reproductive toxicity

Xylene has been found at higher concentrations in cord blood than in maternal blood (Dowty *et al* 1976).

Two studies in mice have reported teratogenic effects of xylene. Nawrot and Staples (1980) dosed CD-1 mice by gavage with 0.3, 0.75 or 1.0 ml/kg/day of pure *ortho-, meta-,* or *para*-xylene on days 6–15 of gestation. Increased incidences of cleft palate and foetal resorptions were found at the two higher dose levels with the *ortho-* and *para*-isomers. In the other study, Marks *et al* (1982) dosed CD-1 mice by gavage with 0.52, 1.03, 2.06, 2.58, 3.10 or 4.13 g/kg/day of a commercial xylene mixture (60.2% *meta*-xylene, 9.1% *ortho*-xylene, 13.6% *para*-xylene and 17% ethylbenzene) in cottonseed oil, on days 6-15 of gestation. A significant increase in the incidence of malformed foetuses was found at the 2.06, 2.58 and 3.10 g/kg dose levels. The major malformation was again cleft palate. Other studies have noted embryotoxic effects, but failed to observe teratogenic effects in pregnant CFY rats exposed by inhalation to xylene isomers at up to 700 ppm on days 7–14 of gestation (Hudak and Ungvary 1978, Ungvary *et al* 1980).

There were no indications of behavioural effects in the offspring of female rats exposed on days 7–16 of gestation to 3500 or 7000 mg/m^3 *para*-xylene by inhalation (Rosen *et al* 1986).

5.5 Discussion

The xylenes have been regularly identified in the atmosphere and in water, but no data appear to be available on levels in food. Xylene is thought to be well absorbed by the gastrointestinal tract, and distributed to the lipid-rich tissues. Metabolism in the liver is rapid, but the pathways do differ slightly, depending on the isomer.

The xylenes are of low acute toxicity in experimental animals. At high doses their principal effects are CNS depression and membrane irritation. The xylenes also appear to be of low chronic toxicity, though they have not been tested by the oral route. The xylenes do not appear to be mutagenic in the Ames test, but there is only limited information available in higher test systems. There also appears to be no information on their carcinogenicity other than two skin-painting studies of inadequate length. There is some evidence that xylene is teratogenic in mice at very high dose levels.

The information available suggests that xylene is of relatively low toxicity and would not appear to present a problem to human health at the concentrations found in water. However, there are several areas in the toxicology of xylene where information is severely lacking.

References

AKIYAMA T, KOGA M, SHINOHARA R, KIDO A and ETOH S (1980) Detection and identification of trace organic substances in the aquatic environment. *Journal of Uoeh* **2,** 285-300.

ANDERSSON K, FUXE K, NILSEN O G, TOFTGARD R, ENEROTH P and GUSTAFSSON J-K (1981) Production of discrete changes in dopamine and noradrenaline levels and turnover in various parts of the rat brain following exposure to xylene, *ortho-*, *meta-*, and *para*-xylene, and ethylbenzene. *Toxicology and Applied Pharmacology* **60,** 535-548.

ASTRAND I, ENGSTROM J and OVRUM P (1978) Exposure to xylene and ethylbenzene. I. Uptake, distribution and elimination in man. *Scandinavian Journal of Work Environment and Health* **4,** 185-194.

BAKKE O M and SCHELINE R R (1970) Hydroxylation of aromatic hydrocarbons in the rat. *Toxicology and Applied Pharmacology* **16,** 691-700.

BERENBLUM I (1941) The carcinogenic action of croton resin. *Cancer Research* **1,** 44-48.

BOS R P, BROUNS R M E, VAN DOORN R, THEUWS J L G and HENDERSON P Th (1981) Non-mutagenicity of toluene, *o-*, *m-* and *p*-xylene, *o*-methylbenzylalcohol and *o*-methylbenzylsulfate in the Ames assay. *Mutation Research* **88,** 273-279.

BRAY H G, HUMPHRIS B G and THORPE W V (1949) Metabolism of derivatives of toluene. III. *o-*, *m-* and *p*-xylene. *Biochemical Journal* **45,** 241-244.

BRUCKNER J V and PETERSON R G (1977) Toxicology of aliphatic and aromatic hydrocarbons. In: Sharp C W and Brehm M L (eds) *Review of inhalants: Euphoria to dysfunction.* NIDA Research monograph 15.

CARPENTER C P, KINKEAD E R, GEARY D L Jr, SULLIVAN L J and KING J M (1975) Petroleum hydrocarbon toxicity studies. V. Animal and human response to vapors of mixed xylenes. *Toxicology and Applied Pharmacology* **33,** 543-558.

DIVINCENZO G D and KRASAVAGE W J (1974) Serum ornithine carbamyl transferase as a liver response test for exposure to organic solvents. *American Industrial Hygiene Association Journal* **35,** 21-29.

DOWTY B J, LASETER J L and STORER J (1976) The transplacental migration and accumulation in blood of volatile organic constituents. *Pediatric Research* **10,** 696-701.

ELOVAARA E, COLLAN Y, PFAFFLI P and VAINIO H (1980) The combined toxicity of technical grade xylene and ethanol in the rat. *Xenobiotica* **10,** 435-445.

ENGSTROM K, HUSMAN K and RIIHIMAKI V (1977) Percutaneous absorption of *m*-xylene in man. *International Archives of Occupational and Environmental*

Health **39,** 181-189.
FABACHER D L and HODGSON E (1977) Hepatic–mixed function oxidase activity in mice treated with methylated benzenes and methylated naphthalenes. *Journal of Toxicology and Environmental Health* **2,** 1143-46.
FABRE R and TRUHAUT R (1954) Le probleme ches solvants de remplacement du benzene dans ses rapports avec l'hygiene industrielle. *Congresso Internazionale de Medicina del Lavoro,* Napoli.
GAMBERALE F, ANNWALL G and HULTENGREN M (1978) Exposure to xylene and ethylbenzene. III. Effects on central nervous functions. *Scandinavian Journal of Work Environment and Health* **4,** 204-211.
GERARDE H W (1960) Toxicology and biochemistry of aromatic hydrocarbons. Elsevier, *Elsevier Monographs.*
GERNER-SMIDT P and FRIEDRICH U (1978) The mutagenic effect of benzene, toluene and xylene studied by the SCE technique. *Mutation Research* **58,** 313-316.
HARPER C, DREW R T and FOUTS J R (1974) Benzene and *p*-xylene: A comparison of inhalation toxicities and *in vitro* hydroxylations. In: Jollow O J, Kocsis J J, Snyder R and Vainio H (eds), *Biological reactive intermediates: formation, toxicity, and inactivation.* New York, Plenum Press, pp 302-311.
HAWORTH S, LAWLOR T, MORTELMANS K, SPECK W and ZEIGER E (1983) Salmonella mutagenicity test results for 250 chemicals. *Environmental Mutagenesis* **5** Suppl 1, 3-142.
HOLZER G, SHANFIELD H, ZLATKIS A, BERTSCH W, JUAREZ P, MAYFIELD H and LIEBICH H M (1977) Collection and analysis of trace organic emissions from natural sources. *Journal of Chromatography* **142,** 755-764.
HUDAK A and UNGVARY G (1978) Embryotoxic effects of benzene and its methyl derivatives: toluene, xylene. *Toxicology* **11,** 55-63.
JENKINS L J Jr, JONES R A and SIEGEL J (1970) Long-term inhalation screening studies of benzene, toluene, *o*-xylene, and cumene on experimental animals. *Toxicology and Applied Pharmacology* **16,** 818-823.
KENNAWAY E L (1924) On the cancer-producing factor in tar. *British Medical Journal* **1,** 564-567.
MACKAY D and LEINONEN P J (1975) Rates of evaporation of low-solubility contaminants from water bodies to atmosphere. *Environmental Science and Technology* **9,** 1178-1180.
MARKS T A, LEDOUX T A and MOORE J A (1982) Teratogenicity of a commercial xylene mixture in the mouse. *Journal of Toxicology and Environmental Health* **9,** 97-105.
MOHTASHAMIPUR E, NORPATH K, WOELKE U and HUBER P (1985) Effects of ethylbenzene, toluene and xylene on the induction of micronuclei in bone marrow polychromatic erythrocytes of mice. *Archives of Toxicology* **58,** 106-109.
NATIONAL ACADEMY OF SCIENCES (1977) Drinking water and health vol 1. Washington DC, National Academy of Sciences.
NATIONAL ACADEMY OF SCIENCES (1980) Drinking water and health vol 3. Washington DC, National Academy Press.
NAWROT P S and STAPLES R E (1980) Embryofetal toxicity and teratogenicity of

isomers of xylene in the mouse. 19th Annual Meeting of the Society of Toxicology, Washington DC, March 9-13 1980, Abstract No 65.

OGATA M, TOMOKUNI K and TAKATSUKA Y (1970) Urinary excretion of hippuric acid and *m*- or *p*-methylhippuric acid in the urine of persons exposed to vapors of toluene and *m*- or *p*-xylene as a test of exposure. *British Journal of Industrial Medicine* **27,** 43-50.

RIIHIMAKI V, SAVOLAINEN K, PFAFFLI P, PEKARI K, SIPPEL H W and LAINE A (1982) Metabolic interaction between *m*-xylene and ethanol. *Archives of Toxicology* **49,** 253-263.

SANDMEYER E E (1981) Aromatic hydrocarbons. In: Clayton G D and Clayton F E (eds), *Patty's industrial hygiene and toxicology,* 3rd Revised Edition, vol 2B, pp 3291-3300.

SAVOLAINEN K (1980) Combined effects of xylene and alcohol on the central nervous system. *Acta Pharmacologica et Toxicologica* **46,** 366-372.

SEDIVEC V and FLEK J (1976) The absorption, metabolism, and excretion of xylenes in man. *International Archives of Occupational and Environmental Health* **37,** 205-217.

SPECK B and MOESCHLIN S (1968) The effect of toluene, xylene, chloramphenicol and thiouracil on bone marrow. *Schweizerische Medizinische Wochenschrift* **98,** 1684-1686.

THORBURN S and COLENUTT B A (1979) A gas chromatographic comparison of volatile organic compounds in urban and rural atmospheres. *International Journal of Environmental Studies* **13,** 265-271.

TSCA INTERAGENCY TESTING COMMITTEE (1977) Initial report of the TSCA interagency testing committee and information dossiers on substances designated. Washington DC, National Science Foundation, PB-275 367.

UNGVARY G, TATRAI E, HUDAK A, BARCZA G and LORINCZ M (1980) Studies on the embryotoxic effects of *ortho-, meta-* and *para*-xylene. *Toxicology* **18,** 61-74.

US ENVIRONMENTAL PROTECTION AGENCY (1975) Analysis of carbon and resin extracts. New Orleans area water supply study. US EPA.

UNITED STATES NATIONAL TOXICOOLOGY PROGRAM (1986) Toxicology and carcinogenesis studies of xylenes (mixed) in F344/N rats and B6C3F1 mice. NTP TR 327, Research Triangle Park.

VAN DOORN R, BOS R P, BROUNS R M E, LEIJDEKKERS Ch-M and HENDERSON P T (1980) Effect of toluene and xylene on liver glutathione and their urinary excretion as mercapturic acids in the rat. *Archives of Toxicology* **43,** 293-304.

VERSCHUEREN K (1977) *Handbook of environmental data on organic chemicals.* Van Nostrand Reinhold Company.

WATER RESEARCH CENTRE (1981) Organic micropollutants in drinking water. Technical Report TR 159.

WILLIAMS R T (1959) *Detoxication mechanisms.* Chapman & Hall.

WOLF M A, ROWE V K, McCOLLISTER D D, HOLLINGSWORTH R L and OYEN F (1956) Toxicological studies of certain alkylated benzenes and benzene. *AMA Archives of Industrial Health* **14,** 387-398.

ZOETEMAN B C J, PIET G J, RUYGROK C T M and HEUVEL R V D (1974) Threshold odour concentrations in water of chemical substances. RID-MEDEDELING, 74-3.

6. THE ALKYLBENZENES

6.1 Introduction

C_3, C_4 and C_5-alkylbenzenes are constituents of fossil fuels. Aromatic hydrocarbons of this type tend to be used in industry as mixture rather than individual compounds. Petroleum products may represent an important source of these chemicals in water.

6.2 Exposure

6.2.1 Air

Holzer *et al* (1977) detected several alkylbenzenes in both urban and rural air of the US.

6.2.2 Food

No information appears to be available on the presence of these compounds in food.

6.2.3 Water

The WRc survey identified eight C_3-alkylbenzene isomers, 12 C_4-alkylbenzene isomers and three C_5-alkylbenzene isomers in the 14 drinking water samples tested (Water Research Centre 1981). The C_3-alkylbenzenes tended to be present in all samples, as were several of the C_4-alkylbenzenes, but the C_5-alkylbenzenes and some of the C_4-alkylbenzenes were much less frequently detected. The more infrequent compounds were primarily found in lowland reservoirs and in other surface waters.

A Japanese study reported the presence of several alkylbenzenes in tap water at levels of 1–6 ng/l (Akiyama *et al* 1980).

6.3 Toxicokinetics

The lipophilic nature of these compounds suggests that they will be readily absorbed by the gastrointestinal tract and subsequently distributed to the lipid-rich tissues.

In the liver, the alkylbenzenes are primarily metabolised by side-chain oxidation to the corresponding alcohol or acid, followed by conjugation of the products with glucuronic acid or glycine. In the case of the polymethylbenzenes (pseudocumene and mesitylene), biotransformation involves the oxidation of only one of the methyl groups to the corresponding benzoic acid and subsequent hippuric acid derivatives (Williams 1959). Oxidation of more than one methyl group can occur (for example, durene), but this is generally only a minor route. Metabolism of those alkylbenzenes with longer side-chains can occur by three mechanisms:

(1) Omega-oxidation to phenyl fatty acids, which can then be broken down by fatty acid beta-oxidation to benzoic acid and phenylacetic acid, depending on the length of the side-chain.
(2) Hydroxylation of the carbon atom adjacent to the aromatic ring to form an alkylphenylcarbinol, which can be subsequently eliminated as a glucuronide conjugate. This pathway is also possible with branched side-chain isomers,

provided that the first carbon atom of the side-chain has a replaceable hydrogen atom.

(3) Hydroxylation of the penultimate carbon atom of the side-chain to form a carbinol.

The extent to which these mechanisms contribute to the overall biotransformation of individual compounds is not clear, although it is largely considered that hydroxylation to carbinols and elimination in the urine as glucuronides is the major route (Williams 1959, Smith *et al* 1954, Elmasry *et al* 1956). If the alkylbenzene has an individual methyl substituent and a larger alkyl group attached to the ring, it appears that the methyl group will be preferentially oxidised to the benzoic acid derivative. Hydroxylation of the aromatic ring itself is known to occur with several alkylbenzenes, but this mechanism is of little quantitative significance. Gerarde and Ahlstrom (1966) have shown that ring oxidation to phenols is more likely to occur with increasing side-chain length and with increasing dose.

6.4 Health effects

6.4.1 Acute and subacute toxicity

The C_3, C_4 and C_5-alkylbenzenes have a low order of acute toxicity. Most members of the group have an oral LD50 in the rat and the mouse of 1–5 g/kg (Gerarde 1960, Wolf *et al* 1956). Several are known to have irritant properties. Sgaragli *et al* (1977) have suggested that 'monocyclic compounds with an aliphatic chain of at least two carbon atoms interact with biomembranes producing solubilisation of proteins'. It is, however, highly unlikely that the irritant properties of the aromatic hydrocarbons are of any concern at current exposure levels from water.

Gerarde (1956) noted CNS depression and membrane irritation, but no significant changes in haematological parameters or growth curves in Wistar rats injected subcutaneously with 1 ml/kg (0.86 g/kg) of *n*-propylbenzene or *n*-butylbenzene in olive oil, daily, for 2 weeks.

Fabacher and Hodgson (1977) found a significant increase in *N*-demethylase activity, but no changes in *O*-demethylase activity or liver weight/body weight ratio in mice given 100 mg/kg body weight/day of 1,2,4,5-tetramethylbenzene or pentamethylbenzene by intraperitoneal injection for 3 days.

6.4.2 Chronic toxicity

The chronic toxicity of the alkylbenzenes is poorly studied, with very little recent information available. The earlier studies which were carried out suggest that these compounds do not possess the haematotoxic or myelotoxic properties of their parent compound, benzene, but membrane irritation and CNS depression have been reported (Wolf *et al* 1956, Gerarde 1956, 1959, 1960).

Ten female rats dosed orally with 462 mg/kg or 769 mg/kg of isopropylbenzene in olive oil, 5 days/week for 6 months, exhibited increased kidney weights but no pathological changes. No effects of any type were observed at 154 mg/kg (Wolf *et al* 1956).

A long-term inhalation study of isopropylbenzene in rats, guinea pigs, dogs and monkeys by Jenkins *et al* (1970) failed to demonstrate significant changes in body weight after 30 repeated 8-hour exposures to 244 ppm or after continuous exposure to 30 ppm for 90 days. Elevated leukocyte numbers were seen in rats after both types of exposure, but little changes in haematocrit or haemoglobin were found in any species. No histopathological changes were observed in the heart, lung, liver, spleen or kidney of any species, or in brain and spinal cord of dogs and monkeys.

6.4.3 Genotoxicity, carcinogenicity and reproductive toxicity

No information appears to be available.

6.5 Discussion

The alkylbenzenes have been detected in the atmosphere and in water. These compounds are lipophilic, and are therefore readily absorbed and distributed to the lipid-rich tissues. They are rapidly metabolised in the liver to alcohols, acids and their conjugates.

Like toluene, xylene and ethylbenzene, the C_3, C_4 and C_5-alkylbenzenes appear to be of low acute and chronic toxicity, but are membrane irritants and CNS depressants at high levels. There is no evidence that these compounds possess the haematotoxic properties of benzene. There appears to be no information available on their genotoxicity, carcinogenicity or reproductive toxicity.

Although there is very little toxicological information on the alkylbenzenes, both the limited information available and the evidence on toluene, xylene and ethylbenzene suggest that a problem to human health is unlikely to exist at the concentrations observed in drinking water.

References

AKIYAMA T, KOGA M, SHINOHARA R, KIDO A and ETOH S (1980) Detection and identification of trace organic substances in the aquatic environment. *Journal of Uoeh* **2,** 285-300.

ELMASRY A M, SMITH J N and WILLIAMS R T (1956) The metabolism of alkylbenzenes: *n*-Propylbenzene and *n*-butylbenzene with further observations on ethylbenzene. *Biochemical Journal* **64,** 50-56.

FABACHER D L and HODGSON E (1977) Hepatic mixed-function oxidase activity in mice treated with methylated benzenes and methylated naphthalenes. *Journal of Toxicology and Environmental Health* **2,** 1143-1146.

GERARDE H W (1956) Toxicological studies on hydrocarbons. II. A comparative study of the effect of benzene and certain mono-*n*-alkylbenzenes on hemopoiesis and bone marrow metabolism in rats. *AMA Archives of Industrial Health* **13,** 468-474.

GERARDE H W (1959) Toxicological studies on hydrocarbons. III. The biochemorphology of the phenylalkanes and the phenylalkenes. *AMA Archives of Industrial Health* **19,** 29-44.

GERARDE H W (1960) Toxicology and biochemistry of aromatic hydrocarbons. *Elsevier monographs,* Elsevier Publishing Company.

GERARDE H W and AHLSTROM D B (1966) Toxicologic studies on hydrocarbons. XI. Influence of dose on the metabolism of mono-*n*-alkyl derivatives of benzene. *Toxicology and Applied Pharmacology* **9,** 185-190.

HOLZER G, SHANFIELD H, ZLATKIS A, BERTSCH W, JUAREZ P, MAYFIELD H and LIEBICH H M (1977) Collection and analysis of trace organic emissions from natural sources. *Journal of Chromatography* **142,** 755-764.

JENKINS L J Jr, JONES R A and SIEGEL J (1970) Long-term inhalation screening studies of benzene, toluene, *o*-xylene, and cumene on experimental animals. *Toxicology and Applied Pharmacology* **16,** 818-823.

SGARAGLI G, CORTE L D, RIZZOTTI-CONTI M and GIOTTI A (1977) Effects of monocyclic compounds on biomembranes. *Biochemical Pharmacology* **26,** 2145-2149.

SMITH J N, SMITHIES R H and WILLIAMS R T (1954) The metabolism of alkylbenzenes. (a) Glucuronic acid excretion following the administration of alkylbenzenes. (b) Elimination of toluene in the expired air of rabbits. *Biochemical Journal* **56,** 317-320.

WATER RESEARCH CENTRE (1981) Organic micropollutants in drinking water. Technical Report TR 159.

WILLIAMS R T (1959) *Detoxication mechanisms.* Chapman & Hall.

WOLF M A, ROWE V K, McCOLLISTER D D, HOLLINGSWORTH R L and OYEN F (1956) Toxicological studies of certain alkylated benzenes and benzene. *AMA Archives of Industrial Health* **14,** 387-398.

7. STYRENE

7.1 Introduction

Styrene (vinylbenzene, phenylethylene, ethenylbenzene, cinnamene) is produced commercially by the dehydrogenation of ethylbenzene or by the demethylation of cumene. World-wide production of styrene was estimated to be 7000 million kg/year in 1977 (International Agency for Research on Cancer 1979). Styrene is used principally in the manufacture of polystyrene, plastics and resins.

CAS Reg. No:	100-42-5
Molecular weight:	140.15
Boiling point:	145.2°C
Solubility:	280 mg/l at 15°C (Verschueren 1977)
Evaporative half-life in water:	No data available
Threshold odour concentration in water:	<1 mg/l (Zoeteman *et al* 1974).

7.2 Exposure

7.2.1 Air

Several studies have detected styrene in the ambient air, though levels were below 1 ppb in all cases (Hoshika 1980, Bos *et al*, Holzer *et al* 1977). Holzer *et al* (1977) found higher levels of styrene in urban air compared to rural air in the US.

Styrene has also been identified in cigarette smoke (Jermini *et al* 1976, Baggett *et al* 1974).

7.2.2 Food

Significant quantities of styrene are present in foodstuffs, particularly in those products which are packaged and stored in polystyrene containers or other styrene-related plastics (Withey 1976). A Canadian survey detected styrene at up to 77.6 μg/

kg in yoghurt, 59.2 μg/kg in butter-fat cream, 22.7 μg/kg in honey, 17.2 μg/kg in homogenised milk, and 9.3 μg/kg in cottage cheese (Withey and Collins 1978). MAFF have calculated an average intake of styrene from food of 1 μg/day with a maximum of 4 μg/day (Ministry of Agriculture, Fisheries and Food 1983).

7.2.3 Water

Styrene was detected at less than 1 μg/l in US finished water (United States Environmental Protection Agency 1975) and at 1 μg/l in the Scheldt river of the Netherlands (Eurocop-Cost 1876. The survey by the WRc identified this compound in 4/14 drinking water samples examined (Water Research Centre 1981).

7.3 Toxicokinetics

7.3.1 Absorption

Fernandez and Caperos (1977) estimated that nearly 90% of inhaled styrene was retained by the lungs of volunteers. This is in contrast to earlier studies which had suggested that 59–66% was retained (Fiserova-Bergerova and Teisinger 1965, Oltramere *et al* 1974). Liquid styrene is quite readily absorbed by the skin, though aqueous solutions are absorbed rather more slowly (Dutkiewicz and Tyras 1968). Styrene has been shown to be readily absorbed by the gastrointestinal tract of rats (Withey 1978, Plotnick and Weigel 1979).

7.3.2 Distribution

Styrene is widely distributed in the body, with the highest concentrations found in the adipose tissue (Withey and Collins 1979, Danishefsky and Willhite 1954, Shugaev 1969).

7.3.3 Metabolism

The relatively rapid metabolism of styrene in the liver occurs primarily by side-chain oxidation followed by conjugation with glucuronic acid, glycine or glutathione. In experimental animals, the principal metabolite of styrene is hippuric acid. Minor metabolites are mandelic acid and phenylglyoxylic acid (Ohtsuji and Ikeda 1971, James and White 1967, Elmasri *et al* 1958, Leibman 1975). In man, however, the major metabolites are mandelic acid and phenylglyoxylic acid, while only trace amounts of hippuric acid are found (Ikeda *et al* 1974). Other minor metabolites of styrene which have also been identified are phenethyl mercapturic acid, 1-phenylethanol, 2-phenylethanol, 4-vinylphenol, hydroxyphenethyl mercapturic acid and phenylethylene glycol glucuronide (Leibman 1975, Pfaffli *et al* 1981).

7.3.4 Excretion

In man, almost all of an absorbed dose of styrene is excreted in the urine as mandelic acid and phenylglyoxylic acid. A small amount is exhaled as carbon dioxide (Fernandez and Caperos 1977, Bardodej and Bardodejova 1966). Rats given a single subcutaneous injection of radiolabelled styrene were found to excrete 71% of the label as metabolites in the urine, 12% was exhaled as carbon dioxide, while 3% was present in the faeces as unchanged styrene (Danishefsky and Willhite 1954).

7.4 Health effects

The health effects of styrene have been reviewed previously (International Agency for Research on Cancer 1979, Leibman 1975, National Academy of Sciences 1977, Harkonen 1978, Bergman 1979, Sandmeyer 1981, Health and Safety Executive 1981).

7.4.1 Acute and subacute toxicity

The most common toxic effects of acute exposure to styrene are CNS depression and irritation of the skin, eyes, nose and respiratory tract. Pathological changes found in experimental animals include haemorrhage, oedema, exudation, leukocytic infiltration, and congestion of the liver, kidneys and lungs (Spencer *et al* 1942). The oral LD50 of styrene in rats is 5.0 g/kg (Wolf *et al* 1956), while the LD50 by intraperitoneal injection in the same species is 2.4 g/kg (Ohtsuji and Ikeda 1971). Styrene-7,8-oxide, proposed as the major intermediate in styrene metabolism, is reported to be of greater acute toxicity than styrene itself (Ohtsuji and Ikeda 1971).

Much recent work on the toxicity of styrene has been related to its biochemical effects, particularly with respect to the enzymes of drug metabolism. Elevated activity of UDP glucuronosyl transferase, epoxide hydrolase, and *p*-nitroanisole *O*-demethylase were found in rat liver following intraperitoneal injection of 3–6 doses of 500 mg/kg body weight of styrene (Parkki *et al* 1976). Lowered activity of benzo-pyrene hydroxylase, styrene oxide hydratase and aldrin epoxidase were reported in rat liver after intraperitoneal injection of 10, 100 or 500 mg/kg body weight of styrene (Lambotte-Vandepaer *et al* 1978). In an oral study (Das *et al* 1981), enhanced aniline hydroxylase and aryl hydrocarbon hydroxylase activities were found in rats given 450 or 900 mg/kg for 7 days. At the higher dose level, inhibition of glutathione *S*-transferase activity and a lowering of hepatic glutathione content were also noted. A depression of non-protein sulphydryl content had previously been reported in mice after intraperitoneal injection of 150–1000 mg/kg body weight of styrene (Vainio and Makinen 1977). A dose-dependent increase in hepatic lipid peroxidation has been found in rats given 0, 50, 100, 200 or 600 mg/kg of styrene by intraperitoneal injection. Depletion of glutathione to a critical level was thought to be the most important factor in the onset of lipid peroxidation (Srivastava *et al* 1983).

Significant increases in serotonin and noradrenaline, decreased activity of monoamine oxidase, but no changes in dopamine or acetylcholinesterase activity were found in the brain tissue of adult male albino rats given oral doses of 1 ml/kg body weight of styrene daily for 15 days (Husain *et al* 1980). In rabbits, subacute inhalation of 1500 ppm of styrene was reported to lower dopamine levels in certain areas of the brain (Mutti *et al* 1984).

Simultaneous oral dosing of ethanol and styrene to rats produced additive effects within the lethal dose range (Hinz *et al* 1980).

7.4.2 Chronic toxicity

The chronic toxicity of styrene in experimental animals, particularly with regard to oral exposure, has been poorly studied.

In guinea pigs exposed by inhalation to 1450 ppm of styrene for 7 hours/day, 5 days/week for 6 months, slightly increased liver and kidney weights and 10% lethality due to pulmonary congestion were observed (Spencer *et al* 1942). No effects were seen in rabbits and primates in the same study, though rats exhibited eye and nasal irritancy. Similar results were found in another inhalation study (Wolf *et al* 1956).

No treatment-related changes were reported in rats exposed to 0, 125 or 250 mg/l of styrene in their drinking water for 2 years (Beliles *et al* 1985).

Chronic human exposure to relatively high levels of styrene in the atmosphere has been described as 'styrene sickness'. The symptoms are nausea, vomiting, loss of appetite, headaches, fatigue, inebriation, lassitude and general weakness (Wilson 1944).

In a study of 494 workers in the US exposed occupationally to styrene, 8.5% of subjects were found to have reduced sensitivity of the lower extremities, prenarcotic symptoms were observable in 13% of cases, and nerve conduction velocities were also decreased in about 13% of workers (Lilis *et al* 1978). Abnormal EEGs have been found in 23 out of 96 workers in a factory making reinforced polyester, and also in several other groups of workers exposed occupationally to styrene (Seppalainen and Harkonen 1976, Klimkova-Deutschova 1962, Roth and Klimkova-Deutschova 1963, Dolmierski *et al* 1974, 1976). An experimental study of five volunteers exposed to 375 ppm of styrene in the atmosphere for 56 minutes found reduced manual dexterity in two of the subjects (Stewart *et al* 1968). In another study, although manual dexterity was reported as normal, a significant deterioration in reaction speed was observed in subjects exposed to 350 ppm of styrene for 30 minutes (Gamberale and Hultegren 1973). A similar slowing of reaction time has been reported in subjects exposed to 50 ppm styrene (Oltramere *et al* 1974), and in a group of workers exposed to styrene-based resin (Cherry *et al* 1981). A study of 98 workers exposed to styrene in a laminating factory found that a reduction of visuo-motor accuracy was the only exposure-related effect in a psychological test battery when compared to a reference group (Lindstrom *et al* 1976). This effect has been reported on another occasion (Harkonen *et al* 1978). Despite a claim (Aldyreva 1972) that chronic exposure to styrene may cause leukopenia, lymphocytosis, toxic hepatitis and disturbance of liver function, little evidence is available to support this. A Polish study of 101 workers exposed occupationally to styrene for about one year failed to find any evidence of haematological abnormalities, apart from a slightly lowered platelet count (Chmielewski and Renke 1976). Similarly, no correlation between the duration of exposure to styrene and haemoglobin, white cell counts or platelet counts was found in 493 workers of a polystyrene factory in the US (Lorimer *et al* 1976).

7.4.3 Genotoxicity

Styrene possesses weak mutagenic activity in the Ames test to *Salmonella typhimurium* TA1530, TA1535 and TA100 when tested in the presence of a metabolising system. These strains are particularly sensitive to base-pair mutagens. No mutagenic activity for styrene has been found in the frameshift-sensitive strains TA1537, TA1538 and TA98 either in the presence or absence of metabolic activation (De Meester *et al* 1977, Vainio *et al* 1976, De Meester *et al* 1981). Styrene-7,8-oxide is mutagenic to the same *Salmonella* strains as styrene, though without the requirement for metabolic activation.

Styrene-7,8-oxide has given positive results in forward mutation tests in Chinese hamster cells and in yeast, in a yeast gene conversion test and in a host-mediated assay. The only positive results for styrene itself were obtained in the host-mediated assay (Loprieno *et al* 1976). Other *in vitro* studies have shown styrene to be genotoxic. Chromosomal aberrations (Linnainmaa *et al* 1978) and sister chromatid exchanges (Norppa *et al* 1980a, Norppa and Vainio 1983) have been reported in cultured human lymphocytes, while in the presence of a metabolising system chromosomal aberrations have been induced in a Chinese hamster cell line (Matsuoki *et al* 1979).

An increased frequency of bone marrow chromosomal aberrations was found in rats exposed by inhalation to 300 ppm of styrene for 2–11 weeks (Meretoja *et al* 1978a). However, no increased incidence of bone marrow chromosomal aberrations was found in two inhalation studies with Chinese hamsters (Norppa *et al* 1979, 1980b), in CD-1 mice given oral doses of 500 mg/kg/day for 4 days or 200 mg/kg/day for 70 days (Sbrana *et al* 1983) or in CD-1 mice given a single oral dose of 500 or 1000 mg/kg of styrene in corn oil (Loprieno *et al* 1978). Norppa (1981) found a significant increase in micronucleated polychromatic erythrocytes in mice given 250 or 1000 mg/kg body weight of styrene by intraperitoneal injection. No such effect was found in a similar study with Chinese hamsters (Penttila *et al* 1980). Styrene has also been reported to induce sister chromatid exchanges in mice exposed by inhalation to between 100 and 900 ppm for 1–4 days (Conner *et al* 1980). Both styrene and styrene oxide were found to induce single strand breaks in DNA of kidney, lung, liver, testis and brain in rats given a range of doses by intraperitoneal injection (Walles and Orsen 1983), and have also been found to induce recessive lethals in Drosophila melanogaster (Donner *et al* 1979).

Several cytogenetic studies of workers exposed occupationally to styrene have shown increased incidences of chromosomal abnormalities. In a group of ten workers manufacturing polyester products, chromosomal aberrations were found in 11–26% of peripheral lymphocytes compared to control values of around 3% (Meretoja *et al* 1977). Similar results were found in workers from two Finnish factories also involved in the manufacture of polyester products (Meretoja *et al* 1978b), and in a group of six men using polyester resin in a Swedish boat-building factory (Hogstedt *et al* 1979). In a larger study of workers exposed to styrene in a Swedish factory making glass fibre reinforced plastics, an average of 7.9% of peripheral lymphocytes were found to contain chromosome aberrations as compared to 3.2% for the matched controls. A slight increase was also noted in the incidence of sister chromatid exchanges (Andersson *et al* 1980). A significant increase in chromosomal aberrations was found in workers from six factories in the reinforced-plastic industry. Sister chromatid exchange frequencies were also significantly increased in four out of the six factories (Camurri *et al* 1983). No increase in chromosomal damage could be found in a German study of 12 male workers who had been exposed to levels of styrene usually below 1 ppm for an average of 44.9 years (Theiss and Fleig 1978).

7.4.4 Carcinogenicity

There is some evidence of a carcinogenic potential for styrene in rats and mice, but the studies involved suffer from severe limitations.

A group of 29 pregnant O(20) strain mice were dosed by stomach tube with 1350 mg/kg body weight of styrene in olive oil on day 17 of gestation. Surviving offspring were then treated weekly with the same dose from weaning for 16 weeks. At the termination of the experiment, when the animals had reached 100 weeks of age, pulmonary tumours (both adenomas and adenocarcinomas) were found in 20/23 males (83%) and 32/32 females. Corresponding figures for vehicle controls were 8/19 in males (42%) and 14/21 in females (67%), while untreated controls gave values of 35/53 in males (64%) and 25/47 in females (53%). The interpretation of this study is difficult in view of the marked decrease in survival time of the animals and the high control incidence of lung tumours (Ponomarkov and Tomatis 1979).

In another experiment, pregnant C57BL mice were dosed by stomach tube with 300 mg/kg body weight of styrene in olive oil on day 17 of gestation. The same dose was given weekly post-weaning to the 27 male and 22 female progeny for 120 weeks. No significant increase in the incidence of any type of tumour was found (Ponomarkov and Tomatis 1979).

In a third experiment, 21 pregnant BDIV rats were dosed by stomach tube with 1350 mg/kg body weight of styrene in olive oil on day 17 of gestation. The 73 male and 71 female progeny were then given 500 mg/kg body-weight weekly for 120 weeks. No statistically significant increase in any type of tumour was noted (Ponomarkov and Tomatis 1979).

In the NCI bioassay, groups of 50 male and 50 female F344 rats were dosed by gavage with 1000 or 2000 mg/kg of styrene in corn oil 5 days/week for 78 weeks. A further group were given 500 mg/kg of styrene in corn oil, 5 days/week for 103 weeks. The only treatment-related effect noted was hepatic necrosis in the high dose group. There was also poor survival of animals at the highest dose level (National Cancer Institute 1979).

Groups of 50 male and 50 female B6C3F1 mice were dosed with 150 or 300 mg/kg of styrene in corn oil, 5 days/week for 78 weeks. Based on surviving animals at 52 weeks, a significant increase in pulmonary tumours was noted in male mice (9/49 in the high dose group and 6/44 in the low dose group, control 0/20). A non-significant increase in pulmonary tumours was observed in females (3/43 in the high dose group and 1/43 in the low dose group, control 0/20). However, the increased incidence of tumours is of doubtful significance in view of historical data on this strain of mice which suggests a 12% (32/271) control incidence of this type of tumour. A non-significant increase in hepatocellular adenomas was also noted in female mice (National Cancer Institute 1979).

Rats exposed to 0, 125 or 500 mg/l of styrene in their drinking water for 2 years showed no treatment-related differences in tumour incidence (Beliles *et al* (1985).

The only major inhalation study carried out concerned groups of 85 male and 85 female Sprague–Dawley rats exposed to 600 ppm of styrene, 6 hours/day, 5 days/ week for 18–21 months. Another group were exposed to 1200 ppm for 2 months, but marked toxicity resulted in reduction of the concentration to 1000 ppm for the remainder of the 18-21-month study. Slightly increased incidences of leukaemias and lymphomas in female rats at both dose levels and a slightly increased incidence of mammary adenocarcinomas at the lower dose level were noted. However, there was also poor survival of animals in this study (Jersey *et al* 1978).

Negative results were obtained in two much earlier mouse studies in which the skin had been painted with styrene oxide, thrice weekly for their lifetime (Van Duuren *et al* 1963, Weil *et al* 1963).

Occupational studies of the carcinogenicity of styrene have suffered from severe methodological difficulties, and provide little evidence for or against an increased tumour incidence related to styrene exposure.

7.4.5 *Reproductive toxicity*

Styrene has been shown to be present in cord blood at similar concentrations to those found in maternal blood, suggesting a relatively free passage across the placenta at low exposure levels (Dowty *et al* 1976).

Embryotoxic effects of styrene have been reported in rats exposed by inhalation to 300 and 600 ppm of styrene for 7 hours/day on days 6–18 of gestation (Murray *et al* 1978), and to 350–1100 ppm for the whole period of gestation (Ragule 1974). Evidence of embryotoxicity has also been found in experiments in mice and rabbits (Murray *et al* 1978). In hamsters exposed to 300–1000 ppm of styrene for 6 hours/day on days 6–16 of gestation, the only reported effect was a marked reduction in litter size (Kankaanpaa *et al* 1980). Injection of 0.5–50 μmol of styrene into the air space of fertilised chicken eggs was found to cause malformations in up to 20% of embryos (Vainio *et al* 1977b).

Styrene was administered to rats in their drinking water at concentrations of 0, 125 or 500 mg/l for three generations. There were no deleterious dose-related effects or decrements in reproductive performance (Beliles *et al* 1985)

Holmberg (1979) documented four cases of CNS defects in children born to mothers who had been exposed to styrene during pregnancy. However, this study is far too small for any conclusions to be drawn.

7.5 Discussion

Styrene has been detected in the atmosphere, food and water, though it appears that food is likely to contribute most to overall exposure. Styrene is readily absorbed by the gastrointestinal tract and extensively distributed throughout the body. The relatively rapid metabolism of this compound is thought to involve the formation of the epoxide intermediate, styrene-7,8-oxide, which may be responsible for some of the toxic effects of styrene.

Styrene is of low acute toxicity, but has been shown to cause nervous system effects, such as reduced nerve conduction velocities, abnormal EEGs, reduced manual dexterity and visuo-motor inaccuracy in workers and volunteers exposed by inhalation. The chronic toxicity of styrene in experimental animals has been quite poorly studied. Styrene has been shown to possess weak mutagenic activity in bacterial assays with metabolic activation and to induce chromosomal aberrations in some *in vitro* and *in vivo* tests. Chromosome aberrations have also been reported in several studies of workers exposed to styrene. Some evidence of a carcinogenic potential for styrene has been documented in rodents, but the studies involved suffer from severe limitations, and better quality studies are necessary before carcinogenicity in rodents can be confirmed. Embryotoxicity of this compound has been reported in rats, rabbits and mice exposed by inhalation to 300–1000 ppm.

Styrene in water may be of concern at higher levels due to its possible carcinogenicity in rodents. With the present low levels of exposure, however, styrene is unlikely to present a hazard.

References

ALDYREVA M V (1972) Styrene, Ethylbenzene. In *Encyclopaedia of Occupational Health and Safety* **2,** pp 1362-1364.

ANDERSSON H C, TRANBERG E A, UGGLA A H, and ZETTERBERG G (1980) Chromosomal aberrations and sister chromatid exchanges in lymphocytes of men occupationally exposed to styrene in a plastic boat factory. *Mutation Research* **73,** 387-401.

BAGGETT M S, MORIE G P, SIMMONS M W and LEWIS J S (1974) Quantitative determination of semivolatile compounds in cigarette smoke. *Journal of Chromatography* **97,** 79-82.

BARDODEJ Z and BARDODEJOVA, E (1966) The metabolism of ethylbenzene, styrene and alphamethyl styrene. 15th International Congress on Occupational Health, Vienna, September 1966, II-I, 457-460.

BELILES R P, BUTALA J H, STACK C R and MAKRIS S (1985) Chronic toxicity and three generation reproduction study of styrene monomer in the drinking water of rats. *Fundamental and Applied Toxicology* **5,** 855-868.

BERGMAN K (1979) Whole body autoradiography and allied tracer techniques in distribution and elimination studies of some organic solvents. *Scandinavian Journal of Work Environment and Health* **5,** 93-104.

BOS R, GUICHERIT R and HOOGEVEEN A (1977) Distribution of some hydrocarbons in ambient air near Delft and the influence on the formation of secondary air pollutants. *Science of the Total Environment* **7,** 269-281.

CAMURRI L, CODELUPPI S, PEDRONI C and SCARDUELLI L (1983) Chromosomal aberrations and sister-chromatid exchanges in workers exposed to styrene. *Mutation Research* **119,** 361-369.

CHERRY N, RODGERS B, VENABLES H, WALDRON H A and WELLS G G (1981) Acute behavioural effects of styrene exposure: a further analysis. *British Journal of Industrial Medicine* **38,** 346-350.

CHMIELEWSKI J and RENKE W (1976) Clinical and experimental studies on the pathogenesis of toxic effects of styrene: 3. Morphology, coagulation and fibrinolysis systems of the blood in persons exposed to the action of styrene during their work. *Bulletin of the Institute of Maritime and Tropical Medicine in Gdynia* **27,** 63-68.

CONNER M K, ALARIE Y and DOMBROSKE R L (1980) Sister chromatid exchanges in murine alveolar macrophages, bone marrow and regenerating liver cells induced by styrene inhalation. *Toxicology and Applied Pharmacology* **55,** 37-42.

DANISHEFSKY I and WILLHITE M (1954) The metabolism of styrene in the rat. *Journal of Biological Chemistry* **211,** 549-553.

DAS M, DIXIT R, MUSHTAQ M, SRIVASTAVA S P and SETH P K (1981) Effect of styrene on hepatic mixed function oxidases, glutathione content and glutathione *S*-transferase activity in rats. *Drug and Chemical Toxicology* **4,** 219-227.

DE MEESTER C, PONCELET F, ROBERFROID M, RONDELET J and MERCIER M (1977) Mutagenicity of styrene and styrene oxide. *Mutation Research* **56**, 147-152.

DE MEESTER C, DUVERGER-VAN BOGAERT M, LAMBOTTE-VANDE-

PAER M, MERCIER M and PONCELET F (1981) Mutagenicity of styrene in the *Salmonella typhimurium* test system. *Mutation Research* **90,** 443-450.

DOLMIERSKI R, KWIATKOWSKI S R and NITKA J (1974) A preliminary evaluation of the studies on the central nervous system in workers exposed to styrene. *Bulletin of the Institute of Maritime and Tropical Medicine in Gdansk* **25**, 399-406.

DOLMIERSKI R, KWIATKOWSKI S R and NITKA J (1976) Clinical and experimental research into the pathogenesis of toxic effects of styrene. 7. Appraisal of the nervous system in the workers exposed to styrene. *Bulletin of the Institute of Maritime and Tropical Medicine in Gdynia* **27,** 193-196.

DONNER M, SORSA M and VAINIO H (1979) Recessive lethals induced by styrene and styrene oxide in Drosophila melanogaster. *Mutation Research* **67,** 373-376.

DOWTY B J, LASETER J L and STORER J (1976) The transplacental migration and accumulation in blood of volatile organic constituents. *Pediatric Research* **10,** 696-701.

DUTKIEWICZ T and TYRAS H (1968) Skin absorption of toluene, styrene and xylene by man. *British Journal of Industrial Medicine* **25,** 243.

ELMASRI A M, SMITH J N and WILLIAMS R T (1958) The metabolism of alkylbenzenes: phenylacetylene and phenylethylene (styrene). *Biochemical Journal* **68,** 199-204.

EUROCOP-COST (1976) A comprehensive list of polluting substances which have been identified in various fresh waters, effluent discharges, aquatic animals and plants, and bottom sediments, 2nd edn, Luxembourg, Commission of the European Communities.

FERNANDEZ J G and CAPEROS J R (1977) Exposition au styrene. 1. Etude experimentale de l'absorption et l'excretion pulmonaires sur des sujets humains. *International Archives of Occupational and Environmental Health* **40,** 1-12.

FISEROVA-BERGEROVA V and TEISINGER J (1965) Pulmonary styrene vapour retention. *Int. Med. Surg.,* **34,** 620-622.

GAMBERALE F and HULTEGREN M (1973) Exposition for styrene. *Psykofysiologiska Funcktioner (Arbete och halsa no. 3) Arbetarskyddsverket* 43-61.

HARKONEN H (1978) Styrene, its experimental and clinical toxicology. *Scandinavian Journal of Work Environment and Health* **4,** 104-113.

HARKONEN H, LINDSTROM K, SEPPALAINEN A M, ASP S and HERNBERG S (1978) Exposure–response relationship between styrene exposure and central nervous functions. *Scandinavian Journal of Work Environment and Health* **4,** 53-59.

HEALTH AND SAFETY EXECUTIVE (1981) Toxicity Review 1. Styrene. HMSO, London.

HINZ G, GOHLKE R and BURCK D (1980) The effect of simultaneous oral application of ethanol and styrene. *Journal of Hygiene, Epidemiology, Microbiology and Immunology* **24,** 262-270.

HOGSTEDT B, HEDNER K, MARK-VENDEL E, MITELMAN F, SCHUTZ A and SKERFVIN S (1979) Increased frequency of chromosome aberrations in workers exposed to styrene. *Scandinavian Journal of Work Environment and Health* **5,** 333-335.

HOLMBERG P C (1979) Central nervous system defects in children born to mothers exposed to organic solvents during pregnancy. *Lancet* **ii,** 177-179.

HOLZER G, SHANFIELD H, ZLATKIS A, BERTSCH W, JUAREZ P, MAYFIELD H and LIEBICH H M (1977) Collection and analysis of trace organic emissions from natural sources. *Journal of Chromatography* **142,** 755-764.

HOSHIKA Y (1980) Gas chromatographic determination of styrene as its dibromide. *Journal of Chromatography* **136,** 95-103.

HUSAIN R, SRIVASTAVA S P, MUSHTAQ M and SETH P K (1980) Effect of styrene on levels of serotonin, noradrenaline, dopamine and activity of acetylcholinesterase and monoamine oxidase in rat brain. *Toxicology Letters* **7,** 47-50.

IKEDA M, IMAMURA T, HAYASHI M, TABUCHI T and HARA I (1974) Evaluation of hippuric, phenylglyoxylic and mandelic acids in urine as indices of styrene exposure. *Internationale Archiv fur Arbeitsmedizin* **32,** 93-101.

INTERNATIONAL AGENCY FOR RESEARCH ON CANCER (1979) IARC Monographs on the evaluation of the carcinogenic risk of chemicals to humans. Vol 19. Some monomers, plastics and synthetic elastomers, and acrolein. IARC, Lyon.

JAMES S P and WHITE D A (1967) The metabolism of phenethyl bromide, styrene and styrene oxide in the rabbit and rat. *Biochemical Journal* **104,** 914-921.

JERMINI C, WEBER A and GRANDJEAN E (1976) Quantitative determination of various gas-phase components of the sidestream smoke of cigarettes in the room air as a contribution to the problem of passive-smoking. *International Archives of Occupational and Environmental Health* **36,** 169-181.

JERSEY G C, BALMER M F and QUAST J F (1978) Two-year chronic inhalation toxicity and carcinogenicity study on monomeric styrene in rats. Toxicology Research Laboratory, Dow Chemical Company, USA.

KANKAANPAA J T J, ELOVAARA E, HEMMINKI K and VAINIO H (1980) The effect of maternally inhaled styrene on embryonal and fetal development in mice and Chinese hamsters. *Acta Pharmacologica et Toxicologica* **47,** 127-129.

KLIMKOVA-DEUTSCHOVA E (1962) Neurologische befunde in der plastikindustrie bei styrol arbeitern. *Internationale Archiv fur Gewerbepathologie and Gewerbehygien* **19,** 35-50.

LAMBOTTE-VANDEPAER M, NOEL G, ROLLMANN B, MERCIER M and ROBERFROID M (1978) Modifying effects of styrene on the catalytic properties of some microsomal enzymes. *Archives of Toxicology* Suppl, 287-290.

LEIBMAN K C (1975) Metabolism and toxicity of styrene. *Environmental Health Perspectives* **11,** 115-119.

LILIS R, LORIMER W V, DIAMOND S and SELIKOFF I J (1978) Neurotoxicity of styrene in production and polymerisation workers. *Environmental Research* **15,** 133-138.

LINDSTROM K, HARKONEN H and HERNBERG S (1976) Disturbances in psychological functions of workers occupationally exposed to styrene. *Scandinavian Journal of Work Environment and Health* **2,** 129-139.

LINNAINMAA K, MERETOJA T, SORSA M and VAINIO H (1978) Cytogenetic effects of styrene and styrene oxide. *Mutation Research* **58,** 277-286.

LOPRIENO N, ABBONDANDOLO A, BARALF R, BARONCELLI S, BONATTI S, BRONZETTI G, CAMMELLINI A, CORSI C, CORTI G,

FREZZA D, LEPORINI C, MAZZACCARO A, NIERI R, ROSELLINI D and ROSSI A M (1976) Mutagenicity of industrial compounds: Styrene and its possible metabolite styrene oxide. *Mutation Research* **40,** 317-324.

LOPRIENO N, PRESCIUTTINI S, SBRANA I, STRETTI G, ZACCARO L, ABBONDANDOLO A, BONATTI S, FIORIO R and MAZZACCARO A (1978) Mutagenicity of industrial compounds. 7. Styrene and styrene oxide. 2. Point mutations, chromosome aberrations and DNA repair induction analyses. *Scandinavian Journal of Work Environment and Health* **4** Suppl 2, 169-178.

LORIMER W V, LILIS R, NICHOLSON W J, ANDERSON H, FISCHBEIN A, DAUM S, ROM W, RICE C and SELIKOFF I J (1976) Clinical studies of styrene workers: Initial findings. *Environmental Health Perspectives,* **17,** 171-181.

MATSUOKI A, HAYASHI M and ISHIDATE M (1979) Chromosomal aberration tests on 29 chemicals combined with S9 mix *in vitro*. *Mutation Research* **66,** 277-290.

MERETOJA T, VAINIO H, SORSA M and HARKONEN H (1977) Occupational styrene exposure and chromosomal aberrations. *Mutation Research* **56,** 193-197.

MERETOJA T, JARVENTAUS H, SORSA M and VAINIO H (1978a) Chromosome aberrations in lymphocytes of workers exposed to styrene. *Scandinavian Journal of Work Environment and Health* **4** Suppl 2, 259-264.

MERETOJA T, VAINIO H and JARVENTAUS H (1978b) Clastogenic effects of styrene exposure on bone marrow cells of rat. *Toxicology Letters* **1,** 315-318.

MINISTRY OF AGRICULTURE, FISHERIES AND FOOD; Working party on styrene (1983) Survey of styrene levels in food contact materials and in foods. Eleventh report of the Steering Group on Food Surveillance. MAFF Food Surveillance Paper No 11, HMSO, London.

MURRAY F J, JOHN J A, BALMER M F and SCHWETZ B A (1978) Teratologic evaluation of styrene given to rats and rabbits by inhalation or by gavage. *Toxicology* **11,** 335-343.

MUTTI A, FALZOI M, ROMANELLI A and FRANCHINI I (1984) Regional alterations of brain catecholamines by styrene exposure in rabbits. *Archives of Toxicology* **55,** 173-177.

NATIONAL ACADEMY OF SCIENCES (1977) Drinking water and health Vol 1. National Academy of Sciences, Washington DC.

NATIONAL CANCER INSTITUTE (1979) Bioassay of styrene for possible carcinogenicity. US National Cancer Institute Rep No NIH 79-1741.

NORPPA H (1981) Styrene and vinyltoluene induce micronuclei in mouse bone marrow. *Toxicology Letters* **8,** 247-251.

NORPPA H and VAINIO H (1983) Induction of sister-chromatid exchanges by styrene analogues in cultured human lymphocytes. *Mutation Research* **116,** 379-387.

NORPPA H, SORSA M, PFAFFLI P and VAINIO H (1980a) Styrene and styrene oxide induce SCEs and are metabolized in human lymhocyte cultures. *Carcinogenesis* **1,** 357-361.

NORPPA H, SORSA M and VAINIO H (1980b) Chromosomal aberrations in bone marrow of Chinese hamster exposed to styrene and ethanol. *Toxicology Letters*

5, 241-244.
NORPPA H, ELOVARAA E, HUSGAFVEL-PURSIAINEN K, SORSA M and VAINIO H (1983) Effects of styrene oxides on chromosomal aberrations, sister chromatid exchanges and hepatic drug biotransformation in Chinese hamsters *in vivo. Chemicobiological Interactions* **26,** 305-315.
OHTSUJI H and IKEDA M (1971) The metabolism of styrene in the rat and the stimulatory effect of phenobarbitol. *Toxicology and Applied Pharmacology* **18,** 321-328.
OLTRAMERE M, DESBAUMES E, IMHOFF C and MICHIELS W (1974) Toxicologie du styrene monomere. Recherches experimentales et cliniques chez l'homme. Editions Medecine et Hygiene, Geneve, 1974.
PARKKI M G, MARNIEMI J and VAINIO H (1976) Action of styrene and its metabolites styrene oxide and styrene glycol on activities of xenobiotic biotransformation enzymes in rat liver *in vivo. Toxicology and Applied Pharmacology* **38,** 59-70.
PENTTILA M, SORSA M and VAINIO H (1980) Inability of styrene to induce nondisjunction in *Drosophila* or a positive micronucleus test in the Chinese hamster. *Toxicology Letters* **6,** 119-123.
PFAFFLI P, HESSO A, VAINIO H and HYVONEN M (1981) 4-Vinyl phenol excretion suggestive of arene oxide formation in workers occupationally exposed to styrene. *Toxicology and Applied Pharmacology* **60,** 85-90.
PLOTNICK H B and WEIGEL W W (1979) Tissue distribution and excretion of C(14)-styrene in male and female rats. *Research Communications in Chemical Pathology and Pharmacology* **24,** 515-524.
PONOMARKOV V and TOMATIS L (1979) Effects of long-term oral administration of styrene to mice and rats. *Scandinavian Journal of Work Environment and Health* **4,** 127-135.
RAGULE N (1974) Embryotoxic action of styrene. *Gigiena i Sanitariia* **11,** 85-86.
ROTH B and KLIMKOVA-DEUTSCHOVA E (1963) The effect of the chronic action of industrial poisons on the electroencephalogram of man. *Reviews of Czechoslovak Medicine* **9,** 217-227.
SANDMEYER E E (1981) Aromatic Hydrocarbons. In: Clayton G D and Clayton F E (eds) *Patty's Industrial Hygiene and Toxicology* 3rd revised edition, Vol 2B, pp 3253–3431.
SBRANA I, LASCIALFARI D, ROSSI A M, LOPRIENO N, BLANCHI M, TORTORETO M and PANTAROTTO C (1983) Bone marrow cell chromosomal aberrations and styrene biotransformation in mice given styrene on a repeated oral schedule. *Chemicobiological Interactions,* **45,** 349-357.
SEPPALAINEN A M and HARKONEN H (1976) Neurophysiological findings among workers occupationally exposed to styrene. *Scandinavian Journal of Work Environment and Health* **2,** 140-146.
SHUGAEV B B (1969) Concentrations of hydrocarbons in tissues as a measure of toxicity. *Archives of Environmental Health* **18,** 878-882.
SPENCER H C, IRISH D D, ADAMS E M and ROWE V K (1942) The response of laboratory animals to monomeric styrene. *Journal of Industrial Hygiene* **24,** 295-301.
SRIVASTAVA S P, DAS M and SETH P K (1983) Enhancement of lipid peroxida-

tion in rat liver on acute exposure to styrene and acrylamide a consequence of glutathione depletion. *Chemicobiological Interactions* **45,** 373-380.

STEWART R D, DODD H C, BARETTA E D and SCHAFFER A W (1968) Human exposure to styrene vapour. *Archives of Environmental Health* **16,** 656-662.

THEISS A M and FLEIG I (1978) Chromosome investigations on workers exposed to styrene/polystyrene. *Journal of Occupational Medicine* **20,** 747-749.

US ENVIRONMENTAL PROTECTION AGENCY (1975) Preliminary assessment of suspected carcinogens in drinking water. Report to Congress, Washington, DC.

VAINIO H and MAKINEN A (1977) Styrene and acrylonitrile induced depression of hepatic non-protein sulphydryl content in various rodent species. *Research Communications in Chemical Pathology and Pharmacology* **17,** 115-124.

VAINIO H, PAAKKONEN R, RONNHOLM K, RAUNIO V and PELKONEN O (1976) A study on the mutagenic activity of styrene and styrene oxide. *Scandinavian Journal of Work Environment and Health* **3,** 147-151.

VAINIO H, HEMMINKI K and ELOVAARA E (1977) Toxicity of styrene and styrene oxide on chick embryos. *Toxicology* **8,** 319-325.

VAN DUUREN B L, NELSON N, ORRIS L, PALMES E D and SCHMITT F L (1963) Carcinogenicity of epoxides, lactones and peroxy compounds. *Journal of the National Cancer Institute* **31,** 2419-2422.

VERSCHUEREN K (1977) *Handbook of environmental data on organic chemicals.* Van Nostrand Reinhold Company.

WALLES S A S and ORSEN I (1983) Single-strand breaks in DNA of various organs of mice induced by styrene and styrene oxide. *Cancer Letters* **21,** 9-15.

WATER RESEARCH CENTRE (1981) Organic micropollutants in drinking water. Technical Report TR 159.

WEIL C S, CONDRA N, HUHN C and STRIEGEL J A (1963) Experimental carcinogenicity and acute toxicity of representative epoxides. *American Industrial Hygiene Association Journal* **24,** 305-325.

WILSON R H ((1944) Health hazards encountered in the manufacture of synthetic rubber. *Journal of the American Medical Association* **124,** 701-703.

WITHEY J R (1976) Quantitative analysis of styrene monomer in polystyrene and foods including some preliminary studies of the uptake and pharmacodynamics of the monomer in rats. *Environmental Health Perspectives* **17,** 125-133.

WITHEY J R (1978) The toxicity of styrene monomer and its pharmacokinetics and distribution in the rat. *Scandinavian Journal of Work Environment and Health* **4** Suppl 2, 31-40.

WITHEY J R and COLLINS P G (1978) Styrene monomer in foods. A limited Canadian survey. *Bulletin of Environmental Contamination and Toxicology* **19,** 86-94.

WITHEY J R and COLLINS P G (1979) The distribution and pharmacokinetics of styrene monomer in rats by the pulmonary route. *Journal of Environmental Pathology and Toxicology* **2,** 1329-1342.

WOLF M A, ROWE V K, McCOLLISTER D D, HOLLINGSWORTH R L and OYEN F (1956) Toxicological studies of certain alkylated benzenes and benzene. *AMA Archives of Industrial Health* **14,** 381-398.

ZOETEMAN B C J, PIET G J, RUYGROK C T M and HEUVEL R V D (1974) Threshold Odour concentrations in water of chemical substances. RID-MEDEDELING 74-3.

8. ISOPROPENYLBENZENE

8.1 Introduction

Isopropenylbenzene (alpha-methylstyrene, 2-phenylpropylene, 1-methyl-1-phenylethene) is primarily derived as a byproduct from the cumene–phenol process. Almost all of that manufactured is used in the synthesis of resins and polymers, which in turn are used in a wide range of products.

The toxicology of this compound has been poorly studied (Gerarde 1960, United States Environmental Protection Agency 1981). Most of the reports available are abstracts or translations of Eastern European studies.

CAS Reg No:	98-83-9
Molecular weight:	118.2
Boiling point:	165.4°C
Solubility:	No data available
Evaporative half-life in water:	No data available
Threshold odour concentration in water:	0.1 mg/l (Zoeteman *et al* 1974)

8.2 Exposure

Isopropenylbenzene was identified in only one of 14 drinking water samples examined in the WRc survey (Water Research Centre 1981). No other information appears to be available on the presence of this compound in air, food or water.

8.3 Toxicokinetics

Although there are no data on the absorption or distribution of isopropenylbenzene, it would be expected to be readily absorbed by the gastrointestinal tract and distributed to the lipid-rich tissues.

The metabolism of isopropenylbenzene has been studied by a Russian group who suggested that biotransformation proceeds via side-chain oxidation to alpha-phenyl-alpha-hydroxypropanol and atrolactic acid (Gadaskina and Aizvert 1979). These two metabolites were also reported to be less toxic than the parent compound, but that phenobarbital-enhanced oxidation of isopropenylbenzene increased its toxicity, while cystamine and methionine-depressed oxidation of isopropenylbenzene lowered its toxicity. The toxicity of isopropenylbenzene may therefore be mediated by a reactive intermediate, probably an epoxide, formed during an initial metabolic step.

8.4 Health effects

8.4.1 Acute and subacute toxicity

The oral LD50 of isopropenylbenzene in rats is 4.9 g/kg (Wolf *et al* 1956) while LD50s of 5.0 g/kg and 10.25 g/kg have been reported in mice (Ogleznev 1964).

A marked irritation and slight necrosis of the skin, and slight conjunctival irritation were found after repeated application of the undiluted compound to the skin and eyes of rabbits (Wolf *et al* 1956). Inflammation, hyperaemia, oedema and sensitisation of the skin of rabbits have also been reported after topical application of a 30% solution of isopropenylbenzene (Mirzoyan and Zhakenova 1972). In man, strong eye and nasal irritation was evident during exposure to 600 ppm of isopropenylbenzene vapour. No irritation was evident at 50 ppm but there was an objectionable odour at 200 ppm (Wolf *et al* 1956). In the Russian literature, oral doses of isopropenylbenzene in rodents have been reported to cause haemodynamic and dystrophic changes in the lung, and morphological changes in the CNS, resembling encephalopathy (Zakharchenko 1969a, Veselova and Ogleznev 1965). Acute inhalation of isopropenylbenzene has been thought to reduce acetylcholine levels in the blood, kidney and liver in rats at 600–1000 ppm (Klimina 1974a), to result in accumulation of ammonia in the brains of mice at 621 ppm for 3 hours (Solov'ev 1969), to induce liver damage in rats at 1035 ppm, and to depress brain tissue respiration in rats at 621 ppm (Solov'ev 1969, Mochkina and Bravve 1969a).

8.4.2 Chronic toxicity

A chronic inhalation study of isopropenylbenzene in four species has been carried out by Wolf *et al* (1956). Slight growth depression and changes in liver and kidney weights were noted in rats and guinea-pigs exposed to 800 ppm for 28, 7-hour, periods. Exposure to 600 ppm for 212 days resulted in slight liver weight changes in rats and guinea-pigs, kidney weight changes in rats, effects on growth and mortality in rabbits, but no effects in rhesus monkeys. No toxic effects were found in any species exposed to 200 ppm for 197 days. There were no histopathological changes reported for any species at any dose level.

Several studies in the Russian literature have described chronic effects of exposure to isopropenylbenzene. These studies have been summarised and reviewed by the US EPA (1981). Effects on the CNS, which have been reported in rats after inhalation, include an increased destruction of brain proteins and uncoupling of brain oxidative phosphorylation at 10 ppm for 6 months (Solov'ev 1974), neuronal damage and vascular disorder in the brain stem at 0.5 ppm for 120 days (Zakharchenko 1969b), and increased brain acetylcholine levels at 8–15 ppm for 1–4 months (Klimina 1974b). Other effects reported in rats after chronic inhalation of isopropenylbenzene include raised hepatic cholesterol at 1–20 ppm for 120 days (Chukreev 1969), damage to the respiratory epithelium and blood vessel permeability at 1 ppm for 4 months (Kuz'min 1969a, b), increased erythrocyte volume and haemolysis (Mochkina and Bravve 1969b), and inhibition of lymphopoiesis at 1 ppm for 120 days (Molodyuk 1969). Another Russian study has suggested that a marked reduction in vital capacity and maximum ventilation of the lungs was found in children living in an area where the air was polluted with isopropenylbenzene and other hydrocarbons from a rubber manufacturing industry (Maslov 1980).

8.4.3 Genotoxicity, carcinogenicity and reproductive toxicity

Isopropenylbenzene has been reported to have only a very weak potential for inducing sister chromatid exchanges in cultured human lymphocytes (Norppa and Vainio 1983).

8.5 Discussion

Isopropenylbenzene was identified in only one of 14 treated water samples examined in the WRc survey. No other data appear to be available on the occurrence of this compound in the environment. Metabolism of isopropenylbenzene is likely to proceed through the side-chain epoxide intermediate.

There appears to be very little information on the toxicity of this compound, and with the exception of the study by Wolf *et al* (1956) very few details are readily available for those studies which have been published.

There is insufficient information available to evaluate the long-term health effects of exposure to isopropenylbenzene.

References

CHUKREEV E F (1969) Effect of the long term action of small concentrations ofalpha-methyl styrene alone and mixed with 1,3-butadiene on the cholesterol level in the liver of animals. *Nauchnye Trudy-Omskii Meditsinskii Institut* **88,** 265-268.

GADASKINA I D and AIZVERT L G (1979) The mechanism of x-methyl styrene toxicity. *Gigiena Truda i Professional'nye Zabolevaniia* **6,** 38-40.

GERARDE H W (1960) Toxicology and biochemistry of aromatic hydrocarbons. *Elsevier Monographs,* Elsevier.

KLIMINA G M (1974a) Study of the single-dose effect of high concentrations of alpha-methyl styrene and acrylonitrile on the cholinergic mediation system. *Narusheniya Metab, Tr Nauch Konf Med Inst Zapadn Sib* **1,** 46-48.

KLIMINA G M (1974b) The effect of chronic inhalation poisoning by alpha-methyl styrene on the cholinergic mediation system. *Narusheniya Metab, Tr Nauchn Konf Med Inst Zapadn Sib* **1,** 291-293.

KUZ'MIN V I (1969a) Changes in the secretion of the epithelium of white rat trachea and bronchi during the action of alpha-methyl styrene vapours. *Nauchnye Trudy-Omskii Meditsinskii Institut* **88,** 209-214.

KUZ'MIN V I (1969b) Pathomorphological and histochemical changes in respiration organs of white rats during the action of alpha-methyl styrene vapours. *Nauchnye Trudy-Omskii Meditsinskii Institut* **88,** 220-225.

MASLOV M L (1980) Effect of various levels of air pollution by emissions from petrochemical plants on the respiratory function of children. *Gigiena i Sanitariia* **1,** 10 12.

MIRZOYAN I M and ZHAKENOVA R K (1972) Effect of alpha-methyl styrene and *t*-dodecyl mercaptan on the skin of animals. *Vop Gig Tr Profzabol, Mater Nauch Konf,* 247-249.

MOCHKINA S E and BRAVVE V N (1969a) Erythrocyte volume in rats subjected to chronic alpha-methyl styrene poisoning. *Tr Krasnoyarsk Gos Med Inst* **9,** 15-17.

MOCHKINA S E and BRAVVE V N (1969b) Vitamin B(12) level in the serum of rats after acute administration of alpha-methyl styrene. *Tr Krasnoyarsk Gos Med Inst* **9,** 13-15.

MOLODYUK A V (1969) Histological and cytochemical study of lymph nodes during chronic poisoning with alpha-methyl styrene. *Nauchnye Trudy-Omskii Meditsinskii Institut* **88,** 226-230.

NORPPA H and VAINIO H (1983) Induction of sister-chromatid exchanges by styrene analogues in cultured human lymphocytes. *Mutation Research* **116,** 379-387.

OGLEZNEV G A (1964) Maximum permissible concentration of alpha-methyl styrene in water supplies. *Gigiena i Sanitariia* **29,** 24-29.

SOLOV'EV I I (1969) The effect of alpha-methyl styrene on brain tissue respiration. *Tr Krasnoyarsk Gos Med Inst* **9,** 9-11.

SOLOV'EV I I (1974) General and particular features of cerebral metabolic failure under the effect of different substances on an organism. *Narusheniya Metab, Tr Nauchn Konf Med Inst Zapadn Sib* **1,** 255-258.

US ENVIRONMENTAL PROTECTION AGENCY (1981) Investigation of Selected Potential Environmental Contaminants: Styrene, Ethylbenzene and Related Compounds. Government Reports Announcements & Index, Issue 01. NTIS/PB81-102659.

VESELOVA V V and OGLEZNEV G A (1965) Morphological changes in the organs of animals in acute and chronic intoxications with alpha-methyl styrene and styrene. *Nauchnye Trudy-Omskii Meditsinskii Institut* **61,** 89-95.

WATER RESEARCH CENTRE (1981) Organic micropollutants in drinking water. Technical Report TR 159.

WOLF M A, ROWE V K, McCOLLISTER D D, HOLLINGSWORTH R L and OYEN F (1956) Toxicological studies of certain alkylated benzenes and benzene. *AMA Archives of Industrial Health,* **14,** 387-398.

ZAKHARCHENKO V I (1969a) Morphological changes in white rat brains during chronic poisoning with alpha-methyl styrene. *Nauchnye Trudy-Omskii Meditsinskii Institut* **88,** 202-208.

ZAKHARCHENKO V I (1969b) Morphohistochemical changes in white rat brain during acute poisoning with alpha-methyl styrene. *Nauchnye Trudy-Omskii Meditsinskii Institut* **88,** 196-201.

ZOETEMAN B C J, PIET G J, RUYGROK C T M and HEUVEL R V D (1974) Threshold odour concentrations in water of chemical substances. RID-MEDEDELING 74-3.

9. THE ALKYLSTYRENES

9.1 Introduction

Methylstyrene (vinyltoluene) is commercially manufactured by the dehydrogenation of ethyltoluene and is used in adhesives, special coatings and latexes. An increased interest in methylstyrene has arisen as a consequence of possible health hazards associated with occupational exposure to styrene. From a toxicological point of view, however, methylstyrene appears to have little merit as a potential replacement for styrene. The addition of a methyl substituent on the aromatic ring of styrene appears to change little in terms of the major route of metabolism and its toxicity.

CAS Reg No:	25013-15-4
Molecular weight:	118.2
Boiling point	171°C
Solubility:	No data available
Evaporative half-life in water:	No data available
Threshold odour concentration in water:	No data available

9.2 Exposure

An unspecified methylstyrene isomer has been identified in rural air of the US (Holzer *et al* 1977).

In the WRc survey, an unspecified methylstyrene isomer was detected in 3/14 drinking water samples tested, three ethylstyrene isomers were identified in 2/14, 3/14 and 4/14 samples respectively, and a dimethylstyrene isomer was detected in one of the 14 samples (Water Research Centre 1981).

9.3 Toxicokinetics

Unlike the saturated di-substituted alkylbenzenes in which oxidation of the smallest alkyl group is the preferred mechanism of biotransformation, methylstyrene is primarily metabolised by oxidation of the larger unsaturated side-chain. Bergemalm-Rynell and Steen (1982) found that the metabolism of methylstyrene in rats closely resembles that of styrene. Most of the metabolites identified in the urine were methyl derivatives of their respective styrene counterparts. The initial metabolic step is therefore the formation of an epoxide intermediate at the vinyl group. A series of compounds were also identified in which the methyl substituent had been oxidised to the alcohol or acid.

In Wistar rats given 50 mg/kg body weight of methylstyrene by intraperitoneal injection, 55% of the dose was recovered as urinary metabolites within 23 hours (Heinonen 1984).

9.4 Health effects

9.4.1 Acute and subacute toxicity

The oral LD50 of methylstyrene in rats has been found to be 4.0 g/kg (Wolf *et al* 1956). Gerarde (1959) noted a 4/10 mortality rate in rats given a single oral dose of 2.5 ml of methylstyrene. Topical application of methylstyrene to rabbits caused slight to moderate irritation and moderate necrosis of the skin, while application to the eyes of rabbits resulted in slight conjunctival irritation, but no corneal injury (Wolf *et al* 1956).

Dose- and time-dependent changes in the glutathione content of rat liver and kidney have been reported in rats after inhalation (Heinonen and Vainio 1981) and intraperitoneal injection (Heinonen and Vainio 1980) of methylstyrene. Enhanced hepatic drug-metabolising activities were also noted in each case.

Inhalation of 400 ppm of methylstyrene (55–70% *meta* and 30–45% *para*-isomer) by human volunteers was found to elicit strong eye and nasal irritation (Wolf *et al* 1956).

9.4.2 Chronic toxicity

In a study by Wolf *et al* (1956), rats, guinea-pigs, rabbits and rhesus monkeys were exposed by inhalation to methylstyrene for a period of 139 days. Moderate mortality and growth depression, increased liver weight and slight histopathological changes in the liver were noted in rats exposed to 1350 ppm. At the same concentration, guinea-pigs exhibited similar though more moderate effects, slight changes in liver histopathology and kidney weight were seen in rabbits, but no effects of any kind were found in rhesus monkeys. No toxic effects were found in any species exposed to 580 ppm.

9.4.3 Genotoxicity

Methylstyrene (mixed isomers) was not found to be mutagenic in the Ames test to *Salmonella typhimurium* TA98, TA100, TA1535, TA1537 and TA1538, either in the presence or absence of metabolic activation, at doses ranging from 1.8 to 1180 μg/plate (Norppa *et al* 1981).

A dose-related induction of sister chromatid exchanges and a significant increase in chromosomal aberrations have been reported in human lymphocytes treated with methylstyrene (mixed isomers) *in vitro* (Norppa *et al* 1981). Induction of sister chromatid exchanges in cultured human lymphocytes has also been found for 2-methylstyrene, 3-methylstyrene, 4-methylstyrene and 3,5-dimethylstyrene (Norppa and Vainio 1983).

Norppa (1981) dosed five male C57BL/6 mice with 500 mg/kg of methylstyrene (60% *meta* and 40% *para*-isomer) by intraperitoneal injection. Increased numbers of micronucleated polychromatic erythrocytes were found in the two surviving animals. Increases in the number of micronuclei were observed at lower dose levels of 200 and 300 mg/kg, though no dose-response was evident. There was some evidence for mitotic delay at 100, 200 and 300 mg/kg, as the ratio of polychromatic to normochromatic cells was lowered at these dose levels.

No increase in the frequency of recessive lethal mutations was found in *Drosophila melanogaster* males exposed to 50, 100 and 300 ppm methylstyrene (mixed isomers) vapour for 5 days, or fed 200 and 500 ppm liquid methylstyrene for 24 hours and 72 hours (Norppa *et al* 1981).

9.4.4 Carcinogenicity

No information appears to be available.

9.4.5 Reproductive toxicity

An increased incidence of foetal resorptions and a change in the foetal sex ratio were found in Sprague–Dawley rats given 250 mg/kg body weight/day of methylstyrene by intraperitoneal injection on days 1–15 of gestation. No maternal toxic effects were noted (Hardin *et al* 1981). A Russian study has reported that methylstyrene was teratogenic in rats by inhalation. Details of this study, however, are limited (Krynskaya *et al* 1969).

9.5 Discussion

There is very little information on the occurrence of alkylstyrenes in the environment. Their metabolism in the liver appears to resemble that of styrene; that is, oxidation of the vinyl side-chain followed by conjugation.

The toxicology of the alkylstyrenes has been quite poorly studied. There is some information for methylstyrene, but almost no information at all for the ethylstyrenes and dimethylstyrene. However, the limited information available suggests that these compounds are likely to have a similar toxic potential to styrene. The methylstyrenes and a dimethylstyrene isomer have been shown to have genotoxic activity in human lymphocytes *in vitro*. Methylstyrene has also been found to induce micronuclei in mice *in vivo*.

Although there is not a great deal of information available on the alkylstyrenes, these compounds would not, in view of their apparent similarity to styrene, appear to represent a hazard to human health at the very low levels encountered through drinking water.

References

BERGEMALM-RYNELL K and STEEN (1982). Urinary metabolites of vinyltoluene in the rat. *Toxicology and Applied Pharmacology* **62,** 19-31.

GERARDE H W (1959) Toxicological studies on hydrocarbons. III. The biochemorphology of the phenylalkanes and the phenylalkenes. *AMA Archives of Industrial Health* **19,** 403-418.

HARDIN B D, BOND G P, SIKOV M R, ANDREW F D, BELILES R P and NIEMEIER R W (1981) Testing of selected workplace chemicals for teratogenic potential. *Scandinavian Journal of Work Environment and Health* **7** (Suppl 4), 66-75.

HEINONEN T H H (1984) Metabolism of vinyltoluene in the rat: effect of induction and inhibition of the cytochrome P-450. *Biochemical Pharmacology* **33,** 1585-1593.

HEINONEN T and VAINIO H (1980) Vinyltoluene induced changes in xenobiotic-metabolizing enzyme activities and tissue glutathione content in various rodent species. *Biochemical Pharmacology* **29,** 2675-2679.

HEINONEN T and VAINIO H (1981) Dose-dependent effects of vinyltoluene inhalation on non-protein thiols and drug biotransformation in liver and kidneys of the rat. *Xenobiotica* **11,** 285-289.

HOLZER G, SHANFIELD H, ZLATKIS A, BERTSCH W, JUAREZ P, MAYFIELD H and LIEBICH H M (1977) Collection and analysis of trace organic emissions from natural sources. *Journal of Chromatography* **142,** 755-764.

KRYNSKAYA I L, PETROVA L I, GURICHEVA Z G, ROBACHEVSKAYA E G and BUKEVICH G M (1969) Toxicity of vinyltoluene and methods for its determination in the air. *Gigiena i Sanitariia* **34,** 334.

NORPPA H (1981) Styrene and vinyltoluene induce micronuclei in mouse bone marrow. *Toxicology Letters* **8,** 247-251.

NORPPA H and VAINIO H (1983) Induction of sister-chromatid exchanges by styrene analogues in cultured human lymphocytes. *Mutation Research* **116,** 379-387.

NORPPA H, SKYTTA E, DONNER M, SORSA M and VAINIO H (1981) Mutagenicity of vinyltoluene. *Mutation Research* **85,** 294.

WATER RESEARCH CENTRE (1981) Organic micropollutants in drinking water. Technical Report TR 159.

WOLF M A, ROWE V K, McCOLLISTER D D, HOLLINGSWORTH R L and OYEN F (1956) Toxicological studies of certain alkylated benzenes and benzene. *AMA Archives of Industrial Health,* **14,** 387-398.

10. BIPHENYL

10.1 Introduction

Biphenyl (diphenyl, phenylbenzene, xenene) is produced by the pyrolytic dehydrogenation of benzene and is used as a fungicide, preservative and as a heat transfer agent.

CAS Reg No:	92-52-4
Molecular weight:	154.2
Boiling point:	255.9°C
Solubility:	7.5 mg/l at 25°C (Verschueren 1977)
Evaporative half-life in water of depth 1m:	7.52 hours at 25°C (Mackay and Leinonen 1975)
Threshold odour concentration in water:	0.5 5μ/l (Van Gemert and Nettenbreijer (1977)

10.2 Exposure

Biphenyl was identified in 7/14 treated water samples of the WRc survey (Water Research Centre 1981). In a Japanese study (Akiyama *et al* 1980), biphenyl was detected at a concentration of 150 ng/l in sewage influent, 3.7 ng/l in sewage effluent and 4 ng/l in tap water.

No data related to levels of biphenyl in air or food appear to be available, though significant quantities may be ingested from biphenyl-treated citrus fruits.

10.3 Toxicokinetics

Biotransformation of biphenyl has been widely studied both *in vivo* and *in vitro.* Numerous phenolic metabolites have been identified, including monohydroxybiphenyls, dihydroxybiphenyls, trihydroxybiphenyls, hydroxymethoxybiphenyls and dihydroxymethoxybiphenyls (Williams 1959, Meyer and Scheline 1976, Meyer *et al* 1976a, Wiebkin *et al* 1976, Willis and Addison 1974, Halpaap-Wood *et al* 1981). Generally, 40–50% of a dose of biphenyl is metabolised to phenols (30% free and 20% conjugated), a further 25–30% to acids (20% free and 5–10% conjugated) and about 1% to biphenylmercapturic acid (Williams 1959, Meyer *et al* 1976a, b, West *et al* 1956).

Meyer *et al* (1976b) found that 92% of an oral dose of 100 mg/kg of biphenyl in rats was eliminated within 96 hours. Of this, 84.8% was found in the urine, 7.3% in the faeces and trace amounts in the expired air. Only 0.6% of the dose remained in the body.

10.4 Health effects

10.4.1 Acute and subacute toxicity

An unspecified oral dose of biphenyl in rabbits induced loss of appetite, depression of body weight, increased respiratory rate, muscular weakness, unsteadiness, coma and death. Little local tissue injury was found, except for some slight irritation, but toxic effects were noted in the liver and kidney. Surviving animals exhibited pulmonary congestion, oedema, lobular and interstitial pneumonitis, some paralysis, and asphyxial convulsions (Deichmann *et al* (1947). Application of 0.5 g/kg of biphenyl to the abdominal skin of rabbits for 2 hours/day, 5 days/week for 4 weeks did not appear to have any dermal effects, but did result in body weight loss (Deichmann *et al* 1947). Oral LD50s of 3.3 g/kg in the rat and 2.4 g/kg in the rabbit have been reported for this compound (Deichmann *et al* 1947).

10.4.2 Chronic toxicity

Histopathological and urinary evidence of kidney damage has been reported in rats fed diets containing 0.5% biphenyl for 120 days. No effects were observed in animals fed 0.1% biphenyl. Rats returned to control diets for 30 and 60 days after 165 days of biphenyl treatment showed regression of the nephrotoxic effects (Booth *et al* 1961). Moderately degenerative changes in the liver and kidney have been reported in rats fed daily oral doses of 50 or 100 mg of biphenyl for 13 months. It was also suggested that thyroid and parathyroid functions were enhanced (Pecchiai and Saffioti 1957). No changes in histopathology or gross pathology were found in dogs fed doses of 25 mg/kg/day of biphenyl, 5 days/week for 52 weeks (Hazleton *et al* 1956).

Rats exposed by inhalation to 0.005, 0.04 and 0.3 mg/m^3 of biphenyl dust, 7 hours/day, 5 days/week for up to 94 days exhibited nasal irritation, respiratory difficulty and significant mortality at the two higher dose levels. There were significant pathological changes in the lung, but only minimal changes in the liver and kidney. In similar experiments with rabbits, no local or systemic toxicity was observed at any exposure level (Deichmann *et al* 1947).

In a study of 24 workers exposed to biphenyl in a Finnish paper mill (Seppalainen and Hakkinen 1975), EEG abnormalities were found in 10 subjects. These abnormalities were also present on re-examination of the subjects 1 and 2 years later. Amongst the 24 workers of this study were also 9 cases of EMG abnormalities, 7 cases of muscular fibrillation and several cases of slowed nerve conduction velocities, particularly those of the slower motor fibres. In an earlier study of this same group of workers (Hakkinen *et al* 1973), common complaints were headaches, gastrointestinal pain and indigestion, numbness and aching of limbs and general fatigue. Also reported were several cases of EEG and EMG abnormalities, elevated levels of serum glutamic oxaloacetic transaminase and serum glutamic pyruvic transaminase in 10/33 workers, plus indications of liver injury in 5 hospitalised workers.

10.4.3 Genotoxicity

Biphenyl is non-mutagenic in the Ames test, both in the presence and absence of metabolic activation, at doses ranging from 1.0 to 100 μg/plate (Haworth *et al* 1983, Probst *et al* 1981, Hirayama *et al* 1981). Negative results were also obtained for inhibition of DNA repair in E. coli WP2, WP2uvrA-, CM571 and WP100 (Hirayama *et al* 1981).

Biphenyl was not found to induce unscheduled DNA synthesis in primary cultures of rat hepatocytes (Probst *et al* 1981) or to increase the incidence of chromosomal aberrations in a Chinese hamster cell line (Ishidate and Odashima 1977).

A single oral dose of 500 mg/kg of biphenyl has been shown to induce mitoses in the adrenal cortex of rats. The significance of this test, however, is not clear (Danz and Urban 1979).

10.4.4 Carcinogenicity

The only information available is from a 13-month rat study in which a group of rats were fed daily oral doses of 50 or 100 mg of biphenyl. Of the 13 animals in the study, two developed papillomata of the forestomach and one a squamous cell carcinoma of the forestomach (Pecchiai and Saffioti 1957).

10.4.5 Reproductive toxicity

No evidence for teratogenicity or embryotoxicity was found in Wistar rats given oral doses of 125–500 mg/kg of technical grade biphenyl on days 6–15 of gestation. Foetotoxic effects and toxicity in the dams were observed at a dose level of 1000 mg/kg (Khera *et al* 1979).

10.5 Discussion

There is little information on the occurrence of biphenyl in the environment. In the liver, biphenyl is rapidly metabolised to a range of phenolic compounds which are eliminated primarily in the urine.

The limited information available suggests that biphenyl is of low acute and chronic toxicity in experimental animals. Toxic effects on the nervous system have been reported in Finnish paper mill workers exposed to biphenyl. This compound does not appear to be mutagenic in bacteria or mammalian cells *in vitro*. There is very little information on carcinogenicity. One study in rats did not give any evidence for teratogenic potential of biphenyl.

WHO has set an unconditional acceptable daily intake for biphenyl of 0–0.05 mg/kg body weight.

Low levels of biphenyl in drinking water would not appear to represent a hazard to human health. However, further information is needed in some areas.

References

AKIYAMA T, KOGA M, SHINOHARA R, KIDD A and ETOH S (1980) Detection and identification of trace organic substances in the aquatic environment. *Journal of Uoeh* **2,** 289-300.

BOOTH A N, AMBROSE A N, DeEDS F and COX A J Jr (1961) The reversible nephrotoxic effects of biphenyl. *Toxicology and Applied Pharmacology* **3,** 560-567.

DANZ M and URBAN H (1979) Carcinogens, promotors and suspicious drugs: Their identical short-term effect in a promoting activity test. *Experimental Pathology* **17,** 181-184.

DEICHMANN W B, KITZMILLER K V, DIERKER M and WITHERUP S (1947) Observations on the effects of diphenyl, *o*- and *p*-aminodiphenyl, *o*- and *p*-nitrodiphenyl and dihydroxyoctachlorodiphenyl upon experimental animals. *Journal of Industrial Hygiene and Toxicology* **29,** 1-13.

HAKKINEN I, SILTANEN E, HERNBERG S, SEPPALAINEN A M, KARLI P and VIKKULA E (1973) Diphenyl poisoning in fruit paper production. *Archives of Environmental Health* **26,** 70-74.

HALPAAP-WOOD K, HORNING E C and HORNING M G (1981) The effect of phenobarbitol and beta-naphthoflavone induction on the metabolism of biphenyl in the rat and mouse. *Drug Metabolism and Disposition* **9,** 97-102.

HAWORTH S, LAWLOR T, MORTELMANS K, SPECK W and ZEIGER E (1983) *Salmonella* mutagenicity test results for 250 chemicals. *Environmental Mutagenesis* **5,** Suppl 1, 3-142.

HAZLETON L W, KUNDZINS W, HOWARD J W and JOHNSTON C O (1956) Studies on biphenyl in the dog. XX International Physiological Congress, Brussels, Belgium, July 30th–Aug 4th 1956.

HIRAYAMA T, NOHARA M, SHINDO H and FUKUI S (1981) Mutagenicity assays of photochemical reaction products of biphenyl (BP) and *o*-phenylphenol (OPP) with NOx. *Chemosphere* **10,** 223-228.

ISHIDATE M Jr and ODASHIMA S (1977) Chromosome tests with 134 compounds on Chinese hamster cells *in vitro* — a screening for chemical carcinogens. *Mutation Research* **48,** 337-354.

KHERA K S, WHALEN C, ANGERS G and TRIVETT G (1979) Assessment of the teratogenic potential of piperonyl butoxide, biphenyl, and phosalone in the rat. *Toxicology and Applied Pharmacology* **47,** 353-358.

MACKAY D and LEINONEN P J (1975) Rates of evaporation of low-solubility contaminants from water bodies to atmosphere. *Environmental Science and Technology* **9,** 1178-1180.

MEYER T and SCHELINE R R (1976) The metabolism of biphenyl. 2. Phenolic metabolites in the rat. *Acta Pharmacologica et Toxicologica* **39,** 419-432.

MEYER T, LARSEN J C, HANSEN E V and SCHELINE R R (1976a) The metabolism of biphenyl. 3. Phenolic metabolites in the pig. *Acta Pharmacologica et Toxicologica* **39,** 433-441.

MEYER T, AARBAKKE J and SCHELINE R R (1976b) The metabolism of biphenyl. 1. Metabolic disposition of C(14)-biphenyl in the rat. *Acta Pharmacologica et Toxicologica* **39,** 412-418.

PECCHIAI L and SAFFIOTI U (1957) Toxicity of biphenyl, diphenyl oxide and their mixtures (Dowtherm). *Medicina del Lavoro* **48,** 247.

PROBST G S, McMAHON R E, HILL L E, THOMPSON C Z, EPP J K and NEAL S B (1981) Chemically induced unscheduled DNA synthesis in primary rat hepatocyte cultures: A comparison with bacterial mutagenicity rising 218 compounds. *Environmental Mutagenesis* **3,** 11-32.

SEPPALAINEN A M and HAKKINEN I (1975) Electrophysiological findings in diphenyl poisoning. *Journal of Neurology, Neurosurgery and Psychiatry* **38,** 248-252.

VAN GEMERT L J and NETTENBREIJER A H (Eds) (1977) Compilation of odour threshold values in air and water. Central Institute for Nutrition and Food Research, National Institute for Water Supply.

VERSCHUEREN K (1977) *Handbook of environmental data on organic chemicals.* Van Nostrand Reinhold Company.

WATER RESEARCH CENTRE (1981) Organic micropollutants in drinking water. Technical Report TR 159.

WEST H D, LAWSON J R, MILLER I H and MATHURA G R (1956) The fate of diphenyl in the rat. *Archives of Biochemistry and Biophysics* **60,** 14-20.

WIEBKIN P, FRY J R, JONES C A, LOWING R and BRIDGES J W (1976) The metabolism of biphenyl by isolated viable rat hepatocytes. *Xenobiotica* **6,** 725-743.

WILLIAMS R T (1959) *Detoxication mechanisms.* Chapman and Hall.

WILLIS D E and ADDISON R F (1974) Hydroxylation of biphenyl *in vitro* by tissue preparations of some marine organisms. *Comparative and General Pharmacology* **5,** 77-81.

11. METHYLBIPHENYL

An unspecified methylbiphenyl isomer was detected in one of the fourteen samples of the WRc survey (Water Research Centre 1981). Methylbiphenyl has also been detected in Japanese tap water, sediment, seawater, river water (filtrate) and rainwater (Akiyama *et al* 1980).

No toxicological information appears to be available on this compound. One could consider, however, that methylbiphenyl and biphenyl are structural analogues of toluene and benzene. In this case, substitution of the methyl group onto the ring of benzene eliminates most of its adverse toxicological properties. Methylbiphenyl is likely to be metabolised by side-chain oxidation in a similar fashion to toluene.

References

AKIYAMA T, KOGA M, SHINOHARA R, KIDD A and ETOH S (1980) Detection and identification of trace organic substances in the aquatic environment. *Journal of Uoeh* **2,** 289-300.

WATER RESEARCH CENTRE (1981) Organic micropollutants in drinking water. Technical Report TR 159.

12. DIPHENYLMETHANE

CAS Reg No:	101-81-5
Molecular weight:	168.3

Diphenylmethane (benzylbenzene, alpha-phenyltoluene, ditan, ditane) was identified in only one of the 14 drinking water samples examined in the WRc survey

(Water Research Centre 1981). This compound has also been detected in Japanese sewage influent (Akiyama *et al* 1980).

In the rat, the principal metabolites of diphenylmethane are benzhydrol, 2-hydroxydiphenylmethane, 4-hydroxydiphenylmethane, 2,2′-dihydroxydiphenylmethane and 4,4′-dihydroxydiphenylmethane (Williams 1959, Deloach *et al* 1978, Stocklinski *et al* 1979, Stocklinski 1981, Gerarde 1960). Adult male rats given 15.3 mg of [^{13}C]diphenylmethane in corn oil were found to excrete 48% of the label in the urine and 18% in the faeces within 24 hours (Stocklinski 1981).

The only toxicological information which appears to be available is that 10/10 male albino rats died after they were given 5 ml/kg of diphenylmethane dissolved in an equal volume of olive oil (Gerarde 1960).

References

AKIYAMA T, KOGA M, SHINOHARA R, KIDD A and ETOH S (1980) Detection and identification of trace organic substances in the aquatic environment. *Journal of Uoeh,* **2,** 289-300.

DELOACH G D, LEARY H W and STOCKLINSKI A W (1978) Identification of *p*-hydroxydiphenylmethane as a urinary metabolite of diphenylmethane in the rat. *Research Communications in Chemical Pathology and Pharmacology* **22,** 419-422.

GERARDE H W (1960) Toxicology and biochemistry of aromatic hydrocarbons. Elsevier Monographs, Elsevier.

STOCKLINSKI A W (1981) Semi-quantitative profile of regioisomeric monohydroxydiphenylmethane metabolites in rat urine, faeces and bile. *Xenobiotica* **11,** 425-432.

STOCKLINSKI A W, DELOACH G D and WILLIAMS H (1979) Identification of benzhydrol as a urinary metabolite of diphenylmethane in the rat. *Research Communications in Chemical Pathology and Pharmacology* **24,** 397-400.

WATER RESEARCH CENTRE (1981) Organic micropollutants in drinking water. Technical Report TR 159.

WILLIAMS R T (1959) Detoxication mechanisms. Chapman and Hall.

6

The halogenated aromatics

1. CHLOROBENZENE

1.1 Introduction

Chlorobenzene (monochlorobenzene) is a widely used industrial chemical involved in the manufacture of phenol, aniline, perfumes, pharmaceuticals, insecticides and dyestuffs.

CAS Reg No:	108-90-7
Molecular weight:	112.6
Boiling point:	132°C
Solubility:	500 mg/l at 20°C (Verschueren 1977)
Evaporative half-life in water:	No data available
Threshold odour concentration in water:	0.1 mg/l (Zoeteman *et al* 1974)

1.2 Exposure

Chlorobenzene has been detected in US drinking water at concentrations of around 5 μg/l (National Academy of Sciences 1977). In the WRc survey, this compound was identified in 5/14 drinking water samples examined (Fielding *et al* 1981).

No other information on the occurrence of chlorobenzene in air, food or water appears to be available.

1.3 Toxicokinetics

Chlorobenzene is readily absorbed by both the gastrointestinal tract and lungs and is distributed primarily to the adipose tissue (Sullivan *et al* 1983, Lindsay Smith *et al* 1972).

In rabbits, the most extensively studied species, oral doses of chlorobenzene are metabolised primarily to *para*-chlorophenylmercapturic acid and glucuronide and sulphate conjugates of 4-chlorocatechol. Minor metabolites include chlorophenols, 4-chlorocatecholmethyl ether and 2-chloroquinol (Lindsay Smith *et al* 1972, Parke and Williams 1955, Spencer and Williams 1950).

Following an oral dose of chlorobenzene in rabbits, about 20% is excreted as metabolites in the urine. Little is excreted in the faeces or is retained in the body. Elimination of unchanged chlorobenzene in the expired air is probably the most important excretory mechanism (Lindsay Smith *et al* 1972).

1.4 Health effects

1.4.1 Acute and subacute toxicity

In experimental animals, chlorobenzene is of relatively low acute toxicity by either the oral or inhalation route of exposure. At high doses the principal toxic effects are hepatic and renal necrosis. Oral LD50s of 1–5 g/kg have been reported for this compound in a range of mammalian species (Deichmann 1981). The mouse appears to be more sensitive than the rat to the acute toxicity of chlorobenzene (Kluwe *et al* 1985).

An increase in hepatic and biliary porphyrins was found in day-old White Leghorn chicks given an oral dose of 800 mg/kg of chlorobenzene in DMSO. Both *para*-dichlorobenzene and 1,2,4-trichlorobenzene were more potent inducers of hepatic porphyria than chlorobenzene (Miranda *et al* 1984).

Intraperitoneal injection of 5 mmol/kg (563 mg/kg) of chlorobenzene in rats led to a tenfold increase in bile duct pancreatic fluid flow. There was no evidence for hepatotoxicity as measured by plasma alanine aminotransferase (Yang *et al* 1979).

Ariyoshi *et al* (1975) found that rat liver microsomal cytochrome P-450 and aminopyrine demethylase levels were lowered after single oral doses of 125, 250, 500 and 1000 mg/kg of chlorobenzene. The activity of delta-ALA synthetase was markedly elevated at all dose levels, while aniline hydroxylase activity was elevated at the highest dose level only. At 250 mg/kg, delta-ALA activity was initially lowered but after 12 hours had returned to normal and by 24 hours had increased markedly. The reverse trend was noted with cytochrome P-450 content. In another study, cytochrome P-450 and glucose-6-phosphatase activities were significantly lowered after oral doses of 800 mg/kg/day for 14 days in male rats. Doses of 200, 400 and 800 mg/kg/day for 14 days were found to increase glucuronyl transferase activity (Carlson and Tardiff 1976). Dalich and Larson (1985) found hepatic centrilobular necrosis, elevated activity of plasma alanine aminotransferase and depression of hepatic cytochrome P-450 and glutathione in Sprague–Dawley rats given a single intraperitoneal dose of 9.8 mmol/kg (1.1 g/kg).

In a study of hepatotoxic mixtures in mice, chlorobenzene and carbon tetrachloride were found to have additive effects. This may indicate a similarity in toxic action (Shelton and Weber 1981).

In man, inhalation of chlorobenzene has been reported to cause CNS depression and narcotic symptoms at 200 ppm and severe toxic effects at 400 ppm (Verschueren 1977).

1.4.2 Chronic toxicity

The limited studies which have been carried out suggest that the toxic effects of chlorobenzene are primarily associated with the liver and kidney.

In a 13-week oral study, reduced survival was found at 500 mg/kg in male and female F-344 rats and at 250 mg/kg in male and female B6C3F1 mice. In surviving female rats exposed to 500 and 750 mg/kg, slight increases in serum alkaline phosphatase and gamma-glutamyl transpeptidase activities were evident. There were no alterations in serum chemistry in male rats or in male and female mice, and there were no significant changes in haematology and urinalyses in any group. A number of dose-dependent histopathological changes were found at and above doses of 250 mg/kg in both sexes of rats and mice. These included hepatic necrosis, degeneration or focal necrosis of the renal proximal tubules, and lymphoid or myeloid depletion of the spleen, bone marrow and thymus (Kluwe *et al* 1985).

Rats fed chlorobenzene in the diet at a dose of 250 mg/kg/day for 93–99 days exhibited retarded growth and elevated liver and kidney weights. Elevated liver and kidney weights were also found in rats given 50 mg/kg but not at 12.5 mg/kg. No histopathological changes were observed at any dose level (Knapp *et al* 1971).

In a Russian study, groups of seven male rats were given 0.001, 0.01 or 0.1 mg/kg/day of chlorobenzene by stomach tube for 9 months. Effects observed in the high-dose animals were inhibition of bone marrow mitosis and erythropoiesis, thrombocytosis, elevated activities of serum transaminase and alkaline phosphatase, lowered activities of liver and kidney alkaline phosphatase and a moderate increase in liver and kidney acid phosphatase activities. Similar though less pronounced effects were found in rats given 0.01 mg/kg, but no effects were observed at 0.001 mg/kg (Varshavskaya 1968).

No effects were seen in dogs given oral doses of 27.25 or 54.5 mg/kg/day of chlorobenzene, 5 days/week over a 93-day period. In a group of eight dogs given 272.5 mg/kg/day, four died after 14–21 doses. The animals which died exhibited gross and/or microscopic pathological changes in the liver, kidney, gastrointestinal tract and haemopoietic system. The pathology of surviving animals was similar, although the changes were on the whole less extensive. Prior to death, clinical studies revealed elevated numbers of immature leukocytes, lowered blood sugar, elevated plasma alanine aminotransferase and alkaline phosphatase activities and in some cases increases in total bilirubin and cholesterol (Knapp *et al* 1971).

Dilley and Lewis (1978) reported increased liver weights in rats and increased lung weights in rabbits after inhalation of 75 or 200 ppm of chlorobenzene vapour, 7 hours/day, 5 days/week for 24 weeks. Other observations in the rat included elevated platelet numbers after 11 weeks, a decrease in plasma aspartate aminotransferase activity, tubular lesions in the kidney, congestion in the liver and kidney, and occasional lesions in the adrenal cortex. No histopathological changes were seen in rabbits. In a Polish study, lowered white blood cell counts were found in Swiss mice exposed by inhalation to 0.1 mg/l of chlorobenzene, 7 hours/day for 3 months (Zub 1978).

1.4.3 Genotoxicity

There is evidence that chlorobenzene can bind covalently to DNA both *in vitro* and *in vivo* (Grilli *et al* 1985). However, chlorobenzene was not found to be mutagenic in the Ames test to *Salmonella typhimurium* TA98, TA100, TA1535 or TA1537, in either the presence or absence of rat liver or hamster liver S-9, at doses ranging from 3.3 to 3333 μg/plate (Haworth *et al* 1983).

It has been reported in the US Federal Register (1984) that chlorobenzene transformed adult rat liver epithelial cells *in vitro*, but was unable to induce unscheduled DNA synthesis in primary cultures of rat hepatocytes.

This compound was found to induce a dose-dependent increase in revertants of *Actinomycetes antibioticus*-400 (Keskinova 1968).

1.4.4 Carcinogenicity

Chlorobenzene has been tested for carcinogenicity in B6C3F1 mice and F-344 rats. Groups of 50 female mice and male and female rats were given 60 or 120 mg/kg body-weight/day in corn oil by gavage, 5 days/week for 2 years. Groups of 50 male mice were given lower doses of 30 and 60 mg/kg body-weight/day. A weak dose-related increase in the incidence of hepatic neoplastic nodules was found in male rats (Kluwe *et al* 1985).

1.4.5 Reproductive toxicity

No teratogenic effects were found in F-344 rats exposed by inhalation to 75, 210 or 590 ppm of chlorobenzene, 6 hours/day on days 6–15 of gestation. An increased incidence of some minor skeletal abnormalities was apparent in the 75 and 590 ppm groups but not in the 210 ppm group. Depression of body weight gain and elevated absolute and relative liver weights were evident in the dams at 590 ppm (John *et al* 1984).

New Zealand White rabbits exposed by inhalation to 10, 30, 75, 210 or 590 ppm of chlorobenzene, 6 hours/day, on days 6–18 of gestation did not give any evidence for teratogenicity or embryotoxicity. Elevated absolute and relative liver weights were observed in the dams at the highest dose level (John *et al* 1984).

1.5 Discussion

There is very little information on the occurrence of chlorobenzene in the environment.

Following oral exposure, most of a dose of chlorobenzene is likely to be exhaled unchanged from the lungs though several metabolites are found in the urine.

The limited studies available suggest that chlorobenzene is of relatively low acute and chronic toxicity. The principal toxic effects are necrosis of the liver and kidney. Chlorobenzene has given negative results for mutagenicity in bacteria, but there is only limited information in higher test systems. There is some evidence for weak carcinogenic potential in male F-344 rats. No carcinogenic effects were found in female rats or in male and female B6C3F1 mice. Chlorobenzene does not appear to be teratogenic in rats or rabbits by the inhalation route.

Although chlorobenzene may possess weak carcinogenic potential to the liver of rats at high dose levels, it is very unlikely that low concentrations of chlorobenzene in drinking water would represent a carcinogenic hazard to man. However, the result of the carcinogenesis bioassay and the evidence for covalent binding to DNA indicate that further studies would be desirable.

References

ARIYOSHI T, IDEGUCHI K, ISHIZUKA Y I, IWASAKI K and ARAKAKI M (1975) Relationship between chemical structure and activity. I. Effects of the number of chlorine atoms in chlorinated benzenes on the components of drug-metabolizing system and the hepatic constituents. *Chemical and Pharmaceutical Bulletin, Tokyo* **23**, 817-823.

CARLSON G P and TARDIFF R G (1976) Effect of chlorinated benzenes on the metabolism of foreign organic compounds. *Toxicology and Applied Pharmacology* **36**, 383-394.

DALICH G M and LARSON R E (1985) Temporal and dose-response features of monochlorobenzene hepatotoxicity in rats. *Fundamental and Applied Toxicology* **5**, 105-116.

DEICHMANN W B (1981) Halogenated cyclic hydrocarbons. In: *Patty's Industrial Hygiene and Toxicology, 3rd Revised Edition*, edited by G D Clayton and F E Clayton Vol 2B, pp. 3603-3769. John Wiley & Sons.

DILLEY J V and LEWIS T R (1978) Toxic evaluation of inhaled chlorobenzene. *Toxicology and Applied Pharmacology* **45**, 327.

FIELDING M, GIBSON T M, JAMES H A, McLOUGHLIN K and STEELE C P (1981) Organic micropollutants in drinking water. WRc Technical Report TR 159.

GRILLI S, ARFELLINI G, COLACCI A, MAZZULLO M and PRODI G (1985) *In vivo* and *in vitro* covalent bindng of chlorobenzene to nucleic acids. *Japanese Journal of Cancer Research (Gann)* **76**, 745-751.

HAWORTH S, LAWLOR T, MORTELMANS K, SPECK W and ZEIGER E (1983) Salmonella mutagenicity test results for 250 chemicals. *Environmental Mutagenesis* **5**, Suppl 1, 3-142.

JOHN J A, HAYES W C, HANLEY T R Jr, JOHNSON K A, GUSHOW T S and RAO K S (1984) Inhalation teratology study on monochlorobenzene in rats and rabbits. *Toxicology and Applied Pharmacology* **76**, 365-373.

KESKINOVA D (1968) The action of dimethylcyclodiazomethane in chlorobenzene solutions on the mutation process in *Actinomycetes antibioticus*-400. *Soviet Genetics* **4,** 1082-1085.

KLUWE W M, DILL G, PERSING R and PETERS A (1985) Toxic responses to acute, subchronic, and chronic oral administrations of monochlorobenzene to rodents. *Journal of Toxicology and Environmental Health* **15**, 745-767.

KNAPP W K Jr, BUSEY W M and KUNDZINS W (1971) Subacute oral toxicity of monochlorobenzene in dogs and rats. *Toxicology and Applied Pharmacology* **19**, 393.

LINDSAY SMITH J R, SHAW B A J and FOULKES D M (1972) Mechanism of mammalian hydroxylation: Some novel metabolites of chlorobenzene. *Xenobiotica* **2**, 215-226.

MIRANDA C L, WANG J-L, HENDERSON M C, NAKAUE H S and BUHLER D R (1984) Effects of chlorobenzenes on hepatic porphyrin and drug metabolism in chick embryo and day-old chick. *Research Communications in Chemical Pathology and Pharmacology* **46**, 13-24.

NATIONAL ACADEMY OF SCIENCES (1977) Drinking Water and Health Vol 1. US National Academy of Sciences, Washington, DC.

PARKE D V and WILLIAMS R T (1955) The metabolism of halogenobenzenes. (a) *Meta*-dichlorobenzene. (b) Further observations on the metabolism of chlorobenzene. *Biochemical Journal* **59**, 415-422.

SHELTON D W and WEBER L J (1981) Quantification of the joint effects of mixtures of hepatotoxic agents: Evaluation of a theoretical model in mice. *Environmental Research* **26**, 33-41.

SPENCER B and WILLIAMS R T (1950) The metabolism of halogenobenzenes. A comparison of the glucuronic acid, ethereal sulphate and mercapturic acid conjugations of chloro-, bromo- and iodo-benzenes and of the *o*-, *m*- and *p*-chlorophenols. Biosynthesis of *o*-, *m*- and *p*-chlorophenyl-glucuronides. *Biochemical Journal* **47**, 279-284.

SULLIVAN T M, BORN G S, CARLSON G P and KESSLER W V (1983) The pharmacokinetics of inhaled chlorobenzene in the rat. *Toxicology and Applied Pharmacology* **71**, 194-203.

US FEDERAL REGISTER (1984) **49**, 18779-18780.

VARSHAVSKAYA S P (1968) Comparative toxicological characteristics of chlorobenzene and dichlorobenzene (*ortho*- and *para*-isomers) in relation to the sanitary protection of water bodies. *Gigiena i Sanitariia* **33**, 17-23.

VERSCHUEREN K (1977) *Handbook of Environmental Data on Organic Chemicals*. Van Nostrand Reinhold Company.

YANG K H, PETERSON R E and FUJIMOTO J M (1979) Increased bile-duct pancreatic fluid flow in benzene and halogenated benzene-treated rats. *Toxicology and Applied Pharmacology* **47**, 505-514.

ZOETEMAN B C J, PIET G J, RUYGROK C T M and HEUVEL R V D (1974) Threshold Odour Concentrations in Water of Chemical Substances. RID-MEDEDELING 74-3.

ZUB M (1978) Reactivity of the white blood cell system to toxic action of benzene and its derivatives. *Acta Biologica Cracoviensic Serie Zoologica* **21**, 163-174.

2. DICHLOROBENZENE

2.1 Introduction

The dichlorobenzenes have been used for a number of years as fumigants, solvents, moth repellants, deodorants, sanitizers, and as intermediates in the manufacture of dyestuffs, insecticides and pharmaceuticals. Most of the toxicological information available relates to the *para*-isomer.

CAS Reg No (mixed):	25321-22-6
Molecular weight:	147.0
Boiling point:	172–179°C
Solubility:	79–145 mg/l at 25°C (Verschueren 1977)
Evaporative half-life in water:	No data available
Threshold odour concentration in water:	0.02 mg/l (Zoeteman *et al* 1974)

2.2 Exposure

2.2.1 Air

The dichlorobenzenes have been detected in the atmosphere on several occasions. Up to 50 ng/m^3 of *ortho*-dichlorobenzene was detected in Los Angeles air (Ware and

West 1977), while *para*-dichlorobenzene has been detected in Tokyo air at a concentration of 1.5–4.2 $\mu g/m^3$ (Morita and Ohi 1975). In the Tokyo study, indoor concentrations were reported to range from 105 to 1700 $\mu g/m^3$. The *meta*-isomer has also been identified in the atmosphere (Holzer *et al* 1977).

2.2.2 Food

There appears to be only limited data on the occurrence of dichlorobenzene in food (Peattie *et al* 1984), though *para*-dichlorobenzene has been found in the tissues of several species of fish (Morita *et al* 1975).

2.2.3 Water

The dichlorobenzenes have been detected in US drinking water at 1–3 μg/l (National Academy of Sciences 1977) and in US surface water at 13 μg/l (World Health Organization 1980). In Japanese tap water, concentrations of 5.8, 4.5 and 0.5 ng/l have been reported for the *para*, *ortho*, and *meta* isomers respectively (Akiyama *et al* 1980). The survey by WRc detected the *para* isomer in all 14 drinking water samples tested. However, the *ortho* isomer was detected in only two samples and the *meta* isomer in only one (Fielding *et al* 1981).

2.3 Toxicokinetics

Hawkins *et al* (1980) demonstrated that *para*-dichlorobenzene is readily absorbed in rats following oral or inhalation exposure, and is distributed primarily to the adipose tissue, liver, kidney and lungs.

In rats, almost all of an oral dose of *para*-dichlorobenzene was eliminated within 5 days, mostly in the urine. It was also reported that 50–60% of the dose had been excreted in the bile within 24 hours. Substantial entero-hepatic recirculation must therefore have taken place. The pattern of metabolites in the urine was similar after both inhalation and oral exposure. The principal products were sulphate and glucuronide conjugates of 2,5-dichlorophenol. Minor metabolites detected were a dihydroxydichlorobenzene and a dichlorobenzene-mercapturic acid. In another study, small amounts of 2,5-dichlorophenyl-methylsulphoxide and 2,5-dichlorophenylmethylsulphone were detected in the urine of rats treated with *para*-dichlorobenzene (Kimura *et al* 1979).

Similar results have been reported for the metabolism of all three isomers in rabbits (Azouz *et al* 1955, Parke and Williams 1955).

2.4 Health effects

2.4.1 Acute and subacute toxicity

The dichlorobenzenes are of relatively low acute toxicity in experimental animals. Oral LD50s of about 500 mg/kg have been reported in rats and rabbits, while much higher figures of 2950 mg/kg and 2800 mg/kg have been reported in mice and guinea-pigs respectively (World Health Organization 1980).

In Sprague–Dawley rats, intraperitoneal injection of either 1.33 mmol/kg (196 mg/kg) of *ortho*-dichlorobenzene or 1.31 mmol/kg (193 mg/kg) of *meta*-dichlorobenzene induced only limited hepatic necrosis. Pretreatment with phenobarbital markedly enhanced the hepatotoxic potential of these two compounds. Intraperitoneal injection of 3.4 mmol/kg (500 mg/kg) of *para*-dichlorobenzene had little effect on the liver. Pretreatment with phenobarbital was not found to enhance the hepatotoxicity of this isomer (Reid *et al* 1973). Hepatic porphyria was reported in rats given oral doses of 900–1000 mg/kg/day of *meta*-dichlorobenzene for 5 days (Poland *et al* 1971). A single oral dose of 800 mg/kg *para*-dichlorobenzene in day-old White Leghorn chicks has also been reported to increase hepatic and biliary porphyrin content (Miranda *et al* 1984).

Unlike *ortho*- and *para*-dichlorobenzene, the *meta* isomer has been shown to enhance liver aminopyrine demethylase and aniline hydroxylase activities in rats given oral doses of 250 mg/kg/day for 3 days. Hepatic cytochrome P-450 content was not altered significantly by treatment with any of the isomers, but hepatic delta-ALA synthetase activity was enhanced by 63, 32 and 42% by *ortho*-, *meta*- and *para*-dichlorobenzene respectively (Ariyoshi *et al* 1984).

Intraperitoneal injection of 5 mmol/kg (735 mg/kg) of *ortho*-dichlorobenzene in rats led to a marked stimulation of bile duct pancreatic fluid flow. This effect was not observed in rats given an identical dose of *para*-dichlorobenzene (Yang *et al* 1979).

There have been many reports in the literature of human poisonings by dichlorobenzene, and these have been reviewed before (United States Environmental Protection Agency 1980). Exposure to sublethal concentrations of dichlorobenzene often causes CNS depression and membrane irritation, though haematotoxicity, liver damage, sensitization and respiratory effects have also been reported.

2.4.2 Chronic toxicity

Slight liver cirrhosis and focal necrosis and elevated liver weight and kidney weight were found in rats dosed orally with 188 and 376 mg/kg of *para*-dichlorobenzene in olive oil, 5 days/week for 138 doses in 192 days. No adverse effects were seen at 18.8 mg/kg (Hollingsworth *et al* 1956). Similar results were found in an identical experiment with *ortho*-dichlorobenzene (Hollingsworth *et al* 1958). In a Russian study, groups of seven male rats were given 0.001, 0.01 and 0.1 mg/kg/day of *ortho*-dichlorobenzene by stomach tube for 9 months. At the high dose, inhibition of bone marrow mitosis and erythropoiesis, thrombocytosis and neutropenia were reported. Biochemical examination revealed increased serum transaminase and alkaline phosphatase levels and lowered liver and kidney alkaline phosphatase activity. No effects were observed at the lowest dose level (Varshavskaya 1968).

In Charles River rats, oral doses of 10–40 mg/kg/day of *para*-dichlorobenzene for 90 days was found to enhance the hepatic detoxification of *O*-ethyl *O*-*p*-nitrophenyl phenylphosphonothioate and to elevate hepatic microsomal benzopyrene hydroxylase and azoreductase activities (Carlson and Tardiff 1976).

Inhalation of 158 ppm of *para*-dichlorobenzene, 7 hours/day, 5 days/week for 5–7 months, was without effect in mice, rabbits and monkeys. Rats and guinea pigs were able to tolerate around 96 ppm without adverse effects. Exposure of rats, rabbits and guinea pigs to 173, 341, and 798 ppm of *para*-dichlorobenzene for up to 6 months produced pronounced toxic effects at the highest dose level, while increases in rat liver and kidney weights and changes in lung and liver histopathology were noted at the lower doses (United States Environmental Protection Agency 1980). No adverse effects were reported in rats, guinea pigs, rabbits and monkeys exposed by inhalation to 93 ppm of *ortho*-dichlorobenzene, 7 hours/day, 5 days/week for 6–7 months

(Hollingsworth *et al* 1958). In studies carried out by ICI (Loeser and Litchfield 1983), groups of 76–79 rats (Alderley Park strain) of both sexes, and groups of 75 female Swiss mice were exposed by inhalation to 75 and 500 ppm of *para*-dichlorobenzene, 5 hours/day, 5 days/week for 57 weeks (mice) or 76 weeks (rats). No treatment-related changes were found at either dose in mice or in the low-dose rats. However, rats exposed to 500 ppm exhibited elevated liver weight and kidney weight, slightly elevated heart and lung weights and slightly increased urinary protein and coproporphyrin output.

2.4.3 Genotoxicity

All three isomers gave negative results in the Ames test with *Salmonella typhimurium* TA98, TA100, TA1535 and TA1537, in both the presence and absence of metabolic activation, at doses ranging from 1.0–100 μg/plate (Haworth *et al* 1983). Unpublished experiments by ICI on *para*-dichlorobenzene found this compound to be non-mutagenic to the Ames strains TA98, TA100, TA1535 and TA1538 when tested in either the liquid or gaseous phase (Loeser and Litchfield 1983).

It has been reported in the US Federal Register (1984) that *ortho*-dichlorobenzene transformed adult rat liver epithelial cells *in vitro*, but was unable to induce unscheduled DNA synthesis in primary cultures of rat hepatocytes.

In a dominant lethal study, groups of 16 male CD-1 mice were exposed by inhalation to 75, 225 or 450 ppm of *para*-dichlorobenzene, 6 hours/day for 5 days. After exposure each male was mated with untreated females each week for 8 weeks. No significant increases were found in pre-implantation egg loss or post-implantation deaths. Fertility, measured by the percentage of female mice becoming pregnant, was also unaffected (Loeser and Litchfield 1983).

No increase in the frequency of bone marrow chromosomal aberrations was found in three *in vivo* cytogenetic experiments of *para*-dichlorobenzene in rats (Loeser and Litchfield 1983). The three types of exposure were:

(a) Inhalation of 299 or 682 ppm for 2 hours.
(b) Inhalation of 75 or 500 ppm, 5 hours/day for 5 days.
(c) Inhalation of 75 or 500 ppm, 5 hours/day, 5 days/week for 3 months.

A Mexican study found chromosomal aberrations in 8.9% of peripheral blood cells taken from 8 male and 18 female subjects who had been accidentally exposed to *ortho*-dichlorobenzene vapours for 4 days. Chromosomal aberrations were found in only 2.0% of cells of 11 unexposed subjects (Zapata-Gayon *et al* 1982).

There is some evidence that *para*-dichlorobenzene can cause genetic damage in plant systems (Srivastava 1966).

2.4.4 Carcinogenicity

The US National Toxicology Program has completed studies of *ortho*-dichlorobenzene and *para*-dichlorobenzene in rats and mice (National Academy of Science 1983, US National Toxicology Program 1985, 1986). Groups of 50 B6C3F1 mice and F-344 rats of both sexes were given doses of 60 or 120 mg/kg body-weight of *ortho*-dichlorobenzene in corn oil by gavage, 5 days/week for 2 years. No evidence for carcinogenicity was found. Groups of 50 B6C3F1 mice and F-344 rats of both sexes were given *para*-dichlorobenzene orally at doses of 150 or 300 mg/kg for male rats and 300 or 600 mg/kg for female rats and male and female mice. An increase in renal tubular cell adenocarcinomas was found in male mice and hepatocellular carcinomas and adenomas in male and female mice.

There was no evidence for increased tumour incidence in the long-term inhalation studies by ICI in mice and rats (Loeser and Litchfield 1983).

2.4.5 Reproductive toxicity

Hayes *et al* (1985) found no evidence for teratogenic effects in New Zealand White rabbits exposed by inhalation to 0, 100, 200 or 400 ppm of *ortho*-dichlorobenzene or 0, 100, 300 or 800 ppm of *para*-dichlorobenzene, 6 hours/day on days 6–18 of gestation. Depression of maternal body weight gain was noted in the high-dose group for both isomers. *Ortho*-dichlorobenzene gave similar results in F-344 rats.

Ruddick *et al* (1983) reported that all three isomers were non-teratogenic in an oral study in Sprague-Dawley rats at dose levels of 50, 100 and 200 mg/kg/day given on days 6–15 of gestation. These results were confirmed in rats given *para*-dichlorobenzen in corn oil at doses of 0–1000 mg/kg/day on days 6–15 of gestation (Giavini *et al* 1986).

Changes in sperm structure and morphology were observed in Sprague-Dawley rats given a single dose of 800 mg/kg of *para*-dichlorobenzene by intraperitoneal injection (Murthy and Doye 1984).

2.5 Discussion

The dichlorobenzenes have been identified in the atmosphere and in drinking water. There are insufficient data, however, to assess relative exposure.

These compounds appear to be readily absorbed by the gastrointestinal tract and distributed primarily to adipose tissue. In the liver, the dichlorobenzenes are metabolised to dichlorophenols and their conjugates.

The dichlorobenzenes have a relatively low order of acute and chronic toxic potential by both the oral and inhalation routes of exposure. They do not appear to be mutagenic in the Ames test and the *para*-isomer has also proved negative in a dominant lethal assay and a mouse bone marrow chromosomal aberration test. An oral carcinogenicity study of *ortho*-dichlorobenzene in rats and mice has given negative results. The positive result for carcinogenicity with para-dichlorobenzene must be interpreted with care in view of the tumour sites. None of the three isomers showed any evidence for teratogenicity and appeared to be of very low embryotoxic potential following oral administration in rats. Similar results were found in inhalation studies of the *ortho* and *para* isomers in rabbits and for the *ortho* isomer in rats.

References

AKIYAMA T, KOGA M, SHINOHARA R, KIDO A and ETOH S (1980) Detection and identification of trace organic substances in the aquatic environment. *Journal of Uoeh* **2**, 285-300.

ARIYOSHI T, IDEGUCHI K, IWASAKI K and ARAKAKI M (1984) Relationship between chemical structure and activity. II. Influences of isomers in dichlorobenzene, trichlorobenzene and tetrachlorobenzene on the activities of drug-metabolizing enzymes. *Chemical and Pharmaceutical Bulletin, Tokyo* **23**, 824-830.

AZOUZ W M, PARKE D V and WILLIAMS R T (1955) The metabolism of halogenobenzenes. *Ortho-* and *para*-dichlorobenzenes. *Biochemical Journal* **59**, 410-415.

CARLSON G P and TARDIFF R G (1976) Effect of chlorinated benzenes on the metabolism of foreign organic compounds. *Toxicology and Applied Pharmacology* **36**, 383-394.

FIELDING M, GIBSON T M, JAMES H A, McLOUGHLIN K and STEELE C P (1981) Organic micropollutants in drinking water. WRc Technical Report TR 159.

GIAVINI E, BROCCIA M L, PRATI M and VISMARA C (1986) Teratologic evaluation of *p*-dichlorobenzene in the rat. *Bulletin of Environmental Contamination and Toxicity* **37**, 164-168.

HAWKINS D R, CHASSEAUD L F, WOODHOUSE R N and CRESSWELL D G (1980) The distribution, excretion and biotransformation of ^{94}C-*p*-dichlorobenzene in rats after repeated inhalation, oral and subcutaneous doses. *Xenobiotica* **10**, 81-95.

HAWORTH S, LAWLOR T, MORTELMANS K, SPECK W and ZEIGER E (1983) Salmonella mutagenicity test results for 250 chemicals. *Environmental Mutagenesis* **5**, Suppl 1, 3-142.

HAYES W C, HANLEY T R Jr, GUSHOW T S, JOHNSON K A and JOHN J A (1985) Teratogenic potential of inhaled dichlorobenzenes in rats and rabbits. *Fundamental and Applied Toxicology* **5**, 190-202.

HOLLINGSWORTH R L, ROWE V K, OYEN F, HOYLE H R and SPENCER H C (1956) Toxicity of paradichlorobenzene. *AMA Archives of Industrial Health* **14**, 138-147.

HOLLINGSWORTH R L, ROWE V K, OYEN F, TORKELSON T R, and ADAMS E M (1958) Toxicity of *o*-dichlorobenzene. *AMA Archives of Industrial Health* **17**, 180-187.

HOLZER G, SHANFIELD H, ZLATKIS A, BERTSCH W, JUAREZ P, MAYFIELD H and LIEBICH H M (1977) Collection and analysis of trace organic emissions from natural sources. *Journal of Chromatography* **142**, 755-764.

KIMURA R, HAYASHI T, SATO M, AIMOTO T and MURATA T (1979) Identification of sulfur-containing metabolites of *p*-dichlorobenzene and their disposition in rats. *Journal of Pharmacobiodymamico* **2**, 237-244.

LOESER E and LITCHFIELD M H (1983) Review of recent toxicology studies on *p*-dichlorobenzene. *Food and Chemical Toxicology* **21**, 825-832.

MIRANDA C L, WANG J-L, HENDERSON M C, NAKAUE H S and BUHLER D R (1984) Effects of chlorobenzenes on hepatic porphyrin and drug metabolism in chick embryo and day-old chick. *Research Communications in Chemical Pathology and Pharmacology* **46**(1), 13-24.

MORITA M and OHI G (1975) *Para*-dichlorobenzene in human tissue and atmosphere in Tokyo metropolitan area. *Environmental Pollution* **8**, 269-274.

MORITA M, MIMURA S, OHI G and YAGYU H (1975) A systematic determination of chlorinated benzenes in human adipose tissue. *Environmental Pollution* **9**, 175-179.

MURTHY R C and DOYE A (1984) Changes in testes of rats exposed to *para*-dichlorobenzene. *Journal of the American College of Toxicology* **3**, 168.

NATIONAL ACADEMY OF SCIENCES (1977) Drinking water and health Vol 1. US National Academy of Sciences, Washington, DC.

NATIONAL ACADEMY OF SCIENCES (1983) Drinking Water and Health Vol 5. National Academy Press, Washington, DC.

PARKE D V and WILLIAMS R T (1955) The metabolism of halogenobenzenes. (a) *Meta*-dichlorobenzene. (b) Further observations on the metabolism of chlorobenzene. *Biochemical Journal* **59**, 415-422.

PEATTIE M E, LINDSAY D G and HOODLESS R A (1984) Dietary exposure of man to chlorinated benzenes in the United Kingdom. *Science of the Total Environment* **34**, 73-86.

POLAND A, GOLDSTEIN J, HICKMAN P and BURSE V W (1971) A reciprocal relationship between the induction of delta-aminolevulinic acid synthetase and drug metabolism produced by *m*-dichlorobenzene. *Biochemical Pharmacology* **20**, 1281-1290.

REID W D, KRISHNA G, GILLETTE J R and BRODIE B B (1973) Biochemical mechanism of hepatic necrosis induced by aromatic hydrocarbons. *Pharmacology* **10**, 193-214.

RUDDICK J A, BLACK W D, VILLENEUVE D C and VALLI V E (1983) A teratological evaluation following oral administration of trichloro- and dichlorobenzene isomers to the rat. *Teratology* **27**, 73A-74A.

SRIVASTAVA L M (1966) Induction of mitotic abnormalities in certain genera of tribe Vicieae by paradichlorobenzene. *Cytologia* **31**, 166-171.

US ENVIRONMENTAL PROTECTION AGENCY (1980) Ambient water quality criteria for dichlorobenzenes. US Department of Commerce NTIS No PB81-117509.

US FEDERAL REGISTER (1984) **49**, 18779-18780.

US NATIONAL TOXICOLOGY PROGRAM (1985) Toxicology and carcinogenesis studies of 1,2-dichlorobenzene in F-344/N rats and B6C3F1 mice (gavage studies). US National Toxicology Program, Technical Report No 255.

US NATIONAL TOXICOLOGY PROGRAM (1986) Toxicology and carcinogenesis studies of 1,4-dichlorobenzene in F-344/N rats and B6C3F1 mice (gavage studies). US National Toxicity Program, Technical Report No 319.

VARSHAVSKAYA S P (1968) Comparative toxicological characteristics of chlorobenzene and dichlorobenzene (*ortho*- and *para*-isomers) in relation to the sanitary protection of water bodies. *Gigiena i Sanitariia* **33**, 17-23.

VERSCHUEREN K (1977) *Handbook of environmental data on organic chemicals*. Van Nostrand Reinhold Company.

WARE S and WEST W L (1977) Investigation of selected potential environmental contaminants: halogenated benzenes, EPA 560/2-77-004.

WORLD HEALTH ORGANISZTION (1980) Toxicological appraisal of halogenated aromatic compounds following groundwater pollution. WHO, Copenhagen.

YANG K H, PETERSON R E and FUJIMOTO J M (1979) Increased bile-duct pancreatic fluid flow in benzene and halogenated benzene-treated rats. *Toxicology and Applied Pharmacology* **47**, 505-514.

ZAPATA-GAYON C, ZAPATA-GAYON N and GONZALEZ-ANGULO A (1982) Clastogenic chromosomal aberrations in 26 individuals exposed to *ortho* dichlorobenzene vapors in the National Medical Center in Mexico City. *Archives of Environmental Health* **37**, 231-235.

ZOETEMAN B C J, PIET G J, RUYGROK C T M and HEUVEL R V D (1974) Threshold odour concentrations in water of chemical substances. *RID-MEDEDELING* **74**-3.

3. TRICHLOROBENZENE

3.1 Introduction

Trichlorobenzene is used as a dielectric fluid, heat transfer medium, solvent, and as an intermediate in the manufacture of insecticides. It has been suggested that small quantities of trichlorobenzenes may be formed during water chlorination (United States Environmental Protection agency (1975).

CAS Reg. No. (1,2,4-isomer):	120-82-1
(1,3,5-isomer):	105-70-3
Molecular weight:	181.4
Boiling point:	209–213°C
Solubility:	<30 mg/l at 20°C (World Health Organization 1980)
Evaporative half life in water:	No data available
Threshold odour concentration in water:	0.005–0.05 mg/l (Zoeteman *et al* 1974).

3.2 Exposure

Trichlorobenzene isomers have been detected in water sources at concentrations of <0.005–13 μg/l (World Health Organization 1980, Akiyama *et al* 1980). The survey by the WRc identified a trichlorobenzene isomer in only one of the 14 drinking water samples examined (Fielding *et al* 1981).

No information could be found concerning the occurrence of this compound in the atmosphere or in food.

3.3 Toxicokinetics

The trichlorobenzenes appear to be readily absorbed by the gastrointestinal tract and distributed primarily to the adipose tissue. They may undergo extensive enterohepatic recirculation (Lingg *et al* 1982).

In rabbits, the major urinary metabolites of trichlorobenzenes are trichlorophenols, 3,4,5-trichlorocatechol and mercapturic acid derivatives (Jondorf *et al* 1955, Kohli *et al* 1976). In rats, 1,2,4-trichlorobenzene is metabolised primarily to 2,3,5- and 2,4,5-trichlorobenzene mercapturic acids. Smaller quantities of trichlorothiophenols and trichlorophenols are also found in the urine (Lingg *et al* 1982). Glucuronide conjugates of two isomers of 3,4,6-trichloro-3,5-cyclo-hexadien-1,2-diol were the principal urinary metabolites of 1,2,4-trichlorobenzene in rhesus monkeys (Lingg *et al* 1982). The presence of mercapturic acids in the urine of rats and rabbits and the dihydrodiol in the urine of rhesus monkeys suggests that reactive arene oxides are important intermediates in the metabolism of trichlorobenzenes.

Rats given an oral dose of 10 mg/kg of ^{14}C-labelled 1,2,4-trichlorobenzene excreted 84% of the dose in the urine and 11% in the faeces by 24 hours (Lingg *et al* 1982). In a similar experiment with rhesus monkeys, only about 40% of the dose was excreted in the urine and <1% in the faeces by 24 hours (Lingg *et al* 1982). Similar qualitative results with some quantitative differences were obtained by Tanaka *et al* (1986) in studies with ^{14}C-labelled 1,2,4-trichlorobenzene in rats. They also presented evidence for reductive dechlorination of 1,2,4-trichlorobenzene by gut microflora
in vivo.

3.4 Health effects

3.4.1 Acute and subacute toxicity

Trichlorobenzenes are of relatively low acute toxicity in experimental animals. Oral LD50s in rodents range from 300 to 800 mg/kg (Brown *et al* 1969, Yamamoto *et al* 1978).

Lethargy and retarded weight gain were reported in rats exposed by inhalation to 200 ppm of 1,2,4-trichlorobenzene, 6 hours/day for 15 days. Similar effects were found in rats exposed to 70 ppm, though no signs of toxicity were evident at 20 ppm. No histopathological changes were found at any concentration (Gage 1970). Female rats given 250 or 500 mg/kg/day of 1,2,4-trichlorobenzene by intraperitoneal injection for 3 days exhibited elevated liver weight and adrenal weight. Lowered body weight and uterus weight were also reported, but there was no evidence that 1,2,4-trichlorobenzene had oestrogenic activity (Robinson *et al* 1981). In rhesus monkeys, daily oral doses of 173.6 mg/kg were lethal within 20–30 days. Doses of up to 25 mg/kg were without effect (Smith *et al* 1978).

A single oral dose of 200 mg/kg of 1,2,4-trichlorobenzene was found markedly to enhance hepatic porphyrins in both adult male Japanese quail and day-old White Leghorn chicks. In a further study, Japanese quail given oral doses of 50 or 200 mg/kg/day for 8 days also exhibited induction of a number of liver constituents and enzymes involved in haem biochemistry and drug metabolism (Miranda *et al* 1983b). Several other studies have shown that 1,2,4-trichlorobenzene readily induces hepatic mixed function oxidase activity (Ariyoshi *et al* 1975, Carlson and Tardiff 1976, Carlson 1978, Miranda 1983a, Miranda 1984). The 1,2,3- and 1,3,5-isomers do not appear to be as potent as the 1,2,4-isomer in this respect (Ariyoshi *et al* 1975).

Intraperitoneal injection of 5 mmol/kg (905 mg/kg) of 1,2,4-trichlorobenzene in rats was found to increase bile-duct pancreatic fluid flow but had no effect on plasma alanine aminotransferase activity. However, in rats given the same dose of 1,3,5-trichlorobenzene, plasma alanine aminotransferase activity was elevated, while there was little effect on bile-duct pancreatic fluid flow (Yang *et al* 1979).

3.4.2 Chronic toxicity

In a comprehensive multigeneration study, Charles River rats were exposed to 1,2,4-trichlorobenzene in their drinking water from birth of the F(0) generation to weaning of the F(2) generation at concentrations of 0, 25, 100 or 400 mg/l. No effects were found on fertility, growth, viability, locomotor activity or blood parameters of either the F(0), F(1) or F(2) generations. Slightly elevated adrenal weights, however, were reported in the F(0) and F(1) generations at 95 days of age at the high dose (Robinson *et al* 1981).

Hepatic cytochrome P-450 and cytochrome *c* reductase were induced by 1,2,4-trichlorobenzene in a 90-day study in which rats were given daily oral doses of 10–40 mg/kg. A slight increase in liver weight/body weight ratio was found at 40 mg/kg but no changes in haemoglobin, haematocrit or liver histopathology were evident at any dose level (Carlson and Tardiff 1976). Daily oral doses of 1–25 mg/kg of 1,2,4-trichlorobenzene for 120 days did not produce any evidence of toxicity in rhesus monkeys. At 125 mg/kg, temporary body-weight loss and some induction of cytochrome P-450 were found (Cragg *et al* 1978).

Histopathological changes were found in the liver and kidney of rats exposed by inhalation to 25, 50 and 100 ppm of 1,2,4-trichlorobenzene, 7 hours/day, 5 days/week, for 4 or 13 weeks. No treatment-related effects were observed in either rats, rabbits or monkeys exposed to 25, 50 or 100 ppm for 26 weeks (Coate *et al* 1977). Rats, rabbits and dogs exposed by inhalation to 30 or 100 ppm of 1,2,4-trichlorobenzene, 7 hours/day, 5 days/week for 30 exposures in 44 days did not exhibit changes in body weight, haematology, clinical chemistry or histopathology. At the high dose, however, there was elevated liver weight in rats and dogs and elevated kidney weight in rats. Increased urinary excretion of uroporphyrin and coproporphyrin was found in rats at both 30 and 100 ppm (Watanabe *et al* 1978, Kociba *et al* 1981). Urinary excretion of porphyrins was also elevated in rats exposed to 10 ppm of 1,2,4-trichlorobenzene for 90 days but not at 3 ppm (Watanabe *et al* 1978). A 90-day inhalation study of 1,3,5-trichlorobenzene in CD rats failed to show significant changes in haematology, clinical chemistry or histopathology at 1.3, 13 or 130 ppm (Sasmore *et al* 1983). In a Polish study, body weight loss and lowered white blood cell counts were found in Swiss mice exposed by inhalation to 0.02 mg/l of trichlorobenzene, 7 hours/day for 3 months (Zub 1978).

3.4.3 Genotoxicity

All three trichlorobenzene isomers have given negative results in the Ames test with *Salmonella typhimurium* TA98, TA100, TA1535 and TA1537, both in the presence and absence of metabolic activation (Schoeny *et al* 1979, Haworth *et al* 1983). The 1,2,3- and 1,2,4-isomers were found to be toxic to the bacteria at concentrations above 100 μg/plate (Haworth *et al* 1983).

It has been reported in the US Federal Register (United States Federal Register 1984) that 1,2,4-trichlorobenzene transformed rat liver epithelial cells *in vitro* but was unable to induce unscheduled DNA synthesis in primary cultures of rat hepatocytes.

No evidence for genotoxicity of 1,3,5-trichlorobenzene was found in a *Drosophila* sex-linked recessive lethal test (Zimmering *et al* 1985).

3.4.4 Carcinogenicity

No information appears to be available.

3.4.5 Reproductive toxicity

There was no evidence of teratogenic effects in groups of Sprague–Dawley rats given oral doses of 75, 150 and 300 mg/kg of 1,2,4-trichlorobenzene or 150, 300 and 600 mg/kg of 1,2,3- and 1,3,5-trichlorobenzene on days 6–15 of gestation (Ruddick *et al* 1983). The absence of teratogenic effects was also found in another study in which Sprague–Dawley rats were given oral doses of 36, 120, 360 and 1200 mg/kg of 1,2,4-trichlorobenzene on days 9–13 of gestation. There was some evidence of delayed growth at 360 mg/kg but maternal deaths occurred in both the 360 mg/kg (2/6) and 1200 mg/kg (6/6) groups (Kitchin and Ebson 1983).

Robinson *et al* (1981) did not report any effects on fertility in rats exposed to 0, 25, 100 or 400 mg/l of 1,2,4-trichlorobenzene in their drinking water from birth of the F(0) generation to weaning of the F(2) generation.

3.5 Discussion

Trichlorobenzenes have been detected in water on several occasions but no information could be found on levels in food or in the atmosphere.

These compounds are readily absorbed by the gastrointestinal tract and distributed primarily to the adipose tissue. The route of metabolism for trichlorobenzenes varies with species. Rats appear to eliminate an oral dose somewhat more quickly than monkeys.

Trichlorobenzenes are of relatively low acute and chronic toxicity in experimental animals. Most of the information relates to the 1,2,4-isomer, which is a potent inducer of hepatic mixed function oxidase activity. Trichlorobenzenes do not appear to be mutagenic in the Ames test, but there are only limited data available in higher test systems. No information appears to be available on carcinogenicity. These compounds do not appear to be teratogenic in rats, and a multigeneration study of 1,2,4-trichlorobenzene failed to observe effects on reproduction at concentrations of up to 400 mg/l in drinking water.

References

AKIYAMA T, KOGA M, SHINOHARA R, KIDO A and ETOH S (1980) Detection and identification of trace organic substances in the aquatic environment. *Journal of Uoeh* **2**, 285-300.

ARIYOSHI T, IDEGUCHI K, IWASAKI K and ARAKAKI M (1975) Relationship between chemical structure and activity. II. Influences of isomers in dichlorobenzene, trichlorobenzene and tetrachlorobenzene on the activities of drug-metabolizing enzymes. *Chemical and Pharmaceutical Bulletin, Tokyo* **23**, 824-830.

BROWN V K H, MUIR C and THORPE E (1969) The acute toxicity and skin irritant properties of 1,2,4-trichlorobenzene. *Annals of Occupational Hygiene* **12**, 209-212.

CARLSON G P (1978) Induction of cytochrome P-450 by halogenated benzenes. *Biochemical Pharmacology* **27**, 361-363.

CARLSON G P and TARDIFF R G (1976) Effect of chlorinated benzenes on the metabolism of foreign organic compounds. *Toxicology and Applied Pharmacology* **36**, 383-394.

COATE W B, SHOENFISCH W H, LEWIS T R and BUSEY W M (1977) Chronic inhalation exposures of rats, rabbits, and monkeys to 1,2,4-trichlorobenzene. *Archives of Environmental Health* **32**, 249-255.

CRAGG S T, WOLFF G F and SMITH C C (1978) Toxicity of 1,2,4-trichlorobenzene in rhesus monkeys: Comparison of two in vivo methods for estimating P-450 activity. *Toxicology and Applied Pharmacology* **45**, 340.

FIELDING M, GIBSON T M, JAMES H A, McLOUGHLIN K and STEELE C P (1981) Organic micropollutants in drinking water. WRc Technical Report TR 159.

GAGE J C (1970) The subacute inhalation toxicity of 109 industrial chemicals. *British Journal of Industrial Medicine* **27**, 1-18.

HAWORTH S, LAWLOR T, MORTELMANS K, SPECK W and ZEIGER E (1983) Salmonella mutagenicity test results for 250 chemicals. *Environmental Mutagenesis* **5**, Suppl 1, 3-142.

JONDORF W R, PARKE D V and WILLIAMS R T (1955) The metabolism of halogenobenzenes. 1:2:3-, 1:2:4- and 1:3:5- trichlorobenzenes. *Biochemical Journal* **61**, 512-521.

KITCHIN K T and EBRON M T (1983) Maternal hepatic and embryonic effects of 1,2,4-trichlorobenzene in the rat. *Environmental Research* **31**, 362-373.

KOCIBA R J, LEONG B K J and HEFNER R E Jr (1981) Subchronic toxicity study of 1,2,4-trichlorobenzene in the rat, rabbit and beagle dog. *Drug and Chemical Toxicology* **4**, 229-249.

KOHLI J, JONES D and SAFE, S (1976) The metabolism of higher chlorinated benzene isomers. *Canadian Journal of Biochemistry* **54**, 203-208.

LINGG R D, KAYLOR W H, PYLE S M, KOPFLER F C, SMITH C C, WOLFE G F and CRAGG S (1982) Comparative metabolism of 1,2,4-trichlorobenzene in the rat and rhesus monkey. *Drug Metabolism and Disposition* **10**, 134-141.

MIRANDA C L, WANG J-L, HENDERSON M C, CARPENTER H M, NAKAUE H S and BUHLER D R (1983a) Differential induction of hepatic drug metabolizing enzymes in Japanese quail by 1,2,4-trichlorobenzene. *Toxicology* **28**, 75-82.

MIRANDA C L, WANG J-L, HENDERSON M C, CARPENTER H M, NAKAUE H S and BUHLER D R (1983b) Studies on the porphyrinogenic action of 1,2,4-trichlorobenzene in birds. *Toxicology* **28**, 83-92.

MIRANDA C L, WANG J-L, HENDERSON M C, NAKAUE H S and BUHLER D R (1984) Effects of chlorobenzenes on hepatic porphyrin and drug metabolism in chick embryo and day-old chick. *Research Communications in Chemical Pathology and Pharmacology* **46**, 13-24.

ROBINSON K S, KAVLOCK R J, CHERNOFF N and GRAY L E (1981) Multigeneration study of 1,2,4-trichlorobenzene in rats. *Journal of Toxicology and Environmental Health* **8**, 489-500.

RUDDICK J A , BLACK W D, VILLENEUVE D C and VALLI V E (1983) A teratological evaluation following oral administration of trichloro- and dichlorobenzene isomers to the rat. *Teratology* **27**, 73A-74A.

SASMORE D P, MITOMA C, TYSON C A and JOHNSON J S (1983) Subchronic inhalation toxicity of 1,3,5-trichlorobenzene. *Drug and Chemical Toxicology* **6**, 241-258.

SCHOENY R S , SMITH C C and LOPER J C (1979) Non-mutagenicity for

Salmonella of the chlorinated hydrocarbons Aroclor 1254, 1,2,4-trichlorobenzene, Mirex and Kepone. *Mutation Research* **68**, 125-132.
SMITH C C, CRAGG S T and WOLFE G F (1978) Subacute toxicity of 1,2,4-trichlorobenzene in sub-human primates. *Federation Proceedings* **37**, 248.
TANAKA A, SATO M, TSUCHIYA T, ADACHI T, NIIMURA T and YAMAHA T (1986) Excretion, distribution and metabolism of 1,2,4-trichlorobenzene in rats. *Archives of Toxicology* **59**, 82-88.
US ENVIRONMENTAL PROTECTION AGENCY (1975) Identification of organic compounds in effluents from industrial sources. EPA.
US FEDERAL REGISTER (1984) **49**, 18779-18780.
WATANABE P G, KOCIBA R J, HEFNER R E Jr, YAKEL H O and LEONG B K J (1978) Subchronic toxicity studies of 1,2,4-trichlorobenzene in experimental animals. *Toxicology and Applied Pharmacology* **45**, 332-33.
WORLD HEALTH ORGANIZATION (1980) Toxicological appraisal of halogenated aromatic compounds following groundwater pollution. WHO, Copenhagen.
YAMAMOTO H, TANIGUCHI Y, IMAI S, OHNO Y and TSUBURA Y (1978) Acute toxicity and local irritation tests of trichlorobenzene. *Journal of the Nara Medical Association* **29**, 569-73.
YANG K H, PETERSON R E and FUJIMOTO J M (1979) Increased bile-duct pancreatic fluid flow in benzene and halogenated benzene-treated rats. *Toxicology and Applied Pharmacology* **47**, 505-514.
ZIMMERING S, MASON J M, VALENCIA R and WOODRUFF R C (1985) Chemical mutagenesis testing in *Drosophila*. II. Results of 20 coded compounds tested for the National Toxicology Program. *Environmental Mutagenesis* **7**, 87-100.
ZOETEMAN B C J, PIET G J, RUYGROK C T M and HEUVEL R V D (1974) Threshold odour concentrations in water of chemical substances. RID-MEDEDELING 74-3.
ZUB M (1978) Reactivity of the white blood cell system to toxic action of benzene and its derivatives. *Acta Biologica Cracoviensia Serie Zoologica* **21**, 163-174.

4. TETRACHLOROBENZENE

4.1 Introduction

This compound is an important intermediate in the synthesis of 2,4,5-trichlorophenol. Tetrachlorobenzene is a metabolite of hexachlorobenzene and lindane. The use of such pesticides may represent an important source of tetrachlorobenzene in the environment.

CAS Reg No (1,2,4,5 isomer):	95-94-3
Molecular weight:	215.9
Boiling point (1,2,4,5 isomer):	246°C
(1,2,3,4 isomer):	254°C
Solubility (1,2,3,4 isomer):	0.16–0.36 mg/l
	(Verschueren 1977)

Evaporative half-life in water:	No data available
Threshold odour concentration in water:	0.01–0.4 mg/l (Zoeteman *et al* 1974).

4.2 Exposure

In the WRc survey, two tetrachlorobenzene isomers were identified in one of the 14 drinking water samples tested (Fielding *et al* 1981).

Tetrachlorobenzenes have been detected in human adipose tissue in Japan (Morita *et al* 1975).

4.3 Toxicokinetics

The metabolism of tetrachlorobenzenes has been studied in rats (Chu *et al* 1984a), rabbits (Jondorf *et al* 1958, Kohli *et al* 1976) and squirrel monkeys (Schwartz *et al* 1985).

In rats, the major metabolites of all three isomers are tetrachlorophenols. Smaller quantities of dechlorinated products, such as trichlorophenols, are also formed. About 50% of oral doses of either 1,2,3,4- or 1,2,3,5-tetrachlorobenzene was excreted within 24 hours. However, only 8% of an oral dose of 1,2,4,5-tetrachlorobenzene was excreted in the same time. The metabolites of 1,2,4,5-tetrachlorobenzene were found largely in the urine, while those of the 1,2,3,5-isomer were present largely in the faeces. The metabolites of the 1,2,3,4-isomer were excreted in similar quantities in both the urine and faeces (Chu *et al* 1984a).

Metabolism in rabbits (Jondorf *et al* 1958, Kohli *et al* 1976) is similar to the rat, but the major urinary metabolite of 1,2,3,4-tetrachlorobenzene in monkeys was *N*-acetyl-*S*-(2,3,4,5-tetrachlorophenyl)cysteine, a modified glutathione conjugate (Schwartz *et al* 1985).

4.4 Health effects

4.4.1 Acute and subacute toxicity

Oral LD50s for tetrachlorobenzenes in the rat and mouse range from 1 to 3 g/kg (World Health Organization 1980, Chu *et al* 1983).

In a subacute study (Chu *et al* 1983), groups of 10 male and 10 female Sprague–Dawley rats were fed diets containing 0.5, 5, 50 or 500 ppm (equivalent to about 0.05, 0.5, 5 and 50 mg/kg body weight/day) of 1,2,3,4-, 1,2,4,5- or 1,2,3,5-tetrachlorobenzene for 28 days. There were no deaths or clinical signs of toxicity in the study. Growth rates and food consumption were also unaffected by the treatment. In animals fed the 1,2,4,5-isomer at 500 ppm, moderate to severe histopathological changes were found in the liver, thyroid, kidneys and lungs. Only mild changes were found at this dose with the 1,2,3,4- and 1,2,3,5-isomers. All three isomers were able to induce hepatic microsomal aminopyrine demethylase activity at 500 ppm. Only the 1,2,4,5-isomer also produced a significant increase in the activity of this enzyme at 50 ppm. The 1,2,4,5-isomer was also found to increase liver weight and serum cholesterol and to induce hepatic microsomal aniline hydroxylase and ethoxyresorufin deethylase activities at 500 ppm. Analysis of tissues revealed that the 1,2,4,5-isomer had been accumulated to much higher levels than the 1,2,3,4- and

1,2,3,5-isomers. This could explain the apparently greater subacute toxic potential of 1,2,4,5-tetrachlorobenzene compared to the 1,2,3,4- and 1,2,3,5-isomers.

Induction of hepatic aminopyrine demethylase and cytochrome P-450, but no effects on aniline hydroxylase activity, were found in rats given oral doses of 250 mg/kg/day for 3 days of either 1,2,3,4-, 1,2,3,5- or 1,2,4,5-tetrachlorobenzene (Ariyoshi *et al* 1975).

4.4.2 Chronic toxicity

Chu *et al* (1984b) fed groups of 15 male and 15 female Sprague–Dawley rats with diets containing 0, 0.5, 5, 50 or 500 ppm of 1,2,3,4-, 1,2,4,5- or 1,2,3,5-tetrachlorobenzene for 90 days. Growth rate and food consumption were not affected by the treatment. The 1,2,4,5-isomer caused elevated liver and kidney weights, elevated serum cholesterol and lowered haemoglobin and haematocrit at 500 ppm. Induction of hepatic microsomal aminopyrine demethylase and aniline hydroxylase activities were reported at both 50 and 500 ppm. Histological changes in the tissues were similar in type and severity to those found in the subacute study (Chu *et al* 1983). Dose-related accumulation in the liver and fat was also reported for 1,2,4,5-tetrachlorobenzene, but little accumulation was found with the 1,2,3,4- and 1,2,3,5-isomers.

Doses of 5 mg/kg/day of 1,2,4,5-tetrachlorobenzene were given in the diet to 2 male and 2 female beagle dogs for 2 years followed by a 20-month recovery period. Although all the clinical chemistry parameters measured were normal after 18 months of treatment, there were slight elevations in serum alkaline phosphatase activity and total bilirubin at 24 months. These parameters had also returned to normal levels within 3 months of cessation of exposure. Histopathological examination of the dogs after the 20-month recovery period did not reveal any treatment-related changes (Braun *et al* 1978).

In a Russian study, 1,2,4,5-tetrachlorobenzene was reported to produce neurotoxic changes in rats and to decrease liver function in rats and rabbits (Fomenko 1965).

4.4.3 Genotoxicity

All three tetrachlorobenzene isomers were non-mutagenic in the Ames test with *Salmonella typhimurium* TA98, TA100, TA1535 and TA1537, either in the presence or absence of rat liver or hamster liver S-9. Toxicity to the tester strains was found at 33 ug/plate for the 1,2,3,4-isomer and at 20 μg/plate for the 1,2,3,5-isomer. The 1,2,4,5-isomer appeared to be non-toxic at concentrations up to 1333 μg/plate (Haworth *et al* 1983).

4.4.4 Carcinogenicity

No information appears to be available.

4.4.5 Reproductive toxicity

No evidence for teratogenicity was found for 1,2,4,5-, 1,2,3,4- and 1,2,3,5-tetrachlorobenzene in Sprague–Dawley rats given oral doses of 50, 100 or 200 mg/kg in corn oil on days 6–15 of gestation. In the dams, the 1,2,4,5-isomer induced mortality in 9/10 animals at 200 mg/kg while elevated serum cholesterol and hepatic mixed function oxidase activities were apparent at 50 and 100 mg/kg. A decrease in the number of foetuses was found at 50 mg/kg with the 1,2,4,5-isomer and at 200 mg/kg for the 1,2,3,4- and 1,2,3,5-isomers. The 1,2,4,5-isomer accumulated in foetal tissues in a dose-dependent manner, with the highest concentrations occurring in the liver and brain. In general, the 1,2,3,4- and 1,2,3,5-isomers were not found to accumulate in foetal tissues (Kacew *et al* 1984).

The toxicity of 1,2,4,5-tetrachlorobenzene to the dams in the above study (Kacew *et al* 1984) appears to conflict with that observed in another study (Kitchin and Ebron 1983a). In this case, no maternal deaths were reported in Sprague–Dawley rats given oral doses of 0, 30, 100, 300 or 1000 mg/kg/day in gum tragacanth on days 9–13 of gestation. Neither were there any effects on maternal liver weight/body weight ratio at any dose level, and body weight gain was decreased only at 1000 mg/kg. Induction of maternal hepatic mixed function oxidase activity was present at all dose levels, while slight hepatic centrilobular hypertrophy was found at 1000 mg/kg. No teratogenic or embryotoxic effects were reported.

In a study of 1,2,3,4-tetrachlorobenzene, Sprague–Dawley rats were given oral doses of 0, 100, 300 or 1000 mg/kg/day in gum tragacanth on days 9–13 of gestation. At the high dose, a number of dams died and there was a decrease in maternal body weight gain in survivors. Some induction of maternal hepatic mixed function oxidase activity was found at 300 and 1000 mg/kg. At 300 mg/kg there were a number of embryotoxic effects, including decreased crown–rump length, head length and yolk sac diameter, and inhibition of growth (Kitchin and Ebron 1983b).

4.5 Discussion

There is very little information on the occurrence of tetrachlorobenzenes in the environment.

In rats and rabbits, tetrachlorobenzenes are metabolised primarily to tetrachlorophenols and smaller quantities of dechlorinated products. In monkeys the principal urinary metabolite of 1,2,3,4-tetrachlorobenzene was a glutathione conjugate. In the rat, 1,2,4,5-tetrachlorobenzene was metabolised far more slowly than the 1,2,3,4- and 1,2,3,5-isomers.

Both 28-day and 90-day studies in rats have shown that the 1,2,4,5-isomer is of greater toxic potential than the 1,2,3,4- and 1,2,3,5-isomers. This would appear to be due to the much longer biological half-life of this compound compared to the other two isomers. The limited data available suggest that this compound is non-mutagenic in the Ames test, but there are no data in higher test systems. A carcinogenicity study has yet to be carried out on any of the tetrachlorobenzene isomers. The tetrachlorobenzenes have given negative results for teratogenicity and are of low embryotoxic potential in rats.

However, two studies appear to have given different results with respect to the effect of the 1,2,4,5-isomer in the dams.

Although the 1,2,3,4- and 1,2,3,5-isomers do not appear to present a risk to human health at the low concentrations encountered in drinking water, the possibility of accumulation of the 1,2,4,5-isomer indicates that further studies would be desirable in this case.

References

ARIYOSHI T, IDEGUCHI K, IWASAKI, K and ARAKAKI M (1975) Relationship between chemical structure and activity. II. Influences of isomers in dichlorobenzene, trichlorobenzene and tetrachlorobenzene on the activities of drug-metabolizing enzymes. *Chemical and Pharmaceutical Bulletin, Tokyo* **23**, 824-830.

BRAUN W H, SUNG L Y, KEYES D G and KOCIBA R J (1978) Pharmacokinetic and toxicological evaluation of dogs fed 1,2,4,5-tetrachlorobenzene in the diet for two years. *Journal of Toxicology and Environmental Health* **4**, 727-734.

CHU I, VILLENEUVE D, SECOURS V and VALLI V E (1983) Comparative toxicity of 1,2,3,4-, 1,2,4,5-, and 1,2,3,5- tetrachlorobenzene in the rat. *Journal of Toxicology and Environmental Health* **11**, 663-677.

CHU I, VILLENEUVE D C, VIAU A, BARNES C R, BENOIT F M and QIN Y H (1984a) Metabolism of 1,2,3,4-, 1,2,3,5-, and 1,2,4,5-tetrachlorobenzene in the rat. *Journal of Toxicology and Environmental Health* **13**, 777-786.

CHU I, VILLENEUVE D C, VALLI V E and SECOURS V E (1984b) Toxicity of 1,2,3,4-, 1,2,3,5- and 1,2,4,5-tetrachlorobenzene in the rat: Results of a 90-day feeding study. *Drug and Chemical Toxicology* **7**, 113-127.

FIELDING M, GIBSON T M, JAMES HA A, McLOUGHLIN K and STEELE C P (1981) Organic micropollutants in drinking water. Technical Report TR 159.

FOMENKO V N (1965) Determination of the maximum permissible concentration of tetrachlorobenzene in water basins. *Hygiene and Sanitation* **30**, 8-15.

HAWORTH S, LAWLOR T, MORTELMANS K, SPECK W and ZEIGER E (1983) Salmonella mutagenicity test results for 250 chemicals. *Environmental Mutagenesis* **5**, Suppl 1, 3-142.

JONDORF W R, PARKE D V and WILLIAMS R T (1958) The metabolism of halogenobenzenes. 1:2:3:4-, 1:2:3:5- and 1:2:4:5- tetrachlorobenzenes. *Biochemical Journal* **69**, 181-189.

KACEW S, RUDDICK J A, PARULEKAR M, VALLI V E, CHU I, and VILLENEUVE D C (1984) A teratological evaluation and analysis of fetal tissue levels following administration of tetrachlorobenzene isomers to the rat. *Teratology* **29**, 21-27.

KITCHIN K T and EBRON M T (1983a) Maternal hepatic effects of 1,2,4,5-tetrachlorobenzene in the rat. *Environmental Research* **32**, 134-144.

KITCHIN K T and EBRON M T (1983b) Maternal hepatic and embryonic effects of 1,2,3,4-tetrachlorobenzene in the rat. *Toxicology* **26**, 243-256.

KOHLI J, JONES D and SAFE S (1976) The metabolism of higher chlorinated benzene isomers. *Canadian Journal of Biochemistry* **54**, 203-208.

MORITA M, MIMURA S, OHI G, YAGYU H and NISHIZAWA T (1975) A systematic determination of chlorinated benzenes in human adipose tissue. *Environmental Pollution* **9**, 175-179.

SCHWARTZ H, CHU I, VILLENEUVE D C, VIAU A and BENOIT F M (1985) Metabolites of 1,2,3,4-tetrachlorobenzene in monkey urine. *Journal of Toxicology and Environmental Health* **15**, 603-607.

VERSCHUEREN K (1977) *Handbook of environmental data on organic chemicals*. Van Nostrand Reinhold Company.

WORLD HEALTH ORGANIZATION (1980) Toxicological appraisal of haloge-

nated aromatic compounds following groundwater pollution. WHO, Copenhagen.
ZOETEMAN B C J, PIET G J, RUYGROK C T M and HEUVEL R V D (1974) Threshold odour concentrations in water of chemical substances. RID-MEDEDELING 74-3.

5. CHLOROTOLUENE

5.1 Introduction
The 2-chlorotoluene isomer is used as a solvent and as an intermediate in the manufacture of pesticides, pharmaceuticals and dyes.

CAS Reg No (2-isomer):	95-49-8
(3-isomer):	108-41-8
(4-isomer):	106-43-4
Molecular weight:	126.6
Boiling point:	159–166°C
Solubility:	No data available
Evaporative half-life in water:	No data available
Threshold odour concentration in water:	No data available

5.2 Exposure
A chlorotoluene isomer was identified in 1/14 drinking water samples in an unpublished survey by WRc (Water Research Centre 1982). An unspecified chlorotoluene isomer has also been detected at low μg/l levels in the Delaware river, USA (Sheldon and Hites 1978).

5.3 Toxicokinetics
Following an oral dose of 1 g/kg of 2-chlorotoluene in rats, only trace amounts remained in the tissues 4 days after dosing. Most of the dose, 85–92%, was excreted in the urine while 5–8% appeared in the faeces and 1.4% was eliminated in the expired air. The major urinary metabolites were derived from oxidation of the methyl group and were 2-chlorohippuric acid, a glucuronide conjugate of 2-chlorobenzylalcohol, and a mercapturic acid derivative (Quistad *et al* 1983). Similar results have been reported in rats given an oral dose of 320 mg/kg (Wold and Emmerson 1974).

5.4 Health effects
It has been reported in the US Federal Register (United States Federal Register 1982) that 2-chlorotoluene gave negative results in the mouse lymphoma forward mutation assay, and in cytogenetic assays in Chinese hamster ovary cells and rat bone marrow.

The results of reproductive studies have also been reported in the US Federal Register (1983a, b). No evidence for teratogenicity was found in rabbits exposed by inhalation to concentrations of up to 10 mg/l or in rats at concentrations of up to 9 mg/l. Maternal toxicity was noted in rabbits at 4 mg/l and 10 mg/l. An increased incidence of skeletal abnormalities was evident in rats at 9 mg/l.

5.5 Discussion

There is insufficient toxicological information for chlorotoluene on which to base an assessment.

References

QUISTAD G B, MULHOLLAND K M and JAMIESON G C (1983) 2-Chlorotoluene metabolism by rats. *Journal of Agricultural and Food Chemistry* **31**, 1158-1162.

SHELDON L S and HITES R A (1978) Organic compounds in the Delaware river. *Environmental Science and Technology* **12**, 1188-1194.

US FEDERAL REGISTER (1982) **47(2**31), 54160-54161.

US FEDERAL REGISTER (1983a) **48**(87), 20132-20133.

US FEDERAL REGISTER (1983b) **48**(228), 53159-53162.

WATER RESEARCH CENTRE (1982) Frequency of occurrence data for compounds identified by GC-MS in XAD-2 samples taken for mutagenic testing survey. WRc Unpublished Report.

WOLD J S and EMMERSON J L The metabolism of 14C *o*-chlorotoluene in the rat. *Pharmacologist* **16**, 196.

6. CHLOROXYLENE

A chloroxylene isomer was identified in 1/14 drinking water samples in an unpublished survey by WRc (Water Research Centre 1982). There appears to be no information available on the environmental occurrence, metabolism or toxicity of chloroxylenes.

Reference

WATER RESEARCH CENTRE (1982) Frequency of occurrence data for compounds identified by GC-MS in XAD-2 samples taken for mutagenic testing survey. WRc Unpublished Report.

7

The halogenated aliphatic compounds

1. THE SATURATED HALOGENATED ALIPHATICS

1.1 Introduction

A group of 48 saturated halogenated aliphatics were identified in surveys of UK drinking water by WRc (Water Research Centre 1981, 1982). The most commonly occurring compounds were the trihalomethanes, and these also tended to occur in the highest concentrations. The trihalomethanes have been reviewed separately. Of the remaining compounds, the halogenated methanes and ethanes are highly volatile and are widely used in industry, hence, air is likely to be a more important source than water of exposure to these compounds. However, the higher molecular weight members of the group are used less extensively and therefore water may be the only source of exposure in these cases.

As a consequence of their industrial usage there is toxicological information available on the halogenated methanes and ethanes. However, there are generally very little toxicological data available for the higher members of this group.

There appears to be no information at all on the metabolism or toxicology of the following compounds:

Chloroiodomethane
Dibromodichloromethane
Bromopentachloroethane
1,1,1-Trichloro-2-methylpropane
2-Bromo-1-chlorobutane
Dichloromethylbutane
Chloropentane
Bromochloropentane
Dichloropentane
1-Bromoheptane
Bromononane
Chlorononane
Bromodecane

1.2 Bromochloromethane

Dihalomethanes in general appear to be metabolised by two different pathways; microsomal oxidation to carbon monoxide and a halide, and by direct conjugation with glutathione, yielding formaldehyde and a halide (Kubic *et al* 1974, Kubic and Anders 1978, Ahmed and Anders 1976, 1978). The rate of production of carbon monoxide from bromochloromethane in isolated rat hepatocytes was slower than that for dibromomethane (Stevens *et al* 1980).

Bromochloromethane is of low acute toxicity, and inhalation studies would suggest that it is also of low chronic toxicity. At high doses, the principal effect is CNS depression.

Inhalation of 1000 ppm, 7 hours/day, 5 days/week for up to 14 weeks was not found to produce toxicity in either rats, rabbits or dogs (Svirbely *et al* 1947). In another inhalation study (Torkelson *et al* 1960), no effects were observed in rats or dogs exposed to 370 ppm for 7 hours/day, 5 days/week for 6 months. However, pathological changes, notably in the liver and testes, were found in guinea-pigs, rabbits, rats and mice exposed to 1000 ppm for 4 months. At a concentration of 500 ppm, moderate hepatotoxicity was observed in female rats, and a small increase in liver weight was apparent in male rats. At this concentration there were no effects in guinea-pigs or rabbits. A later study (MacEwen *et al* 1966) found no pathological changes in rats or dogs exposed by inhalation to 500 or 1000 ppm, 6 hours/day for 124 exposures over 6 months, though depression of body weight gain was observed in rats. In the two latter studies, increased blood bromide was reported.

Unpublished mutagenicity studies by Dow Chemical Company gave negative results in both yeast and the Ames test (Torkelson and Rowe 1981). However, Simmon *et al* (1977) found that bromochloromethane was a potent mutagen to *Salmonella typhimurium* TA100 when tested in a desiccator. This compound has also given positive results in spot tests with *S. typhimurium* and *Escherichia coli* (Osterman-Golkar *et al* 1983).

No data were found on carcinogenicity or reproductive toxicity of bromochloromethane.

1.3 Dibromomethane

Dibromomethane is of low acute toxicity in rodents, but its chronic toxicity has been poorly studied. Several limited subchronic studies have been carried out (Torkelson and Rowe 1981). No effects were reported in a small number of rabbits given 60 doses of 300 mg/kg spread over 92 days, but anaesthesia was produced in animals given 400 mg/kg. CNS effects and degenerative changes in the lung, liver and kidneys of rats, and toxicity to the liver and kidneys of rabbits, were found following exposure by inhalation to 1000 ppm for 73 days (54 exposures). Inhalation of 200 ppm for 114 days (79 exposures) also produced histological changes in the liver and kidneys of rats and rabbits. However, 6-hour daily exposures of 25, 75 or 125 ppm over 90 days (60–70 exposures) were not found to produce pathological changes in either rats or dogs, although blood bromide and carboxyhaemoglobin were markedly elevated in this study.

In unpublished mutagenicity studies by Dow Chemical Company, dibromomethane was reported to be weakly mutagenic in yeast, but negative in the Ames test

(Torkelson and Rowe 1981). However, Van Bladeren *et al* (1980) found it to be mutagenic to *S. typhimurium* TA100 in a modified Ames test in which the compound was pre-incubated with the indicator organisms for 15 minutes. Although dibromomethane was directly mutagenic, addition of either a metabolising enzyme system or glutathione led to increased activity. This compound was also reported to be a potent mutagen in *S. typhimurium* TA100 when tested in a desiccator (Simmon *et al* 1977) and in spot tests with *E. coli* and *S. typhimurium* (Osterman-Golkar *et al* 1983).

There appear to be no data on the carcinogenicity or reproductive toxicity of dibromomethane.

1.4 Tetrachloromethane (carbon tetrachloride)

Tetrachloromethane is a widely used industrial chemical that has been extensively studied. The health effects of this compound have been reviewed on a number of previous occasions (National Academy of Sciences 1977, International Agency for Research on Cancer 1979, US Environmental Protection Agency 1980, 1984, World Health Organization 1984, Torkelson and Rowe 1981). Tetrachloromethane has frequently been detected in air, food and water samples. Typical concentrations found in drinking water are 2–3 μg/l. However, air is thought to represent the major source of environmental exposure (US Environmental Protection Agency 1984).

This compound is readily taken up by the lungs and more slowly by the gastrointestinal tract and skin. Distribution is dependent on the route of exposure, but is primarily to the lipid-rich tissues and bone-marrow. Most of a dose of tetrachloromethane is exhaled unchanged from the lungs, but some is metabolised by the liver. Early studies found that chloroform and to a lesser extent carbon dioxide were metabolites of tetrachloromethane (Butler 1961, Paul and Rubinstein 1963). The first step in the biotransformation of tetrachloromethane is thought to involve the production of a trichloromethyl radical, CCl_3. (Poyer *et al* 1980, Albano *et al* 1982). This may then be converted to chloroform, dichloromethylcarbene (Pohl and George 1983) and phosgene (Kubic and Anders 1980, Waller and Recknagel 1982) or may react with molecular oxygen to form the highly reactive trichloromethyl peroxy radical CCl_3O_2. (Slater 1982, Symons *et al* 1982, Monig *et al* 1983). This radical may play an important role in the toxicity of tetrachloromethane to the liver.

Tetrachloromethane is of moderate acute toxicity in experimental animals. Lethal doses can induce death very rapidly by CNS depression or more slowly through massive liver damage. Hepatic changes are characterised by accumulation of fat, and cell necrosis in the centrilobular region. Tetrachloromethane also stimulates hepatic lipid peroxidation and depletes hepatic glutathione and glutathione-related enzymes (Yalcin *et al* 1986). There is evidence to suggest that there is an age difference in susceptibility to tetrachloromethane hepatotoxicity in experimental animals (Cagen and Klaassen 1979) but the mechanism of action of tetrachloromethane in the liver is not fully understood.

Acute studies have also shown this compound to be toxic to the kidney (Zimmerman and Norbach 1980) and adrenal glands (Brogan *et al* 1984), and able to modify hepatic, adrenal and pulmonary mono-oxygenase activities (Smuckler *et al* 1967, Head *et al* 1981, Colby *et al* 1981, Malendowicz and Colby 1982). In subacute studies, high doses of tetrachloromethane were shown to be toxic to the testis in rats (Chatterjee 1966, Kalla and Bansal 1975).

In a subchronic study (Bruckner *et al* 1986), groups of 15 adult male Sprague–Dawley rats were dosed by gavage with 0, 1, 10 and 33 mg/kg body weight/day of tetrachloromethane in corn oil, 5 days/week for 12 weeks. Animals in the highest dose group exhibited marked pathological changes in the liver, depression of body weight gain and increased liver weight/body weight ratios. Elevated activities of serum sorbitol dehydrogenase, ornithine-carbamyl transferase and glutamic-pyruvic transaminase were found throughout the treatment period. In the 10 mg/kg dose group, the only effects noted were mild centrilobular vacuolisation in the liver and a slight elevation of serum sorbitol dehydrogenase activity. No effects were found in animals given 1 mg/kg and there were no pathological changes in the kidney in any dose group.

There have been two recent subchronic studies of tetrachloromethane in mice. In the first (Hayes *et al* 1986), groups of 20 male and female CD-1 mice were dosed by gavage with 0, 12, 120, 540 and 1200 mg/kg body weight/day in corn oil for 90 days. Pathological changes in the liver, increased liver and spleen weights and organ to body weight ratios, and changes in serum chemistry were evident in all dose groups, though there was a dose response with respect to severity. There were no pathological changes in the kidney in any dose group. In the other study (Condie *et al* 1986), groups of 12 male and female CD-1 mice were dosed by gavage with 0, 1.2, 12 and 120 mg/kg body-weight/day in either corn oil or aqueous suspension (1% Tween 60), 5 days/week over a 90-day period. The animals were examined for effects on serum enzyme activities and histopathology of the liver. There were no effects in the low-dose animals other than increased fatty deposits in the corn oil vehicle group compared to the aqueous vehicle group. At 12 mg/kg, hepatocellular cytomegaly and necrosis were evident in the corn oil vehicle group but not in the aqueous vehicle group. Severe hepatotoxicity was apparent in all the high-dose groups, but again the incidence was greater in the corn oil vehicle group. In this study it would appear that the hepatotoxicity of tetrachloromethane was enhanced by the use of corn oil as a vehicle compared to an aqueous suspension.

Metabolites of tetrachloromethane have been reported to bind to hepatic nuclear and mitochondrial DNA *in vivo* (Diaz-Gomez and Castro 1980, Levy and Brabec 1984), but bacterial mutagenicity tests have largely proved negative. Tetrachloromethane also gave negative results for induction of unscheduled DNA synthesis in rat hepatocytes *in vivo* (Mirsalis and Butterworth 1980, Mirsalis *et al* 1982). However, positive results have been reported in yeast (Callen *et al* 1980).

Epidemiological data for carcinogenicity are sparse, though three cases of human liver cancer have been reported several years after poisoning with tetrachloromethane. However, a number of studies have shown that prolonged administration of high doses of tetrachloromethane by the oral or subcutaneous routes can induce liver tumours in rats, mice and hamsters (Della Porta *et al* 1961, Reuber and Glover 1970, National Cancer Institute 1976). In the National Cancer Institute study, groups of 50 male and 50 female Osborne–Mendel rats were dosed by gavage with either 47 and 94 mg/kg body weight/day (males) or 80 and 160 mg/kg body-weight/day (females), in corn oil on 5 days/week for 78 weeks. Surviving animals were then fed a control diet and killed at 110 weeks. There appeared to be a slightly increased incidence of hepatocellular carcinomas and liver neoplastic nodules. Groups of 50 male and 50 female mice of the B6C3F1 strain were dosed by gavage with 1250 and 2500 mg/kg body weight/day in corn oil on 5 days/week for 78 weeks. Hepatocellular carcinomas developed in nearly all the treated animals. The incidence of hepatocellular carcinomas in the pooled controls was 5/77 in males and 1/80 in females. Using these data and a linearised multistage model, the US EPA have calculated an increased risk of one additional cancer for every 100 000 people at a tetrachloromethane concentration of 4 μg/l. However, the relevance of the model is questionable in view of the uncertainty surrounding the mechanism of carcinogenic action of tetrachloromethane. Moreover, the data used may be inappropriate for assessing risk from drinking water, as a recent subchronic study (Condie *et al* 1986) has shown that the vehicle of administration has an important influence on toxicity and hence possibly on carcinogenicity also.

The small number of studies that have looked at the reproductive toxicology of tetrachloromethane suggest that this compound is embryotoxic at high doses, but is not teratogenic (Schwetz *et al* 1974).

1.5 Tetrabromomethane

Little has been published on the metabolism of tetrabromomethane. There is some evidence that bromide radicals are produced *in vitro* (Mico *et al* 1982).

Equally there are only sparse toxicological data for this compound. Tetrabromomethane is severely irritating to the rabbit eye and can cause permanent damage to the cornea. The acute oral LD50 in rats is 1800 mg/kg (Torkelson and Rowe 1981). Intraperitoneal injection of a single dose of 25–125 μl/kg in male rats was found to cause marked toxicity to the kidney but no toxicity to the liver. Dietary chlordecone treatment for 15 days after dosing abolished nephrotoxicity (Agarwal *et al* 1983).

No effects were observed in rats exposed to 0.1 ppm of tetrabromomethane vapour, 7 hours/day, 5 days/week for 6 months. Concentrations above 5 ppm were reported to inhibit growth and cause fatty and degenerative changes in the liver (Torkelson and Rowe 1981). Another study found metabolic changes in the liver and irritation of the eyes and respiratory tract of rats exposed by inhalation to 0.07–74 ppm, 4 hours/day for 4 months (Torkelson and Rowe 1981).

The limited information available would suggest that tetrabromomethane is probably of greater chronic toxic potential than most of the other halomethanes. No data on mutagenicity, carcinogenicity or reproductive toxicity appear to be available for this compound.

1.6 Bromoethane

There appear to be no data available on the metabolism of bromoethane.

This compound is of low acute toxicity, but there are very little data on its long-term effects. A limited study on rabbits reported no apparent toxicity after oral doses of 200 mg/kg/day for 61 days (Torkelson and Rowe 1981). Some evidence of hepatotoxicity was found in rats exposed to 540 ppm in the air, 4 hours/day for 6 months (Karimullina and Gizatullina 1969). Chronic inhalation studies in mice and rats are currently being conducted by the US National Toxicology Program.

Several studies have shown that bromoethane has mutagenic activity. It is a potent mutagen in *S. typhimurium* TA100 and TA1535 when the assay is modified to take into account the volatility of the compound (Torkelson and Rowe 1981, Simmon and Poirier 1976, Barber *et al* 1981, 1983). It is also mutagenic to *E. coli*

WP2 (Simmon and Poirier 1976), weakly mutagenic in yeast (Torkelson and Rowe 1981), but gave negative results in an early *Drosophila* study (Vogel and Chandler 1974).

Intraperitoneal injection of 1200, 3000 or 6000 mg/kg, three times per week for 24 doses in strain A mice, was not found to significantly increase the number of mice with lung tumours (Poirier *et al* 1975). Single subcutaneous injections of doses up to 1400 mg/kg body weight were not found to produce local sarcomas in rats (Dipple *et al* 1981).

Information from long-term carcinogenicity studies and data on reproductive toxicity are not available.

1.7 Iodoethane

No information could be found on the metabolism of iodoethane, and there are very little data on acute or chronic toxic effects. Two rabbits survived an oral dose of 100 mg/kg, but 3/3 died after a dose of 300 mg/kg (Torkelson and Rowe 1981). Inhalation of 120 ppm for 7 hours was tolerated by mice, but exposure to 150 ppm for 24 hours or 290 ppm for 3 hours proved fatal (Torkelson and Rowe 1981).

Iodoethane has been used for the treatment of fungal infections in man. It can cause CNS depression, skin lesions, peripheral neuritis and toxicity to the liver, kidney, lung and thyroid.

Iodoethane was found to be mutagenic to *S. typhimurium* TA1535 and TA100 both with and without metabolic activation (Simmon and Poirier 1976, Barber *et al* 1981) and to *E. coli* WP2 (hcr^-) (Simmon and Poirier 1976). There is also evidence from *in vitro* studies that iodoethane has alkylating activity. However, in accord with bromoethane this compound proved negative for induction of lung tumours in a short-term test in strain A mice (Poirier *et al* 1975).

1.8 1,1-Dichloroethane

Groups of rats and mice were dosed by gavage with either the maximum tolerated dose or 1/4 of the maximum tolerated dose of 1,1-dichloroethane for 4 weeks. For rats the maximum tolerated dose was 700 mg/kg, while for mice it was 1800 mg/kg. The animals were then given a single dose of radiolabelled compound, and its metabolism was followed for 48 hours. This compound was primarily excreted unchanged in the expired air. Metabolites in the urine accounted for only 7% and 29% of the dose in rats and mice respectively (Mitoma *et al* 1985).

No adverse effects were observed in rats, guinea-pigs, cats and rabbits exposed to 500 ppm of 1,1-dichloroethane vapour, 6 hours/day, 5 days/week for 13 weeks. An additional 13 weeks at 1000 ppm was tolerated by rats, guinea-pigs and rabbits, but cats showed histological evidence of nephrotoxicity and elevated blood urea (Hofmann *et al* 1971). An unpublished study by Dow Chemical Company in which rats, guinea-pigs, rabbits and dogs were exposed to either 500 or 1000 ppm in the air, 7 hours/day, 5 days/week for 6 months found no evidence of exposure-related effects (Torkelson and Rowe 1981).

Colacci *et al* (1985) demonstrated covalent binding to rat and mouse DNA both *in vivo* and *in vitro* following treatment with radiolabelled 1,1-dichloroethane. However, Simmon *et al* (1977) reported that this compound was non-mutagenic to

S. typhimurium in the Ames test.

A carcinogenicity study of 1,1-dichloroethane in mice and rats has been carried out by the National Cancer Institute. The animals were dosed by gavage with 382 and 764 mg/kg/day (male rats), 475 and 950 mg/kg/day (female rats), 1442 and 2885 mg/kg/day (male mice) and 1665 and 3331 mg/kg/day (female mice) for 78 weeks. Although marginal increases in some tumours were noted, animal survival was very poor. The study was therefore inconclusive (Weisburger 1977).

No teratogenic effects were found in a study of pregnant rats exposed to 3800 or 6000 ppm in the air on days 6-15 of gestation. However, depression of body-weight gain in the dams and delayed bone ossification in the foetus were observed (Schwetz *et al* 1974).

1.9 1,2-Dichloroethane

1,2-Dichloroethane (ethylene dichloride) is an important industrial chemical, its major usage being in the manufacture of vinyl chloride. There are considerably more toxicological data on this compound than on 1,1-dichloroethane.

1,2-Dichloroethane has been identified in air, food and water, mostly at point emission sources. The relative contribution of each to overall exposure is unclear.

The gastrointestinal absorption of 1,2-dichloroethane is rapid and complete. Most of either an oral dose or intraperitoneal dose of 1,2-dichloroethane in rats or mice was excreted as metabolites in the urine. The remainder was exhaled unchanged or as carbon dioxide (Yllner 1961, Mitoma *et al* 1985). However, the precise pathways of biotransformation are not fully clear. One is thought to involve the dehalogenation of 1,2-dichloroethane to 2-chloroethanol, followed by oxidation to 2-chloroethanoic acid and subsequent conjugation. Direct conjugation with glutathione is also thought to be a quantitatively important pathway.

This halogenated hydrocarbon appears to be of moderate acute toxicity in experimental animals; the main effect at high doses is CNS depression.

Chronic inhalation studies indicate that the main target organs for toxicity are the liver, kidneys and adrenals. Heppel *et al* (1946) found no pathological changes in a range of species exposed to 100 ppm for several months. At higher doses, rats, mice and guinea-pigs proved the more sensitive species. Monkeys and rabbits appeared to tolerate prolonged exposure to 200 ppm quite well, while only slight changes in the liver were found in dogs exposed to 400 ppm for 8 months. Similar results have been obtained in other chronic inhalation studies (Hofmann *et al* 1971, Spencer *et al* 1951).

Groups of 18 male and 18 female rats fed diets containing 250 or 500 ppm 1,2-dichloroethane (corresponding to daily doses of about 20 and 40 mg/kg body-weight) for 2 years showed no effects on body weight, reproductive performance and blood chemistry (Alumot *et al* 1976a). Chickens fed similar diets also showed no effects on growth, fertility and blood chemistry, but there was an effect on egg production at the higher dose, and a slight decrease in egg weight was evident at both dose levels (Alumot *et al* 1976b).

Several studies have shown that 1,2-dichloroethane is a direct-acting base-pair mutagen in bacterial systems (Rannug 1980, Davidson *et al* 1982). Rannug *et al* (1978) demonstrated that mutagenic activity was enhanced both by metabolising systems and by glutathione. There is conflicting evidence that a glutathione conjugate may be the actual mutagen (Storer and Conolly 1985, Lin *et al* 1985, Inskeep *et al* 1986).

1,2-Dichloroethane has also given positive results for genotoxicity in cultured human lymphocytes (Perocco and Prodi 1981), CHO/HGPRT system (Tan and Hsie 1981), human lymphoblastoid cell lines (Crespi *et al* 1985), yeast (Simmon 1980) and *Drosophila* (King et al 1979), but two *in vivo* mouse micronucleus assays have proved negative (King *et al* 1979, Jenssen and Ramel 1980).

There is evidence that 1,2-dichloroethane is carcinogenic in rats and mice. Groups of 50 male and female Osborne–Mendel rats and B6C3F1 mice were dosed by gavage with time-weighted average doses of 47 and 95 mg/kg/day for male and female rats, 97 and 195 mg/kg/day for male mice, and 149 and 299 mg/kg/day for female mice in corn oil. Statistically significant increases were observed for malignant stomach tumours and haemangiosarcomas in male rats, for mammary adenocarcinomas in both female rats and mice, and for lung adenomas in male and female mice (Weisburger 1977). An 18-month inhalation study in Sprague–Dawley rats and Swiss mice at doses of 5, 10, 50 and 150–250 ppm found no increased incidence of malignant tumours (Maltoni *et al* 1980).

No teratogenic or embryotoxic effects were found in pregnant rats and rabbits exposed by inhalation to 0, 100 or 300 ppm on days 6–15 and 6–18 of gestation respectively. Maternal toxicity was evident at both doses in rabbits, and in rats at 300 ppm but not 100 ppm (Rao *et al* 1980). A multigeneration study in mice by Lane *et al* (1982) also gave negative results for effects on fertility and teratogenicity. The mice received 0, 30, 90 or 290 mg/l in the drinking water, corresponding to daily doses of 0, 5, 15 and 50 mg/kg body weight.

1.10 1,1,1-Trichloroethane

1,1,1-Trichloroethane (methyl chloroform) is widely used as a solvent in cleaning, degreasing, cosmetic manufacture and aerosols. It is generally present at around 1 ppb in the atmosphere, and has been identified on several occasions in water samples. It has also been found in a variety of foodstuffs. The US FDA approves this compound as a constituent of food packaging.

In mammals, the majority of a dose of 1,1,1-trichloroethane is exhaled unchanged (Mitoma *et al* 1985). A small proportion is metabolised to trichloroethanol and trichloroacetic acid. Dechlorination does not appear to be a significant pathway of metabolism for this compound.

Many cases of acute human exposure to very high doses of 1,1,1-trichloroethane have been reported in the literature. Most deaths are caused by oedema and congestion of the lungs, though in the case of solvent abusers, some deaths may have resulted from heart failure.

This compound is of low acute toxicity in experimental animals; the oral LD50s for mice and rats are of the order of 11 g/kg (Torkelson *et al* 1958).

There is little experimental evidence available to suggest that chronic exposure to other than near lethal doses of 1,1,1-trichloroethane can cause toxic effects. The toxic effects generally reported are CNS depression, liver and kidney damage (Torkelson *et al* 1958, Prendergast *et al* 1967, MacEwan *et al* 1974, McNutt *et al*

1975, National Cancer Institute 1977).

Several studies have reported that this compound is non-mutagenic in bacterial tests, though some studies designed specifically for volatile compounds have found weak activity in *S. typhimurium* TA100 and TA1535 (Simmon *et al* 1977, Nestmann *et al* 1984, Shimada *et al* 1985). There is equivocal evidence for unscheduled DNA synthesis *in vitro* (Milman *et al* 1984, Shimada *et al* 1985), but negative results have been reported for sister chromatid exchange in *Drosophila*, the micronucleus assay and the dominant lethal assay. Only very limited covalent binding was found in mouse and rat liver DNA in both *in vitro* and *in vivo* experiments (Turina *et al* 1986).

The data from the first NCI carcinogenesis bioassay of technical grade 1,1,1-trichloroethane were insufficient to indicate a carcinogenic or non-carcinogenic potential for this compound (National Cancer Institute 1977). In a repeat test, doses of 1500 and 3000 mg/kg in mice and 375 and 750 mg/kg in rats were given in corn oil for 2 years. No evidence of carcinogenicity was found in rats, but an increased incidence of hepatocellular carcinomas was observed in mice (US National Toxicology Program 1982). In an inhalation study, no increased tumour incidence was found in rats exposed by inhalation to 875 or 1750 ppm for 6 hours/day, 5 days/week for one year (Rampy *et al* 1977).

1,1,1-trichloroethane does not appear to be teratogenic in rodents (Schwetz *et al* 1975, York *et al* 1982). No toxic signs or effects on fertility were observed in a mouse multigeneration study at reported concentrations of 580, 1750 and 5800 mg/l in the drinking water (Lane *et al* 1982).

1.11 1,1,2-Trichloroethane

1,1,2-Trichloroethane (vinyl trichloride) is used as a solvent for chlorinated rubber, fats, oils and resins, and in the manufacture of 1,1-dichloroethylene. There is rather less information available on this compound than on the 1,1,1-isomer.

1,1,2-Trichloroethane has been identified in drinking water on several occasions. No other exposure-related data appear to be available.

Yllner (1971b) found that of an intraperitoneal dose of 100–200 mg/kg body weight in mice, 73–87% was eliminated in the urine and 16-22% in the expired air after 3 days. In urine, the major metabolites were chloroacetic acid and glutathione conjugates. Minor metabolites were 2,2-dichloroethanol, 2,2,2-trichloroethanol, oxalic acid and trichloroacetic acid. The quantity eliminated in the expired air was composed of carbon dioxide (60%) and unchanged compound (40%). In an oral study in both rats and mice, Mitoma *et al* (1985) also found that most of a dose of 1,1,2-trichloroethane was eliminated as metabolites in the urine. Biotransformation of 1,1,2-trichloroethane by rat liver microsomes has been found to result in mono- and dichloroacetic acid and mono- and dichloroethanol (Van Dyke and Wineman 1971, Ivanetich and Van den Honert 1981).

This compound is of low acute toxicity in experimental animals. Oral LD50s of 835 mg/kg, 378 mg/kg and 491 mg/kg have been reported for the rat, male mouse and female mouse respectively (Smyth *et al* 1969, White *et al* 1985). The principal acute effects are CNS depression and toxicity to the liver and kidney. 1,1,2-Trichloroethane appears to be of greater hepatotoxic potential than the 1,1,1-isomer, but is much less hepatotoxic than carbon tetrachloride and chloroform (Plaa *et al* 1958, Klaassen and Plaa 1966, 1967, 1969). In terms of its potential to induce kidney damage, it is more toxic than 1,1,1-trichloroethane and carbon tetrachloride but less toxic than chloroform (Plaa and Larson 1965, Klaassen and Plaa 1966, 1967, Watrous and Plaa 1972).

In a subacute study, no effects on body weight, organ to body weight ratios and haematology were evident in CD-1 mice dosed by gavage with 0, 3.8 or 38 mg/kg body-weight/day in an Emulphor solution for 14 days. There was a slight depression of serum lactate dehydrogenase activity in the high-dose group (White *et al* 1985). No alterations in humoral or cell-mediated immune function were found in male CD-1 mice treated in exactly the same way as those in the previous study (Sanders *et al* 1985).

CD-1 mice were exposed to 1,1,2-trichloroethane in their drinking water at concentrations of 0.02, 0.2 and 2 g/l for 90 days. The time-weighted average doses were calculated to be 4.4, 46 and 305 mg/kg body weight/day for the male mice and 3.9, 44 and 384 mg/kg body weight/day for the female mice. Fluid consumption, body weight, organ weights, haematology, serum chemistry and liver glutathione and mixed function oxidase activity were assessed, but there was no histopathology. In male mice, lowered liver glutathione and elevated serum alkaline phosphatase were the only clear dose-related effects. In female mice, however, glutathione levels were elevated along with serum alkaline phosphatase, alanine aminotransferase, aspartic aminotransferase, fibrinogen and liver weight. Depression of hepatic microsomal cytochrome P-450 and aniline hydroxylase activity were also noted. Although most changes were found at the higher dose levels, elevated serum alkaline phosphatase and aspartic aminotranferase were evident in female mice even at 0.02 g/l (White *et al* 1985). CD-1 mice treated in exactly the same way but evaluated for effects on immune function gave no indication of changes in cell-mediated immunity, but humoral immune status was depressed in both sexes at 0.2 and 2 g/l (Sanders *et al* 1985).

Simmon *et al* (1977) reported that 1,1,2-trichloroethane was non-mutagenic at doses up to 5 mg/plate (or up to a dose that gave a toxic response) in the Ames test to *S. typhimurium* TA1535, TA1537, TA1538, TA98 or TA100, either with or without metabolic activation. Rannug *et al* (1978) also found this compound to be non-mutagenic to *S. typhimurium* TA1535 at doses ranging from 20 to 60 μmol/plate. However, 1,1,2-trichloroethane exhibited greater covalent binding to rat and mouse liver DNA *in vivo* than the 1,1,1-isomer. Covalent binding to mouse liver DNA was much higher than with rat liver DNA (Mazzullo *et al* 1986). This compound has also been reported to induce unscheduled DNA synthesis *in vitro* (Milman *et al* 1984).

A 78-week oral carcinogenicity study of 1,1,2-trichloroethane gave inconclusive results in rats, but induced significant increases in hepatocellular carcinomas and adrenal phaeochromocytomas in both male and female mice. The dose regimen for mice was 150 or 300 mg/kg body weight of technical grade 1,1,2-trichloroethane in corn oil for 8 weeks and then 200 or 400 mg/kg body weight for 70 weeks. The surviving animals were sacrificed after a further 12-week observation period. The rats were given 35 or 70 mg/kg body weight for 20 weeks followed by 50 or 100 mg/kg body weight for 58 weeks. The observation period in this case was 34–35 weeks (Weisburger 1977).

No information on the reproductive toxicology of this compound appears to be available.

1.12 Tetrachloroethane

Tetrachloroethane exists in two isomeric forms, the 1,1,2,2- and 1,1,1,2-isomers. This compound is widely used in industry as a solvent and also in the manufacture of vinylidene chloride, insecticides and bleach. There is little information available on the occurrence of tetrachloroethane in the environment. It occurred only infrequently in the WRc survey (Water Research Centre 1981).

Tetrachloroethane is readily absorbed by all routes and is distributed to the fatty tissue, heart, brain, blood and liver. Mitoma *et al* (1985) found that oral doses of 1,1,1,2- or 1,1,2,2-tetrachloroethane in rats and mice were mostly eliminated as metabolites in the urine. In mice given 210–320 mg/kg of 1,1,2,2-tetrachloroethane by intraperitoneal injection, 84% of the dose had been eliminated by 3 days. Half of the dose was expired by the lungs, mainly as carbon dioxide, while 28% was excreted in the urine. The major urinary metabolites identified were dichloroacetic acid, trichloroacetic acid, trichloroethanol and oxalic acid (Yllner 1971d). Incubation with rat liver microsomes was found to produce largely dichloroacetic acid. This metabolic pathway is thought to proceed through the reactive dichloroacetyl chloride (Ivanetich and Van den Honert 1981). Of a single subcutaneous dose of 1.2–2.0 g/kg of the 1,1,1,2-isomer in mice, about half was expired unchanged and around 30% excreted as metabolites in the urine after 3 days. The major urinary metabolite was trichloroacetic acid (Yllner 1971c). In guinea-pigs and rabbits, the major urinary metabolites were trichloroethanol and its glucuronide conjugate (Truhaut and Phu Lich 1973). Incubation of this isomer with rat liver microsomes resulted in the production of 1,1-dichloroethylene and 1,1,2-trichloroethane (Thompson *et al* 1984, Town and Leibman 1984).

1,1,2,2-tetrachloroethane is of relatively low acute toxicity after oral or intraperitoneal administration in rodents. 1,1,1,2-Tetrachloroethane appears to be some two to three times less toxic than the 1,1,2,2-isomer. The primary acute toxic effects of both compounds are CNS depression and hepatotoxicity (Plaa *et al* 1958, Truhaut *et al* 1974). The chronic effects of tetrachloroethane have been very poorly studied. Inhalation experiments have been carried out in rabbits and rats, but these have provided extremely little information. Possible effects on the liver were reported in rabbits inhaling 100 mg/m^3 for 7–11 months (Navrotskii *et al* 1971), while an effect on antibody formation was also reported in rabbits inhaling 2 mg/m^3 for 8–10 months (Shmuter 1972). Occupational exposure to tetrachloroethane vapour has been shown to affect the nervous system, gastrointestinal system and liver. There is very little information as to the concentrations that can cause these effects.

1,1,2,2-Tetrachloroethane was weakly mutagenic in the Ames test to *S. typhimurium* TA1530 and TA1535. It was also shown to inhibit the growth of DNA polymerase-deficient *E. coli* (Brem *et al* 1974). The same isomer induced mitotic gene conversions in the yeast *Saccharomyces cerevisiae* D7 (Callen *et al* 1980).

An oral carcinogenicity study of 1,1,2,2-tetrachloroethane by the NCI has given positive results in mice. Groups of 50 male and 50 female B6C3F1 mice were given time-weighted average doses of 142 and 284 mg/kg body weight/day for 78 weeks. A significant dose-related increase in the incidence of hepatocellular carcinomas was found for both sexes. Osborne–Mendel rats given time-weighted average doses of 62 and 108 mg/kg/day in males and 43 and 76 mg/kg/day in females for 78 weeks did not produce significant increases in tumour yields (National Cancer Institute 1978).

A study in which strain A mice were given thrice-weekly intraperitoneal injections of 80–400 mg/kg of 1,1,2,2-tetrachloroethane for 5–16 doses failed to produce a significant increase in lung adenomas (Theiss *et al* 1977).

Schmidt (1976) has reported that 1,1,2,2-tetrachloroethane was embryotoxic and weakly teratogenic in mice following intraperitoneal injection of 300–400 mg/kg/day during organogenesis.

1.13 Hexachloroethane

This compound is used as an intermediate in the manufacture of a wide range of industrial chemicals. There is very little information available on its environmental occurrence.

Hexachloroethane is readily absorbed and distributed to the lipid-rich tissues. In a recent study (Mitoma *et al* 1985), groups of rats and mice were dosed by gavage with either the maximum tolerated dose or 1/4 of the maximum tolerated dose of hexachloroethane for 4 weeks. The maximum tolerated dose for rats was 500 mg/kg, while for mice it was 1000 mg/kg. The animals were then given a single dose of radiolabelled compound, and its metabolism was followed for 48 hours. About 2/3 of the dose was exhaled unchanged, while most of the remainder was eliminated as metabolites in the urine. However, this compound appears to be eliminated more slowly in rabbits. Three days after rabbits were fed 500 mg/kg, only 14–24% and 5% of the dose had been eliminated in the expired air and urine respectively. The principal metabolites of this compound were trichloroethylene, tetrachloroethylene, pentachloroethane and tetrachloroethane (Jondorf *et al* 1957). In rats fed 62 mg/kg body weight/day of hexachloroethane for 8 weeks, the highest concentrations were found in the fat, with smaller concentrations in the kidney. Higher levels were found in the kidneys of males than females. The rate of clearance of hexachloroethane from the fat suggested a half-life of 2–3 days (Gorzinski *et al* 1985).

Hexachloroethane is of low acute oral toxicity in experimental animals. At high doses its primary effects are CNS depression and hepatotoxicity. Subacute oral administration of hexachloroethane in rabbits produced histological changes in the liver at 320 and 1000 mg/kg/day. No effects were found at 100 mg/kg/day (Weeks *et al* 1979). In a subchronic study, groups of 10 male and 10 female F–344 rats were fed hexachloroethane in the diet at dose levels equivalent to 1, 15 and 62 mg/kg body weight/day for 16 weeks. An increase in kidney weight and pathological changes in this organ were found at the higher dose levels, particularly in males. At the high dose there was also an increase in liver weight and some evidence of toxicity to hepatocytes, again particularly in the males. No effects were reported in either males or females at 1 mg/kg (Gorzinski *et al* 1985). A much earlier study found no effects on body weight, clinical chemistry or tissue histology in male rats and male and female rabbits given oral doses of 50 μg/kg/day for $5\frac{1}{2}$ months (Tugarinova *et al* 1963).

Negative results for mutagenic activity have been reported in the Ames test and in yeast (Weeks *et al* 1979).

In an NCI carcinogenesis bioassay, groups of 50 male and 50 female B6C3F1 mice were dosed by gavage with 590 and 1179 mg/kg/day of hexachloroethane (time-weighted average doses) in corn oil, 5 days/week for 78 weeks. A significant increase in hepatocellular carcinomas was evident in both male and female mice. There was, however, very poor survival in the control and low-dose males. Equivocal results were obtained in Osborne–Mendel rats given time-weighted average doses of 212 and 423 mg/kg/day over 77 weeks (Weisburger 1977).

No teratogenic effects were found in Sprague–Dawley rats given daily oral doses of 50, 100, or 500 mg/kg on days 6–16 of gestation. At the highest dose level, depression of body weight gain was apparent in the dams, foetal resorption was increased, and gestation indices were lowered (85).

1.14 Bromopropane

Of a single intraperitoneal dose of 200 mg/kg of 1-bromopropane in rats, 56% of the dose was expired unchanged within 2 hours. By 48 hours, only a further 4% was expired unchanged, 1.4% was exhaled as carbon dioxide and around 40% was excreted as metabolites in the urine. The urinary metabolites were mercapturic acids resulting from conjugation with glutathione (Jones and Walsh 1979).

No acute or chronic toxicological information appear to be available for bromopropane. Barber *et al* (1981) reported that 1-bromopropane was mutagenic in the Ames test at 9–20 μmol/plate to *S. typhimurium* TA100 and TA1535, but not TA98. Activity was similar in both the presence and absence of metabolic activation. The assays were conducted in a closed, inert incubation system, designed for testing volatile compounds. 1–Bromopropane gave negative results in a dominant lethal assay in rats (Saito–Suzuki *et al* 1982).

A single subcutaneous injection of either 102, 344 or 1021 mg/kg of 2-bromopropane in rats failed to produce sarcomas at the injection site by 90 weeks (Dipple *et al* 1981).

1.15 Bromochloropropane

Four bromochloropropane isomers were detected in UK drinking water by WRc. The only data that appear to be available on these compounds are oral LD50s for the 1-bromo-3-chloro- isomer of 930 mg/kg in the rat and 1290 mg/kg in the mouse and an oral LD50 of 1326 mg/kg in the rat for a mixture of 1-bromo-2-chloropropane and 1-chloro-2-bromopropane (Registry of Toxic Effects of Chemical Substances).

1.16 1-Bromobutane

The metabolism of 1-bromobutane is similar to that of 1-bromopropane. Direct conjugation with glutathione and oxidation prior to conjugation are the two major pathways (James *et al* 1968).

There are very few toxicity data for this compound. LD50s, by the intraperitoneal route, of 4450 and 6680 mg/kg have been reported for the rat and mouse respectively. 1–Bromobutane was mutagenic in the Ames test to *S. typhimurium* TA1535 and TA100 at 10–28 μmol/plate when tested in a closed system (Barber *et al* 1981). Simmon *et al* (1977) also reported that 1-bromobutane was mutagenic in the Ames test when tested in a closed system. No significant increases in lung tumours were found in strain A mice given 16 intraperitoneal injections of 33 or 82 mg/kg or 13 intraperitoneal injections of 164 mg/kg and followed until 24 weeks after the first injection (Poirier *et al* 1975).

1.17 Chlorobutane

The acute toxicity of both 1- and 2-chlorobutane isomers in experimental animals is low. In subacute feeding studies, rats given 2 mg/kg for 6 months showed increased serum inorganic phosphate and altered alkaline phosphatase, cholinesterase and succinate dehydrogenase levels. No effects on brain electrical activity, heart rate or blood enzyme or phosphate levels were found at 0.02 or 0.2 mg/kg (Rudnev *et al* 1979). It has also been suggested that rats became 'sensitised to antibodies' after treatment with 110 mg/kg for one month (Rudnev *et al* 1979) and 'autosensitised' following 30 daily oral exposures of 0.0022 mg/kg (Vinogradov 1979). In a 13-week study carried out for the US National Toxicology Program (1986) groups of 10 male and 10 female rats were dosed by gavage with up to 500 mg/kg body weight/day of 1-chlorobutane in corn oil. Similar groups of mice received doses of up to 1000 mg/kg body weight/day. In the rats, there were deaths at 500 mg/kg and convulsions and depression of body weight gain at 250 mg/kg. In the mice, the only compound-related effects noted were convulsions in two females at 1000 mg/kg.

1-Chlorobutane gave negative results in the Ames test, either in a modified liquid suspension assay (Eder *et al* 1980) or when tested in a sealed container (Barber *et al* 1981). However, Simmon (1981) reported that this compound was directly mutagenic to *S. typhimurium* TA100 when tested in a desiccator. 1-Chlorobutane was found to be mutagenic in the mouse lymphoma assay in the absence of S-9 but did not induce sister chromatid exchanges or chromosome aberrations in CHO cells either in the presence or absence of S-9 (US National Toxicology Program 1986).

In a carcinogenicity study, groups of 50 male and 50 female F-344 rats were dosed by gavage with 0, 60 or 120 mg/kg body weight/day of 1-chlorobutane in corn oil, 5 days/week for 103 weeks. Similar size groups of B6C3F1 mice were dosed with 0, 500 or 1000 mg/kg body weight/day on 5 days/week, but all the female animals given 1000 mg/kg had died by week 52. Hence, further groups of mice were started at concentrations of 0 and 250 mg/kg/day. In all high-dose groups there was reduced survival compared to vehicle controls. Some marginal increases in tumour incidence were observed, but these were not thought to be due to administration of the compound (US National Toxicology Program 1986). The 1-isomer was not found to induce lung tumours in strain A mice after 24 intraperitoneal injections of 1200–6000 mg/kg, but 2-chlorobutane significantly increased the average number of lung tumours/mouse after 13 injections of 3240 mg/kg (Poirier *et al* 1975).

1-Chlorobutane was reported to be embryotoxic (Leonskaya 1980) and teratogenic (Rudnev *et al* 1979) in rats only at near lethal doses.

1.18 Dibromopentane

1,5-Dibromopentane has been shown to be mutagenic in the Ames test to *S. typhimurium* TA1530 and TA1535 but not TA1538. It also inhibited the growth of DNA polymerase-deficient *E. coli* (Brem *et al* 1974).

1.19 Bromohexane

The only information available on this compound is from a study in which bromohexane was reported to be mutagenic and embryotropic in rats, though the activity was lower than that for bromobutane (Oktyabr'skii 1977).

1.20 Bromooctane

The only toxicological data on bromooctane are an oral LD50 of 5020 mg/kg in the rat and a dermal LD50 of 8944 mg/kg in the rabbit for the 1-isomer (Smyth *et al* 1969).

1.21 Chlorooctane

Chlorooctane was not found to increase the incidence of lung tumours in strain A mice after thrice-weekly injection of 160 or 400 mg/kg for 24 doses or 800 mg/kg for 5 doses (Theiss *et al* 1977).

1.22 Discussion

Almost all the information available on mammalian metabolism relates to the halogenated methanes and ethanes. For most of these compounds, elimination in the expired air either in an unchanged form or as carbon dioxide would appear to be a quantitatively important pathway at high doses. It may not be as important at low doses, but there are little data available to confirm this. With respect to the biotransformation of halogenated alkanes, the route of metabolism is different, depending on the degree of halogen substitution. Compounds with few halogen atoms are generally rapidly metabolised by aliphatic oxidation, whereas highly substituted compounds are often metabolised in the first instance by dechlorination, which is a much slower pathway. The halogen substituent itself is also important, as iodine atoms are more readily lost than bromine atoms, which are in turn more readily lost than chlorine atoms.

The availability of toxicological data for individual compounds in this group varies markedly. Some compounds have been studied extensively, but for most compounds there is either little or no information. In terms of assessing toxic hazard, it is particularly difficult to compare the lower members of the group with the higher members, as there is very little toxicological information available on the latter compounds.

The data that are available on the halogenated methanes and ethanes suggest that these compounds are of moderate to low acute toxicity in experimental animals. Most long-term studies have been carried out using the inhalation route of exposure. In subchronic oral studies, tetrachloromethane, 1,1,2-trichloroethane and hexachloroethane were found to produce toxic effects at doses in the low mg/kg range. The target organ for toxicity is almost always the liver.

A number of the compounds in this group have been shown to be mutagenic in bacterial tests, particularly if the assay is carried out in an enclosed system to offset the problem of volatility. These compounds are often direct-acting mutagens; that is, they do not require metabolism in order to express their mutagenic activity, and probably act as alkylating agents.

Several of the compounds have also been shown to be carcinogenic in rodents, although none have been satisfactorily demonstrated to be human carcinogens. These compounds are not particularly potent carcinogens in experimental animals, and when considered individually no compound would appear to present a significant risk to human health. However, it is possible that these compounds may have additive or synergistic effects.

The data available on reproductive toxicity indicate that the halogenated alkanes may be embryotoxic at high doses, but there is little evidence for teratogenic potential.

2. THE UNSATURATED HALOGENATED ALIPHATICS

2.1 Introduction

Several halogenated aliphatic alkenes were detected in surveys of drinking water by WRc (Water Research Centre 1981, 1982); trichloroethylene and tetrachloroethylene (which have been considered previously), plus 1,2-dichloroethylene, five chloromethylbutene isomers, bromotrichloroethylene and one tetrachlorobutadiene isomer. Apart from trichloroethylene and tetrachloroethylene, the remaining compounds occurred infrequently in drinking water. Only one halogenated aliphatic alkyne, a dichloropropyne isomer, was identified in UK drinking water.

2.2 The halogenated alkenes

The most important metabolic step for the halogenated alkenes is probably conversion to epoxides by mono-oxygenases (Leibman and Ortiz 1977). Epoxides can be very reactive intermediates, which may be responsible for some of the toxic effects of this group of compounds. Detoxication of epoxides generally occurs through epoxide hydrase or by conjugation with glutathione.

For 1,2-dichloroethylene, it appears that both the *cis* and *trans* isomers are metabolised to dichloroacetic acid and dichloroethanol, via an epoxide intermediate. The epoxide then undergoes molecular rearrangement, with migration of a chlorine atom (Bonse *et al* 1975, Bolt *et al* 1982). Inhalation studies have shown that the *cis* isomer is metabolised more rapidly than the *trans* isomer (Filser and Bolt 1979).

There is some toxicological information available for 1,2-dichloroethylene, but there are almost no data on the remaining compounds.

The acute toxicity of 1,2-dichloroethylene in experimental animals appears to be low. The oral LD50 for the *trans* isomer has been reported to be 1260 mg/kg in the rat (Freundt *et al* 1977) and 2120–2390 mg/kg in the mouse (Barnes *et al* 1985). At sublethal doses, this compound has narcotic properties, and can also result in toxicity to the liver and kidney (Jenkins *et al* 1972).

In a 90-day study, *trans*-1,2-dichloroethylene induced only minimal effects in CD-1 mice receiving drinking water containing 100, 1000 or 2000 mg/l of the test compound dissolved in 1% Emulphor. The average doses consumed were calculated to be 17, 175 and 387 mg/kg body weight/day for the males and 23, 224 and 452 mg/kg body weight/day for the females. There was a slight increase in liver weight in male mice receiving 1000 mg/l. In the females there was a decrease in lung weight at the high dose and a decrease in thymus weight at both 1000 mg/l and 2000 mg/l. There were some slight changes in haematology and clinical chemistry, notably elevation of blood glucose at all three dose levels in both species, decreased liver glutathione in high-dose males, decreased serum alanine aminotransferase and aspartate aminotransferase at all dose levels in females, and reduced activity of hepatic aniline hydroxylase also in females. Microscopic pathology was not assessed (Barnes *et al*

1985). In groups of CD–1 mice receiving identical treatments to those above, there were no changes in cell-mediated immunity in either males or females or in the humoral immune status of females. At all three dose levels in males there was a reduced ability of spleen cells to produce antibody against sheep erythrocytes, but this did not appear to depress the function of the humoral immune system (Shopp *et al* 1985).

Rats, rabbits, guinea pigs and dogs exposed by inhalation to 500 or 1000 ppm of a 60 : 40 *cis–trans* mixture of 1,2-dichloroethylene, 7 hours/day, 5 days/week for 6 months showed no changes in mortality, growth, organ and body weights, haematology, clinical chemistry and gross and microscopic pathology of the major organs (Torkelson and Rowe 1981). However, Freundt *et al* (1977) reported pathological changes in the liver and lung of rats exposed by inhalation to 200 ppm of the *trans*-isomer, 8 hours/day, 5 days/week for 16 weeks.

Both the *cis* and *trans* isomers of 1,2-dichloroethylene have given negative results in the Ames test (Greim *et al* 1975, Neudecker *et al* 1986, Mortelmans *et al* 1986), but the *cis* isomer proved positive for induction of unscheduled DNA synthesis in rat hepatocytes *in vitro*, whereas the *trans* isomer was without effect (Costa and Ivanetich 1984). Both isomers were found to be weak inducers of mitotic crossing over in suspension assays with the yeast, *S. cerevisiae* D7, particularly in the presence of S-9, but there was little evidence for mitotic gene conversion or point mutation. The *cis* isomer also showed evidence of mutagenic activity in host-mediated assays using the same strain of yeast (Bronzetti *et al* 1984).

The mutagenicity of two chloromethylbutene isomers has been investigated by Neudecker *et al* (1980) as part of a structure/activity study on allyl chloride (3-chloro-1-propene). The main findings were that allylic structures (C=C–C–Cl) exhibited alkylating activity in the nitrobenzyl pyridine alkylation test, and were directly mutagenic to *S. typhimurium* TA100 in the Ames test. The presence of S-9 appeared to reduce mutagenic activity. Addition of one or two methyl groups to the structure, for example in the case of compounds such as 3-chloro-2-methyl-1-butene and 1-chloro-2-methyl-2-butene, tended to increase direct mutagenic potential. If the allylic structure itself was disturbed by movement of the chlorine atom onto a different carbon atom or by inserting an extra carbon atom between the chlorine atom and the double bond, direct mutagenic activity and alkylating activity were lost. Addition of S-9 tended to increase mutagenic potential for these compounds.

There appear to be no data available on carcinogenicity or reproductive toxicity.

2.3 The halogenated alkynes

A dichloropropyne isomer was detected in 5/14 drinking water samples in an unpublished survey by WRc (Water Research Centre 1982). There appears to be no toxicological information available on this compound.

2.4 Discussion

As a chemical group, the halogenated alkenes are thought to be metabolised to reactive epoxides that may be responsible for the toxicological effects of these compounds. In the case of the chloromethylbutenes, at least two of the possible isomers appear to have direct mutagenic activity in bacteria.

There is insufficient toxicological information available for these compounds on which to base an assessment.

REFERENCES

AGARWAL A K, BERNDT W O and MEHENDALE H M (1983) Possible nephrotoxic effect of carbon tetrabromide and its interaction with chlordecone. *Toxicology Letters* **17**, 57-62.

AHMED A E and ANDERS M W (1976) Metabolism of dihalomethanes to formaldehyde and inorganic halide. I. *In vitro* studies. *Drug Metabolism and Disposition* **4**, 357-361.

AHMED A E and ANDERS M W (1978) Metabolism of dihalomethanes to formaldehyde and inorganic halide. II. Studies on the mechanism of the reaction. *Biochemical Pharmacology* **27**, 2021-2025.

ALBANO E, LOTT K A K, SLATER T F, STIER A, SYMONS M C R and TOMASI A (1982) Spin-trapping studies on the free-radical products formed by metabolic activation of carbon tetrachloride in rat liver microsomal fractions, isolated hepatocytes and *in vivo* in the rat. *Biochemical Journal* **204**, 593-603.

ALUMOT E, NACHTOMI E, MANDEL E, HOLSTEIN P, BONDI A and HERZBERG M (1976a) Tolerance and acceptable daily intake of chlorinated fumigants in the rat diet. *Food and Cosmetics Toxicology* **14**, 105-110.

ALUMOT E, MEIDLER M, HOLSTEIN P and HERZBERG M (1976b) Tolerance and acceptable daily intake of ethylene dichloride in the chicken diet. *Food and Cosmetics Toxicology* **14**, 111-114.

BARBER E D, DONISH W H and MUELLER K R (1981) A procedure for the quantitative measurement of the mutagenicity of volatile liquids in the Ames Salmonella/microsome assay. *Mutation Research* **90**, 31-48.

BARBER E D, DONISH W H and MUELLER K R (1983) The relationship between growth and reversion in the Ames Salmonella plate incorporation assay. *Mutation Research* **113**, 89-101.

BARNES D W, SANDERS V M, WHITE K L Jr, SHOPP G M Jr and MUNSON A E (1985) Toxicology of *trans*-1,2-dichloroethylene in the mouse. *Drug and Chemical Toxicology* **8**, 373-392.

BOLT H M, LAIB R J and FILSER J G (1982) Reactive metabolites and carcinogenicity of halogenated ethylenes. *Biochemical Pharmacology* **31**, 1-4.

BONSE G, URBAN T, REICHERT D and HENSCHLER D (1975) Chemical reactivity, metabolic oxirane formation and biological reactivity of chlorinated ethylenes in the isolated perfused rat liver preparation. *Biochemical Pharmacology* **24**, 1829-1834.

BREM H, STEIN A B and ROSENKRANZ H S (1974) The mutagenicity and DNA-modifying effects of haloalkanes. *Cancer Research* **34**, 2576-2579.

BROGAN W C III, EACHO P I, HINTON D E and COLBY H D (1984) Effects of carbon tetrachloride on adrenocortical structure and function in guinea pigs. *Toxicology and Applied Pharmacology* **75**, 118-127.

BRONZETTI G, BAUER C, CORSI C, DEL CARRATORE R, GALLI A,

NIERI R, PAOLINI M, CUNDARI E, FORTI G C and CRENSHAW J (1984) Comparative genetic activity of *cis-* and *trans-* 1,2-dichloroethylene in yeast. *Teratogenesis, Carcinogenesis and Mutagenesis* **4**, 365-375.

BRUCKNER J V, MACKENZIE W F, MURALIDHARA S, LUTHRA R, KYLE G M and ACOSTA D (1986) Oral toxicity of carbon tetrachloride: Acute, subacute, and subchronic studies in rats. *Fundamental and Applied Toxicology* **6**, 16-34.

BUTLER T C (1961) Reduction of carbon tetrachloride *in vivo* and reduction of carbon tetrachloride and chloroform *in vitro* by tissues and tissue constituents. *Journal of Pharmacology and Experimental Therapeutics* **134**, 311-319.

CAGEN S Z and KLAASSEN C D (1979) Hepatotoxicity of carbon tetrachloride in developing rats. *Toxicology and Applied Pharmacology* **50**, 347-354.

CALLEN D F, WOLF C R and PHILPOT R M (1980) Cytochrome P-450 mediated genetic activity and cytotoxicity of seven halogenated aliphatic hydrocarbons in *Saccharomyces cerevisiae. Mutation Research* **77**, 55-63.

CHATTERJEE A (1966) Testicular degeneration in rats by carbon tetrachloride intoxication. *Experientia* **22**, 395-396.

COLACCI A, ARFELLINI G, MAZZULLO M, PRODI G and GRILLI S (1985) Genotoxicity of 1,1-dichloroethane. *Research Communications in Chemical Pathology and Pharmacology* **49**, 243-254.

COLBY H D, BROGAN W C III and MILES P R (1981) Carbon tetrachloride-induced changes in adrenal microsomal mixed-function oxidases and lipid peroxidation. *Toxicology and Applied Pharmacology* **60**, 492-499.

CONDIE L W, LAURIE R D, MILLS T, ROBINSON M and BERCZ J P (1986) Effect of gavage vehicle on hepatotoxicity of carbon tetrachloride in CD-1 mice: corn oil versus Tween-60 aqueous emulsion. *Fundamental and Applied Toxicology* **7**, 199-206.

COSTA A K and IVANETICH K M (1984) Chlorinated ethylenes: their metabolism and effect on DNA repair in hepatocytes. *Carcinogenesis* **5**, 1629-1636.

CRESPI C L, SEIXAS G M, TURNER T R, RYAN C G and PENMAN B W (1985) Mutagenicity of 1,2-dichloroethane and 1,2-dibromoethane in two human lymphoblastoid cell lines. *Mutation Research* **142**, 133-140.

DAVIDSON I W F, SUMNER D D and PARKER J C (1982) Ethylene dichloride: A review of its metabolism, mutagenic and carcinogenic potential. *Drug and Chemical Toxicology* **5**, 319-388.

DELLA PORTA G, TERRACINI B and SHUBIK P (1961) Induction with carbon tetrachloride of liver cell carcinomas in hamsters. *Journal of the National Cancer Institute* **26**, 855-863.

DIAZ-GOMEZ M I and CASTRO J A (1980) Binding of carbon tetrachloride metabolites to liver nuclear DNA, proteins, and lipids. *Toxicology and Applied Pharmacology* **56**, 199-206.

DIPPLE A, LEVY L S and LAWLEY P D (1981) Comparative carcinogenicity of alkylating agents: Comparisons of a series of alkyl and aralkyl bromides of differing chemical reactivities as inducers of sarcoma at the site of a single injection in the rat. *Carcinogenesis* **2**, 103-107.

EDER E, NEUDECKER T, LUTZ D and HENSCHLER D (1980) Mutagenic potential of allyl and allylic compounds. Structure–activity relationship as determined by alkylating and direct *in vitro* mutagenic properties. *Biochemical Pharmacology* **29**, 993-998.

FILSER J G and BOLT H M (1979) Pharmacokinetics of halogenated ethylenes in rats. *Archives of Toxicology* **42**, 123-136.

FREUNDT K J, LIEBALDT G P and LIEBERWIRTH E (1977) Toxicity studies on *trans*-1,2-dichloroethylene. *Toxicology* **7**, 141-153.

GORZINSKI S J, NOLAN R J, McCOLLISTER S B, KOCIBA R J and MATTSSON J L (1985) Subchronic oral toxicity, tissue distribution and clearance of hexachloroethane in the rat. *Drug and Chemical Toxicology* **8**, 155-169.

GREIM H, BONSE G, RADWAN Z, REICHERT D and HENSCHLER D (1975) Mutagenicity *in vitro* and potential carcinogenicity of chlorinated ethylenes as a function of metabolic oxirane formation. *Biochemical Pharmacology* **24**, 2013-2017.

HAYES J R, CONDIE L W and BORZELLECA J F (1986) Acute, 14-day repeated dosing and 90-day subchronic studies of carbon tetrachloride in CD-1 mice. *Fundamental and Applied Toxicology* **7**, 454-463.

HEAD B, MOODY D E, WOO C H and SMUCKLER E A (1981) Alterations of specific forms of cytochrome P-450 in rat liver during acute carbon tetrachloride intoxication. *Toxicology and Applied Pharmacology* **61**, 286-295.

HEPPEL L A, NEAL P A, PERRIN T L, ENDICOTT K M and PORTERFIELD V T (1946) The toxicology of 1,2-dichloroethane (ethylene dichloride). V. The effects of daily inhalations. *Journal of Industrial Hygiene and Toxicology* **28**, 113-120.

HOFMANN H T, BIRNSTIEL H and JOBST P (1971) On the inhalation toxicity of 1,1- and 1,2-dichloroethane. *Archives of Toxicology* **27**, 248-265.

INSKEEP P B, KOGA N, CMARIK J L and GUENGERICH F P (1986) Covalent binding of 1,2-dihaloalkanes to DNA and stability of the major DNA adduct, *S*-[2-(N7-guanyl)ethyl]glutathione. *Cancer Research* **46**, 2839-2844.

INTERNATIONAL AGENCY FOR RESEARCH ON CANCER (1979) IARC Monographs on the Evaluation of the Carcinogenic Risk of Chemicals to Humans. Some Halogenated Hydrocarbons. IARC, Lyon, Vol 20, 371–399.

IVANETICH K M and VAN DEN HONERT L H (1981) Chloroethanes: Their metabolism by hepatic cytochrome P-450 *in vitro*. *Carcinogenesis* **2**, 697-702.

JAMES S P, JEFFERY D A, WARING R H and WOOD P B (1968) Some metabolites of 1-bromobutane in the rabbit and the rat. *Biochemical Journal* **109**, 727-736.

JENKINS L J Jr, TRABULUS M J and MURPHY S D (1972) Biochemical effects of 1,1-dichloroethylene in rats: comparison with carbon tetrachloride and 1,2-dichloroethylene. *Toxicology and Applied Pharmacology* **23**, 501-510.

JENSSEN D and RAMEL C (1980) The micronucleus test as a part of a short-term mutagenicity test program for the prediction of carcinogenicity evaluated by 143 agents tested. *Mutation Research* **75**, 191-202.

JONDORF W R, PARKE D V and WILLIAMS R T (1957) The metabolism of [^{14}C]hexachloroethane. *Biochemical Journal* **65**, 14P-15P.

JONES A R and WALSH D A (1979) The oxidative metabolism of 1-bromopropane in the rat. *Xenobiotica* **9**, 763-772.

KALLA N R and BANSAL M P (1975) Effect of carbon tetrachloride on gonadal physiology in male rats. *Acta Anatomica* **91**, 380-385.

KARIMULLINA N K and GIZATULLINA A A (1969) Effects of ethyl bromide on the liver. *Farmakologiia i Toksikologiia* **32**, 165. (*Chemical Abstracts* **70**, 113460p).

KING M T, BEIKIRCH H, ECKHARDT K, GOCKE E and WILD D (1979) Mutagenicity studies with X-ray-contrast media, analgesics, antipyretics, antirheumatics and some other pharmaceutical drugs in bacterial, *Drosophila* and mammalian test systems. *Mutation Research* **66**, 33-43.

KLAASSEN C D and PLAA G L (1966) Relative effects of various chlorinated hydrocarbons on liver and kidney function in mice. *Toxicology and Applied Pharmacology* **9**, 139-151.

KLAASSEN C D and PLAA G L (1967) Relative effects of various chlorinated hydrocarbons on liver and kidney function in dogs. *Toxicology and Applied Pharmacology* **10**, 119-131.

KLAASSEN C D and PLAA G L (1969) Comparison of the biochemical alterations elicited in livers from rats treated with carbon tetrachloride, chloroform, 1,1,2-trichloroethane and 1,1,1-trichloroethane. *Biochemical Pharmacology* **18**, 2019-2027.

KUBIC V L and ANDERS M W (1978) Metabolism of dihalomethanes to carbon monoxide–III. *Biochemical Pharmacology* **27**, 2349-2355.

KUBIC V A and ANDERS M W (1980) Metabolism of carbon tetrachloride to phosgene. *Life Sciences* **26**, 2151-2155.

KUBIC V L, ANDERS M W, ENGEL R R, BURLOV C H and CAUGHEY W S (1974) Metabolism of dihalomethanes to carbon monoxide. *Drug Metabolism and Distribution* **2**, 53-57.

LANE R W, RIDDLE B L and BORZELLECA J F (1982) Effects of 1,2-dichloroethane and 1,1,1-trichloroethane in drinking water on reproduction and development in mice. *Toxicology and Applied Pharmacology* **63**, 409-421.

LEIBMAN K C and ORTIZ E (1977) Metabolism of halogenated ethylenes. *Environmental Health Perspectives* **21**, 91-97.

LEONSKAYA G (1980) Evaluation of the embryotoxic and teratogenic effect of butyl and benzyl chlorides in a determination of their hygienic standards in reservoir water. *Gigiena Naselennykh Mest, Kiev* **19**, 40-43.

LEVY G N and BRABEC M J (1984) Binding of carbon tetrachloride metabolites to rat hepatic mitochondrial DNA. *Toxicology Letters* **22**, 229-234.

LIN E L C, MATTOX J K and PEREIRA M A (1985) Glutathione plus cytosol- and microsome-mediated binding of 1,2-dichloroethane to polynucleotides. *Toxicology and Applied Pharmacology* **78**, 428-435.

MacEWEN J D, McNERNEY J M, VERNOT E H and HARPER D T (1966) Chronic inhalation toxicity of chlorobromomethane. *Journal of Occupational Medicine* **8**, 251-256.

MacEWAN J, KINKEAD E and HAUN C (1974) A study of the biological effect of continuous inhalation exposure of 1,1,1-trichloroethane (methyl chloroform) in animals. NASA Contract Report 134232.

MALENDOWICZ L K and COLBY H D (1982) Effects of carbon tetrachloride on adrenocortical function in rats. *Toxicology and Applied Pharmacology* **65**, 32-37.

MALTONI C, VALGIMIGLI L and SCARNATO C (1980) Banbury Report 5. Ethylene dichloride: A potential health risk? Cold Spring Harbor Laboratory, 3.

MAZZULLO M, COLACCI A, GRILLI S, PRODI G and ARFELLINI G (1986) 1,1,2-Trichloroethane: evidence of genotoxicity from short-term tests. *Japanese Journal of Cancer Research* (Gann) **77**, 532-539.

McNUTT N S, AMSTER R L, McCONNELL E E and MORRIS F (1975) Hepatic lesions in mice after continuous inhalation exposure to 1,1,1-trichloroethane. *Laboratory Investigation* **32**, 642-654.

MICO B A, BRANCHFLOWER R V, POHL L R, PUDZIANOWSKI A T and LOEW G H (1982) Oxidation of carbon tetrachloride, bromotrichloromethane and carbon tetrabromide by rat liver microsomes to electrophilic halogens. *Life Sciences* **30**, 131-137.

MILMAN H A, MITOMA C, TYSON C, RICCIO E S, SIVAK A, TU A S, WILLIAMS G M and TONG C (1984) Comparative pharmacokinetics/metabolism, carcinogenicity and mutagenicity of chlorinated ethanes and ethylenes. In *Abstracts of the International Conference on Organic Solvent Toxicity,* Stockholm, Sweden, October 15-17.

MIRSALIS J C and BUTTERWORTH B E (1980) Detection of unscheduled DNA synthesis in hepatocytes isolated from rats treated with genotoxic agents: an *in vivo–in vitro* assay for potential carcinogens and mutagens. *Carcinogenesis* **1**, 621-625.

MIRSALIS J C, TYSON C K and BUTTERWORTH B E (1982) Detection of genotoxic carcinogens in the *in vivo–in vitro* hepatocyte DNA repair assay. *Environmental Mutagenesis* **4**, 553-562.

MITOMA C, STEEGER T, JACKSON S E, WHEELER K P, ROGERS J H and MILMAN H A (1985) Metabolic disposition study of chlorinated hydrocarbons in rats and mice. *Drug and Chemical Toxicology* **8**, 183-194.

MONIG J, BAHNEMANN D and ASMUS K D (1983) One electron reduction of CCl_4 in oxygenated aqueous solutions: A CCl_3O_2.-free radical mediated formation of Cl^- and CO_2. *Chemicobiological Interactions* **45**, 15-27.

MORTELMANS K, HAWORTH S, LAWLOR T, SPECK W, TAINER B and ZEIGER E (1986) Salmonella mutagenicity tests: II. Results from the testing of 270 chemicals. *Environmental Mutagenesis* **8**, Suppl 7, 1-119.

NATIONAL ACADEMY OF SCIENCES (1977) Drinking Water and Health. Safe Drinking Water Committee, National Academy of Sciences, Washington, DC, 703-707.

NATIONAL CANCER INSTITUTE (1976) Carcinogenesis bioassay of trichloroethylene. NCI CG-TR-2.

NATIONAL CANCER INSTITUTE (1977) Bioassay of 1,1,1-trichloroethane for possible carcinogenicity. NTIS PB-265 082.

NATIONAL CANCER INSTITUTE (1978) Bioassay of 1,1,2,2-tetrachloroethane for possible carcinogenicity. NTIS PB-277 453.

NAVROTSKII V K, KASHIN L M, KULINSKAYA I L, MIKHAILOVSKAYA L F, SHMUTER L M, BURLAKA-VOVK Z I and ZADOROZHNYI B V (1971) Tr S'ezde Gig Vkr SSR **8**, 224 (*Chemical Abstracts* **77**, 071060v).

NESTMANN E R, OTSON R, KOWBEL D J, BOTHWELL P D and HARRINGTON T R (1984) Mutagenicity in a modified Salmonella assay of fabricprotecting products containing 1,1,1-trichloroethane. *Environmental Mutagenesis* **6**, 71-80.

NEUDECKER T, LUTZ D, EDER E and HENSCHLER D (1980) Structure–activity relationship in halogen and alkyl substituted allyl and allylic compounds: Correlation of alkylating and mutagenic properties. *Biochemical Pharmacology* **29**, 2611-2617.

NEUDECKER T, DEKANT W, JORNS M, EDER E and HENSCHLER D (1986) Mutagenicity of chloroolefins in the Salmonella/mammalian microsome test - II. Structural requirements for the metabolic activation of non-allylic chloropropenes and methylated derivatives via epoxide formation. *Biochemical Pharmacology* **35**, 195-200.

OKTYABR'SKII O N (1977) Mutagenic and embryotropic effect of alkyl chlorides. *Gig Aspekty Okhr Zdorov'ya Naseleniya* 125-126.

OSTERMAN-GOLKAR S, HUSSAIN S, WALLES S, ANDERSTAM B and SIGVARDSSON K (1983) Chemical reactivity and mutagenicity of some dihalomethanes. *Chemicobiological Interactions* **46**, 121-130.

PACKER J E, SLATER T F and WILSON R L (1978) Reactions of the carbon tetrachloride-related peroxy free radical (CCl_3O_2) with amino acids: Pulse radiolysis evidence. *Life Sciences* **23**, 2617-2620.

PAUL B B and RUBINSTEIN D (1963) Metabolism of carbon tetrachloride and chloroform by the rat. *Journal of Pharmacology and Experimental Therapeutics* **141**, 141-148.

PEROCCO P and PRODI G (1981) DNA damage by haloalkanes in human lymphocytes cultured *in vitro*. *Cancer Letters* **13**, 213-218.

PLAA G L and LARSON R E (1965) Relative nephrotoxic properties of chlorinated methane, ethane, and ethylene derivatives in mice. *Toxicology and Applied Pharmacology* **7**, 37-44.

PLAA G L, EVANS E A and HINE C H (1958) Relative hepatotoxicity of seven halogenated hydrocarbons. *Journal of Pharmacology and Experimental Therapeutics* **123**, 224-229.

POHL L R and GEORGE J W (1983) Identification of dichloromethyl carbene as a metabolite of carbon tetrachloride. *Biochemical and Biophysical Research Communications* **117**, 367-371.

POIRIER L A, STONER G D and SHIMKIN M B (1975) Bioassay of alkyl halides and nucleotide base analogs by pulmonary tumor response in strain A mice. *Cancer Research* **35**, 1411-1415.

POYER J L, McCAY P B, LAI E K, JANZEN E G and DAVIS E R (1980) Confirmation of assignment of the trichloromethyl radical spin adduct detected by spin trapping during ^{13}C-carbon tetrachloride metabolism *in vitro* and *in vivo*. *Biochemical and Biophysical Research Communications* **94**, 1154-1160.

PRENDERGAST J A, JONES R A, JENKINS L J Jr and SIEGEL J (1967) Effects on experimental animals of long-term inhalation of trichloroethylene, carbon tetrachloride, 1,1,1-trichloroethane dichlorodifluoromethane and 1,1-dichloroethylene. *Toxicology and Applied Pharmacology* **10**, 270-289.

RAMPY L W, QUAST J F, LEONG B K J and GEHRING P J (1977) Results of long-term inhalation toxicity studies on rats of 1,1,1-trichloroethane and perchloroethylene formulations. In *Proceedings of the International Congress on*

Toxicology (Abstracts), Toronto, 27.
RANNUG U (1980) Genotoxic effects of 1,2-dibromoethane and 1,2-dichloroethane. *Mutation Research* **76**, 269-295.
RANNUG U, SUNDVALL A and RAMEL C (1978) The mutagenic effect of 1,2-dichloroethane on *Salmonella typhimurium*. I. Activation through conjugation with glutathione *in vitro*. *Chemicobiological Interactions* **20**, 1-16.
RAO K S, MURRAY J S, DEACON M M, JOHN J A, CALHOUN L L and YOUNG J T (1980) Banbury Report 5. Ethylene dichloride: A potential health risk? Cold Spring Harbor Laboratory, 149.
REGISTRY OF TOXIC EFFECTS OF CHEMICAL SUBSTANCES National Institute for Occupational Safety and Health, Cincinnati, Ohio.
REUBER M D and GLOVER E L (1970) Cirrhosis and carcinoma of the liver in male rats given subcutaneous carbon tetrachloride. *Journal of the National Cancer Institute* **44**, 419-427.
RUDNEV M I, TOMASHEVSKAYA L A and VINOGRADOV G I (1979) Hygienic substantiation of the permissible content of benzyl and butyl chlorides in reservoir water. *Gigiena i Sanitariia* **3**, 11-15.
SAITO-SUZUKI R, TERAMOTO S and SHIRASU Y (1982) Dominant lethal studies in rats with 1,2-dibromo-3-chloropropane and its structurally related compounds. *Mutation Research* **101**, 321-327.
SANDERS V M, WHITE K L Jr, SHOPP G M Jr and MUNSON A E (1985) Humoral and cell-mediated immune status of mice exposed to 1,1,2-trichloroethane. *Drug and Chemical Toxicology* **8**, 357-372.
SCHMIDT R (1976) The embryotoxic and teratogenic effect of tetrachloroethane – experimental investigations. *Biologische Rundschau* **14**, 220-223.
SCHWETZ B A, LEONG B K J and GEHRING P J (1974) Embryo and fetotoxicity of inhaled carbon tetrachloride, 1,1-dichloroethane and methyl ethyl ketone in rats. *Toxicology and Applied Pharmacology* **28**, 452-464.
SCHWETZ B A, LEONG B K J and GEHRING P J (1975) The effect of maternally inhaled trichloroethylene, perchloroethylene, methyl chloroform, and methylene chloride on embryonal and fetal development in mice and rats. *Toxicology and Applied Pharmacology* **32**, 84-96.
SHIMADA T, SWANSON A F, LEBER P and WILLIAMS G M (1985) Activities of chlorinated ethane and ethylene compounds in the Salmonella/rat microsome mutagenesis and rat hepatocyte/DNA repair assays under vapor phase exposure conditions. *Cell Biology and Toxicology* **1**, 159-179.
SHMUTER L M (1972) Effects of chronic action of small concentrations of chlorinated hydrocarbons on the production of various classes of immunoglobulins. *Gigiena i Sanitariia* **37**, 36-40.
SHOPP G M Jr, SANDERS V M, WHITE K L Jr and MUNSON A E (1985) Humoral and cell-mediated immune status of mice exposed to *trans*-1,2-dichloroethylene. *Drug and Chemical Toxicology* **8**, 393-407.
SIMMON V F (1980) Review of nonbacterial tests of the genotoxicity of ethylene dichloride. Banbury Report 5. Ethylene dichloride: A potential health risk? Cold Spring Harbor Laboratory, 97.
SIMMON V (1981) Applications of the Salmonella/microsome assay. In *Short-term tests for Chemical Carcinogens* edited by H Stich *et al*, New York, Springer-

Verlag, pp. 120-126.

SIMMON V F and POIRIER L A (1976) Mutagenicity of alkyl halides to *S. typhimurium* TA 1535 and TA 100 and to *E. coli* WP2(hcr-). *Proceedings of the American Association for Cancer Research* **17**, 85.

SIMMON V F, KAUHANEN K and TARDIFF R G (1977) Mutagenic activity of chemicals identified in drinking water. In *Progress in Genetic Toxicology* edited by D Scott, B A Bridges and F H Sobels. Elsevier/North-Holland Biomedical Press, 249-258.

SLATER T F (1982) Activation of carbon tetrachloride: Chemical principles and biological significance. In *Free Radicals, Lipid Peroxidation and Cancer* edited by D C H McBrien and T F Slater, Academic Press, pp. 243-270.

SMUCKLER E A, ARRHENIUS E and HULTIN T (1967) Alterations in microsomal electron transport, oxidative *N*-demethylation and azo-dye cleavage in carbon tetrachloride and dimethylnitrosamine-induced liver injury. *Biochemical Journal* **103**, 55-64.

SMYTH H F Jr, CARPENTER C P, WEIL C S, POZZANI U C, STRIEGEL J A and NYCUM J S (1969) Range-finding toxicity data: List VII. *American Industrial Hygiene Association Journal* **30**, 470-476.

SPENCER H C, ROWE V K, ADAMS E M, McCOLLISTER D D and IRISH D D (1951) Vapor toxicity of ethylene dichloride determined by experiments on laboratory animals. *Archives of Industrial Hygiene and Occupational Medicine* **4**, 482-493.

STEVENS J L, RATNAYAKE J H and ANDERS M W (1980) Metabolism of dihalomethanes to carbon monoxide. IV. Studies in isolated hepatocytes. *Toxicology and Applied Pharmacology* **55**, 484-489.

STORER R D and CONOLLY R B (1985) An investigation of the role of microsomal oxidative metabolism in the *in vivo* genotoxicity of 1,2-dichloroethane. *Toxicology and Applied Pharmacology* **77**, 36-46.

SVIRBELY J L, HIGHMAN B, ALFORD W C and VON OETTINGEN W F (1947) The toxicity and narcotic action of monochloromonobromomethane with special reference to inorganic and volatile bromide in blood, urine and brain. *Journal of Industrial Hygiene and Toxicology* **29**, 382-389.

SYMONS M C R, ALBANO E, SLATER T F and TOMASI A (1982) Radiolysis of tetrachloromethane. *Journal of the Chemical Society Faraday Transactions I* **78**, 2205-2214.

TAN E-Y and HSIE A W (1981) Mutagenicity and cytotoxicity of haloethanes as studied in the CHO/HGPRT system. *Mutation Research* **90**, 183-191.

THEISS J C, STONER G D, SHIMKIN M B and WEISBURGER E K (1977) Tests for carcinogenicity of organic contaminants of United States drinking waters by pulmonary tumor response in strain A mice. *Cancer Research* **37**, 2717-2720.

THOMPSON J A, HO B and MASTOVICH S L (1984) Reductive metabolism of 1,1,1,2-tetrachloroethane and related chloroethanes by rat liver microsomes. *Chemicobiological Interactions* **51**, 321-333.

TORKELSON T R and ROWE V K (1981) Halogenated aliphatic hydrocarbons containing chlorine, bromine and iodine. In *Patty's Industrial Hygiene and Toxicology* edited by G D Clayton and F E Clayton, 3rd Revised Edition, Vol 2B. John Wiley & Sons, New York, pp. 3433-3601.

TORKELSON T R, OYEN F, McCOLLISTER D D and ROWE V K (1958) Toxicity of 1,1,1-trichloroethane as determined on laboratory animals and human subjects. *American Industrial Hygiene Association Journal* **19**, 353-362.

TORKELSON T R, OYEN F and ROWE V K (1960) The toxicity of bromochloromethane (methylene chlorobromide) as determined on laboratory animals. *American Industrial Hygiene Association Journal* **21**, 275-286.

TOWN C and LEIBMAN K C (1984) The *in vitro* dechlorination of some polychlorinated ethanes. *Drug Metabolism and Disposition* **12**, 4-8.

TRUHAUT R and PHU LICH N (1973) Transformations metaboliques du tetrachloro 1,1,1,2 ethane chez le rat, le cobaye et le lapin. *Journal Europeen de Toxicologie* No 4-5, 211-217.

TRUHAUT R, PHU LICH N, DUTERTRE-CATELLA H, MOLAS G and NGOC HUYEN V (1974) Contribution to the toxicological study of 1,1,1,2-tetrachloroethane. *Archives des Maladies Professionelles, de Medicine, du Travail et de Securite Sociale* **35**, 593-608.

TUGARINOVA V I, MIKLASHEVSKII V E, ALEKSEEVA N P and YAKOVLEVA G P (1963) Experimental determination of limits of allowable tetrachloroethane (TCLE) and hexachloroethane (HCLE) concentrations in water. *USSR Literature on Water Supply and Pollution Control* **5**, 145-154.

TURINA M P, COLACCI A, GRILLI S, MAZZULLO M, PRODI G and LATTANZI G (1986) Short-term tests of genotoxicity for 1,1,1-trichloroethane. *Research Communications in Chemical Pathology and Pharmacology* **52**, 305-320.

UNITED STATES ENVIRONMENTAL PROTECTION AGENCY (1980) Ambient Water Quality Criteria for Carbon Tetrachloride. EPA-440/5-80-026.

UNITED STATES ENVIRONMENTAL PROTECTION AGENCY (1984) Health Assessment Document for Carbon Tetrachloride. Final Report. EPA-600/8-82/001F.

UNITED STATES NATIONAL TOXICOLOGY PROGRAM (1982) Bioassay of 1,1,1-trichloroethane for possible carcinogenicity (final report in preparation). National Toxicology Program, Bethesda, Maryland.

UNITED STATES NATIONAL TOXICOLOGY PROGRAM (1986) Toxicology and carcinogenesis studies of *n*-butyl chloride in F344/N rats and B6C3F1 mice. National Toxicology Program Technical Report No 312, NIH Publication No 86-2568.

VAN BLADEREN P J, BREIMER D D, ROTTEVEEL-SMIJS G M T and MOHN G R (1980) Mutagenic activation of dibromomethane and diiodomethane by mammalian microsomes and glutathione-*S*-transferases. *Mutation Research* **74**, 341-346.

VAN DYKE R A and WINEMAN C G (1971) Enzymatic dechlorination. Dechlorination of chloroethanes and propanes *in vitro*. *Biochemical Pharmacology* **20**, 463-470.

VINOGRADOV G I (1979) Autosensitizing effect in the per os administration of chemical substances to animals. *Vrachebnoe Delo* **9**, 100-102.

VOGEL E and CHANDLER J L R (1974) Mutagenicity testing of cyclamate and some pesticides in *Drosophila melanogaster*. *Experientia* **30**, 621.

WALLER R L and RECKNAGEL R O (1982) Evaluation of a role for phosgene

production in the hepatotoxic mechanism of action of carbon tetrachloride and bromotrichloromethane. *Toxicology and Applied Pharmacology* **66**, 172-181.
WATER RESEARCH CENTRE (1981) Organic micropollutants in drinking water. Water Research Centre Technical Report TR 159.
WATER RESEARCH CENTRE (1982) Frequency of occurrence data for compounds identified by GC-MS in XAD-2 samples taken for mutagenic testing survey. WRc unpublished report.
WATROUS W M and PLAA G L (1972) The nephrotoxicity of single and multiple doses of aliphatic chlorinated hydrocarbon solvents in male mice. *Toxicology and Applied Pharmacology* **23**, 640-649.
WEEKS M H, ANGERHOFER R A, BISHOP R, THOMASINO J and POPE C R (1979) The toxicity of hexachloroethane in laboratory animals. *American Industrial Hygiene Association Journal* **40**, 187-199.
WEISBURGER E K (1977) Carcinogenicity studies on halogenated hydrocarbons. *Environmental Health Perspectives* **21**, 7-16.
WHITE K L Jr, SANDERS V M, BARNES D W, SHOPP G M Jr and MUNSON A E (1985) Toxicology of 1,1,2-trichloroethane in the mouse. *Drug and Chemical Toxicology* **8**, 333-355.
WORLD HEALTH ORGANIZATION (1984) Carbon tetrachloride. In Guidelines for Drinking-Water Quality Vol 2. Health Criteria and Other Supporting Information. WHO Geneva.
YALCIN A S, KOCAK-TOKER N, UYSAL M, AYKAC G, SIVAS A and OZ H (1986) Stimulation of lipid peroxidation and impairment of glutathione-dependent defence system in the liver of rats repeatedly treated with carbon tetrachloride. *Journal of Applied Toxicology* **6**, 303-306.
YLLNER S (1971a) Metabolism of 1,2-dichloroethane-^{14}C in the mouse. *Acta Pharmacologica et Toxicologica* **30**, 257-265.
YLLNER S (1971b) Metabolism of 1,1,2-trichloroethane-1,2-[^{14}C] in the mouse. *Acta Pharmacologica et Toxicologica* **30**, 248-256.
YLLNER S (1971c) Metabolism of 1,1,1,2-tetrachloroethane in the mouse. *Acta Pharmacologica et Toxicologica* **29**, 471-480.
YLLNER S (1971d) Metabolism of 1,1,2,2-tetrachloroethane-94C in the mouse. *Acta Pharmacologica et Toxicologica* **29**, 499-512.
YORK R G, SOWRY B M, HASTINGS L and MANSON J M (1982) Evaluation of teratogenicity and neurotoxicity with maternal inhalation exposure to methyl chloroform. *Journal of Toxicology and Environmental Health* **9**, 251-266.
ZIMMERMAN S W and NORBACH D H (1980) Nephrotoxic effects of long-term carbon tetrachloride administration in rats. *Archives of Pathology and Laboratory Medicine* **104**, 94-99.

8

The miscellaneous halogenated compounds

1. INTRODUCTION

This group is composed of 25 compounds identified by gas chromatography–mass spectrometry in two surveys of UK drinking water by WRc. It is in the nature of this group that it contains a diversity of compounds, hence, general statements on the toxicological properties of the miscellaneous halogenated compounds are not possible. The structures of some of the compounds are shown in Figure 1.

Probably all the chemicals in this group are of anthropogenic origins. Many of the compounds can be produced during water chlorination, several may have an industrial source, while dicamba is used as a herbicide and clofibrate as a pharmaceutical. Although it is likely that water may be a major environmental source of exposure to most of the compounds in this group, many of these compounds occurred infrequently in drinking water, and then only at very low concentrations.

The information available on the metabolism of the miscellaneous halogenated compounds is generally poor, though not unsurprisingly clofibrate has been well studied.

2. THE HALOGENATED ACETONITRILES

2.1 Introduction

Halogenated acetonitriles have only recently been recognised as common micropollutants in treated waters. This discovery has led to the initiation of research projects on the potential health effects of these compounds, the results of which are just beginning to become available.

2.2 Exposure

Dichloroacetonitrile was the first member of the group to be identified in drinking water (McKinney *et al* 1976). In a survey of three drinking waters in the US, dichloroacetonitrile was identified in all samples at an average concentration of 2 μg/l. Dibromoacetonitrile was also identified in all three samples, though at a

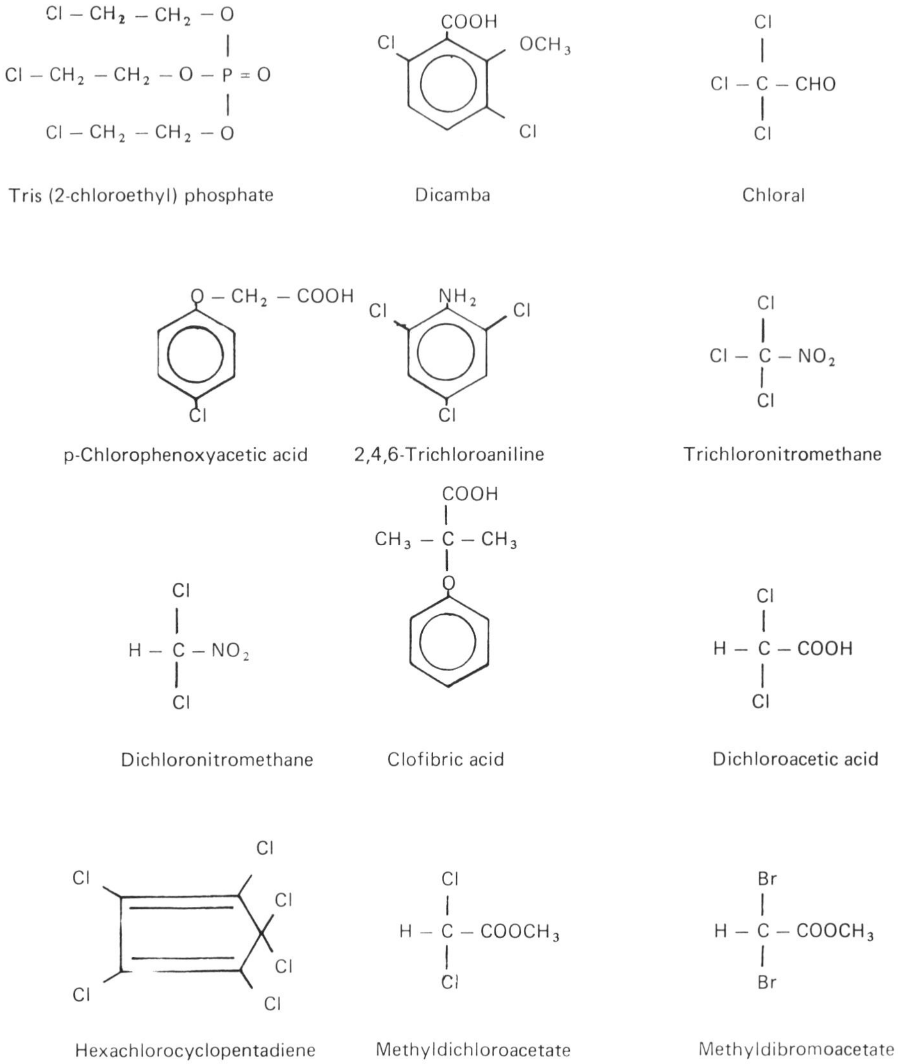

Fig. 8.1 — Structures of some of the miscellaneous halogenated compounds identified in drinking water.

higher average concentration of around 10 μg/l. Trichloroacetonitrile was detected at generally less than 1 μg/l (Keith *et al* 1983). The highest total halogenated acetonitrile concentration reported to date is 40μ g/l in a chlorinated well water in the US (Bieber and Trehy 1983). Dichloroacetonitrile has also consistently been identified in drinking water samples from southern Ontario, Canada, at concentrations ranging from 0.3 to 8.1 μg/l. In the same survey, bromochloroacetonitrile was present at levels generally below 1 μg/l (Oliver 1983). In the WRc survey, dichloroacetonitrile was identified in 11/14 drinking water samples, dibromoacetonitrile in 8/

14, bromochloroacetonitrile in 7/14, and chlorophenoxyacetonitrile in 5/14 (Water Research Centre 1981).

A number of experiments have been performed which suggest that halogenated acetonitriles are produced from the reaction of chlorine with natural organic materials in water. Bieber and Trehy (1983) demonstrated the production of dichloroacetonitrile following the aqueous chlorination of some amino acids, particularly aspartic acid. Although free amino acid levels in water are rather low, significant quantities of aspartic acid and other amino acids are found associated with humic matter. Dichloroacetonitrile was also produced following the chlorination of fulvic acid at pH 7 and of two species of algae at pH 6–8 (Oliver 1983). In the Canadian survey, the highest levels of halogenated acetonitriles were found in those waters containing high total organic carbon and which received high chlorine doses. In laboratory experiments, the yield of halogenated acetonitriles and trihalomethanes from the chlorination of natural waters was dependent on the free chlorine concentration and the contact time (Bieber and Trehy 1983). Bieber and Trehy have proposed that halogenated acetonitriles are formed by a stepwise halogenation reaction mechanism at the N-terminals of polypeptides. Helz *et al* (1983) also suggest that sensitive amino acids may be attacked independently of the stepwise mechanism, thereby severing the polypeptide at this point and creating another N-terminal peptide suitable for stepwise oxidation. Although chloroform was produced from the hydrolysis of trichloroacetonitrile at pH 9 and has also been detected after dichloroacetonitrile was allowed to stand for a few days with NaOCl, the yields were very small, suggesting that most chloroform in drinking water is not derived from the breakdown of halogenated acetonitriles (Keith *et al* 1983).

In the US, where residual levels of chlorine are present at the tap, there has been concern that reactive chlorinated compounds may be formed in the gastrointestinal tract. In a study by Mink *et al* (1983), dichloroacetonitrile was detected in the upper gastrointestinal tract of both fasted and non-fasted rats after treatment with NaOCl. Following treatment with NaOCl and KBr, dichloroacetonitrile and dibromoacetonitrile were produced. These compounds, however, were not detected in the blood.

2.3 Toxicokinetics

In rats, 7.7–12.8% of oral doses of dibromoacetonitrile, dichloroacetonitrile or bromochloroacetonitrile were excreted in the urine as thiocyanate within 24 hours (Pereira *et al* 1984).

2.4 Health effects

The only data available at present relate to the genotoxic potential of the halogenated acetonitriles and their carcinogenicity in short-term assays.

Dichloroacetonitrile has been shown to be mutagenic in the Ames test to *Salmonella typhimurium* TA100, TA98, and TA1535, both in the presence and absence of metabolic activation (Simmon *et al* 1977, Bull 1982a). It did not, however, increase mitotic recombination in the yeast *S. cerevisiae* (Simmon *et al* 1977). Bromochloroacetonitrile was directly mutagenic to *S. typhimurium* TA100 and TA1535 (Bull 1982a). Chloroacetonitrile, trichloroacetonitrile and dibromoacetonitrile were negative in the Ames test, though toxicity limited the concentration of the latter two compounds that could be tested (Bull 1982a).

Halogenated acetonitriles have been reported to bind to calf thymus DNA and to react with *p*-nitrobenzopyridine, a nucleophilic trapping agent (Daniel *et al* 1983, 1986). Trichloroacetonitrile, dibromoacetonitrile, bromochloroacetonitrile and dichloroacetonitrile have been shown to induce DNA breaks in cultured human lymphocytes, though the test with chloroacetonitrile was inconclusive (Bull 1982a). All five compounds significantly increased the incidence of sister chromatid exchanges in Chinese hamster ovary cells *in vitro*, but gave negative results in the mouse micronucleus assay (Bull 1984).

Halogenated acetonitriles have been tested for tumour-initiating activity in mouse skin. Doses of 200, 400 and 800 mg/kg in 0.2 ml acetone were applied to the shaved backs of female Sencar mice thrice weekly for 2 weeks. Two weeks after the last dose the animals began receiving 1 μg of the tumour promoter TPA in 0.2 ml acetone thrice weekly for 20 weeks. Significantly increased tumour incidences were found with chloroacetonitrile, dibromoacetonitrile and bromochloroacetonitrile. Dichloroacetonitrile and trichloroacetonitrile gave equivocal results (Bull 1986, 1982b, Bull and Robinson 1985, Bull *et al* 1985, Meier *et al* 1983, United States Environmental Protection Agency 1983).

Strain A/J mice were given 10 mg/kg of several halogenated acetonitriles by intraperitoneal injection, thrice weekly for 8 weeks. At 9 months of age, increased incidences of lung tumours were found with chloroacetonitrile, bromochloroacetonitrile and trichloroacetonitrile (Bull 1984).

2.5 Discussion

It is now apparent that halogenated acetonitriles are common organic micropollutants in drinking water, and their presence is clearly associated with the process of water chlorination.

Dichloroacetonitrile and bromochloroacetonitrile are mutagenic in the Ames test. Most of the compounds have given some indication of genotoxicity in mammalian cells *in vitro* and initiating activity *in vivo*.

There are insufficient data available for the halogenated acetonitriles on which to base an assessment of the hazard to consumers from the presence of these compounds in drinking water.

References

BIEBER T I and TREHY M L (1983) Dihaloacetonitriles in chlorinated natural waters. In Jolley R L *et al* (eds) *Water chlorination: environmental impact and health effects,* Vol. 4 Book 1, Ann Arbor Science, Michigan, pp 85–96.

BULL R J (1982a) Toxicological problems associated with alternative methods of disinfection. *Journal of the American Water Works Association* **74**, 642–648.

BULL R J (1982b) Experimental methods for evaluating the health risks associated with organic chemicals in drinking water. *Toxicological and Environmental Chemistry Reviews* **6**, 1–17.

BULL R J (1986) Toxicological data on selected hazardous chemicals and possible extrapolation to man. Paper presented at the IARC Workshop on the Evaluation of methods for assessing human health hazards from chemicals in drinking water. IARC Internal Technical Report No 86/001. Lyon, France.

BULL R J and ROBINSON M (1985) Carcinogenic activity of haloacetonitriles andhaloacetone derivatives in the mouse skin and lung. In *Water Chlorination: Chemistry, Environmental Impact and Health Effects,* Vol 5, edited by R L Jolley. Lewis Publishers Inc, Chelsea, Mich, pp 221–227.

BULL R J, MEIER J R, ROBINSON M, RINGHAND H P, LAURIE R D and STOBER J A (1985) Evaluation of mutagenic and carcinogenic properties of brominated and chlorinated acetonitriles: by-products of chlorination. *Fundamental and Applied Toxicology* **5**, 1065–1074.

DANIEL F B, PEREIRA M A, LIN E H C, HAAS D L and MATTOX J K (1983) Genotoxicity of haloacetonitriles. *Toxicologist* **3**, 37.

DANIEL R B, SCHENK, K M, MATTOX J K, LIN E L C, HAAS D L and PEREIRA M A (1986) Genotoxic properties of haloacetonitriles: drinking water by-products of chlorine disinfection. *Fundamental and Applied Toxicology* **6**, 447–453.

HELZ G R, DOTSON D A and SIGLEO A C (1983) Chlorine demand: Studies concerning its chemical basis. In JOLLEY R L *et al* (eds) *Water chlorination: environmental impact and health effects,* Vol. 4, Book 1, Ann Arbor Science, Michigan.

KEITH L H, HALL R C, HANISCH R C, HENDERSON J E and LANDOLT R G (1983) New methods for gas chromatographic analysis of water pollutants. In JOLLEY R L *et al* (eds) *Water chlorination: environmental impact and health effects,* Vol. 4 Book 2, Ann Arbor Science, Michigan, pp 563–582.

McKINNEY J D, MAURER R R, HASS J R and THOMAS R O (1976) Possible factors in the drinking water of laboratory animals causing reproductive failure. In Keith L H (ed) *Identification and analysis of organic pollutants in water,* Ann Arbor Science, Michigan, pp 417–432.

MEIER J R, BAKER K L, BULL R J and ROBINSON M R (1983) Mutagenicity and tumor initiating activity of halogenated acetonitriles. *Environmental Mutagenesis* **5**, 447–448.

MINK F L, COLEMAN W E, MUNCH J W, KAYLOR W H and RINGHAND H P (1983) *In vivo* formation of halogenated reaction products following peroral sodium hypochlorite. *Bulletin of Environmental Contamination and Toxicology,* **30**, 394–399.

OLIVER B G (1983) Dihaloacetonitriles in drinking water: Algae and fulvic acid as precursors. *Environmental Science and Technology,* **17**, 80–83.

PEREIRA M A, LIN L C and MATTOX J K (1984) Haloacetonitrile excretion as thiocyanate and inhibition of dimethylnitrosamine demethylase: a proposed metabolic scheme. *Journal of Toxicology and Environmental Health,* **13**, 633–641.

SIMMON V F, KAUHANEN K and TARDIFF R G (1977) Mutagenic activity of chemicals identified in drinking water. In Scott D, Bridges B A and Sobels F H (eds), *Progress in genetic toxicology,* Elsevier/North-Holland Biomedical Press.

UNITED STATES ENVIRONMENTAL PROTECTION AGENCY (1983) Progress report, July–Oct 1983.

WATER RESEARCH CENTRE (1981) Organic micropollutants in drinking water. WRc Technical Report TR 159.

3. CHLORAL

3.1 Introduction

Chloral (trichloroethanal) has been regularly identified in finished waters. Its hydrate, 2,2,2-trichloro-1,1-ethanediol, is used occasionally as a sedative hypnotic (in cases where patients are intolerant to barbiturates) and in industry in the production of polyurethanes. Chlorination of dissolved organic materials during water treatment would appear to be the primary source of chloral in drinking water.

Chloral Hydrate	CAS Reg. No:	302-17-0
	Molecular weight:	165.4

3.2 Exposure

An EPA survey (United Stated Environmental Protection Agency 1975) identified chloral in 6/10 water supplies at levels of up to 5 μg/l. More recently, levels of up to 12 μg/l were detected in tap water samples taken immediately following water treatment at two sites in the US. The concentrations of chloral were found to increase if the samples were allowed to stand for 24 hours before the chlorine residual was neutralised. Chloral was not detectable in the reservoir waters supplied to the treatment plants (Uden and Miller 1983). This compound was identified in only one of 14 drinking water samples tested in the WRc survey (Water Research Centre 1981).

In laboratory experiments, Miller and Uden (1983) showed that choral was formed during the chlorination of humic substances. Production of chloral was not as quantitatively significant, however, as that of chloroform, dichloroacetic acid or trichloroacetic acid. Christman *et al* (1983) have also reported the production of chloral following the chlorination of fulvic acid.

3.3 Toxicokinetics

Chloral is readily metabolised by alcohol dehydrogenase to trichloroethanol. Biotransformation can occur in several tissues and red blood cells (Butler 1949).

3.4 Health effects

3.4.1 Acute and subacute toxicity

Chloral is of relatively low acute toxicity in experimental animals. Oral LD50s of 285 mg/kg, 1100 mg/kg and 1000 mg/kg have been reported for the rat, mouse and dog respectively (National Academy of Sciences 1977). Motor incoordination was demonstrated in half of a group of CD-1 mice given oral doses of 84 mg/kg of chloral. The peak effect was observed 5 minutes after dosing, and recovery occurred within 2–3 hours (Kallman *et al* 1984). In a 14-day range-finding study, male CD-1 mice were given 14.4 or 144 mg/kg body weight of chloral hydrate by gavage. A significant increase in liver weight and a reduction in spleen weight were found at the high dose level. Similar effects were seen at the low dose level, but these were not statistically significant. A significant decrease in serum lactate dehydrogenase activity was also reported in the high-dose group (Sanders *et al* 1982).

Intraperitoneal injection of unspecified doses of either chloral or its hydrate to mice for 5 days was found to inhibit pulmonary mixed function oxidase activity by around 50%. No changes were observed in hepatic mixed function oxidase activity (Saunders and Harper 1981). *In vitro* experiments have shown that chloral hydrate is a reversible inhibitor of rat erythrocyte and dog kidney microsomal ATPases (Bergese *et al* 1983).

Chloral is also of low acute toxicity to man, though at very high doses dyspnoea, deep stupor, vasodilation, lowering of blood pressure, cyanosis, lowered body temperature and sometimes death due to respiratory depression are seen. Although an adult death has been reported after a dose of 1.2 g of chloral hydrate and an infant death after only 180 mg, doses prescribed are normally 0.3–2 g/day for adults and 50 mg/kg body weight/day for small children (Martindale 1972). Chloral is irritant to mucous membranes and the skin.

In man, there appears to be an interaction between ethanol and chloral hydrate, resulting in prolonged pharmacological activity on the CNS. The mechanism of interaction is not clear, though modification of the rate of metabolism of ethanol and/or chloral is suspected (Owen and Taberner 1980, Sharkawi *et al* 1983).

3.4.2 Chronic toxicity

Three 90-day toxicity studies of chloral hydrate in mice have recently been published. In each case, CD-1 mice were exposed to chloral hydrate at 1/10 and 1/100 of the LD50 (oral LD50s were 1442 and 1265 mg/kg for male and female mice respectively) via their drinking water. These dose levels corresponded to concentrations in the drinking water of 70 and 700 mg/l (Kallman *et al* 1984, Sanders *et al* 1982, Kauffman *et al* 1982).

Sanders *et al* (1982) reported slightly elevated body weight gain in male mice but not female mice. Liver weight/body weight ratio was also increased in male mice, though spleen weight was not found to be affected. Of the haematological parameters measured, some reduction in erythrocyte counts was seen in females of the high-dose group, while elevated fibrinogen levels were reported in high-dose males and low-dose females. Although microsomal protein was elevated by 10% in high-dose females, no such change was found in the males. Cytochrome b_5 levels were found to be significantly elevated in treated males, but somewhat decreased in females. Microsomal aminopyrine-*N*-demethylase activity was also elevated in males, but not females, while aniline hydroxylase activity was increased in both sexes. The effects of chloral hydrate on clinical chemistry also differed for the two sexes. A 45% increase in lactate dehydrogenase activity and a 48% increase in serum aspartate aminotransferase activity observed in males were not found in females. Also noted in the high-dose males were decreased serum calcium, sodium and phosphorus, and a reduction in blood urea nitrogen. In females, serum potassium, phosphorus, glucose and cholesterol were elevated.

In a similar study, Kauffmann *et al* (1982) failed to observe any changes in the immune status of male mice exposed to 70 or 700 mg/l of chloral hydrate in their drinking water for 90 days. In female mice, however, spleen cells from treated animals were found to have a lowered ability to produce antibody against sheep erythrocytes. This would indicate a depression in humoral immune function.

Kallman *et al* (1984) did not find changes in behaviour, swimming endurance or locomotor activity in CD-1 mice exposed to 70 or 700 mg/l of chloral hydrate in their drinking water for 90 days. There was, however, some depression of body weight gain and lowered body temperature when measured on day 91.

In a study of 1618 patients treated with 0.5–1.0 g/day of chloral hydrate, reversible side-effects were found in 2.3% of patients. CNS depression and gastrointestinal symptoms were the most common effects, though skin rash was evident in 5 patients (Shapiro *et al* 1969). Symptoms of chronic poisoning with chloral in man are similar to those seen for chronic alcoholism.

3.4.3 Genotoxicity

Chloral hydrate is mutagenic in the Ames test to *Salmonella typhimurium* TA100 at concentrations of around 10 mg/plate. Although it is a weak direct-acting mutagen, the presence of a metabolising system tends to enhance its activity. Chloral hydrate has given negative results with the TA98, TA1535 and TA1537 strains, both in the presence and absence of metabolic activation (Waskell 1978, Bignami *et al* 1980, Haworth *et al* 1983).

Chloral hydrate has been found to be weakly positive for the induction of mitotic gene conversion in the yeast *Saccharomyces cerevisiae* D7 both *in vitro* and in a host-mediated assay (Bronzetti *et al* 1984). This compound has also given positive results for reversion in *Saccharomyces cerevisiae* XV185-14C (Nestmann and Lee 1985). Chloral hydrate is a weak inducer of sister chromatid exchanges in human lymphocytes *in vitro* (Gu *et al* 1981).

Effects of chloral hydrate on the mitotic spindle have been reported in mouse secondary spermatocytes (Russo *et al* 1984), grasshopper spermatocytes (Ris 1949), *Pleurodeles waltlii* eggs (Sentein and Ates 1974), *Aspergillus nidulans* (Mercer and Morris 1975) and in plant systems (Levan 1938).

3.4.4 Carcinogenicity

No information appears to be available.

3.4.5 Reproductive toxicity

No information appears to be available on the reproductive toxicity of chloral. However, this compound is thought to cross the placenta (Dentkos 1966).

3.5 Discussion

Chloral has been regularly identified in drinking water. It appears to be formed by chlorination during water treatment.

Chloral is of relatively low acute and chronic toxicity in the mouse. At high doses, the liver appears to be the main target organ. Some evidence for altered immune competence has also been reported. Chloral hydrate is weakly mutagenic in the Ames test, but is well known to have effects on the mitotic spindle in several systems.

Although the information available suggests that low levels of chloral in drinking water would not present a hazard to human health, there are no long-term studies available in a species other than the mouse, and there are no data available on carcinogenicity and reproductive toxicity.

References

BERGESE J R, DOMENECH C E and BALEGNO H F (1983) Chloral hydrate inhibition *in vitro* of ATPase in membrane of rat erythrocytes and in microsomes of dog kidney external medulla. *Biochemical Pharmacology* **32**, 3221–3225.

BIGNAMI M, CONTI G, CONTI L, CREBELLI R, MISURACA F, PUGLIA A M, RANDAZZO R, SCIANDRELLO G and CARERE A (1980) Mutagenicity of halogenated aliphatic hydrocarbons in *Salmonella typhimurium, Streptomyces coelicolor* and *Aspergillus nidulans. Chemicobiological Interactions* **30**, 9–23.

BRONZETTI G, GALLI A, CORSI C, CUNDARI E, DEL CARRATORE R, NIERI R and PAOLINI M (1984) Genetic and biochemical investigation on chloral hydrate *in vitro* and *in vivo*. *Mutation Research* **141**, 19–22.

BUTLER T C (1949) Reduction and oxidation of chloral hydrate by isolated tissues *in vitro*. *Journal of Pharmacology and Experimental Therapeutics* **95**, 360–372.

CHRISTMAN R F, NORWOOD D L, MILLINGTON D S, JOHNSON J D and STEVENS A A (1983) Identity and yields of major halogenated products of aquatic fulvic acid chlorination. *Environmental Science and Technology* **17**, 625–628.

DENTKOS M C (1966) Passage of drugs across the placenta. *American Journal of Hospital Pharmacy* **23**, 139–144.

GU Z W, SELE B, CHMARA D, JALBERT P, VINCENT M, VINCENT F, MARKA C and FAURE J (1981) Effets du trichloroethylene at de ses metabolites sur le taux d'echanges de chromatides-soeurs. *Annales de Genetiques* **24**, 105–106.

HAWORTH S, LAWLOR T, MORTELMANS K, SPECK W and ZEIGER E (1983) Salmonella mutagenicity test results for 250 chemicals. *Environmental Mutagenesis* **5**, Suppl 1, 3–142.

KALLMAN M J, KAEMPF G L and BALSTER R L (1984) Behavioral toxicity of chloral in mice: An approach to evaluation. *Neurobehavioural Toxicology and Teratology* **6**, 137–146.

KAUFFMANN B M, WHITE K L Jr, SANDERS V M, DOUGLAS K A, SAIN L E, BORZELLECA J F and MUNSON A E (1982) Humoral and cell-mediated immune status in mice exposed to chloral hydrate. *Environmental Health Perspectives* **44**, 147–151.

LEVAN A (1938) The effect of colchicine on root mitosis in Allium. *Hereditas* **24**, 471–486.

MARTINDALE (1972) *The Extra Pharmacopoeia*. Twenty-sixth Edition. The Pharmaceutical Press, London.

MERCER B and MORRIS N R (1975) The effect of chloral hydrate upon mitosis in *Aspergillus nidulans*. *Journal of General Microbiology* **88**, 197–199.

MILLER J W and UDEN P C (1983) Characterization of nonvolatile aqueous chlorination products of humic substances. *Environmental Science and Technology* **17**, 150–157.

NATIONAL ACADEMY OF SCIENCES (1977) Drinking water and health Vol 1. National Academy of Sciences, Washington, DC.

NESTMANN E R and LEE E G-H (1985) Genetic activity in *Saccharomyces cerevisiae* of compounds found in effluents of pulp and paper mills. *Mutation Research* **155**, 53–60.

OWEN B E and TABERNER P V (1980) Studies on the hypnotic effects of chloral hydrate and ethanol and their metabolism *in vivo* and *in vitro*. *Biochemical*

Pharmacology **29**, 3011–3016.
RIS H (1949) The anaphase movement of chromosomes in the spermatocytes of the grasshopper. *Biological Bulletin* **96**, 90–106.
RUSSO A, PACCHIEROTTI F and METALLI P (1984) Nondisjunction induced in mouse spermatogenesis by chloral hydrate, a metabolite of trichloroethylene. *Environmental Mutagenesis* **6**, 695–703.
SANDERS V M, KAUFFMANN B M, WHITE K L Jr, DOUGLAS K A, BARNES D W, SAIN L E, BRADSHAW T J, BORZELLECA J F and MUNSON A E (1982) Toxicology of chloral hydrate in the mouse. *Environmental Health Perspectives* **44**, 137–146.
SAUNDERS D S and HARPER C (1981) Pulmonary toxicity of chloral hydrate and trichloroacetaldehyde. *Federation Proceedings* **40** (3 Part 1), 698 Abstract 2681.
SENTEIN P and ATES Y (1974) Action de l'hydrate de chloral sur les mitoses de segmentation de l'oeuf de pleurodele. Etude cytologique et ultrastructurale. *Chromosoma* **45**, 215–244.
SHAPIRO S, SLONE D, LEWIS G P and JICK H (1969) Clinical effects of hypnotics. II. An epidemiologic study. *Journal of the American Medical Association* **209**, 2016–2020.
SHARKAWI M, DE SAINT BLANQUAT G and ELFASSY B (1983) Inhibition of alcohol dehydrogenase by chloral hydrate and trichloroethanol: possible role in the chloral hydrate–ethanol interaction. *Toxicology Letters* **17**, 321–328.
UDEN P C and MILLER J W (1983) Chlorinated acids and chloral in drinking water. *Journal of the American Water Works Association* **75**, 524–527.
UNITED STATES ENVIRONMENTAL PROTECTION AGENCY (1975) Preliminary assessment of suspected carcinogens in drinking water. US EPA, Washington, DC. EPA-56014-75-005.
WASKELL L (1978) A study of the mutagenicity of anesthetics and their metabolites. *Mutation Research* **57**, 141–153.
WATER RESEARCH CENTRE (1981) Organic micropollutants in drinking water. WRc Technical Report TR 159.

4. CHLORO-ISO-PROPYLPHENOL

Chloro-iso-propylphenol was identified in one of 14 drinking water samples in a survey by WRc (Water Research Centre 1982).

No information appears to be available for this compound.

Reference

WATER RESEARCH CENTRE (1982) Frequency of occurrence data for compounds identified by GC–MS in XAD-2 samples taken for mutagenic testing survey. WRc unpublished report.

5. THE CHLOROPHENOLS

5.1 Introduction

Chlorinated phenols are used as fungicides, disinfectants, flea repellants and wood preservatives, and as intermediates in the manufacture of pesticides, herbicides and dyes. They all appear to be relatively soluble in water, though they may undergo photolysis in aqueous solution and are readily broken down by microbiological action. Compounds with a *meta*-substituted chlorine atom (for example 2,4,5-trichlorophenol), appear to be rather more resistant to biodegradation.

The occurrence of chlorophenols in drinking water can cause problems with taste and odour. Odour thresholds in water are of the order of 0.5–20 μg/l for dichlorophenols and 11–1000 μg/l for trichlorophenols. These compounds also appear to cause tainting of fish flesh at similar concentrations.

Both the US EPA (United Stated Environmental Protection Agency 1980a,b) and the Canadian National Research Council (National Research Council of Canada 1982) have recently reviewed the chlorophenols.

5.2 Exposure

Several surveys throughout the world have identified chlorophenols in water samples (Ahlborg and Thunberg 1980). Occurrence is primarily associated with industrial and sewage effluents, though they may also be present as breakdown products following the use of phenoxyacid herbicides. Chlorophenols can be produced during the chlorination of water, particularly where phenol levels are high and ammonia levels are low.

In a survey of treated water by WRc (Water Research Centre 1981), a trichlorophenol isomer was detected in only one of 14 samples tested. In a further (unpublished) survey, isomers of both dichlorophenol and trichlorophenol were identified, though again in only a small number of samples.

Chlorophenols have also been identified in food, air, soil and in the tissues of both aquatic and terrestrial organisms.

5.3 Toxicokinetics

Chlorophenols are weak acids and have been shown to permeate human skin *in vitro* (Roberts *et al* 1977). They would be expected to be readily absorbed by the gastrointestinal tract. Chlorophenols are thought to be distributed primarily to the liver and kidney (Somani and Khalique 1982). Excretion via the urine is rapid, either as unchanged chlorophenols or as conjugates, particularly glucuronides (Somani *et al* 1981, Korte *et al* 1978). There is evidence that chlorinated methoxy-phenol metabolites may also be formed (Somani *et al* 1984).

5.4 Health effects

5.4.1 Acute and subacute toxicity

Chlorophenols appear to be of moderate to low acute toxicity in experimental animals. Oral LD50s in the rat of 580–2940 mg/kg and 820–3000 mg/kg have been reported for dichlorophenols and trichlorophenols respectively (Registry of toxic effects of chemical substances 1983).

Borzelleca *et al* (1985a) determined the acute oral LD50s of mono- and dichlorophenols in mice as follows:

	Acute oral LD50 (mg/kg)	
	Male	Female
2-Chlorophenol	347	345
3-Chlorophenol	521	530
4-Chlorophenol	1373	1422
2,3-Dichlorophenol	2585	2376
2,4-Dichlorophenol	1276	1352
2,5-Dichlorophenol	1600	946
2,6-Dichlorophenol	2198	2120
3,4-Dichlorophenol	1685	2046
3,5-Dichlorophenol	2643	2389

A 28-day rabbit study in which the animals were given 20 oral doses of 1.0–500 mg/kg of 2,4,5-trichlorophenol (purity 97–98%) showed slight changes in the liver and kidney at the highest dose. No effects other than an initial body weight loss and a slight increase in kidney weight were observed in rats fed up to 1 g/kg of 2,4,5-trichlorophenol on 18 occasions over a 24-day period (McCollister *et al* 1961). In a range-finding experiment prior to the NCI carcinogenicity study, 2,4,6-trichlorophenol was given in the diet to F344 rats for 7 weeks. The minimum toxic dose was reported to be 500 mg/kg body weight/day (National Cancer Institute 1979). In a subacute study of 2,4-dichlorophenol, all mice dosed orally with 667 mg/kg/day for 10 days survived the treatment (Kobayashi *et al* 1972). However, pathological investigations appear not to have been carried out in these studies.

McCollister *et al* (1961) reported that 2,4,5-trichlorophenol was not particularly irritating to rabbit skin. A 5% solution of 2,4,5-trichlorophenol in sesame oil was mildly irritating to a few human subjects, though most gave no response. No evidence for sensitisation was found.

The acute toxicity of chlorophenols in man is characterised by increased respiratory rate, sweating, nausea and vomiting.

5.4.2 Chronic toxicity

Groups of 10 male and 10 female Wistar rats fed diets containing 0, 0.01, 0.03 or 0.1% 2,4,5-trichlorophenol (purity 99%) for 98 days showed no adverse effects. Assuming that on average these animals consumed a quantity of feed equivalent to 10% of their body weight daily, the dietary concentrations would correspond to doses of 0, 10, 30, and 100 mg/kg body weight/day. At higher dietary concentrations of 0.3% and 1.0% (300 and 1000 mg/kg body weight/day), slight changes in the liver and kidney were found. Slight body weight depression in high-dose females was also observed (McCollister *et al* 1961).

No toxic effects were reported in male mice given 45 or 100 mg/kg/day of 2,4-dichlorophenol for 6 months. At a dose level of 230 mg/kg/day, slight changes were noted in hepatocyte morphology (Kobayashi *et al* 1972). In a very recent 90-day study, no clear treatment-related or dose-dependent effects were found in CD-1 mice given drinking water containing 200, 600 or 2000 mg/ml of 2,4-dichlorophenol (corresponding to doses of about 50, 150 and 500 mg/kg body weight/day). Gross pathology, body weights, organ weights, haematology, clinical chemistry and hepatic mixed function oxidase activity were all assessed, but no histopathology was carried out (Borzelleca *et al* 1985b).

In a recent study by Exon and Koller (1985), groups of female Sprague–Dawley rats were given drinking water containing 3, 30 or 300 mg/l of 2,4-dichlorophenol or 2,4,6-trichlorophenol. The animals were exposed from weaning through breeding to parturition. Eight of the resulting pups were randomly selected from each group, and after weaning were continued on the treatments for 12–15 weeks. No effects on body weight were found in any group, though elevated liver weights were apparent in rats exposed to 30 and 300 mg/l of 2,4,6-trichlorophenol and also in those exposed to 300 mg/l of 2,4-dichlorophenol. Elevated spleen weights were found in rats given the highest doses of 2,4-dichlorophenol and 2,4,6-trichlorophenol. Although thymus weights were not significantly altered from controls, a consistent decrease in the weight of this organ was evident in the 2,4-dichlorophenol-treated rats. No significant change in immunocompetence was found in rats exposed to 2,4,6-trichlorophenol. An increase in humoral immunity (as indicated by anti-keyhole limpet haemocyanin antibody) was found for 2,4-dichlorophenol at the highest dose level. This compound also caused a dose-related lowering of cell-mediated immune function. In rats which were continued on the treatments for 2 years rather than 12–15 weeks, elevated packed cell volume, haemoglobin and red blood cell numbers were noted in those exposed to 300 mg/l of 2,4-dichlorophenol.

5.4.3 Biochemical toxicity

The trichlorophenols and 2,4-dichlorophenol have been reported to inhibit oxidative phosphorylation in rat liver mitochondria and rat brain homogenate (Mitsuda *et al* 1963, Farquharson *et al* 1958)). Weinbach and Garbus (1965) demonstrated that 0.05 mM 2,4,5-trichlorophenol completely uncoupled mitochondrial oxidative phosphorylation *in vitro*. Korte *et al* (1976) found that 3,4-dichlorophenol produced swelling of the bovine lens *in vitro* and reduced ATP, ADP and the activities of malate dehydrogenase, glucose-6-phosphate dehydogenase and pyruvate kinase. 2,4,5-Trichlorophenol also reduced ATP, ADP and the activity of glucose-6-phosphate dehydrogenase, but had no effect on the other enzymes examined.

Arrhenius *et al* (1977) have suggested that 2,4-dichlorophenol and 2,4,6-trichlorophenol selectively inhibit the coupling of the flavin and cytochrome P-450 in the drug-metabolising oxidation cycle.

5.4.4 Genotoxicity

Rasanen *et al* (1977) found a whole range of chlorophenols to be non-mutagenic in the Ames test to *Salmonella typhimurium* TA98, TA100, TA1535 and TA1537 when tested at 5 μg/plate either in the presence or absence of metabolic activation. Similar findings have been reported by other workers (Lawlor and Haworth 1979, Haworth *et al* 1983, Rapson *et al* 1980, Kinae *et al* 1981).

2,4,6-Trichlorophenol has been reported to be genotoxic in the *Bacillus subtilis* rec assay (Kinae *et al* 1981) and in *Saccharomyces cerevisiae* (Fahrig *et al* 1978). There is also evidence for mutagenic activity in Chinese hamster V79 cells where induction of resistance to 6-thioguanine was the genetic marker (Hattula and Knuutinen 1985). Other chlorophenols have been found to be genotoxic in the *Escherichia coli* WP100 rec assay (Lawlor and Haworth 1979).

2,4-Dichlorophenol was not found to induce unscheduled DNA synthesis in primary cultures of rat hepatocytes (Probst *et al* 1981).

No cytogenetic effects were found in a group of workers who had been exposed during an accident 10 years previously to crude 2,4,5-trichlorophenol which contained a 'higher than normal concentration of the impurity TCDD (2,3,7,8-tetrachlorodibenzo-*p*-dioxin)' (Blank *et al* 1983).

5.4.5 Carcinogenicity

Four oral carcinogenicity studies have been carried out on 2,4,6-trichlorophenol; the first two, in mice, gave equivocal results, whilst the third and fourth, in rats and mice respectively, gave positive results.

In the earlier mouse studies, 18 male and 18 female mice of both the B6C3F1 and B6AKF1 strains were dosed daily by stomach tube with 100 mg/kg body weight of 2,4,6-trichlorophenol (commercial grade) in 0.5% gelatin from 7 days old to 4 weeks. The mice were then given 260 mg/kg/day until 78 weeks of age. In the B6C3F1 strain, if the numbers of tumours in both males and females are combined, a statistically significant increase in hepatomas and reticulum cell sarcomas is derived. If, however, males and females are considered separately, no such significant increase in tumours is found. Survival in the study was good, apart from male B6C3F1 mice, of which 8/18 died during the experiment (National Cancer Institute 1968).

In the more recent studies, groups of 50 male and 50 female F344 rats were fed 2,4,6-trichlorophenol (purity unspecified) at 5000 or 10 000 mg/kg in the diet for 106 weeks. Groups of 50 male B6C3F1 mice were similarly dosed with 5000 or 10 000 mg/kg in the diet for 105 weeks, whilst groups of 50 female mice were begun on 10 000 and 20 000 mg/kg diet, but this was reduced to 2500 and 5000 mg/kg diet at 38 weeks. The time-weighted average doses for the female mice were 5214 and 10 428 mg/kg diet. Significant dose-related increases of lymphoma and leukaemia in male rats, and hepatocellular carcinomas or adenomas in male and female mice, were found. Leukocytosis and monocytosis of the peripheral blood and hyperplasia of the bone marrow were also evident in male rats without tumours (National Cancer Institute 1979).

Incidence of hepatocellular carcinomasor adenomas in B6C3F1 mice

	Control	Low dose	High dose
Male	4/20	32/49	39/47
Female	1/20	12/50	24/48

Incidence of lymphoma or leukaemia in F344 rats

	Control	Low dose	High dose
Male	4/20	25/50	29/50
Female	3/20	11/50	13/50

Exon and Koller (1985) found that exposure of Sprague–Dawley rats to 3, 30 or 300 mg/l of 2,4-dichlorophenol in their drinking water for 2 years did not result in an increased macroscopically observable tumour incidence.

Subcutaneous studies have also been carried out on commercial grade 2,4,6- and

2,4,5-trichlorophenol. Groups of 18 male and 18 female mice of both the B6C3F1 and B6AKF1 strains were given a single subcutaneous injection of either 464 mg/kg body weight of 2,4,6-trichlorophenol or 1000 mg/kg body weight of 2,4,5-trichlorophenol at 28 days of age. The animals were observed to 78 weeks of age, at which point no increase in tumour incidence was found (National Cancer Institute 1968).

Boutwell and Bosch (1959) investigated the tumour-promoting activity of a series of chlorophenols in female Sutter mice initiated with 75 μg of dimethylbenzanthracene. For each chlorophenol studied, 25 μl of a 20% solution was applied to the skin twice weekly for 15 or 24 weeks. An increase in the number of surviving mice with skin papillomas and the average number of papillomas per animal was found with 2,4-dichlorophenol and 2,4,5-trichlorophenol. For 2,4-dichlorophenol, the percentage of surviving animals with carcinomas was also increased. Negative results were obtained in this test with 2,4,6-trichlorophenol.

A small Swedish study has suggested that occupational exposure to chlorophenols gave an increased risk of 6.6 for soft-tissue sarcomas. However, the subjects were also exposed to chlorinated dioxins and chlorinated dibenzofurans as impurities (Hardell and Sandstrom 1979).

5.4.6 Reproductive toxicity

Two studies have looked at the reproductive toxicity of chlorophenols. In the first, mice were treated by gavage with either a single dose of 800–900 mg/kg of 2,4,5-trichlorophenol during gestation on one of days 8–15, or three consecutive doses of 250–300 mg/kg on days 7–9, 10–12 or 13–15 in a 1:1 solution of honey:water. No effects on foetal mortality, foetal weight or incidence of malformations were found (Hood *et al* 1979). In the second study, female Sprague–Dawley rats were given drinking water containing 3, 30 or 300 mg/l of 2,4-dichlorophenol or 2,4,6-trichlorophenol from weaning to breeding with untreated males at 90 days and through parturition. Litter sizes of females exposed to 300 mg/l of 2,4-dichlorophenol and 300 mg/l of 2,4,6-trichlorophenol were significantly smaller than controls. Although increased numbers of stillborn pups were observed with both compounds, this was found to be statistically non-significant. Survival to weaning was significantly reduced in rats given 30 mg/l of 2,4-dichlorophenol, but not in any other group.

5.5 Discussion

The occurrence of chlorophenols in water samples tends to be associated with industrial and sewage effluents. Chlorophenols are readily absorbed by the body, but are rapidly eliminated in the urine unchanged or as simple conjugates.

Although toxicological information for some of the dichlorophenol isomers is sparse, both the dichlorophenols and trichlorophenols appear to be of relatively low acute and chronic toxicity. There is a question mark, however, concerning the carcinogenicity of 2,4,6-trichlorophenol. Increased numbers of tumours have been found in rats and mice fed high concentrations of this compound. However, the very high dose levels used resulted in toxicity, which may well have had a very important bearing on tumour development. These studies may be unrepresentative of the carcinogenic potential of this compound at lower doses, which do not result in tissue damage.

References

AHLBORG U G and THUNBERG T M (1980) Chlorinated phenols: occurrence, toxicity, metabolism and environmental impact. *CRC Critical Reviews in Toxicology* **7**, 1–35.

ARRHENIUS E, RENBERG L, JOHANSSON L and ZETTERQVIST M A (1977) Disturbance of microsomal detoxication mechanisms in liver by chlorophenol pesticides. *Chemicobiological Interactions* **18**, 35–46.

BLACKBURN K, ZENICK H, HOPE E, MANSON J M, GEORGE E L and SMITH M K (1986) Evaluation of the reproductive toxicology of 2,4,6-trichlorophenol in male and female rats. *Fundamental and Applied Toxicology* **6**, 233–239.

BLANK C E, COOKE P and POTTER A M (1983) Investigations for genotoxic effects after exposure to crude 2,4,5-trichloro-phenol. *British Journal of Industrial Medicine* **40**, 87–91.

BORZELLECA J F, HAYES J R, CONDIE L W and EGLE J L Jr (1985a) Acute toxicity of monochlorophenols, dichlorophenols and pentachlorophenol in the mouse. *Toxicology Letters* **29**, 39–42.

BORZELLECA J F, HAYES J R, CONDIE L W and EGLE J L Jr (1985b) Acute and subchronic toxicity of 2,4-dichlorophenol in CD-1 mice. *Fundamental and Applied Toxicology* **5**, 478–486.

BOUTWELL R K and BOSCH D K (1959) The tumor-promoting action of phenol and related compounds for mouse skin. *Cancer Research* **19**, 413–424.

EXON J H and KOLLER L D (1985) Toxicity of 2-chlorophenol, 2,4-dichlorophenol and 2,4,6-trichlorophenol. In: *Water chlorination: environmental impact and health effects* Vol 5, edited by R L Jolley *et al.* Lewis Publishers Inc, Chelsea, Mich, pp 317–330.

FAHRIG R, NILSSON C A and RAPPE C (1978) Genetic activities of chlorophenols and chlorophenol impurities. In: RAO K R (ed) *Pentachlorophenol: chemistry, pharmacology and environmental toxicology.* Plenum Press, New York, pp 325–338.

FARQUHARSON M E, GAGE J C and NORTHOVER J (1958) The biological action of chlorophenols. *British Journal of Pharmacology* **13**, 20–24.

HARDELL L and SANDSTROM A (1979) Case-control study: soft-tissue sarcomas and exposure to phenoxyacetic acids or chlorophenols. *British Journal of Cancer* **39**, 711–717.

HATTULA M L and KNUUTINEN J (1985) Mutagenesis of mammalian cells in culture by chlorophenols, chlorocatechols and chloroguaiacols. *Chemosphere* **14**, 1617–1625.

HAWORTH S, LAWLOR T, MORTELMANS K, SPECK W and ZEIGER E (1983) Salmonella mutagenicity test results for 250 chemicals. *Environmental Mutagenesis* **5**, Suppl 1, 3–142.

HOOD R D, PATTERSON B L, THACKER G T, SLOAN G L and SZCZECH G M (1979) Prenatal effects of 2,4,5-T, 2,4,5-trichlorophenol, and phenoxyacetic acid in mice. *Journal of Environmental Science and Health* **13**, 189–204.

KINAE N, HASHIZUME T, MAKITA T, TOMITA I, KIMURA I and KANAMORI H (1981) Studies on the toxicity of pulp and paper mill effluents – I. Mutagenicity of the sediment samples derived from kraft paper mills. *Water*

Research **15**, 17–24.
KOBAYASHI S, TOIDA S, KAWAMURA H, CHANG H S, FUKUDA T and KAWAGUCHI K (1972) Chronic toxicity of 2,4-dichlorophenol in mice. *Journal of the Medical Society of Toho University Japan* **19**, 356.
KORTE F, FREITAG D, GEYER H, KLEIN W, KRAUS A G and LAHANIATIS E (1978) Ecotoxicologic profile analysis. A concept for establishing ecotoxicologic priority list for chemicals. *Chemosphere* **7**, 79–102.
KORTE I, ISMAIL R M, HOCKWIN O and KLEIN W (1976) Studies on the influences of some environmental chemicals and their metabolites on the content of free adenine nucleotides, intermediates of glycolysis on the activities of certain enzymes of bovine lenses *in vitro*. *Chemosphere* **5**, 131–136.
LAWLOR T and HAWORTH S R (1979) Evaluation of the genetic activity of nine chlorinated phenols, seven chlorinated benzenes, and three chlorinated hexanes. *Environmental Mutagenesis* **1**, 143.
McCOLLISTER D D, LOCKWOOD D T and ROWE V K (1961) Toxicologic information on 2,4,5-trichlorophenol. *Toxicology and Applied Pharmacology* **3**, 63–70.
MITSUDA H, MURAKAMI K and KAWAI F (1963) Effect of chlorophenol analogues on the oxidative phosphorylation in rat liver mitochondria. *Agricultural and Biological Chemistry* **27**, 366.
NATIONAL CANCER INSTITUTE (1968) Evaluation of carcinogenic, teratogenic, and mutagenic activities of selected pesticides and industrial chemicals. Vol 1. Carcinogenic study. US Department of Commerce, National Technical Information Service, August 1968. PB–223 159.
NATIONAL CANCER INSTITUTE (1979) Bioassay of 2,4,6-trichlorophenol for possible carcinogenicity. US Department of Health, Education and Welfare, National Cancer Institute, Technical Report No. 155.
NATIONAL RESEARCH COUNCIL OF CANADA (1982) Chlorinated phenols: criteria for environmental quality. NRC Associate Committee on Scientific Criteria for Environmental Quality, NRC No. 18578.
PROBST G S, McMAHON R E, HILL L E, THOMPSON C Z, EPP J K and NEAL S B (1981) Chemically-induced unscheduled DNA synthesis in primary rat hepatocyte cultures: a comparison with bacterial mutagenicity using 218 compounds. *Environmental Mutagenesis* **3**, 11–32.
RAPSON W H, NAZAR M A and BUTSKY V V (1980) Mutagenicity produced by aqueous chlorination of organic compounds. *Bulletin of Environmental Contamination and Toxicology* **24**, 590–596.
RASANEN L, HATTULA M L and ARSTILA A U (1977) The mutagenicity of MCPA and its soil metabolites, chlorinated phenols, catechols and some widely used slimicides in Finland. *Bulletin of Environmental Contamination and Toxicology* **18**, 565–571.
REGISTRY OF TOXIC EFFECTS OF CHEMICAL SUBSTANCES (1983) National Institute for Occupational Safety and Health, Cincinnati, Ohio, April 1983.
ROBERTS M S, ANDERSON R A and SWARBRICK J (1977) Permeability of human epidermis to phenolic compounds. *Journal of Pharmacy and Pharmacology* **29**, 677–683.

SOMANI S M and KHALIQUE A (1982) Distribution and metabolism of 2,4-dichlorophenol in rats. *Journal of Toxicology and Environmental Health* **9**, 889–897.
SOMANI S M, KAKA J S and SMART T A (1981) Disposition of 2,4-dimethylphenol and 2,4-dichlorophenol in rat. *Federation Proceedings* **40**, 698.
SOMANI S M, SMART T and KHALIQUE A (1984) Metabolism of 2,4-dichlorophenol by isolated perfused rat liver. *Journal of Toxicology and Environmental Health* **13**, 787–798.
US ENVIRONMENTAL PROTECTION AGENCY (1980a) Ambient water quality criteria for chlorinated phenols, EPA-440/5-80-032.
US ENVIRONMENTAL PROTECTION AGENCY (1980b) Ambient water quality criteria for 2,4-dichlorophenol, EPA-440/5-80-042.
WATER RESEARCH CENTRE (1981) Organic micropollutants in drinking water. WRc Technical Report TR 159.
WEINBACH E C and GARBUS J (1965) The interaction of uncoupling phenols with mitochondria and with mitochondrial protein. *Journal of Biological Chemistry* **210**, 1811.

6. *p*-CHLOROPHENOXYACETIC ACID

p-Chlorophenoxyacetic acid (Tomato Fix, Tomatotone, Sure-Set, CPA) was found in a preliminary survey of treated water by WRc (Water Research Centre 1981). This compound has been used as a herbicide.

CAS Reg. No: 122-88-3
Molecular weight: 186.6

The only toxicological data which appear to be available are an oral LD50 in the rat of 850 mg/kg (Bailey and White 1965) and an intraperitoneal LD50 in the mouse of 680 mg/kg (Maccari *et al* 1970).

References

BAILEY G W and WHITE J L (1965) Herbicides: a compilation of their physical, chemical, and biological properties. *Residue Reviews* **10**, 97–122.
MACCARI M, MILANI C and GATTI M T (1970) Proprietes pharamacologiques de quelques sels d'aminopyrine. *Chimica Therapeutica* **5**, 211–215.
WATER RESEARCH CENTRE (1981) Organic micropollutants in drinking water. WRc Technical Report TR 159.

7. 2-(*p*-CHLOROPHENOXY)-2-METHYLPROPIONIC ACID (CLOFIBRIC ACID)

7.1 Introduction

Clofibric acid is the pharmacologically active form of the hypolipidaemic drug clofibrate (its ethyl ester). Clinical trials with clofibrate have demonstrated its ability to reduce serum cholesterol and triglyceride levels, resulting in a lowering of nonfatal myocardial infarctions. Clofibrate is recommended in cases of severe hyperlipidaemia where control by other dietary means are found to be ineffective.

The pharmacology and toxicology of hypolipidaemic drugs is an area under extensive research, but which remains very complex and difficult to evaluate in view of the wide range of biochemical systems affected by these compounds. An added problem with clofibrate is the absence of a suitable model species. Changes seen in the liver of rats treated with clofibrate do not appear to occur in the monkey and man.

Clofibric acid	CAS Reg No:	882-09-7
	Molecular weight:	214.7
Clofibrate	CAS Reg No:	637-07-0
	Molecular weight:	242.7
	Boiling point:	148–150°C

7.2 Exposure

Clofibric acid was identified in both raw and treated water in a preliminary survey by WRc (Water Research Centre 1981). This compound has also been identified at an average concentration of 7 μg/l in treated sewage effluent from a plant in Kansas City, Missouri (Hignite and Azarnoff 1977).

With the exception of patients prescribed clofibrate (dose of about 0.5–2.0 g/day taken in two to four portions), water-derived clofibric acid may represent the major source of exposure to this drug.

7.3 Toxicokinetics

Following oral doses of clofibric acid and clofibrate in rats, an essentially similar pharmacokinetic pattern is seen. In the dog, however, approximately 40% higher clofibric acid levels are found in the plasma following clofibric acid dosing compared to clofibrate dosing. The situation with man tends to correspond to that of the rat (Cayen *et al* 1977).

The half-life of clofibric acid in the rat is 8.3 hours (Baldwin *et al* 1980), a somewhat lower value than that found in man (Mannisto *et al* 1975). This variation is probably due to differences in plasma protein binding, which has been shown to vary with serum concentration and species (plasma protein binding in man > dog > rat).

A study of the metabolism of clofibric acid in several species has indicated that there are roughly two types of metabolisers (Emudianughe *et al* 1983):

(1) Rat, rabbit, guinea-pig and man. These species tend to eliminate 60–90% of a dose in the urine within 24 hours as a combination of the free acid and glucuronide conjugate. Other minor metabolites have been reported following incubation with human and rat liver microsomes, but these metabolites have yet to be identified (Houin *et al* 1975). Both the rabbit and man eliminate the drug primarily as the glucuronide conjugate.

(2) Dog, cat and ferret. These species only eliminate 23–39% of a dose of clofibric acid in the urine within 24 hours; the major metabolite for all three species is a taurine conjugate.

In a study of bile-duct cannulated rats (Emudianughe *et al* 1983), 67% of a dose of clofibrate was eliminated in the bile and 21% in the urine within 24 hours. For both routes almost all of the drug was found as the glucuronide conjugate. This suggests that in the rat, clofibric acid is rapidly conjugated with glucuronic acid and eliminated primarily in the bile. The conjugate may then be hydrolysed back to the free acid by gut bacteria and reabsorbed into the blood. This recirculation would appear to be very proficient, for in the rat 96% of a dose of clofibric acid is eliminated in the urine within 24 hours.

Pretreatment of rats with phenobarbital does not appear to influence the metabolism of clofibrate (Hignite and Azarnoff 1977).

Thorp (1962), in studies with monkeys, suggested that the volume of distribution of clofibric acid corresponded to the plasma and extracellular fluid only. At doses greater than 100 mg/kg, detectable levels of clofibric acid were found in the liver. The compound was not detected in the fat, heart, spleen or muscle.

7.4 Pharmacological mechanism of action of clofibrate

Several mechanisms have been suggested for the hypolipidaemic activity of clofibrate, though as yet a completely satisfactory explanation is lacking. One of the earliest theories proposed that clofibric acid displaces the hormone, thyroxine, from plasma binding proteins (Chang *et al* 1967). There is a good deal of evidence linking thyroid hormones and lipid biochemistry, but the action of clofibrate on this system is not clear.

Other suggestions for the mechanism of action of clofibrate include: induction of peroxisomal fatty acid oxidative enzymes and peroxisomal catalase (Heller 1981), inhibition of the mobilisation of fatty acids from fat storage depots, and inhibition of cholesterol biosynthesis (Witiak *et al* 1971). Although many hypolipidaemic compounds produce peroxisomal proliferation in rats, this is by no means seen for all compounds. Further, clofibrate has hypolipidaemic activity in species such as man which do not exhibit these hepatic changes.

7.5 Health effects

The major target organ for clofibrate in rats is the liver. The characteristic hepatic changes generally seen are:

(1) Hepatomegaly (probably due to hypertrophy).
(2) Proliferation of smooth endoplasmic reticulum (SER).
(3) A large increase in the number of peroxisomes and elevation of peroxisomal enzyme activities, for example fatty acid beta-oxidative enzymes and carnitine acetyltransferase.
(4) Induction of a cytochrome P-450 specific for lauric acid hydroxylation.

Although peroxisomal proliferation is almost invariably found with hepatomegaly, some experiments have suggested that these may in fact be separate events. Clofibrate-induced liver enlargement has been found without reports of peroxisomal proliferation (Svoboda *et al* 1967). Two weeks after the cessation of clofibrate treatment, peroxisomal proliferation had persisted, but liver weight had apparently returned to normal (Svoboda *et al* 1967, Hess *et al* 1965). Actinomycin C has been shown to impair clofibrate-induced peroxisomal proliferation, but had no effect on liver weight (Svoboda *et al* 1967).

In chronic studies, clofibrate has been shown to induce hepatocellular tumours in rats. In the monkey and man, however, there is no evidence for the liver changes or liver tumours seen in rats.

7.5.1 *Acute and subacute toxicity*

Male Wistar rats given oral doses of 20–600 mg/kg/day of clofibrate for 1 week exhibited hepatomegaly, with an increase in peroxisomal numbers and sizes. Depressed microsomal coumarin hydroxylase and aminopyrine demethylase activities were seen at 200 mg/kg (Cohen and Grasso 1981). Male rats dosed orally with 30 mg/kg/day of clofibrate for 10 days exhibited proliferation of both hepatic SER and rough endoplasmic reticulum (RER), plus a large increase in the number of peroxisomes and elevation of some microsomal enzyme activities (Elek and Jambor 1981).

An increase in hepatic microsomal cytochrome P–450 lauric acid hydroxylation was found in rats and mice, but not in the marmoset, fed clofibrate for 14 days (Orton and Parker 1982). Induction of lauric acid hydroxylation has also been found in primary cultures of rat hepatocytes (Lake *et al* 1983).

Oral LD50s for clofibrate are 1650 mg/kg in the rat and 1280 mg/kg in the mouse (Metz *et al* 1977).

7.5.2 *Chronic toxicity*

In a 90-day study, Sprague–Dawley rats exposed to 250 mg/kg body weight/day of clofibrate via the diet exhibited similar hepatic changes to those seen in short-term studies, though cytoplasmic granularity, ribosomal detachment, glycogen depletion, disarrangement of RER and pleomorphic mitochondria were also observed (Barnard *et al* 1980).

In rhesus monkeys fed diets containing 0.5–2% clofibrate for 2 years, no effects were noted other than a slight increase in liver weight in the high-dose group after 3 months (Platt and Thorp 1966). Similarly, no effects on hepatocytes were found in monkeys given oral doses of 200 mg/kg/day of clofibrate for 1 year (Blane and Pinaroli 1980) and in one squirrel monkey given oral doses of 75 mg/kg/day for 22 days (Svoboda *et al* 1967).

Studies on patients prescribed clofibrate also suggest that the liver changes seen in rats do not occur in primates (Schwandt *et al* 1978, Hanefield *et al* 1980). There does appear to be a correlation, however, between clofibrate therapy and an increased incidence of gallstones (Coronary Drug Research Group 1975, Cooper *et al* 1975, Committee of Principal Investigators 1978, Bateson *et al* 1978). Clofibrate treatment tends to increase biliary cholesterol, but lowers bile acids.

7.5.3 *Sex-dependent effects of clofibrate*

Sex-dependent effects have been reported on a number of occasions. In beagle dogs, oral doses of 35–45 mg/kg of clofibrate on alternate days for 3 months resulted in liver enlargement in females but not in males (Platt and Thorp 1966). In rats, clofibrate-related liver changes tend to be seen in males rather than females. Dependency on the male sex hormone was indicated when castrated males given clofibrate and oestradiol benzoate did not produce peroxisomal proliferation and when ovariectomised females given clofibrate and testosterone propionate did develop this change (Svoboda *et al* 1967, 1969).

7.5.4 Genotoxicity

Clofibrate does not appear to be mutagenic in the Ames test when tested in either the presence or absence of metabolic activation (Warren *et al* 1980).

Clofibrate was found to inhibit the incorporation of tritiated thymidine into the DNA of replicating mouse splenic lymphocytes. However, this was reversible on removal of the compound, suggesting no covalent binding to DNA (Warren *et al* 1980).

This compound was not found to induce sister chromatid exchanges in the peripheral lymphocytes of rats or in the bone marrow cells of Chinese hamsters given oral doses of 200 mg/kg/day for 2 weeks. Negative results were also found with Chinese hamster ovary cells *in vitro* at clofibrate concentrations of 0.01–1.0 mM (Linnainmaa 1984). Similarly, no evidence for mutagenic activity was found in a hepatocyte-mediated V79 cell test where induction of resistance to ouabain and 6-thioguanine were the genetic markers (Dayan *et al* 1985).

7.5.5 Carcinogenicity

Clofibrate fed at 0.5% (v/w) in the diet for up to 28 months to 15 Fischer 344 rats produced one or more hepatocellular carcinomas in 10/11 animals surviving to 24–28 months. Other tumours seen were pancreatic exocrine acinar carcinomas (2/11), a dermatofibrosarcoma and an intestinal leiomyoma. No hepatocellular carcinomas or the other tumour types mentioned above were found in 14 surviving control animals (Reddy and Qureshi 1979). In another study, 25 Fischer 344 rats were fed clofibrate at 0.5% in the diet for 72–97 weeks. Ten of the animals exhibited malignant tumours. Hepatocellular carcinomas (4/25), a pancreatic exocrine acinar carcinoma, pancreatic exocrine acinar adenomas (3/25), and a low incidence of a variety of other tumour types were found only in the treated animals (Svoboda and Azarnoff 1979).

In view of the absence of genotoxic activity for clofibrate, it would not appear that its carcinogenicity in rats is determined by this mechanism. It has been suggested that the changes seen in the liver of rats may lead to liver nodules and subsequently tumours (Cohen and Grasso 1981). The biochemical mechanism of this process could involve the formation of active oxygen species which lead to genetic damage or non-specific hepatic damage followed by hyperplasia.

Unpublished studies in CD–1 mice and C57BL/10J mice have failed to demonstrate any carcinogenic potential for clofibrate. Hepatomegaly was present, but the other hepatic changes found in rats were not (Cohen and Grasso 1981).

Treatment with clofibrate after exposure of F–344 rats to *N*-nitrosodiethylamine was found to enhance the number of liver tumours produced by nitrosamine treatment alone. However, little interpretation can be made of this experiment, as treatment with clofibrate alone was not investigated (Reddy and Rao 1978). In another study, clofibrate produced only a slight enhancement of liver foci and no increase in neoplasms in rats pretreated with *N*-2-fluorenylacetamide (Numoto *et al* 1984).

A clinical trial conducted by WHO found that there were significantly more deaths in a clofibrate-treated group compared to a high-cholesterol control group (162/5331 v 127/5296) during the period of treatment (Committee of Principal Investigators 1978, 1984). Many of the excess deaths were due to cancer (58 v 42), but no individual organ appeared to be of particular importance. There is some evidence to suggest that the cancer death rate of the control group may have been abnormally low. Several other trials with clofibrate have failed to observe an increase in cancer incidence (Coronary Drug Project Research Group 1975, Group of Physicians of the Newcastle upon Tyne Region 1971, Krasno and Kidera 1972, Research Committee of the Scottish Society of Physicians 1971).

7.5.6 Reproductive toxicity

Placental transfer of clofibrate and passage into milk have been reported in rats (Chhabra and Kurup 1978).

There appears to be relatively little information on the reproductive toxicity of clofibrate. However, the limited studies available have given no evidence for teratogenic potential (Chhabra and Kurup 1978, Pantaleoni and Valeri 1974, Dange *et al* 1975).

7.6 Discussion

Despite much interest in clofibrate and other hypolipidaemic drugs, both the pharmacological and toxicological mechanism of action of these compounds remains unclear. In rats treated with clofibrate a well defined series of hepatic changes are seen, principally characterised by a large increase in the number of peroxisomes. Although clofibrate does not appear to have genotoxic activity, it is a liver carcinogen in rats. It has therefore been suggested that hepatic peroxisomal proliferation induces a large increase in reactive oxygen species which either damage DNA or result in general cellular damage which leads to hyperplasia, foci, nodules and ultimately tumours. In man and the monkey, however, clofibrate does not appear to induce these liver changes, and therefore the carcinogenic scenario described above is unlikely to be relevant. Data from clinical trials provide very little evidence for hepatic carcinogenic activity of clofibrate in man.

In view of the absence of toxic effects in monkeys exposed to high levels of clofibrate in the diet and the little evidence for deleterious effects in patients prescribed 0.5–2.0 g/day of clofibrate, exposure to low concentrations of clofibrate through drinking water would not appear to represent a hazard to human health.

References

BALDWIN J R, WITIAK D T and FELLER D R (1980) Disposition of clofibrate in the rat: acute and chronic administration. *Biochemical Pharmacology* **29**, 3143–3154.

BARNARD S D, MOLELLO J A, CALDWELL W J and LeBEAU J E (1980) Comparative ultrastructural study of rat hepatocytes after treatment with the hypolipidaemic agents probucol, clofibrate and fenofibrate. *Journal of Toxicology and Environmental Health* **6**, 547–557.

BATESON M C, MACLEAN D, ROSS P E and BOUCHIER I A D (1978) Clofibrate therapy and gallstone induction. *American Journal of Digestive Diseases* **23**, 623–628.

BLANE G F and PINAROLI F (1980) Fenofibrate: etudes de toxicologie animale en rapport avec les effets secondaires chez les malades. *Nouvelle Press Medicale* **9**, 3737.

CAYEN M N, FERDINANDI E S, GRESELIN E, ROBINSON W T and DVORNIK D (1977) Clofibrate and clofibric acid: comparison of the metabolic disposition in rats and dogs. *Journal of Pharmacology and Experimental Therapeutics* **200**, 33–43.

CHANG Y H, PINSON R Jr and MALONE M H (1967) Displacement of l-thyroxine from its binding proteins in human, dog, and rat plasma by alpha-(*p*-chlorophenoxy)-isobutyric acid. *Biochemical Pharmacology* **16**, 2053–2055.

CHHABRA S and KURUP C K R (1978) Maternal transport of chlorophenoxyisobutyrate at the foetal and neonatal stages of development. *Biochemical Pharmacology* **27**, 2063–2065.

COHEN A J and GRASSO P (1981) Review of the hepatic response to hypolipidaemic drugs in rodents and assessment of its toxicological significance to man. *Food and Cosmetics Toxicology* **19**, 585–605.

COMMITTEE OF PRINCIPAL INVESTIGATORS (1978) A cooperative trial in the primary prevention of ischaemic heart disease using clofibrate. *British Heart Journal* **40**, 1069–1118.

COMMITTEE OF PRINCIPAL INVESTIGATORS (1984) WHO cooperative trial on primary prevention of ischaemic heart disease with clofibrate to lower serum cholesterol: final mortality follow-up. *Lancet* **ii**, 600–604.

COOPER J, GEIZEROVA H and OLIVER M F (1975) Clofibrate and gallstones. *Lancet* **i**, 1083.

CORONARY DRUG PROJECT RESEARCH GROUP (1975) Clofibrate and niacin in coronary heart disease. *Journal of the American Medical Association* **231**, 360–381.

DANGE M, JUNGHANI J, NACHBAUR J, PERRAUD J and REINERT H (1975) Postnatal thrombosis (PNT) in newborn rats by hypolipemic agents. *Teratology* **12**, 328.

DAYAN J, DEGUINGAND S and TRUZMAN C (1985) Study of the mutagenic activity of 6 hepatotoxic pharmaceutical drugs in the *Salmonella typhimurium* microsome test, and the HGPRT and Na^+/K^+ ATPase system in cultured mammalian cells. *Mutation Research* **157**, 1–12.

ELEK S J and JAMBOR E (1981) The effects of hypolipidaemic agents on the hepatic drug metabolism of the rat. In: Plaa G L and Duncan W A M (eds) *Proceedings of the First International Congress on Toxicology: Toxicology as a Predictive Science.* New York, Academic Press, p 641.

EMUDIANUGHE T, CALDWELL J, SINCLAIR K A and SMITH R L (1983) Species differences in the metabolic conjugation of clofibric acid and clofibrate in laboratory animals and man. *Drug Metabolism and Disposition* **11**, 97–102.

GROUP OF PHYSICIANS OF THE NEWCASTLE UPON TYNE REGION (1971) Trial of clofibrate in the treatment of ischaemic heart disease. *British Medical Journal* Dec 25 1971, 767–775.

HANEFIELD M, KEMMER C, LEONHARDT W, KUNZE K D, JAROSS W and HALLER H (1980) Effects of *p*-chlorophenoxyisobutyric acid (CPIB) on the human liver. *Atherosclerosis* **36**, 159.

HELLER R F (1981) Coronary heart disease, cancer, lipoproteins, and the effects of clofibrate: is enzyme induction a common link and are lipoproteins red herrings? *Lancet* **ii**, 1258–1260.

HESS R, STAUBLI W and RIESS W (1965) Nature of the hepato-megalic effect produced by ethyl-chlorophenoxyisobutyrate in the rat. *Nature* **208**, 856–858.

HIGNITE C and AZARNOFF D L (1977) Drugs and drug metabolites as environmental contaminants: chlorophenoxyisobutyrate and salicylic acid in sewage water effluent. *Life Sciences* **20**, 337–342.

HOUIN G, THEBAULT J J, D'ATHIS Ph, TILLEMENT J P and BEAUMONT J L (1975) A GLC method for estimation of chlorophenoxy-isobutyric acid in plasma. Pharmacokinetics of a single oral dose of clofibrate in man. *European Journal of Clinical Pharmacology* **8**, 433–437.

KRASNO L R and KIDERA G J (1972) Clofibrate in coronary heart disease. Effects on morbidity and mortality. *Journal of the American Medical Association* **219**, 845–851.

LAKE B G, GRAY T J B, STUBBERFIELD C R, BEAMAND J A and GANGOLLI S D (1983) Induction of lauric acid hydroxylation and maintenance of cytochrome P-450 content by clofibrate in primary cultures of rat hepatocytes. *Life Sciences* **33**, 249–254.

LINNAINMAA K (1984) Induction of sister chromatid exchanges by the peroxisome proliferators 2,4-D, MCPA, and clofibrate *in vivo* and *in vitro*. *Carcinogenesis* **5**, 703–707.

MANNISTO P T, TUOMISTO J, JOUNELA A and PENTTILA O (1975) Pharmacokinetics of clofibrate and chlorophenoxy isobutyric acid. I Cross-over studies on human volunteers. *Acta Pharmacologica et Toxicologica* **36**, 353–365.

METZ G, SPECKER M, STERHER W, HEISLER E and GRAHWIT G (1977) 1-(Theophyllin-7-yl)-ethyl-2-[2-(*p*-chlorophenoxy)-2-methyl propionate] (ML 1024), a new hypolipemic agent. *Arzneimittel Forschung* **27**, 1173–1177.

NUMOTO S, FURUKAWA K, FURUYA K and WILLIAMS G M (1984) Effects of the hepatocarcinogenic peroxisome-proliferating hypolipidemic agents clofibrate and nafenopin on the rat liver cell membrane enzymes γ-glutamyltranspeptidase and alkaline phosphatase and on the early stages of liver carcinogenesis. *Carcinogenesis* **5**, 1603–1611.

ORTON T C and PARKER G L (1982) The effect of hypolipidemic agents on the hepatic microsomal drug-metabolizing enzyme system of the rat. Induction of Cytochrome(s) P-450 with specificity toward terminal hydroxylation of lauric acid. *Drug Metabolism and Disposition* **10**, 110–115.

PANTALEONI G C and VALERI P (1974) Investigations on the interactions of clofibrate with reproductive function. *Clinica Terapeutica* **69**, 321–328.

PLATT D S and THORP J M (1966) Changes in the weight and composition of the liver in the rat, dog and monkey treated with ethyl chlorophenoxyisobutyrate. *Biochemical Pharmacology* **15**, 915–925.

REDDY J K and QURESHI S A (1979) Tumorigenicity of the hypolipidaemic peroxisome proliferator clofibrate in rats. *British Journal of Cancer* **40**, 476–482.

REDDY J K and RAO M S (1978) Enhancement by Wy-14,643, a hepatic peroxisome proliferator, of diethylnitrosamine-initiated hepatic tumorigenesis in the rat. *British Journal of Cancer* **38**, 537–543.

RESEARCH COMMITTEE OF THE SCOTTISH SOCIETY OF PHYSICIANS (1971) Ischaemic heart disease: a secondary prevention trial using clofibrate. *British Medical Journal* Dec 25 1971, 775–784.
SCHWANDT P, KLINGE O and IMMICH H (1978) Clofibrate and the liver. *Lancet* **ii**, 325.
SVOBODA D J and AZARNOFF D L (1979) Tumors in male rats fed ethylchlorophenoxybutyrate, a hypolipidaemic drug. *Cancer Research* **39**, 3419–3428.
SVOBODA D, GRADY H and AZARNOFF D (1967) Microbodies in experimentally altered cells. *Journal of Cell Biology* **35**, 127.
SVOBODA D, AZARNOFF D and REDDY J (1969) Microbodies in experimentally altered cells. II. The relationship of microbody proliferation to endocrine glands. *Journal of Cell Biology* **40**, 734–746.
THORP J M (1962) Experimental evaluation of an orally active combination of androsterone with ethyl chlorophenoxyisobutyrate. *Lancet* **i**, 1323–1326.
WARREN J R, SIMMON V F and REDDY J K (1980) Properties of hypolipidemic peroxisome proliferators in the lymphocyte [^{3}H] thymidine and Salmonella mutagenesis assays. *Cancer Research* **40**, 36–41.
WATER RESEARCH CENTRE (1981) Organic micropollutants in drinking water. WRc Technical Report TR 159.
WITIAK D T, FELLER D R, STRATFORD E S, HACKNEY R E, NAZARETH R and WAGNER G (1971) Inhibitory action of alpha-(4-chlorophenoxy)-alpha-methylpropionic acid analogs on cholesterol biosynthesis and lipolysis *in vitro*. *Journal of Medicinal Chemistry* **14**, 754–757.

8. DICHLOROACETIC ACID

8.1 Introduction

As the sodium salt, dichloroacetic acid has been used to treat lactic acidosis, while in the form of a di-isopropylammonium salt it is available to the general public in the US as ‘vitamin B15’ (pangamic acid). Most experiments on this compound have been performed with the sodium salt; in these cases the compound will be referred to as dichloroacetate.

CAS Reg No:	79-43-6
Molecular weight:	128.9
Boiling point:	194°C
Solubility:	86.3 g/l (Verschueren 1983)

8.2 Exposure

Dichloroacetic acid has been detected at levels of 63 and 123 μg/l in tap water samples taken immediately following water treatment at two sites in the US. If the samples were allowed to stand for 24 hours before the chlorine residual was neutralised, dichloroacetic acid concentrations were found to increase to 80 and 133 μg/l respectively. This compound was not detected in the raw water (Uden and Miller 1983). Dichloroacetic acid was identified in an initial survey of treated water by WRc (Water Research Centre 1981).

Miller and Uden (1983) have demonstrated that chlorination of humic substances in the laboratory can give rise to dichloroacetic acid. Christman *et al* (1983) have also reported the production of dichloroacetic acid following the chlorination of fulvic acid.

8.3 Toxicokinetics

The major metabolites of dichloroacetate in mammals are thought to be oxalate and glyoxylate (Yount *et al* 1982).

8.4 Biochemical effects

The principal effect of dichloroacetate on intermediary metabolism is to reduce circulating lactate levels. This is achieved by direct stimulation of pyruvate dehydrogenase, the enzyme which catalyses the rate-limiting step in the oxidation of lactate to pyruvate, and by the inhibition of pyruvate carboxylase and pyruvate kinase by oxalate, a metabolite of dichloroacetate (Demaugre *et al* 1983). High levels of oxalate lower the mitochondrial $NADH/NAD^+$ ratio and reduce Krebs cycle substrate concentrations (Demaugre *et al* 1983). Stimulation of pyruvate dehydrogenase also results in increased bicarbonate formation, and hence in a higher arterial pH (Stacpoole *et al* 1983).

8.5 Health effects

8.5.1 Acute and subacute toxicity

Oral LD50s for dichloroacetic acid are 2.8–>5 g/kg in the rat (Smythe *et al* 1951, Woodard *et al* 1941, Traina *et al* 1977) and 4.8–>5 g/kg in the mouse (Yount *et al* 1982, Woodard *et al* 1941, Traina *et al* 1977). Acute oral doses of up to 1 g/kg were not found to induce mortality in dogs (Traina *et al* 1977). It has been reported that intravenous administration of 34 g of dichloroacetate at 8–12 g/hour to a 71-year-old patient succeeded in treating lactic acidosis without complications (Irsigler *et al* 1979).

8.5.2 Chronic toxicity

In a 3-month study by Katz *et al* (1981), Sprague–Dawley rats of both sexes were treated by gavage with 125, 500 or 2000 mg/kg/day of an aqueous solution of dichloroacetate, while beagle dogs of both sexes were dosed orally with 50, 75 or 100 mg/kg/day in gelatin capsules. Of 15 male and 15 female rats in the high-dose group, four (two of each sex) died during the experiment. In the dog study, 1/3 females at 75 mg/kg and 1/4 males at 100 mg/kg also died during treatment. A number of treatment-related effects were common to both rats and dogs and were generally found at all dose levels. These were suppression of food consumption and body weight gain, hind-limb weakness, testicular degeneration, vacuolation of white matter myelin of the cerebrum, and reduced plasma glucose, pyruvate, lactate and triglycerides. Depression of red blood cells, haemoglobin and haematocrit, plus the presence of haemosiderin in the kupffer cells, suggest haemolytic anaemia. Dogs also exhibited atrophy of the prostate gland, cystic mucosal hyperplasia in the gall bladder, plus a number of ocular lesions. Male rats of the high-dose group often exhibited aspermatogenesis.

In an unpublished study by Katz *et al* (1977) of dogs given 10, 40 and 100 mg/kg/day of dichloroacetate for one month by intravenous injection, the ocular, testicular, CNS or prostate changes reported in the above study were not observed.

Rats fed diets containing 6000 ppm of dichloroacetate for 12 weeks exhibited depressed food consumption and body weight gain, hind-limb weakness, lowered nerve conduction velocities and testicular degeneration. Organ weight/body weight ratios for the liver, adrenals, kidney and brain were all elevated compared to controls. Approximate dosages varied from 600 mg/kg body weight/day at the beginning of the study to about 380 mg/kg body weight/day at the end of the study (Yount *et al* 1982).

In conjunction with the CNS changes observed in animals following subchronic exposure to dichloroacetate, neuropathy has been reported in a small number of patients prescribed this compound (Stacpoole *et al* 1979, Moore *et al* 1979, Coude *et al* 1979).

8.5.3 Genotoxicity

In the Ames test, dichloroacetate gave a dose-related response in *Salmonella typhimurium* TA98, but a doubling in the number of revertants over control was not seen. Addition of S-9 slightly increased the number of revertants seen (Herbert *et al* 1980).

8.5.4 Carcinogenicity

No information appears to be available.

8.5.5 Reproductive toxicity

No information appears to be available.

8.6 Discussion

Chlorination appears to be responsible for the occurrence of dichloroacetic acid in drinking water. For a micropollutant, quite high levels of this compound have been detected in treated water in the US. Dichloroacetate and its metabolite, oxalate, have profound effects on intermediary metabolism. However, exposure to relatively low levels through drinking water is very unlikely to produce significant effects.

In rats and dogs, subchronic exposure to dichloroacetate has been shown to induce a range of toxic effects including haemolytic anaemia, testicular degeneration, neurological changes and ocular toxicity.

There are insufficient data available for dichloroacetic acid on which to base an assessment.

References

CHRISTMAN R F, NORWOOD D L, MILLINGTON D S, JOHNSON J D and STEVENS A A (1983) Identity and yields of major halogenated products of aquatic fulvic acid chlorination. *Environmental Science and Technology* **17**, 625–628.

COUDE F X, SAUDUBRAY J M, DeMAUGRE F, MARSAC C and LEROUX J

P (1979) Dichloroacetate as treatment for congenital lactic acidosis. *New England Journal of Medicine* **299**, 1365–1366.
DEMAUGRE F, BUC H A, CEPANEC C, MONCION A and LEROUX J P (1983) Comparison of the effects of 2-chloropropionate and dichloroacetate on ketogenesis and lipogenesis in isolated rat hepatocytes. *Biochemical Pharmacology* **32**, 1881–1885.
HERBERT V, GARDNER A and COLMAN N (1980) Mutagenicity of dichloroacetate, an ingredient of some formulations of pangamic acid (trade-named 'vitamin B15'). *American Journal of Clinical Nutrition* **33**, 1179–1182.
IRSIGLER K, BRANDLE J, KASPAR L, KRITZ H, LAGEDER H and RETAL H (1979) Treatment of biguanide-induced lactic acidosis with dichloroacetate. *Arzneimittel Forschung,* **29**, 555–559.
KATZ R, DIENER R and THOMPSON S (1977) CGS 7937A (Sodium Dichloroacetate): 30-day intravenous administration to dogs. Report No. 7–77, Sec.C p52, CIBA-GEIGY Pharmaceuticals Division, Summit, New Jersey.
KATZ R, TAI C N, DIENER R M, McCONNELL R F and SEMONICK D E (1981) Dichloroacetate, Sodium: 3-month oral toxicity studies in rats and dogs. *Toxicology and Applied Pharmacology* **57**, 273–287.
MILLER J W and UDEN P C (1983) Characterization of nonvolatile aqueous chlorination products of humic substances. *Environmental Science and Technology* **17**, 150–157.
MOORE G W, SWIFT L L, RABINOWITZ D R, CROFFORD O B, OATES J A and STACPOOLE P W (1979) Reduction of serum cholesterol in two patients with homozygous familial hypercholesterolemia by dichloroacetate. *Atherosclerosis* **33**, 285–293.
SMYTHE H F Jr, CARPENTER C P and WEIL C S (1951) Range finding toxicity data: List IV. *Archives of Industrial Hygiene and Occupational Medicine* **4**, 119–122.
STACPOOLE P W, MOORE G W and KORNHAUSER D M (1979) Toxicity of chronic dichloroacetate. *New England Journal of Medicine* **300**, 372.
STACPOOLE P W, HARMAN E M, CURRY S H, BAUMGARTNER T G and MISBIN R I (1983) Treatment of lactic acidosis with dichloroacetate. *New England Journal of Medicine* **309**, 390–396.
TRAINA V, KATZ R, DIENER R and THOMPSON S (1977) CGS 7937A (Sodium Dichloroacetate): acute and subacute toxicity studies in mice, rats and dogs. Unpublished Report no. 7–77, CIBA-GEIGY Pharmaceuticals Division, Summit, New Jersey.
UDEN P C and MILLER J W (1983) Chlorinated acids and chloral in drinking water. *Journal of the American Water Works Association* **75**, 524–527.
VERSCHUEREN K (1983) *Handbook of Environmental Data on Organic Chemicals.* Second Edition. Van Nostrand Reinhold Company, 1983.
WATER RESEARCH CENTRE (1981) Organic micropollutants in drinking water. WRc Technical Report TR 159.
WOODARD G, LANGE S W, NELSON K W and CALVERY H O (1941) Acute oral toxicity of acetic, chloroacetic, dichloroacetic, and trichloroacetic acids. *Journal of Industrial Hygiene and Toxicology* **23**, 78–81.
YOUNT E A, FELTEN S Y, O'CONNOR B L, PETERSON R G, POWELL R S,

YUM M N and HARRIS R A (1982) Comparison of the metabolic and toxic effects of 2-chloropropionate and dichloroacetate. *Journal of Pharmacology and Experimental Therapeutics* **222**, 501–508.

9. DICHLOROCYCLOPENTADIENE

Dichlorocyclopentadiene was identified in one of 14 drinking water samples in a survey by WRc (Water Research Centre 1982).

No information appears to be available for this compound.

Reference

WATER RESEARCH CENTRE (1982) Frequency of occurrence data for compounds identified by GC–MS in XAD-2 samples taken for mutagenic testing survey. WRc unpublished report.

10. 3,6-DICHLORO-2-METHOXYBENZOIC ACID (DICAMBA)

10.1 Introduction

Dicamba (Banvel, Dianate, 3,6-dichloro-*ortho*-anisic acid, Mediben, 3,6-dichloro-2-methoxybenzoic acid) was introduced as a herbicide in 1965 by the Velsicol Chemical Corporation. It is produced by hydrolysis of 1,2,4-trichlorobenzene followed by treatment with carbon dioxide and dimethyl sulphate. Dicamba is normally used as the potassium, sodium or amine salt in combination with other herbicides such as dichlorprop, mecoprop, benazolin, 2,4,5-T, TBA and MCPA. These formulations are particularly employed as pre-emergence herbicides for broad-leaved weeds in cereal crops, grass seed crops and grasslands. Dicamba is fairly resistant to oxidation and hydrolysis, and after application can persist in the soil for around 7–10 months. However, it is degraded by plants to 2,5-dichloro-3-hydroxy-6-methoxybenzoic acid and by uv light to 3,6-dichlorosalicylic acid. Dicamba is not readily absorbed onto soils, and therefore tends to be leached by runoff waters.

CAS Reg No:	1918-00-9
Molecular weight:	221.0
Solubility:	7900 mg/l at 25°C (Verschueren 1983)
Threshold odour concentration in water:	200 mg/l (Golovan 1970)

10.2 Exposure

Dicamba was detected in an initial survey of treated water by WRc (Water Research Centre 1981). No other data on occurrence in water, food or air appear to be available.

10.3 Toxicokinetics

^{14}C-carboxyl-labelled dicamba administered by three different routes to CD rats was found to be eliminated primarily in the urine, with small amounts in the faeces. Over

90% of the dose was eliminated in the first 24 hours. Rats fed 1000 or 10 000 ppm of dicamba in the diet eliminated most of the dose unchanged. About 20% was excreted as the glucuronide conjugate (Tye and Engel 1967).

10.4 Health effects

10.4.1 Acute and subacute toxicity

Dicamba has a relatively low order of acute toxicity in the rat, mouse, guinea-pig, hen and pheasant. Oral LD50s in these species range from 566 to 1414 mg/kg. Toxicity is characterised by muscular spasms, urinary incontinence and dyspnoea (Edson and Sanderson 1965).

No significant effects on growth rate were found in weanling CD rats fed 658–23 500 ppm of Banvel D (41.3% dicamba, 44.1% water, 14.6% dimethylamine) in the diet for 3 weeks (National Academy of Sciences 1977).

10.4.2 Chronic toxicity

No treatment-related pathological changes were found in Wistar rats given dicamba in the diet at 0, 32, 100, 316, 1000 or 3162 ppm for 15 weeks. A significant increase in liver weight/body weight ratio was found at the top two dose levels. The highest no-effect level in this study, 316 ppm, corresponds to a dose of 19 mg/kg body weight/day (Edson and Sanderson 1965). In Sprague–Dawley rats fed 1000 ppm of Banvel D for 13 weeks (National Academy of Sciences 1977), hypersensitivity and moderate hepatic necrosis and vacuolisation were noted. Slight liver changes were observed in animals at 800 ppm, but no adverse effects were reported at 500 ppm, which corresponds to 206 ppm of dicamba (National Academy of Sciences 1977). Exposure of Sprague–Dawley rats to diets containing 5, 50, 100, 250 or 500 ppm of technical grade dicamba (90% dicamba) for 2 years did not appear to produce adverse effects (National Academy of Sciences 1977).

In beagle dogs fed diets containing 100 or 250 ppm of dicamba for 90 days, only yellowish coloration of the liver was found. Exposure of beagles to 5, 25 or 50 ppm of technical grade dicamba in the diet for 2 years was not found to affect mortality, growth, organ weights, haematology or histopathology (National Academy of Sciences 1977).

10.4.3 Genotoxicity

Dicamba has given negative results for mutagenicity in the Ames test with *Salmonella typhimurium* TA98 and TA100, either in the presence or absence of metabolic activation (National Academy of Sciences 1977, Anderson *et al* 1972, Moriya *et al* 1983). Waters *et al* (1982) have indicated positive results for this compound in two prokaryote DNA damage assays, *E. coli* polA and *B. subtilis* rec.

10.4.4 Carcinogenicity

No evidence for tumour induction has been found in long-term chronic toxicity studies in rats and dogs (National Academy of Sciences 1977).

10.4.5 Reproductive toxicity

In multigeneration studies, no effects were found in CD rats fed diets containing up to 500 ppm of Banvel D (206 ppm of dicamba) or in Sprague–Dawley rats fed diets containing 500 ppm of dicamba (National Academy of Sciences 1977).

Injection of 200 ppm of dicamba into chicken eggs was reported to cause a 20% reduction in hatchability (Dunachie and Fletcher 1967).

10.5 Discussion

Dicamba has a short half-life in the body, and is eliminated in the urine unchanged or as a glucuronide conjugate. It is of relatively low toxicity to experimental animals after both acute and chronic exposure.

This compound would not appear to represent a hazard to human health at very low concentrations in drinking water.

References

ANDERSEN K J, LEIGHTY E J and TAKAHASHI M T (1972) Evaluation of herbicides for possible mutagenic properties. *Journal of Agricultural and Food Chemistry* **20**, 649–656.

DUNACHIE J F and FLETCHER W W (1967) Effects of some herbicides on the hatching rate of hen's eggs. *Nature* **215**, 1406–1407.

EDSON E F and SANDERSON D M (1965) Toxicity of the herbicides, 2-methoxy-3,6-dichlorobenzoic acid (dicamba) and 2-methoxy-3,5,6-trichlorobenzoic acid (tricamba). *Food and Cosmetics Toxicology* **3**, 299–304.

GOLOVAN D J (1970) Experimental validation of permissible concentration of dianate (Dicamba) and 2,3,6-trichlorobenzoic acid in water bodies. *Hygiene and Sanitation* (cover to cover translation of *Gigiena i Sanitariia*) **35**, 14–18.

MORIYA M, OHTA T, WATANABE K, MIYAZAWA T, KATO K and SHIRASU Y (1983) Further mutagenicity studies on pesticides in bacterial reversion assay systems. *Mutation Research* **11**, 185–216.

NATIONAL ACADEMY OF SCIENCES (1977) *Drinking water and health* **1**. US National Academy of Sciences, Washington, DC.

TYE R and ENGEL R (1967) Distribution and excretion of dicamba by rats as determined by radiotracer technique. *Journal of Agricultural and Food Chemistry* **15**, 837–840.

VERSCHUEREN K (1983) *Handbook of environmental data on organic chemicals.* Second Edition. Van Nostrand Reinhold Company.

WATER RESEARCH CENTRE (1981) Organic micropollutants in drinking water. WRc Technical Report TR 159.

WATERS M D, SANDHU S S, SIMMON V F, MORTELMANS K E, MITCHELL A D, JORGENSON T A, JONES D C L, VALENCIA R and GARRETT N E (1982) Study of pesticide genotoxicity. *Basic Life Sciences* **21**, 275–326.

11. DICHLORONITROMETHANE

Dichloronitromethane was identified in only one of 14 drinking water samples tested in the WRc survey (Water Research Centre 1981).

No information appears to be available for this compound.

Reference

WATER RESEARCH CENTRE (1981) Organic micropollutants in drinking water. WRc Technical Report TR 159.

12. ETHYLCHLOROACETATE

CAS Reg No:	105-39-5
Molecular weight:	122.6
Boiling point:	143°C

Ethylchloroacetate was identified in one of 14 drinking water samples in a survey by WRc (Water Research Centre 1982).

An LD50 of 230 mg/kg by skin application has been reported for the rabbit (Vernot *et al* 1977).

This compound gave negative results for both gene conversion and reversion in *Saccharomyces cerevisiae* D7 and XV185-14C respectively (Nestmann and Lee 1985).

References

NESTMANN E R and LEE EG-H (1985) Genetic activity in *Saccharomyces cerevisiae* of compounds found in effluents of pulp and paper mills. *Mutation Research* **155**, 53–60.

VERNOT E H, MACEWAN J D, HAUN C C and KINKEAD E R (1977) Acute toxicity and skin corrosion data for some organic and inorganic compounds and aqueous solutions. *Toxicology and Applied Pharmacology* **42**, 417–423.

WATER RESEARCH CENTRE (1982) Frequency of occurrence data for compounds identified by GC–MS in XAD-2 samples taken for mutagenic testing survey. WRc unpublished report.

13. HEXACHLOROCYCLOPENTADIENE

13.1 Introduction

Hexachlorocyclopentadiene (HCCPD) is widely used as a chemical intermediate in the manufacture of chlorinated cyclodiene insecticides and flame-retardant chemicals. Interest in this compound was aroused when toxic effects of the insecticide chlordecone were found to be related to HCCPD as a contaminant. There is evidence for photodecomposition of HCCPD in water (Atallah *et al* 1981, Benoit and Williams 1981).

CAS Reg No:	77-47-4
Molecular weight:	272.8
Boiling point:	234°C
Threshold odour concentration in water:	14–16 μg/l (Vershueren 1983)

13.2 Exposure

Benoit and Williams (1981) detected HCCPD at levels of 57–110 ng/l in Ottowa treated waters. HCCPD was not detectable in the raw water. Earlier, Thruston

(1978) identified HCCPD in the drinking water of Georgia, US, also at ng/l levels. This compound was detected in only one of 14 drinking water samples examined in the WRc survey (Water Research Centre 1981).

HCCPD has been identified in effluents from two chemical plants in the US, and also in the atmosphere near one of the plants (United States Environmental Protection Agency 1978).

13.3 Toxicokinetics

Lawrence and Dorough (1981) found that around 84% of an inhaled dose of HCCPD was retained by Sprague–Dawley female rats. Three days after exposure, the highest levels of the compound were found in the lungs, trachea and kidneys. The same workers also studied the metabolism of HCCPD in female Sprague–Dawley rats following inhalation, oral and intravenous administration (1982). Treatment by each route with equivalent doses of the compound resulted in the excretion of 68.2% of the oral dose, 23.1% of the inhaled dose and 31.4% of the intravenous dose in the faeces within 72 hours. Urinary excretion in the same period accounted for 24.4%, 23.1% and 31.4% of the oral, inhaled and intravenous doses respectively. Biliary excretion was between 9% and 18% for all three routes. In view of the low biliary excretion of HCCPD and the high levels found in the faeces, it would appear that this compound is poorly absorbed from the gastrointestinal tract. Mehendale (1977), however, has reported that only 10% of a single oral dose of HCCPD was eliminated in the faeces in male Sprague–Dawley rats, while more than 50% was eliminated in the expired air.

El Dareer *et al* (1983) found that 39% of an intravenous dose, 11.5% of an inhaled dose, but only 2.4% of an oral dose remained in the tissues of male Fischer 344 rats 72 hours after dosing. Three days after single oral doses of HCCPD in rats and mice, the tissues which contained the highest concentrations were the liver, kidneys, fat and ovaries (Dorough and Ranieri 1984).

There appears to be no information available on metabolites of HCCPD.

13.4 Health effects

13.4.1 Acute and subacute toxicity

In general, it appears that HCCPD is of greater toxicity following exposure by inhalation than after oral or cutaneous administration. The lung is the principal target organ. An oral LD50 of 505 mg/kg has been reported for the male rat (Treon *et al* 1955).

Following the dumping of a large volume of HCCPD in a US municipal sewage system, a number of toxic effects were observed in sewage workers (Morse *et al* 1979, Kominsky *et al* 1980). Eye irritation, headaches and throat irritation were the most frequently reported effects, occurring in 59%, 45% and 27% of workers respectively. Plasma lactate dehydrogenase activity was elevated in 11/41 workers, and proteinuria was found in 6/41 workers.

13.4.2 Chronic toxicity

Oral doses of 0, 10, 19, 38, 75 and 150 mg/kg/day of HCCPD were given to groups of 10 male and 10 female F344 rats, 5 days/week for 13 weeks. Some mortality was noted at the top two dose levels. Depression of body weight gain was found at doses of 38 mg/kg in males and 75 mg/kg in females. At doses of 38 mg/kg and above, nephrosis was observed in both males and females, while at 19 mg/kg proliferative and inflammatory changes were found in the forestomach of females (Abdo *et al* 1984).

Groups of 10 male and 10 female B6C3F1 mice were given oral doses of 0, 19, 38, 75, 150 and 300 mg/kg/day of HCCPD, 5 days/week for 13 weeks. Depression of body weight gain was apparent at 150 and 300 mg/kg. There were also some deaths at the highest dose level. Nephrosis was evident in females at 38 mg/kg, while proliferative and inflammatory changes in the forestomach were found in females at 19 mg/kg and in males at 38 mg/kg. Elevated liver and kidney weights were found in female mice at all dose levels (Abdo *et al* 1984).

No treatment-related effects were found in rats fed diets containing 30, 100 or 300 ppm of HCCPD for 90 days (United States Environmental Protection Agency 1978).

Inhalation of up to 0.2 ppm of HCCPD by monkeys or rats for 90 days was reported to produce no detectable lung changes (Rand *et al* 1982a). Further study using electron microscopy, however, indicated dose-related ultrastructural changes in the Clara cells of the bronchiolar epithelium. These changes were characterised by an increased incidence of intracellular inclusion bodies (Rand *et al* 1982b).

13.4.3 Genotoxicity

HCCPD was not found to be mutagenic in the Ames test to *Salmonella typhimurium* TA98, TA100, TA1535, TA1537, in either the presence or absence of metabolic activation (United States Environmental Protection Agency 1978, Haworth *et al* 1983). Negative results have also been found in *E. coli* K12 (Goggelman *et al* 1978).

HCCPD has also proved negative in the mouse lymphoma assay, dominant lethal assay and BALB/3T3 cell transformation assay (United States Environmental Protection Agency 1978), but gave inconclusive results in a *Drosophila* sex-linked recessive lethal test (Zimmering *et al* 1985).

13.4.4 Carcinogenicity

No information appears to be available.

13.4.5 Reproductive toxicity

Oral doses of 3, 10, 30 or 100 mg/kg/day of HCCPD to Charles River rats on days 6–15 of gestation was not found to produce abnormalities in the offspring. All dams of the high-dose group died before day 10 of gestation (United States Environmental Protection agency 1978). No evidence for teratogenicity was found in CF-1 mice given 5, 25 or 75 mg/kg/day of HCCPD by gavage on days 6–15 of gestation, or in New Zealand white rabbits given the same doses on days 6–18 of gestation. Maternal toxicity was observed in rabbits at the highest dose level, but no embryotoxic effects were seen at any dose level in either species (Murray *et al* 1980).

13.5 Discussion

HCCPD is poorly absorbed by the oral route, and most of a dose is eliminated primarily in the faeces within 72 hours.

Subchronic studies in rats and and mice have shown that HCCPD can produce toxic effects at 19 mg/kg. The principal target organs appear to be the kidney and gastrointestinal tract. HCCPD has given negative results for genotoxicity in several assays. There is no information on carcinogenicity, but it does not appear to be teratogenic in rats, mice or rabbits.

HCCPD appears to be of greater toxicity in experimental animals than do most of the other compounds in this group. Further chronic toxicity studies are required to identify no-effect levels for HCCPD in different species.

References

ABDO K M, MONTGOMERY C A, KLUWE W M, FARNELL D R and PREJEAN J D (1984) Toxicity of hexachlorocyclopentadiene: subchronic (13-week) administration by gavage to F344 rats and B6C3F1 mice. *Journal of Applied Toxicology* **4**, 75–81.

ATALLAH Y H, WHITACRE D M and BUTZ R G (1981) Fate of hexachlorocyclopentadiene in the environment. In: Kham M A Q and Stanton R H (eds) *Toxicology of halogenated hydrocarbons.* Pergamon Press, pp 344–355.

BENOIT F M and WILLIAMS D T (1981) Determination of hexachlorocyclopentadiene at the nanogram per litre level in drinking water. *Bulletin of Environmental Contamination and Toxicology* **27**, 303–308.

DOROUGH H W and RANIERI T A (1984) Distribution and elimination of hexachlorocyclopentadiene in rats and mice. *Drug and Chemical Toxicology* **7**, 73–89.

EL DAREER S M, NOKER P E, TILLERY K F and HILL D L (1983) Investigations on the basis for the differential toxicity of hexachlorocyclopentadiene administered to rats by various routes. *Journal of Toxicology and Environmental Health* **12**, 203–211.

GOGGELMAN W, BONSE G, HENSCHLER D and CREIM H (1978) Mutagenicity of chlorinated cyclopentadienes due to metabolic activation. *Biochemical Pharmacology* **27**, 2927–2929.

HAWORTH S, LAWLOR T, MORTELMANS K, SPECK W and ZEIGER E (1983) Salmonella mutagenicity test results for 250 chemicals. *Environmental Mutagenesis* **5**, Suppl 1, 3–142.

KOMINSKY J R, WISSEMAN C L and MORSE D L (1980) Hexachlorocyclopentadiene contamination of a municipal wastewater treatment plant. *American Industrial Hygiene Association Journal* **41**, 552–556.

LAWRENCE L J and DOROUGH H W (1981) Retention and fate of inhaled hexachlorocyclopentadiene in the rat. *Bulletin of Environmental Contamination and Toxicology* **26**, 663–668.

LAWRENCE L J and DOROUGH H W (1982) Fate of inhaled hexachlorocyclopentadiene in albino rats and comparison to the oral and iv routes of administration. *Fundamental and Applied Toxicology* **2**, 235–240.

MEHENDALE H M (1977) Chemical reactivity – absorption, retention, metabolism, and elimination of hexachlorocyclopentadiene. *Environmental Health Perspectives* **21**, 275–278.

MORSE D L, KOMINSKY J R, WISSEMAN C L and LANDRIGAN P J (1979) Occupational exposure to hexachlorocyclopentadiene. How safe is sewage?

Journal of the American Medical Association **241**, 2177–2179.

MURRAY F J, SCHWETZ B A, BALMER M F and STAPLES R E (1980) Teratogenic potential of hexachlorocyclopentadiene in mice and rabbits. *Toxicology and Applied Pharmacology* **53**, 497–500.

RAND G M, NEES P O, CALO C J, ALEXANDER D J and CLARK G C (1982a) Effects of inhalation exposure to hexachlorocyclopentadiene on rats and monkeys. *Journal of Toxicology and Environmental Health* **9**, 743–760.

RAND G M, NEES P O, CALO C J, CLARKE G C and EDMONDSON N A (1982b) The Clara cell: an electron microscopy examination of the terminal bronchioles of rats and monkeys following inhalation of hexachlorocyclopentadiene. *Journal of Toxicology and Environmental Health* **10**, 59–72.

THRUSTON A D Jr (1978) High pressure liquid chromatography techniques for the isolation and identification of organics in drinking water extracts. *Journal of Chromatographic Science* **16**, 254–259.

TREON J F, CLEVELAND F P and CAPPEL J (1955) The toxicity of hexachlorocyclopentadiene. *Archives of Industrial Health* **11**, 459–472.

UNITED STATES ENVIRONMENTAL PROTECTION AGENCY (1978) Reviews of the environmental Effects of Pollutants. XII. Hexachlorocyclopentadiene. US EPA, EPA-600/1-78-047.

VERSCHUEREN K (1983) *Handbook of environmental data on organic chemicals.* Second Edition. Van Nostrand Reinhold Company.

WATER RESEARCH CENTRE (1981) Organic micropollutants in drinking water. WRc Technical Report TR 159.

ZIMMERING S, MASON JM, VALENCIA R and WOODRUFF R C (1985) Chemical mutagenesis testing in *Drosophila.* II. Results of 20 coded compounds tested for the National Toxicology Program. *Environmental Mutagenesis* **7**, 87–100.

14. METHYLDIBROMOACETATE

This compound was identified in one of 14 drinking water samples examined in a survey by WRc (Water Research Centre 1982).

No information appears to be available for this compound.

Reference

WATER RESEARCH CENTRE (1982) Frequency of occurrence data for compounds identified by GC–MS in XAD-2 samples taken for mutagenic testing survey. WRc unpublished report.

15. METHYLDICHLOROACETATE

CAS Reg No:	116-54-1
Molecular weight:	143.0
Boiling point:	143–145°C

Methyldichloroacetate was detected in 2/14 drinking water samples in a survey by WRc (Water Research Centre 1982).

In an inhalation study, groups of five Wistar rats were exposed to methyldichloroacetate for 0.5–7 hours at concentrations of 1000–4000 ppm. Exposure of one group to 4000 ppm for 1 hour and another group to 2000 ppm for 4 hours resulted in 100% mortality in both cases. No deaths were seen in a group exposed to 1000 ppm for 7 hours. The compound was found to be irritant to the eyes and lungs of the animals, and evidence of kidney congestion was obtained in rats exposed to 2000 ppm (Torkelson *et al* 1971).

Methyldichloroacetate gave negative results for both gene conversion and reversion in *Saccharomyces cerevisisae* D7 and XV185-14C respectively (Nestmann and Lee 1985).

There are insufficient data on methyldichloroacetate on which to base an assessment. However, this compound may have similar biochemical and toxicological properties to dichloroacetic acid, as the ester linkage should be easily broken by intestinal hydrolases and/or gastrointestinal microorganisms.

References

NESTMANN E R and LEE E G-H (1985) Genetic activity in *Saccharomyces cerevisiae* of compounds found in effluents of pulp and paper mills. *Mutation Research* **155**, 53–60.

TORKELSON T R, KARY C D, CHENOWETH M B and LARSEN E R (1971) Single exposure of rats to the vapors of trace substances in methoxyflurane. *Toxicology and Applied Pharmacology* **19**, 1–9.

WATER RESEARCH CENTRE (1982) Frequency of occurrence data for compounds identified by GC–MS in XAD-2 samples taken for mutagenic testing survey. WRc unpublished report.

16. POLYCHLORINATED TERPHENYLS

16.1 Introduction

Polychlorinated terphenyls (PCTs) are heat stable, non-flammable resins containing three aromatic rings in either *ortho, meta* or *para* configurations. Any hydrogen atom of the three rings can be substituted with chlorine. PCTs have similar properties, and hence similar uses, to the polychlorinated biphenyls (PCBs), for example as plasticisers, hydraulic fluid or lubricant, sealants, flame retardants, and as components of adhesives, paints and waxes. PCTs appear to have long half-lives in the environment, though they are less resistant to biodegradation and photodegradation than the PCBs.

16.2 Exposure

Although PCTs have been detected on many occasions in environmental samples, they are invariably found at much lower levels than the PCBs (Jensen and Jorgensen 1983, Doguchi 1977, Kimbrough 1980). In most instances it would appear that PCT contamination of the environment is related to nearby industrial manufacture or usage. Stratton and Sosebee (1976) detected PCT isomers at up to 13 ppm in the soil near a factory in Chicago, Illinois, which uses PCTs in waxes for investment casting. At a similar plant in Michigan, concentrations of up to 7.5 μg/l of PCTs were found in wastewater from the industrial estate, and levels of up to 5 ppm dry-weight in sludge deposits within the sewer. In West Germany, Buchert *et al* (1981) have detected PCTs in sewage sludge and in lake sediments. PCTs have been identified in Rhine water at 70 ng/l (Freudenthal and Greve 1973), but were not detected in a Japanese 1974 survey of 60 water samples or 1976 survey of 194 water samples. They were identified, however, in 20/145 sediment samples at levels of 0.5–330 ppt in the latter survey (Jensen and Jorgensen 1983). PCTs were identified in only one of 14 drinking water samples in a survey by WRc (Water Research Centre 1982).

In a Canadian survey of 73 samples of foodstuffs, 5.5% of the samples were found to contain PCT levels of 0.01–0.05 ppm (Villeneuve *et al* 1973). A study of 445 samples of food packaging materials identified PCTs in every sample. Concentrations of 10 ppm were found in 4% of the samples (Villeneuve *et al* 1973). PCTs have also been identified in Japanese vegetable products, the human intake from this source being estimated as 0.05 μg/day (Doguchi 1977).

PCTs have been detected in fish, birds, terrestrial species and in human adipose tissue on many occasions (Jensen and Jorgensen 1983, Doguchi 1977, Kimbrough 1980, Wright *et al* 1978, Fukano and Doguchi 1977, Doguchi and Fukano 1975, Doguchi *et al* 1974, Hassell and Holmes 1977). It appears that although environmental levels of PCTs are rather lower than the PCBs, PCT levels in human fat are comparable to those of the PCBs. The reason for this discrepancy is not clear.

16.3 Toxicokinetics

PCTs have been found to accumulate in the livers of mice fed 20–200 ppm of PCTs in the diet for 3–6 months. The levels of PCTs in the liver rose to 4–10-fold greater than the daily dose received in the diet (Sekita *et al* 1975). The liver was again found to contain the highest concentrations of PCTs following oral administration of Aroclor 5460 (a PCT mixture) to rats for 1 week. PCT residues were also found in all other tissues analysed (Sosa-Lucero *et al* 1973).

16.4 Effects on hepatic drug metabolising enzyme activities

High doses of PCTs appear to induce hepatic microsomal drug metabolism. PCTs induce both the 3-methylcholanthrene and phenobarbital forms of cytochrome P-450 (Sosa-Lucero *et al* 1973, Nilsen and Toftgard 1981).

16.5 Health effects

Generally, there is little information on the toxicology of the PCTs. That which is available suggests a similar toxic potential to the PCBs, that is, relatively low acute and chronic toxicity. The liver is the principal target organ at high doses.

16.5.1 Acute and subacute toxicity

The acute toxicity of PCT mixtures in rodents is very low. Oral LD50s in rats range from 10 to 20 g/kg (Fishbein 1974).

16.5.2 Chronic toxicity

Allen and Norback (1973) reported reduction in body weight, hair loss, subcutaneous oedema, liver hypertrophy, oedematous thickening of the stomach wall plus hypertrophy and hyperplasia of the pyloric and gastric mucosa in male rhesus monkeys fed diets containing 5000 ppm of PCTs for 3 months.

16.5.3 Genotoxicity
No information appears to be available on the mutagenicity of PCTs. PCBs are at best only weakly mutagenic, and one would expect similar activity for PCTs.

16.5.4 Carcinogenicity
In a study by Shirai *et al* (1978), groups of ICR mice were fed diets containing 250 ppm Kanechlor C (95% PCT + 5% PCB), 500 ppm Kanechlor C, or 250 ppm Kanechlor C + 50 ppm of hexachlorobenzene, for 24 weeks. Depression of body weight gain was seen in all groups. The PCT mixture, Kanechlor C, was found to induce hyperplastic nodules in the livers of 3/35 animals of the low-dose group and 6/35 animals of the high-dose group. Hepatocellular carcinomas were also observed in 3/35 animals of the high-dose group, but none were found in the low-dose group. No hepatic hyperplastic nodules or hepatocellular carcinomas were observed in controls. Co-administration of the PCT mixture with hexachlorobenzene resulted in a large increase in the numbers of animals with liver hyperplastic nodules and hepatocellular carcinomas.

16.5.5 Reproductive toxicity
Environmental reproductive effects of PCBs have been reported in a range of species (Jensen and Jorgensen 1983). However, no such ecological data are available for the PCTs. A laboratory investigation of White Leghorn chickens fed 20 ppm of Aroclor 5460 in the diet has suggested an increased number of dead or abnormal embryos. No change was found in hatchability (Cecil *et al* 1974).

16.6 Discussion
The EEC directive of 1976 (Commission of the European Communities 1976) restricted the use of PCTs to closed systems only. This is in line with the regulations for PCBs. However, from June 1986 an amendment to the directive (Commission of the European Communities 1985) will prohibit most uses of PCBs and PCTs.

PCTs do occur in the environment, but generally at lower levels than the PCBs. The toxicology of the PCTs is not well studied, though they do seem to have similar properties to the PCBs. At high doses, PCTs appear to be able to induce hepatic microsomal enzyme activities in rodents, and there is evidence that they can induce liver tumours in mice. The major consideration with PCTs is their persistence, though as their use is now severely restricted, levels in water should not rise to sufficient concentrations to present a problem.

References
ALLEN J R and NORBACK D H (1973) Polychlorinated biphenyl- and triphenyl-induced gastric mucosal hyperplasia in primates. *Science* **179**, 498–499.

BUCHERT H, BIHLER S, SCHOTT P, ROPER H P, PACHUR H J and BALLSCHMITER K (1981) Organochlorine pollutant anlysis of contaminated and uncontaminated lake sediment by high resolution gas chromatography. *Chemosphere* **10**, 945–956.

CECIL H C, BITMAN J, LILLIE R J and VERRET J (1974) Embryotoxic and teratogenic effects in unhatched fertile eggs from hens fed polychlorinated

biphenyls (PCBs). *Bulletin of Environmental Contamination and Toxicology* **11**, 489–495.
COMMISSION OF THE EUROPEAN COMMUNITIES (1976) Council Directive 76/769/EEC
COMMISSION OF THE EUROPEAN COMMUNITIES (1985) Council Directive 85/467/EEC 1st October 1985.
DOGUCHI M (1977) Polychlorinated terphenyls as an environmental pollutant in Japan. *Ecotoxicology and Environmental Safety* **1**, 239–248.
DOGUCHI M and FUKANO S (1975) Residue levels of polychlorinated terphenyls, polychlorinated biphenyls and DDT in human blood. *Bulletin of Environmental Contamination and Toxicology* **13**, 57–63.
DOGUCHI M, FUKANO S and USHIO F (1974) Polychlorinated terphenyls in the human fat. *Bulletin of Environmental Contamination and Toxicology* **11**, 157–158.
FISHBEIN L (1974) Toxicity of chlorinated biphenyls. *Annual Reviews in Pharmacology* **14**, 139–156.
FREUDENTHAL J and GREVE P A (1973) Polychlorinated terphenyls in the environment. *Bulletin of Environmental Contamination and Toxicology* **10**, 108–111.
FUKANO S and DOGUCHI M (1977) PCT, PCB and pesticide residues in human fat and blood. *Bulletin of Environmental Contamination and Toxicology* **17**, 613–617.
HASSELL K D and HOLMES D C (1977) Polychlorinated terphenyls in some British birds. *Bulletin of Environmental Contamination and Toxicology* **17**, 618–621.
JENSEN A A and JORGENSEN K J (1983) Polychlorinated terphenyls (PCTs) use, levels and biological effects. *Science of the Total Environment* **27**, 231–250.
KIMBROUGH R D (1980) Environmental pollution of air, water and soil. In: Kimbrough R D (ed) *Topics in environmental health volume 4. Halogenated biphenyls, terphenyls, naphthalenes, dibenzodioxins and related products.* Elsevier/North-Holland, Amsterdam.
NILSEN O G and TOFTGARD R (1981) Effects of polychlorinated terphenyls and paraffins on rat liver microsomal cytochrome P-450 and *in vitro* metabolic activities. *Archives of Toxicology* **47**, 1–11.
SEKITA H, TAKEDA M and USHIYAMA M (1975) Accumulation of PCT in tissues of mice after long-term feeding of Kanechlor-C. *Journal of Hygienic Chemistry (Tokyo)* **21**, 307–312.
SHIRAI T, MIYATA Y, NAKANISHI K, MURASAKI G'I and ITO N (1978) Hepatocarcinogenicity of polychlorinated terphenyl in ICR mice and its enhancement by hexachlorobenzene. *Cancer Letters* **4**, 271–275.
SOSA-LUCERO J C, DE LA IGLESIA F A and THOMAS G H (1973) Distribution of a polychlorinated terphenyl (Aroclor 5460) in rat tissues and effects on hepatic microsomal mixed function oxidases. *Bulletin of Environmental Contamination and Toxicology* **10**, 248–256.
STRATTON C L and SOSEBEE J B Jr (1976) PCB and PCT contamination of the environment near sites of manufacture and use. *Environmental Science and Technology* **10**, 1229–1233.

VILLENEUVE D C, REYNOLDS L M, THOMAS G H and PHILLIPS W E J (1973) Polychlorinated biphenyls and polychlorinated terphenyls in Canadian food packaging materials. *Journal of the Association of Official Analytical Chemists* **56**, 999–1001.

WATER RESEARCH CENTRE (1982) Frequency of occurrence data for compounds identified by GC–MS in XAD-2 samples taken for mutagenic testing survey. WRc unpublished report.

WRIGHT L H, LEWIS R G, CRIST H L, SOVOCOOL G W and SIMPSON J M (1978) The identification of polychlorinated terphenyls at trace levels in human adipose tissue by gas chromatography/mass spectrometry. *Journal of Analytical Toxicology* **2**, 76–79.

17. TRICHLOROACETONE

Trichloroacetone was identified in 10/14 drinking water samples in a survey by WRc (Water Research Centre 1982). 1,1,1-Trichloroacetone has been identified in drinking water on several other occasions (Suffet *et al* 1976, Akiyama *et al* 1980, Gurol *et al* 1983).

Both 1,1,1- and 1,1,3-trichloroacetone gave positive results for gene conversion in *Sacccharomyces cerevisiae* D7 in the absence of metabolic activation (Nestmann and Lee 1985). These compounds are direct-acting mutagens in the Ames/*Salmonella* assay and cause structural aberrations in the chromosomes of CHO cells when tested *in vitro*. However, they were not clastogenic when tested *in vivo* and did not adversely affect several indicators of testicular function in mice *in vivo* (Blazak *et al* 1987).

References

AKIYAMA T, KOGA M, SHINOHARA R, KIDO A and ETOH S (1980) Detection and identification of trace organic substances in the aquatic environment. *Journal of Uoeh* **2**, 285–300.

BLAZAK W F, MEIER J R, STEWART B E, BLACHMAN D C and DEAHL J T (1987) Genotoxicity studies of 1,1,1- and 1,1,3-trichloroacetones (TCA). *Environmental Mutagenesis* **9**, Suppl 8, 16.

GUROL M D, WOWK A, MYERS S and SUFFET I H (1983) Kinetics and mechanism of haloform formation: chloroform formation from trichloroacetone. In: Jolley R L *et al* (eds) *Water chlorination: environmental impact and health effects,* Vol 4 Book 1, Ann Arbor Science, Michigan.

NESTMANN E R and LEE E G-H (1985) Genetic activity in *Saccharomyces cerevisiae* of compounds found in effluents of pulp and paper mills. *Mutation Research* **155**, 53–60.

SUFFET I H, BRENNER L and SILVER B (1976) Identification of 1,1,1-trichloroacetone (1,1,1-trichloropropanone) in two drinking waters: a known precursor in haloform reaction. *Environmental Science and Technology* **10**, 1273–1275.

WATER RESEARCH CENTRE (1982) Frequency of occurrence data for compounds identified by GC–MS in XAD-2 samples taken for mutagenic testing survey. WRc unpublished report.

18. TRICHLOROANILINE

18.1 Introduction

Trichloroaniline is used as an intermediate in the manufacture of dyestuffs.

CAS Reg No:	634-93-5
Molecular weight:	196.47
Boiling point:	262.4°C

18.2 Exposure

Trichloroaniline was detected in only one of 14 drinking water samples in a survey by WRc (Water Research Centre 1982).

18.3 Toxicokinetics

No information appears to be available.

18.4 Health effects

Zimmer *et al* (1980) found that trichloroaniline gave negative results in the Ames test with *Salmonella typhimurium* TA100 and TA98, in either the presence or absence of metabolic activation.

Carcinogenicity studies on trichloroaniline have been carried out in rats and mice (Weisburger *et al* 1978). Male and female CD-1 mice were fed diets containing 6000 and 12000 mg/kg of trichloroaniline for 18 months. Male Charles River rats were begun on diets containing 3000 and 6000 mg/kg, but due to toxicity and early deaths in the high-dose group these concentrations were lowered to 1500 and 3000 mg/kg diet after 5 months. At the conclusion of the experiments, there was no significant increase in tumour incidence in the rats or female mice, but an increase in vascular and liver tumours was found in male mice compared to controls.

	High dose	Low dose	Controls
Liver tumours	1/16	5/18	7/99
Vascular tumours	12/16	10/18	5/99

18.5 Discussion

There is very little information available on the environmental occurrence, metabolism and toxicity of trichloroaniline. This compound has given a positive result for carcinogenicity in a high-dose feeding study in mice.

References

WATER RESEARCH CENTRE (1982) Frequency of occurrence data for compounds identified by GC–MS in XAD-2 samples taken for mutagenic testing survey. WRc unpublished report.

WEISBURGER E K, RUSSFIELD A B, HOMBURGER F, WEISBURGER J H, BOGER E, VAN DONGEN C G and CHU K C (1978) Testing of twenty-one environmental aromatic amines or derivatives for long-term toxicity or carcinogenicity. *Journal of Environmental Pathology and Toxicology* **2**, 325–356.

ZIMMER D, MAZUREK J, PETZOLD G and BHUYAN B K (1980) Bacterial mutagenicity and mammalian cell DNA damage by several substituted anilines. *Mutation Research* **77**, 317–326.

19. TRICHLORONITROMETHANE

19.1 Introduction

Trichloronitromethane (chloropicrin, nitrochloroform) has been used as a fumigant for the control of pest infestation of foods, as a fungicide, as a war poison gas, and in dyestuffs. It appears that low levels of chloropicrin residues remain in foodstuffs for some time after treatment (Getzendaner *et al* 1965).

CAS Reg No:	76-06-2
Molecular weight:	164.4
Boiling point:	112°C
Solubility:	2000 mg/l (Verschueren 1983)
Threshold odour concentration in water:	7.3 μg/l (Verschueren 1983)

19.2 Exposure

The survey by WRc detected this compound in 3/14 drinking water samples tested. All three samples were derived from river waters (Water Research Centre 1981).

19.3 Toxicokinetics

No information appears to be available.

19.4 Health effects

19.4.1 Acute and subacute toxicity

In man, inhalation of chloropicrin can cause skin irritation, lacrimation and pulmonary irritation, particularly affecting the smaller bronchi. Inhalation of around 15 ppm for 1 minute can be intolerable, while exposure to 119 ppm for 30 minutes may cause death (Stokinger 1982).

The oral LD50 in the rat has been reported to be 250 mg/kg. An intraperitoneal LD50 of 25 mg/kg for the mouse has also been reported (Registry of toxic effects of chemical substances 1978).

19.4.2 Chronic toxicity

The only information that appears to be available is that in the carcinogenicity studies (National Cancer Institute 1978).

19.4.3 Genotoxicity

Ames tests carried out at two independent laboratories have given conflicting results (Haworth *et al* 1983). One laboratory found chloropicrin to be mutagenic to *Salmonella typhimurium* TA100, TA1535 and TA98 in the presence of a metabolising system. The other laboratory, however, found positive results in only the TA100 strain. Moriya *et al* (1983) have also reported that chloropicrin is mutagenic to TA100 in the presence of S-9, though they also found it had weak direct-acting mutagenicity in *Salmonella typhimurium* TA98 and in *E. coli* WP2.

19.4.4 Carcinogenicity

Although carcinogenicity bioassays have been carried out in rats and mice, the studies provide little information, due to severe toxicity problems which resulted in high mortality rates (National Cancer Institute 1978).

Groups of 50 male and 50 female Osborne–Mendel rats were given time-weighted average daily doses of 25 mg/kg (males) and 20 mg/kg (females) by gavage on 5 days/week from weeks 1 to 33 and cyclically (four treated weeks followed by an untreated week) from weeks 34 to 78. Other groups of rats were given time-weighted average daily doses of 26 mg/kg (males) and 22 mg/kg (females) by gavage on 5 days/week from weeks 1 to 17, weeks 31 to 33 and cyclically (four treated weeks followed by an untreated week) from weeks 34 to 78. Although no significantly increased tumour incidence was found, there was a very high incidence of early deaths.

Groups of 50 male and 50 B6C3F1 mice were given time-weighted average daily doses of 33 and 66 mg/kg by gavage on 5 days/week for 78 weeks. No significant increase in tumour incidence was found, but there was a rapid decrease in survival of high-dose animals after the first year of the study.

19.4.5 Reproductive toxicity

No information appears to be available.

19.5 Discussion

There appears to be very little information available on the environmental occurrence and mammalian metabolism of chloropicrin.

The limited information available suggests that chloropicrin is of moderate acute toxicity. Chloropicrin has been shown to be mutagenic in the Ames test, but bioassays carried out in rats and mice were inadequate to assess carcinogenic potential. Those studies demonstrate, however, that chloropicrin is of quite high chronic toxicity.

There is insufficient information available to assess the significance to health of low levels of chloropicrin in drinking water.

References

GETZENDANER M E, WAGONER E T and LAMBERT M (1965) Chloropicrin residues in food commodities after chamber fumigations. *Journal of Agricultural and Food Chemistry* **13**, 565–568.

HAWORTH S, LAWLOR T, MORTELMANS K, SPECK W and ZEIGER E (1983) Salmonella mutagenicity test results for 250 chemicals. *Environmental Mutagenesis* **5**, Suppl 1, 3–142.

MORIYA M, OHTA T, WATANABE K, MIYAZAWA T, KATO K and SHIRASU Y (1983) Further mutagenicity studies on pesticides in bacterial reversion assay systems. *Mutation Research* **116**, 185–216.

NATIONAL CANCER INSTITUTE (1978) Bioassay of chloropicrin for possible

carcinogenicity. *National Cancer Institute Carcinogenesis Technical Reports Series Bethesda,* Maryland, NCI-CG-TR-65.
REGISTRY OF TOXIC EFFECTS OF CHEMICAL SUBSTANCES (1978) National Institute for Occupational Safety and Health, Cincinnati, Ohio, 1978.
STOKINGER H E (1982) Aliphatic nitro compounds, nitrates, nitrites. In: Clayton G D and Clayton F E (eds) *Patty's industrial hygiene and toxicology,* 3rd revised edition, Vol 2C, John Wiley and Sons, pp 4141–4208.
VERSCHUEREN K (1983) *Handbook of environmental data on organic chemicals,* second edition. Van Nostrand Reinhold Company.
WATER RESEARCH CENTRE (1981) *Organic micropollutants in drinking water.* WRc Technical Report TR 159.

20. TRI-(HALOALKYL)PHOSPHATES

20.1 Introduction

Tris(2-chloroethyl)phosphate, (Flame Retardant 3CF, Fyrol CEF, Celluflex) is used as a flame retardant for textiles.

CAS Reg No:	115-96-8
Molecular weight:	285.5

20.2 Exposure

Tris(2-chloroethyl)phosphate was detected in only one of 14 drinking water samples in a survey by WRc (Water Research Centre 1981). In a further, unpublished survey (Water Research Centre 1982), tris(2-chloroethyl)phosphate was identifed in 5/14 drinking water samples tested. Two unspecified tri(haloalkyl)phosphates were also detected in one of the samples in this survey.

A tap water survey of 29 sites across Canada revealed the presence of tris(2-chloroethyl)phosphate at levels ranging from <0.1 to 52 ng/l. Levels of up to 9 ng/l were also found in raw water (Williams and LeBel 1981).

20.3 Toxicokinetics

No information appears to be available on the mammalian metabolism of tris(2-chloroethyl)phosphate.

20.4 Health effects

A good deal of the information available on the toxicology of tris(2-chloroethyl)-phosphate has been generated by the Stauffer Chemical Company. Their data has been reported in a review by Ulsamer *et al* (1980).

20.4.1 Acute and subacute toxicity

The acute oral LD50 of tris(2-chloroethyl)phosphate in rats ranges from 430 to 1230 mg/kg. Animals given the highest doses exhibited acute depression and spasmodic contractions (Ulsamer *et al* 1980). This compound is of low ophthalmotoxicity in rabbits, but is a primary skin irritant in the same species.

Tris(2-chloroethyl)phosphate had no insecticidal activity to houseflies, but it did cause a 50% inhibition of Southern armyworm microsomal *N*-demethylase activity. It was also reported to have weak anticholinesterase activity in electric ray preparations (Eldefrawi *et al* 1977). Inhibition of plasma cholinesterase and neurotoxic esterase has also been found in hens given 10 ml/kg of tris(2-chloroethyl)phosphate (Sprague et al 1981). Hens treated twice with 10 ml/kg of tris(2-chloroethyl)phosphate and observed for 6 weeks did not exhibit delayed neurotoxicity (Sprague *et al* 1981).

No gross or histopathological changes were found in rats fed diets containing 0.5% tris(2-chloroethyl)phosphate for 30 days (Ulsamer *et al* 1980).

20.4.2 Chronic toxicity
No information appears to be available.

20.4.3 Genotoxicity
Tris(2-chloroethyl)phosphate has given negative results for mutagenicity in the Ames test with *Salmonella typhimurium* TA1535, TA1537, TA1538, TA98 and TA100, in both the presence and absence of metabolic activation (Ulsamer *et al* 1980, Prival *et al* 1977, Haworth *et al* 1983). However, Nakamura *et al* (1979) reported that tris(2-chloroethyl)phosphate was mutagenic to TA1535 in the presence of S-9.

This compound gave negative results in the mouse lymphoma forward mutation assay but positive results in the mouse BALB/3T3 cell transformation assay (Ulsamer *et al* 1980). Sala *et al* (1982) similarly found that tris(2-chloroethyl)phosphate was able to transform Syrian hamster embryo cells, whereas it gave negative results for mutation in V79 cells. These workers also found that this compound induced sister chromatid exchanges in V79 cells, but gave equivocal results in the Chinese hamster micronucleus assay and was negative in a mouse skin initiation test (Sala *et al* 1982).

20.4.4 Carcinogenicity
No information appears to be available.

20.4.5 Reproductive toxicity
No information appears to be available.

20.5 Discussion
There is little information available on the metabolism and toxicology of tris(2-chloroethyl)phosphate. It does not appear to be mutagenic in the Ames test, but has given positive results for cell transformation and sister chromatid exchange in mammalian cells *in vitro*.

There are insufficient data available for tris(2-chloroethyl) phosphate on which to base an assessment.

References
ELDEFRAWI A T, MANSOUR N A, BRATTSTEN L B, AHRENS V D and LISK D J (1977) Further toxicologic studies with commercial and candidate

flame retardant chemicals. Part II. *Bulletin of Environmental Contamination and Toxicology* **17**, 720–726.

HAWORTH S, LAWLOR T, MORTELMANS K, SPECK W and ZEIGER E (1983) Salmonella mutagenicity test results for 250 chemicals. *Environmental Mutagenesis* **5**, Suppl 1, 3–142.

NAKAMURA A, TATENO N, KOJIMA S, KANIWA M A and KAWAMURA T (1979) The mutagenicity of halogenated alkanols and their phosphoric acid esters for *Salmonella typhimurium*. *Mutation Research* **66**, 373–380.

PRIVAL M J, McCOY E C, GUTTER B and ROSENKRANZ H S (1977) Tris(2,3-dibromopropyl)phosphate: mutagenicity of a widely used flame-retardant. *Science* **195**, 76–78.

SALA M, GU Z G, MOENS G and CHOUROULINKOV I (1982) *In vivo* and *in vitro* biological effects of the flame retardants tris(2,3-dibromopropyl)phosphate and tris(2-chlorethyl)ortho phosphate. *European Journal of Cancer and Clinical Oncology* **18**, 1337–1344.

SPRAGUE G L, SANDVIK L L, BROOKINS-HENDRICKS M J and BICKFORD A A (1981) The neurotoxicity of two organophosphorous ester flame retardants in hens. *Journal of Toxicology and Environmental Health* **8**, 507–518.

ULSAMER A G, OSTERBERG R E and McLAUGHLIN J Jr (1980) Flame-retardant chemicals in textiles. *Clinical Toxicology* **17**, 101–131.

WATER RESEARCH CENTRE (1981) Organic micropollutants in drinking water. WRc Technical Report TR 159.

WATER RESEARCH CENTRE (1982) Frequency of occurrence data for compounds identified by GC–MS in XAD-2 samples taken for mutagenic testing survey. WRc unpublished report.

WILLIAMS D T and LeBEL G L (1981) A national survey of tri(haloalkyl)-, trialkyl-, and triarylphosphates in Canadian drinking water. *Bulletin of Environmental Contamination and Toxicology* **27**, 450–457.

9

Halogenated ethers

1. INTRODUCTION

Some halogenated ethers have been widely used in industry as solvents, in textile treatment and in the manufacture of ion exchange resins and pesticides. Particularly important members of this group are bis-(chloromethyl)ether, chloromethyl methyl ether, bis-(2-chloroisopropyl)ether and bis-(2-chloroethyl)ether. The industrial use of both bis-(chloromethyl)ether and chloromethyl methyl ether has been linked with respiratory cancer.

Of the halogenated ethers identified in drinking water by WRc, there appears to be toxicological information available only for one compound, bis-(2-chloroethyl)-ether. All the information documented in this review is therefore concerned with this compound.

Bis-(2-chloroethyl)ether is prepared commercially as a byproduct from the manufacture of ethylene oxide. It has been used as a solvent, soil fumigant, insecticide, acaricide and as an intermediate in the manufacture of medicines and pharmaceuticals.

CAS Reg No:	111-44-4
Molecular weight:	143.0
Boiling point:	178°C
Solubility:	10.2 g/l (Verschueren 1983)
Threshold odour concentration in water:	0.36 mg/l (Verschueren 1983)

2. EXPOSURE

Four halogenated ethers have been detected in drinking water by WRc (Water Research Centre 1981). These were bis-(2-chloroethyl)ether and unspecified isomers of bromopropyl methyl ether, bromoethyl chloroethyl ether and chloroethyl propyl ether. Bromopropyl methyl ether and chloroethyl propyl ether were only detected in the treated water from one particular groundwater source. Although bis-

(2-chloroethyl)ether and bromoethyl chloroethyl ether were not detected in any of the 14 samples, they were both found in an initial survey of treated water. Bis-(2-chloroethyl)ether was also identified in raw water.

In the US, bis-(2-chloroethyl)ether has been detected in the finished water of 13/113 cities at concentrations of less than 1 μg/l (Dressman *et al* 1977). This compound has also been identified in river water (Rosen *et al* 1963) and in the treated effluent from rubber manufacturing plants (Webb *et al* 1973). Bis-(2-chloroisopropyl)ether has also been regularly identified in raw water and drinking water in the US (Rosen *et al* 1963, Kleopfer and Fairless 1972).

There appears to be no information on the occurrence of bis-(2-chloroethyl)ether in food or air.

Very little is known about the environmental fate of halogenated ethers. Alpha-haloethers (compounds in which the halogen is attached to the carbon atom immediately next to the ether oxygen) are very reactive and would not remain in water for any longer than a few seconds. Other halogenated ethers, however, are more stable and may persist in water for several days or weeks (Durkin *et al* 1975).

3. TOXICOKINETICS

Oral doses of bis-(2-chloroethyl)ether are rapidly metabolised in the rat (Lingg *et al* 1979, 1982, Muller *et al* 1979). Biotransformation proceeds by cleavage at the ether linkage to give thiodiglycolic acid and a number of minor metabolites. Following an oral dose of 40 mg/kg in rats, about 65% was excreted in the urine within 48 hours. A further 12% of the dose was eliminated in the expired air as carbon dioxide.

4. HEALTH EFFECTS

The toxicology of bis-(2-chloroethyl)ether has been reviewed previously (Durkin *et al* 1975, United States Environmental Protection Agency 1980, National Academy of Sciences 1980, International Agency for Research on Cancer 1975).

4.1 Acute and subacute toxicity

Oral LD50s for bis-(2-chloroethyl)ether of 75-150, 136 and 126 mg/kg have been reported in the rat, mouse and rabbit respectively (Registry of Toxic Effects of Chemical Substances 1983).

In a study of guinea-pigs exposed to bis-(2-chloroethyl)ether, inhalation of 100 ppm for a short period resulted in eye and nose irritation, while exposure to 500–1000 ppm was lethal. Irritation of the nasal passage was found in animals continuously exposed to 35 ppm for 13 hours (Schrenk *et al* 1933). Human volunteers found brief exposure to 550 ppm of bis-(2-chloroethyl)ether vapour to be extremely irritating to the eyes and nasal passage. Irritation was also found at 100 and 260 ppm, though these concentrations were reported to be tolerable. At 35 ppm, no irritation was apparent, but the odour of bis-(2-chloroethyl)ether was still detectable (Schrenk *et al* 1933).

4.2 Chronic toxicity

Rats and guinea-pigs exposed by inhalation to 69 ppm of bis-(2-chloroethyl)ether, 7 hours/day, 5 days/week for about 19 weeks exhibited no adverse effects in gross appearance, behaviour, mortality, haematology or tissue histology. Depression of growth, particularly in males, and some inconsistent differences in organ weights were found (Kirwin *et al* 1981).

4.3 Genotoxicity

Bis-(2-chloroethyl)ether is a potent direct-acting mutagen in bacterial systems, particularly *Salmonella typhimurium* TA100 and TA1535, when tested in suspension or in a desiccator (United States Environmental Protection Agency 1980, Simmon *et al* 1977, Simmon and Tardiff 1978). This compound was not found to be mutagenic in a host-mediated assay (United States Environmental Protection Agency 1980).

Bis-(2-chloroethyl)ether has also given negative results in the mouse heritable translocation test (Jorgenson *et al* 1978). In this study, groups of adult male mice were treated daily by gavage with three (unspecified) dose levels of bis-(2-chloroethyl)ether for a period of 8 weeks. At this point, each treated male was then mated with two untreated virgin females to produce an F1 generation. When the males from the F1 generation had reached maturity, 100 animals per dose group were each mated with three virgin females. The pregnant females were evaluated to identify suspect F1 males. Each suspect male was rebred with three virgin females to assess breeding efficiency. The F1 males, after two breedings, were examined cytogenetically.

4.4 Carcinogenicity

In oral carcinogenicity studies, bis-(2-chloroethyl)ether has given positive results in mice but not in rats. Groups of 18 male and 18 female mice of two hybrid strains received a dose of 100 mg/kg body weight/day by gavage at 7 days of age. This absolute dose (not adjusted for increasing body weight) was then given each day until the animals had reached 28 days of age. After this time the compound was incorporated in the diet at 300 ppm (about 45 mg/kg body weight) for 80 weeks. Male mice of both strains and female mice of one strain exhibited an increased incidence of liver tumours (Innes *et al* 1969). In the rat study, groups of 26 male and 26 female animals of the Charles River CD strain were given twice-weekly doses of 25 or 50 mg/kg body weight by gavage for 18 months, followed by an untreated observation period of 6 months. There was no evidence for increased tumour incidence (Weisburger *et al* 1981).

Of 30 female Swiss mice given a weekly subcutaneous injection of 1 mg of bis-(2-chloroethyl)ether in paraffin oil for lifetime, 2 mice developed sarcomas at the injection site. No sarcomas occurred in a control group of 60 animals which received paraffin oil alone (Van Duuren *et al* 1972).

A single application of 1 mg of bis-(2-chloroethyl)ether in 0.1 ml of benzene to the skin of 20 female Swiss mice followed by phorbol myristate treatment, thrice weekly for 590 days, was not found to induce skin carcinomas. Skin papillomas were observed in 3 mice treated with bis-(2-chloroethyl)ether and in 2/20 control mice (Van Duuren *et al* 1972).

Strain A mice given intraperitoneal injections of 8 or 20 mg/kg, three times/week for 8 weeks, or 4 injections of 40 mg/kg, did not exhibit an increased incidence of lung tumours (Theiss *et al* 1977).

4.5 Reproductive toxicity

No information appears to be available.

5. DISCUSSION

Both the WRc survey and several studies from the US indicate that the halogenated ethers, particularly bis-(2-chloroethyl)ether, are fairly common micropollutants in drinking water, though concentrations are probably below 1 μg/l. Bis-(2-chloroethyl)ether may be formed during water chlorination if sufficient ethyl ether is present, but the major source of this compound in water is probably industrial.

The only toxicological information available on the halogenated ethers detected in drinking water by WRc relates to bis-(2-chloroethyl)ether. This compound appears to be of moderate acute toxicity, but its chronic toxicity has been poorly studied. Bis(2-chloroethyl)ether is mutagenic in bacterial systems and has given positive results in an oral carcinogenicity study in the mouse. An oral study in rats failed to show any carcinogenic potential for bis-(2-chloroethyl)ether. There appears to be no information on reproductive toxicity.

Although there is insufficient information available to assess the hazard to human health, bis-(2-chloroethyl)ether has been shown to be mutagenic in bacterial systems and gave positive results in a mouse carcinogenicity bioassay. These compounds must therefore be viewed with caution as micropollutants in drinking water.

REFERENCES

DRESSMAN R C, FAIR J and McFARREN E F (1977) Determinative method for analysis of aqueous sample extracts for bis(2-chloro)ethers and dichlorobenzenes. *Environmental Science and Technology* **11,** 719-721.

DURKIN P R, HOWARD P H and SAXENA J (1975) Investigation of selected potential environmental contaminants: Haloethers. US EPA, EPA-560/2-75-006.

INNES J R M, ULLAND B M, VALERIO M G, PETRUCELLI L, FISHBEIN L, HART E R, PALLOTTA A J, BATES R R, FALK H L, GART J J, KLEIN M, MITCHELL I and PETERS J (1969) Bioassay of pesticides and industrial chemicals for tumorigenicity in mice: A preliminary note. *Journal of the National Cancer Institute* **42,** 1101-1114.

INTERNATIONAL AGENCY FOR RESEARCH ON CANCER (1975) IARC Monographs on the evaluation of carcinogenic risk of chemicals to man. Volume 9. Some aziridines, *N*-, *S*- & *O*-mustards and selenium. IARC, Lyon.

JORGENSON T A, RUSHBROOK C J, NEWELL G W and TARDIFF R G (1978) Study of the mutagenic potential of bis(2-chloroethyl) and bis(2-chloroisopropyl) ethers in mice by the heritable translocation test. *Mutation Research* **53,** 124.

KIRWIN C J Jr and SANDMEYER E E (1981) Ethers. In: Clayton G D and

Clayton F E (eds) *Patty's industrial hygiene and toxicology,* 3rd revised edition, vol 2A. John Wiley & Sons, Inc, pp 2517-2519.

KLEOPFER R D and FAIRLESS B J (1972) Characterization of organic components in a municipal water supply. *Environmental Science and Technology* **6,** 1036-1037.

LINGG R D, KAYLOR W H, PYLE S M and TARDIFF R G (1979) Thiodiglycolic acid: A major metabolite of bis(2-chloroethyl) ether. *Toxicology and Applied Pharmacology* **47,** 23.

LINGG R D, KAYLOR W H, PYLE S M, DOMINO M M, SMITH C C and WOLFE G F (1982) Metabolism of bis(2-chloroethyl)ether and bis(2-chloroisopropyl)ether in the rat. *Archives of Environmental Contamination and Toxicology* **11,** 173-183.

MULLER G, NORPOTH K and ECKARD R (1979) Identification of *S*-(carboxymethyl)-L-cysteine and thiodiglycolic acid, urinary metabolites of 2,2′-bis-(chloroethyl)ether in the rat. *Cancer Letters* **7,** 299.

NATIONAL ACADEMY OF SCIENCES (1980) Drinking water and health volume 1. Washington DC, National Academy Press.

REGISTRY OF TOXIC EFFECTS OF CHEMICAL SUBSTANCES (1983) National Institute for Occupational Safety & Health, Cincinnati, Ohio.

ROSEN A A, SKEEL R T and ETTINGER M B (1963) Relationship of river water odor to specific organic contaminants. *Journal of the Water Pollution Control Federation* **35,** 777-782.

SCHRENK H H, PATTY F A and YANT W P (1933) Acute response of guinea-pigs to vapors of some new commercial organic compounds. *Public Health Reports* **48,** 1389.

SIMMON V F, KAUHANEN K and TARDIFF R G (1977) Mutagenic activity of chemicals identified in drinking water. In: Scott D, Bridges B A and Sobels F H (eds) *Progress in genetic toxicology.* Elsevier/North-Holland Biomedical Press, pp 249-258.

SIMMON V F and TARDIFF R G (1978) The mutagenic activity of halogenated compounds found in chlorinated drinking water. In: JOLLEY R L *et al* (eds) *Water chlorination. Environmental impact and health effects* vol 2. Ann Arbor, pp 417-431.

THEISS J C, STONE G D, SHIMKIN M B and WEISBURGER E K (1977) Test for carcinogenicity of organic contaminants of United States drinking waters by pulmonary tumor response in strain A mice. *Cancer Research* **37,** 2717-2720.

US ENVIRONMENTAL PROTECTION AGENCY (1980) Ambient water quality criteria for chloroalkyl ethers. US EPA, EPA-440/5-80-030.

VAN DUUREN B L, KATZ C, GOLDSCHMIDT B M, FRENKEL K and SIVAK A (1972) Carcinogenicity of halo-ethers. II. Structure–activity relationships of analogs of bis(chloromethyl)ether. *Journal of the National Cancer Institute* **48,** 1431-1439.

VERSCHUEREN K (1983) *Handbook of environmental data on organic chemicals.* 2nd edn. Van Nostrand Reinhold Company.

WATER RESEARCH CENTRE (1981) Organic micropollutants in drinking water. Technical Report TR 159.

WEBB R G, GARRISON A W, KEITH L H and MgGUIRE J M (1973) Current

practice in GC–MS analysis of organics in water. US EPA, EPA-R2-73-277.
WEISBURGER E K, ULLAND B M, NAM J -M, GART J J and WEISBURGER J H (1981) Carcinogenicity tests of certain environmental and industrial chemicals. *Journal of the National Cancer Institute* **67**, 75-88.

10

The polycyclic aromatic hydrocarbons

1. OVERVIEW

The polycyclic aromatic hydrocarbons (PAH) are a large group of compounds occurring widely in the environment from both natural and anthropogenic sources. Studies by WRc have identified some 20 PAH in drinking water in the UK. The structures of several of these compounds are shown in Figure 1.

About two thirds of the PAH found in raw water appears to be bound to particulate matter which is removed by flocculation, sedimentation and filtration processes. The remaining third may be significantly removed by oxidation. Contact with coal-tar-based pipe linings during distribution is known to lead to elevated concentrations of some PAH, particularly fluoranthene. Estimates of exposure to PAH indicate that drinking water is a very minor source, with a typical contribution of less than 1%.

PAH are highly lipid-soluble and readily absorbed from the gastrointestinal tract of mammals. They are rapidly distributed to a wide variety of tissues, with a particular tendency for localisation in body fat.

Metabolism of PAH is via the cytochrome P-450 mediated mixed function oxidase system with oxidation or hydroxylation as the first step. The resultant epoxides or phenols may then go through a detoxification reaction to produce glucuronides, sulphates or glutathione conjugates. Some of the epoxides, however, may be metabolised to dihydrodiols, which in turn may undergo conjugation to form soluble detoxification products or oxidation to diol-epoxides. These latter compounds are thought to be the ultimate carcinogens in cases where carcinogenicity has been demonstrated. The metabolites of PAH are primarily eliminated in the urine and faeces as water-soluble compounds.

PAH can induce the synthesis of the enzymes responsible for their own metabolism. This in turn means that the efficiency of metabolism of PAH will increase with continued exposure. However, the effects of various exogenous and endogenous inducers, genetic factors, age, sex and nutritional status, which have been shown to influence these enzyme systems, make it difficult to predict whether the carcinogenicity of PAH will be increased or decreased with time.

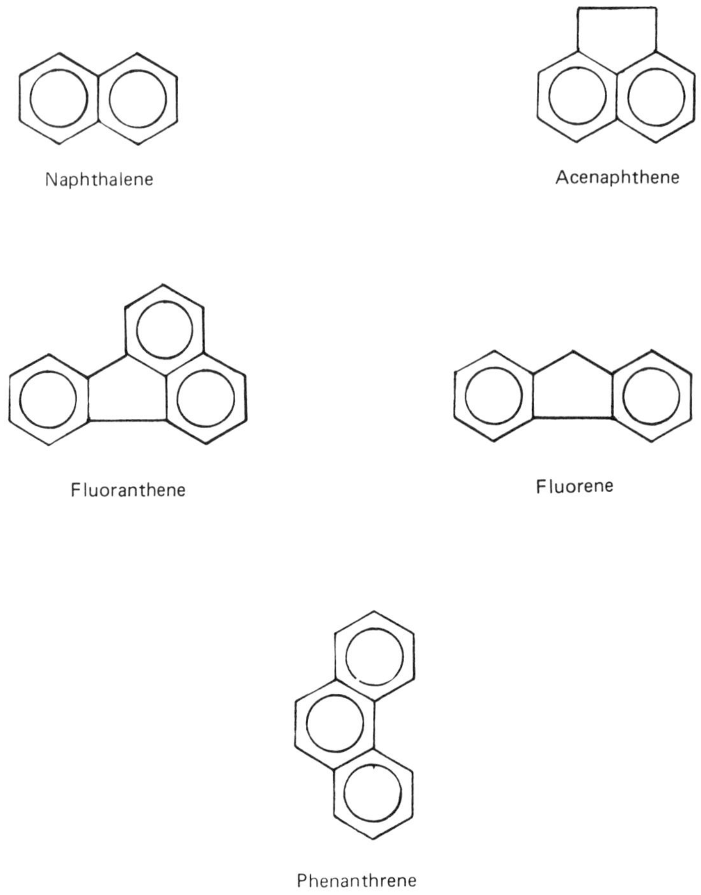

Fig. 1 — Structures of some of the polycyclic aromatic hydrocarbons identified in drinking water.

Numerous studies show that, despite their high lipid solubility, PAH have little tendency for bio-concentration in the fatty tissues of animals or man, primarily because PAH are rapidly and extensively metabolised.

Little information is available on the acute, subacute and chronic toxicity of PAH after ingestion. This is reflected by the limited data reported for the PAH identified in drinking water by WRc.

The most frequently expressed concern regarding the health effects of PAH is carcinogenicity. Epidemiological studies of some occupation-associated skin cancers in man provide strong presumptive evidence of the role of PAH in certain kinds of human cancer. Many PAH are capable of producing tumours in skin and other epithelial tissues in numerous test species, though only benzo(*a*)pyrene appears to have been well studied with regard to oral exposure. Malignant tumours can often be induced by very small quantities of certain PAH and with very short latency periods.

Although there is very little information available on the carcinogenicity of the PAH encountered in drinking water, there is no evidence for the potent activity found with some PAH such as benzo(*a*)pyrene. Naphthalene is the subject of a US National Toxicology Program carcinogenicity bioassay.

Naphthalene, fluorene and the methyl fluorenes have so far proved negative in *in vitro* mutagenicity assays, the alkyl naphthalenes and phenanthrenes have been shown to be mutagenic under special conditions, fluoranthene and some methyl phenanthrenes have been shown to be mutagens, while acenaphthene does not appear to have been tested. Fluoranthene was positive in a mouse lung adenoma bioassay, the significance of which is unclear. There is some evidence for phenanthrene being a weak initiator in skin, and some evidence for the alkyl naphthalenes and fluoranthene being co-carcinogens. However, the significance of these findings in relation to environmental exposure, particularly at the low concentrations detected in drinking water, is not clear. PAH are rarely encountered singly in the environment, and many interactions can occur with mixtures of PAH whereby the potency of known carcinogenic PAH may be modified, usually enhanced. These interactions are not well understood, and their role in the possible effects of PAH under circumstances of environmental exposure is uncertain.

In view of the lack of evidence for their carcinogenicity and the low concentrations of the PAH in drinking water, it would seem unlikely that they would present a significant risk to human health. This must also be considered against the background of discontinued use of coal-tar linings to distribution systems and their gradual replacement by other materials or linings, thereby removing one of the major sources of PAH in drinking water. The role of PAH in drinking water in relation to overall environmental exposure to PAH is likely to be negligible, since other sources such as food contain very much greater quantities of PAH and a much wider range of compounds.

2. NAPHTHALENE

2.1 Introduction

Naphthalene is principally produced by petroleum refining and coal-tar distillation. It is used in the manufacture of a wide range of products including pesticides, fungicides, detergents, dyes, resins and motor fuel. It has also been used in moth balls, as an antiseptic and as an antihelminthic.

CAS Reg No:	91-20-3
Molecular weight:	128.2
Boiling point:	218°C
Solubility:	30 mg/l at 25°c (Verschueren 1983)
Evaporative half life in water of depth 1 m:	7.15 hours at 25°C (Verschueren 1983)
Threshold odour concentration in water:	0.001-0.5 mg/l (Verschueren 1983)

2.2 Exposure

Naphthalene has been frequently identified in both raw and treated water samples. It was detected at 0.6–7.5 ng/l in the final water from five water treatment plants in Canada (Benoit *et al* 1979), and at 2.2 ng/l in Japanese tap water (Akiyama *et al* 1980). Both of these studies also reported the presence of naphthalene in raw waters. Levels of up to 1.4 μg/l have been detected in US drinking water (United States Environmental Protection Agency 1980). This compound was identified in all 14 drinking water samples in the WRc survey (Water Research Centre 1981). The major sources of naphthalene in the aquatic environment are thought to be industrial effluents and oil spills (United States Environmental Protection Agency 1980).

Little information is available on the occurrence of naphthalene in air or food, though it has been identified in cigarette smoke (Schmeltz *et al* 1976).

Naphthalene was found in 6/8 samples of mother's milk (Pellizzari *et al* 1982).

2.3 Toxicokinetics

The biotransformation of naphthalene has been quite widely studied (Corner and Young 1954, Boyland *et al* 1961, Jerina *et al* 1970, Oesch and Daly 1972). It is clear that the first metabolic step is oxidation by cytochrome P-450 to naphthalene-1,2-oxide. This is followed by either conjugation with glutathione, rearrangement to give 1-naphthol and smaller quantities of 2-naphthol, or action by epoxide hydrolase to give naphthalene-1,2-dihdrodiol. One study (Horning *et al* 1980) has indicated that a whole range of epoxide metabolites, including di-epoxides and dihydriol-epoxides, can be formed in the rat *in vivo*. Both *in vivo* and *in vitro* experiments indicate that around 50% of a dose of naphthalene is conjugated with glutathione (Chen and Dorough 1979). Naphthalene may undergo entero-hepatic recirculation in the rat (Pue *et al* 1982).

Using isolated rat hepatocytes, Schwarz *et al* (1980) found that a rise in the naphthalene concentration of the incubate from 400 to 1200 μM resulted in a two-fold increase in the formation of water-soluble metabolites but a ten-fold increase in irreversible binding to cellular macromolecules. Inhibition of both glucuronide and sulphate conjugation led to increased binding to macromolecules, although the quantity of water-soluble metabolites formed remained the same. It would appear that conjugative capacity may have a very important bearing on the covalent binding of naphthalene.

2.4 Health effects

The principal acute effects of naphthalene in laboratory animals, ophthalmotoxicity and pulmonary necrosis, are quite well studied. However, there are little data on chronic exposure available for this compound.

2.4.1 Acute and subacute toxicity

Oral LD50s of 1.8–2.4 g/kg and 0.5–1.0 g/kg have been reported for the rat and mouse respectively. Intravenous and intraperitoneal LD50s in the mouse range from 100 to 150 mg/kg (Registry of Toxic Effects of Chemical Substances).

There are several reports of the cataractogenic activity of naphthalene in laboratory animals (Gehring 1971). The pathogenesis of the lesion is thought to begin with swelling of the lens cortex, followed by epithelial proliferation and discoloration. The mature cataract is composed of a liquid cortex encapsulated by layers of lens epithelium. One study has reported elevated alkaline phosphatase and lipid peroxidation in the eyes of male albino rats following oral administration of 1 g/kg/day of naphthalene in groundnut oil for 10 days (Rao and Pandya 1981). The mechanism of action of naphthalene in the eye is thought to be due to metabolites, possibly the 1,2- and/or 1,4-naphthoquinones (Van Heyningen and Pirie 1967, Rees and Pirie 1967, Cohen *et al* 1983, Thornalley *et al* 1984, Doherty *et al* 1984). At present, the action of these metabolites in the eye is unclear, although it may involve covalent binding and/or the propagation of active oxygen species by redox cycling.

Rao and Pandya (1981) found a number of hepatic changes in rats dosed orally with 1 g/kg/day of naphthalene for 10 days. Increased liver weight, elevated alkaline phosphatase and aniline hydroxylase activity, and increased lipid peroxidation were observed. Little or no hepatic effects were reported in male Sprague–Dawley rats given 30 mg of naphthalene by intraperitoneal injection. Pretreatment with phenobarbital was not found to significantly influence the lack of hepatotoxicity (Brodie *et al* 1971).

Following up a study by Reid *et al* (1973) in which selective toxicity of naphthalene for the non-ciliated (Clara) cells of the bronchiolar epithelium had been observed, Mahvi *et al* (1977) examined in more detail the pulmonary lesion produced by the injection of 1–2 mmol/kg of naphthalene to C57BL/6J mice. Under the electron microscope the Clara cells appeared to expand and subsequently exfoliate. Abnormalities were also observed in the bronchiolar ciliated cells following exfoliation of the Clara cells. It is unclear, however, whether this was due to a direct effect of the chemical on the ciliated cells, or, in view of the proposed secretory role of the Clara cell, merely a response to the change in the bronchiolar environment. Tong *et al* (1981) also found that naphthalene was selectively toxic to Clara cells in C57BL/6J mice. They further reported significant reductions in several pulmonary microsomal enzyme activities, an effect not reproduced in the liver. Swiss Webster mice given intraperitoneal injections of 300–400 mg/kg of naphthalene also exhibited dose-dependent bronchiolar epithelial necrosis (Warren *et al* 1982). Pretreatment with diethylmaleate (to deplete glutathione) increased the pulmonary toxicity of naphthalene to this strain, whereas prior injection of piperonyl butoxide (a P-450 inhibitor) decreased toxicity. Pretreatment with SKF 525-A (another P-450 inhibitor) had no effect. Studies on the effects of the above pretreatments on the covalent binding of naphthalene in the lung corresponded well with the observed toxic responses. Maximal covalent binding was found to occur before the onset of necrosis. Covalent binding, however, was greater in the liver and kidney than in the lung (Warren *et al* 1982). These experiments would suggest that the selective toxicity of naphthalene to the Clara cell may relate to the cytochrome P-450 and glutathione content of these cells. It has been reported that there is a well-developed mixed-function oxidase system present in the Clara cell but not in other lung cell types. If naphthalene is preferentially metabolised in the lung by the relatively small number of Clara cells, these cells would therefore be exposed to far higher levels of reactive metabolites than would be possible for individual hepatocytes, which all possess a well-developed mixed-function oxidase capability.

No evidence for immunotoxicity was found in CD-1 mice given 27, 53 or 267 mg/kg of naphthalene by gavage for 14 days. Parameters measured were humoral immune response, response to mitogens, delayed hypersensitivity response, popliteal lymph node response, bone marrow stem cell number and DNA synthesis. However, at the high dose there was a decrease in male thymus weight, a decrease in female lung and spleen weights, and depression of body weight gain in both sexes. There were no effects on serum enzymes or electrolytes (Shopp *et al* 1984).

Naphthalene is also an inhibitor of mitochondrial respiration. It has been shown to inhibit oxygen consumption by monkey kidney and human larynx carcinoma cell lines, primary turkey fibroblasts, and isolated cardiac mitochondria (Harmon and Sanborn 1982). It appears to affect both ubiquinone reduction and reduced ubiquinone oxidation (Harmon and Sanborn 1982, Struble and Harmon 1983).

Acute human poisoning with naphthalene is characterised by gastrointestinal and neurological disturbances and toxicity to the eye at very high doses. It has been reported that haemolytic anaemia and nephrotoxicity may follow in some cases (Sandmeyer 1981).

2.4.2 Chronic toxicity

Early studies of repeated exposure to naphthalene found nephritis and haemolytic anaemia in dogs, and cataracts in rabbits and rats (Gerarde 1960).

The only effects observed in CD-1 mice given 5.3, 53 or 133 mg/kg/day of naphthalene for 90 days were decreased spleen weight in females and lowered hepatic aryl hydrocarbon hydroxylase activity in both sexes at the high dose. The other parameters measured were body weight, organ weights, serum enzymes and electrolytes, immunological competence, and several hepatic drug-metabolising enzymes (Shopp *et al* 1984).

In man, dermal and ophthalmological changes have been seen in workers occupationally exposed to naphthalene (Sandmeyer 1981).

2.4.3 Genotoxicity

Bacterial mutagenicity studies of naphthalene have to date all proved negative (Kraemer *et al* 1974, McCann *et al* 1975, Kaden *et al* 1979, Florin *et al* 1980, Mamber *et al* 1983).

2.4.4 Carcinogenicity

Naphthalene has been shown to inhibit the induction of skin tumours by benzo(*a*)-pyrene in female S-D mice and in MRC/H mice (Schmeltz et al 1978, Crabtree 1946).

Naphthalene is currently being tested in a US National Toxicology Program carcinogenesis bioassay.

2.4.5 Reproductive toxicity

Naphthalene has been reported to cross the human placenta and cause neonatal toxicity (Ansiulewicz *et al* 1959).

No evidence for teratogenicity was found in Sprague–Dawley rats given 395 mg/kg of naphthalene by intraperitoneal injection on days 1–15 of gestation (Hardin *et al* 1981). Naphthalene was administered to CD-1 mice at a dose of 300 mg/kg body weight by gavage on days 7–14 of gestation. This was a dose considered to be just below the threshold of adult lethality. There was a significant reduction in live pups per litter (Plasterer *et al* 1985).

2.5 Discussion

Naphthalene is a common micropollutant in drinking water. Its acute toxicity in animals is low, the principal effects at high doses being toxicity to the lung and eye. There are very little data, however, on chronic toxicity, carcinogenicity and reproductive toxicity. This compound does not appear to be mutagenic in bacterial assays, but there are no data in higher test systems.

References

AKIYAMA T, KOGA M, SHINOHARA R, KIDO A and ETOH S (1980) Detection and identification of trace organic substances in the aquatic environment. *Journal of Uoeh* **2**, 285-300.

ANSIULEWICZ J A, DICK H J and CHIARVILI E E (1959) Transplacental naphthalene migration. *American Journal of Obstetrics and Gynecology* **78**, 519-521.

BENOIT F M, LeBEL G L and WILLIAMS D T (1979) Polycyclic aromatic hydrocarbons in Eastern Ontario drinking waters, 1978. *Bulletin of Environmental Contamination and Toxicology* **23**, 774-778.

BOYLAND E, RAMSAY G S and SIMS P (1961) The secretion of metabolites of naphthalene, 1:2-dihydronaphthalene and 1:2-epoxy-1:2:3:4-tetrahydronaphthalene in rat bile. *Biochemical Journal* **78**, 376-384.

BRODIE B B, REID W D, CHO A K, SIPES G, KRISHNA G and GILLETTE J R (1971) Possible mechanism of liver necrosis caused by aromatic organic compounds. *Proceedings of the National Academy of Sciences* **68**, 160-164.

CHEN K-C and DOROUGH H W (1979) Glutathione and mercapturic acid conjugations in the metabolism of naphthalene and 1-naphthyl *N*-methylcarbamate (Carbaryl). *Drug and Chemical Toxicology* **2**, 331-354.

COHEN G M, WILSON G D, GIBBY E M, SMITH M T, DOHERTY M A and CONNORS T A (1983) 1-Naphthol: A potential selective antitumour agent. *Biochemical Pharmacology* **32**, 2363-2365.

CORNER E D S and YOUNG L (1954) The metabolism of naphthalene in animals of different species. *Biochemical Journal* **58**, 647-655.

CRABTREE H G (1946) Some effects of aromatic hydrocarbons on sulfur metabolism and tumor induction in mice. *Cancer Research* **6**, 553-559.

DOHERTY M A, COHEN G M and SMITH M T (1984) Mechanisms of toxic injury to isolated hepatocytes by 1-naphthol. *Biochemical Pharmacology* **33**, 543-549.

FLORIN I, RUTBERG L, CURVALL M and ENZELL C R (1980) Screening of tobacco smoke constituents for mutagenicity using the Ames' test. *Toxicology* **18**, 219-232.

GEHRING P J (1971) The cataractogenic activity of chemical agents. *CRC Critical Reviews in Toxicology* **1**, 93-118.

GERARDE H W (1960) Toxicology and biochemistry of aromatic hydrocarbons. Elsevier Monographs.

HARDIN B D, BOND G P, SIKOV M R, ANDREW F D, BELILES R P and NIEMEIER R W (1981) Testing of selected workplace chemicals for teratogenic potential. *Scandinavian Journal of Work Environment and Health* **7**, Suppl 4, 66-75.

HARMON H J and SANBORN M R (1982) Effect of naphthalene on respiration in heart mitochondria and intact cultured cells. *Environmental Research* **29**, 160-173.

HORNING M G, STILLWELL W G, GRIFFIN G W and TSANG W-S (1980) Epoxide intermediates in the metabolism of naphthalene by the rat. *Drug Metabolism and Disposition* **8**, 404-414.

JERINA D M, DALY J W, WITKOP B, ZALTZMAN-NIRENBERG P and UDENFRIEND S (1970) 1,2-Naphthalene oxide as an intermediate in the microsomal hydroxylation of naphthalene. *Biochemistry* **9**, 147-156.

KADEN D A, HITES R A and THILLY W G (1979) Mutagenicity of soot and associated polycyclic aromatic hydrocarbons to *Salmonella typhimurium*. *Cancer Research* **39**, 4152-4159.

KRAEMER M, BIMBOES D and GREIM H (1974) *S. typhimurium* and *E. coli* to detect chemical mutagens. *Naunyn-Schmiedebergs Archives of Pharmacology* **284**, R46.

MAHVI D, BANK H and HARLEY R (1977) Morphology of a naphthalene-induced bronchiolar lesion. *American Journal of Pathology* **86**, 559-567.

MAMBER S W, BRYSON V and KATZ S E (1983) The *Escherichia coli* WP2/WP100 rec assay for detection of potential chemical carcinogens. *Mutation Research* **119**, 135-144.

McCANN J, CHOI E, YAMASAKI E and AMES B N (1975) Detection of carcinogens or mutagens in the *Salmonella*/microsome test: Assay of 300 chemicals. *Proceedings of the National Academy of Science* **72**, 5135-5139.

OESCH F and DALY J (1972) Conversion of naphthalene to *trans*-naphthalene dihydrodiol: Evidence for the presence of a coupled aryl monooxygenase-epoxide hydrase system in hepatic microsomes. *Biochemical and Biophysical Research Communications* **46**, 1713-1720.

PELLIZZARI E D, HARTWELL T D, HARRIS B S H, WADDELL R D, WHITAKER D A and ERICKSON M D (1982) Purgeable organic compounds in mother's milk. *Bulletin of Environmental Contamination and Toxicology* **28**, 322-328.

PLASTERER M R, BRADSHAW N S, BOOTH G M, SCHULER R L and HARDIN B D (1985) Developmental toxicity of nine selected compounds following prenatal exposure in the mouse: napthalene, *p*-nitrophenol, sodium selenite, dimethylphthalate, ethylenethiourea and four glycol ether derivatives. *Journal of Toxicology and Environmental Health* **15**, 25-38.

PUE M A, FROST G S and HIROM P C (1982) The enterohepatic circulation of a glutathione conjugate of naphthalene in the rat. *Biochemical Society Transactions* **10**, 112.

RAO G S and PANDYA K P (1981) Biochemical changes induced by naphthalene after oral administration in albino rats. *Toxicology Letters* **8**, 311-315.

REES J R and PIRIE A (1967) Possible reactions of 1,2-naphthoquinone in the eye. *Biochemical Journal* **102**, 853-863.

REGISTRY OF TOXIC EFFECTS OF CHEMICAL SUBSTANCES National Institute for Occupational Safety & Health, Cincinnati, Ohio.

REID W D, ILETT K F, GLICK J M and KRISHNA G (1973) Metabolism and binding of aromatic hydrocarbons in the lung: Relationship to experimental bronchiolar necrosis. *American Review of Respiratory Diseases* **107,** 539-551.

SANDMEYER E E (1981) Aromatic hydrocarbons. In: Clayton G D and Clayton F E (eds) *Patty's industrial hygiene and toxicology*, 3rd edn, vol 2B, pp 3333-3343.

SCHMELTZ I, TOSK J and HOFFMANN D (1976) Formation and determination of naphthalenes in cigarette smoke. *Analytical Chemistry* **48**, 645-650.

SCHMELTZ I, TOSK J, HILFRICH J, HIROTA N, HOFFMANN D and WYNDER E L (1978) Bioassays of naphthalene and alkylnaphthalenes for co-carcinogenic activity. Relation to tobacco carcinogenesis. In: Jones P W and Freudenthal R I (eds) *Carcinogenesis, Polynuclear Aromatic Hydrocarbons*, vol 3. New York, Raven Press, pp 47-60.

SCHWARZ L R, MEZGER M and HESSE S (1980) Effect of decreased glucuronidation and sulfation on covalent binding of naphthalene in isolated rat hepatocytes. *Toxicology* **17**, 119-122.

SHOPP G M, WHITE K L Jr, HOLSAPPLE M P, BARNES D W, DUKE S S, ANDERSON A C, CONDIE L W Jr, HAYES J R and BORZELLECA J F (1984) Naphthalene toxicity in CD-1 mice: General toxicology and immunotoxicology. *Fundamental and Applied Toxicology* **4**, 406-419.

STRUBLE V G and HARMON H J (1983) Molecular basis for inhibition of mitochondrial respiration by naphthalene. *Bulletin of Environmental Contamination and Toxicology* **31**, 644-648.

THORNALLEY P J, DOHERTY M A, SMITH M T, BANNISTER J V and COHEN G M (1984) The formation of active oxygen species following activation of 1-naphthol, 1,2- and 1,4-naphthoquinone by rat liver microsomes. *Chemicobiological Interactions* **48**, 195-206.

TONG S S, HIROKATA Y, TRUSH M A, MIMNAUGH E G, GINSBURG E, LOWE M C and GRAM T E (1981) Clara cell damage and inhibition of pulmonary mixed-function oxidase activity by naphthalene. *Biochemical and Biophysical Research Communications* **100**, 944-950.

US ENVIRONMENTAL PROTECTION AGENCY (1980) Ambient water quality criteria for naphthalene. US EPA, EPA-440/5-80-059.

VAN HEYNINGEN R and PIRIE A (1967) The metabolism of naphthalene and its toxic effect on the eye. *Biochemical Journal* **102**, 842-852.

VERSCHUEREN K (1983) *Handbook of environmental data on organic chemicals*. 2nd edn, New York, Van Nostrand Reinhold Company.

WARREN D L, BROWN D L Jr and BUCKPITT A R (1982) Evidence for cytochrome P-450 mediated metabolism in the bronchiolar damage by naphthalene. *Chemicobiological Interactions* **40**, 287-303.

WATER RESEARCH CENTRE (1981) Organic micropollutants in drinking water. WRc Technical Report TR 159.

3. THE ALKYLNAPHTHALENES

3.1 Introduction

Short-chain alkylnaphthalenes are constituents of coal tar, motor exhaust fumes and cigarette smoke. Of this group only the metabolism and acute toxicity of one particular compound, 2-methylnaphthalene, has been studied in any depth.

3.2 Exposure

In the WRc survey, 1-methylnaphthalene and 2-methylnaphthalene were found in all treated water samples and in raw water, six dimethylnaphthalene isomers and one ethylnaphthalene isomer were identified in treated water, and three dimethylnaphthalene isomers were found in raw water (Water Research Centre 1981). Alkylnaphthalenes have also been detected in Canadian drinking water at low ng/l levels (Benoit *et al* 1979) and in a range of Japanese waters (Akiyama *et al* 1980).

Significant levels of alkylnaphthalenes are present in cigarette smoke (Schmeltz *et al* 1976). These compounds have also been detected in food and motor vehicle exhaust fumes.

3.3 Toxicokinetics

There are several studies on the mammalian metabolism of 2-methylnaphthalene, but almost no information for any of the other compounds. It is clear, however, that a parallel may exist with the more widely studied alkylbenzenes in which the small alkyl side-chain renders these compounds amenable to rapid aliphatic hydroxylation. Metabolism by ring oxidation can occur, but is generally of less quantitative significance than side-chain oxidation. The data available for 2-methylnaphthalene would support this.

The early study by Grimes and Young (1956) reported several urinary metabolites of 2-methylnaphthalene in rats, mice, rabbits and guinea-pigs. These included naphthoic acid, the glycine conjugate of naphthoic acid (naphthuric acid), 7-methyl-1-naphthol, 7-methyl-2-naphthol, and 1,2-dihydro-7-methylnaphthalene-1,2-diol.

In guinea-pigs given an oral dose of 10 mg/kg of radiolabelled 2-methylnaphthalene, nearly 80% was excreted as metabolites in the urine while 10% was recovered in the faeces in the first 24 hours. Side-chain oxidation products accounted for 76% of the total urinary radioactivity, whilst glucuronide and sulphate conjugates of 7-methyl-1-naphthol and *S*-(7-methyl-1-naphthyl)cysteine amounted to 18% (Teshima *et al* 1983). In rats, 55% of the total dose from two subcutaneous injections of radiolabelled 2-methylnaphthalene was eliminated in the urine after 3 days. About 3–5% of the urinary radiolabel was found to be unchanged 2-methylnaphthalene, whilst 30–35% was naphthuric acid (Melancon *et al* 1982).

Breger *et al* (1983) identified three isomeric dihydrodiols following incubation of 2-methylnaphthalene with rat liver microsomes. Further work revealed that these were in fact the 3,4-, 5,6- and 7,8-dihydrodiols of 2-methylnaphthalene (Breger *et al* 1983). With both hepatic and pulmonary microsomes from male C57BL/6J mice, Griffin *et al* (1981) detected three dihydrodiol and three mono-hydroxylated metabolites of 2-methylnaphthalene. Kidney microsomes produced only trace quantities of metabolites.

3.4 Health effects

Very little toxicological information is available for these compounds. Two recent studies have looked in some detail at the acute toxicity of 2-methylnaphthalene in mice, but chronic studies are completely lacking.

3.4.1 *Acute and subacute toxicity*

In C57BL/6J mice, a single intraperitoneal dose of 200 mg/kg of 2-methylnaphthalene was found to induce selective necrosis of the bronchiolar epithelium, specifically the non-ciliated (Clara) cells. Toxicity was not seen at lower doses, but at higher doses upper respiratory tract damage was also evident. No effects were observed in the liver or kidney at doses up to 1000 mg/kg (Griffin *et al* 1982). In further studies, pretreatment with the cytochrome P-450 inhibiting agents piperonyl butoxide and SKF 525-A had no effect on toxicity, while pretreatment with the P-450 inducing agents 3-methylcholanthrene and phenobarbital decreased the toxicity of 2-methylnaphthalene (Griffin *et al* 1983). This would suggest that the inducing agents used in this study tended to induce those forms of cytochrome P-450 which detoxify 2-methylnaphthalene in preference to those forms which activate the compound. DBA/2J mice also exhibit pulmonary toxicity following an acute intraperitoneal dose of 200 mg/kg of 2-methylnaphthalene. Again, no toxicity to the liver or kidney was found at doses up to 1000 mg/kg. A dose-dependent increase in covalent binding in the lung, liver and kidney was found at 25-500 mg/kg. Similar levels of irreversible binding (in nmol 2-methylnaphthalene/mg protein) were seen in all three organs. In this strain, pretreatment with cytochrome P-450 inducing agents such as phenobarbital and 3-methylcholanthrene, or inhibitors such as SKF 525-A and piperonyl butoxide, failed to have any effect on toxicity. Phenobarbital pretreatment, however, did result in a doubling of covalent binding in the liver (Griffin *et al* 1983). It has been suggested that pulmonary toxicity may not occur in the rat or hamster (Griffin *et al* 1983).

Fabacher and Hodgson (1977) examined the induction of hepatic mixed function oxidase activities in male mice given 100 mg/kg/day of various akylnaphthalenes by intraperitoneal injection for 3 days. Liver weight/body weight ratio and hepatic *O*-demethylase activity were significantly elevated in the case of one compound, 1,4,6,7-tetramethylnaphthalene, but all the other compounds proved negative.

3.4.2 *Chronic toxicity*

No data appear to be available.

3.4.3 *Genotoxicity*

In the Ames test, 1-methylnaphthalene, 2-methylnaphthalene and 1,4-dimethylnaphthalene were all non-mutagenic to *Salmonella typhimurium* TA98 and TA100. All three compounds were toxic at a concentration of 3 μmol/plate (Florin *et al* 1980). In a forward mutation assay in *Salmonella typhimurium* TM677 where resistance to 8-azaguanine was the genetic marker, 1-methylnaphthalene was weakly mutagenic, while 2,6-dimethylnaphthalene proved negative (Kaden *et al* 1979).

3.4.4 *Carcinogenicity*

Two studies have looked at the effects of alkylnaphthalenes on the induction of carcinogenesis by other PAHs. Schmeltz *et al* (1978) found that most alkylnaphthalenes inhibited the induction of mouse skin tumours by benzo(*a*)pyrene. However, 2,3-dimethyl-, a trimethyl- and tetramethylnaphthalene enhanced the carcinogenicity of benzo(*a*)pyrene. 1,4-Dimethylnaphthalene has been found to inhibit the development of 7,12-dimethylbenz(*a*)anthracene-induced hamster buccal pouch carcinomas (Malament and Shklar 1981).

3.4.5 Reproductive toxicity

No data appear to be available.

3.5 Discussion

Alkylnaphthalenes are ubiquitous micropollutants in drinking water. Other sources of exposure are food and cigarette smoking. Metabolism by the liver is rapid and occurs primarily by oxidation of the aliphatic side-chain. 2-Methylnaphthalene is of relatively low acute toxicity, though at high doses it is selectively toxic to the Clara cells of the lung. No chronic toxicity, carcinogenicity or reproductive toxicity data appear to be available for these compounds.

There are insufficient data for the alkylnaphthalenes on which to base an assessment.

References

AKIYAMA T, KOGA M, SHINOHARA R, KIDO A and ETOH S (1980) Detection and identification of trace organic substances in the aquatic environment. *Journal of Uoeh* **2**, 285-300.

BENOIT F M, LeBEL G L and WILLIAMS D T (1979) Polycyclic aromatic hydrocarbons in Eastern Ontario drinking waters, 1978. *Bulletin of Environmental Contamination and Toxicology* **23**, 774-778.

BREGER R K, FRANKLIN R B and LECH J J (1981) Metabolism of 2-methylnaphthalene to isomeric dihydrodiols by hepatic microsomes of rat and rainbow trout. *Drug Metabolism and Disposition* **9**, 88-93.

BREGER R K, NOVAK R F, FRANKLIN R B, RICKERTS D and LECH J J (1983) Further structural analysis of rat liver microsomal metabolites of 2-methylnaphthalene. *Drug Metabolism and Disposition* **11**, 319-323.

FABACHER D L and HODGSON E (1977) Hepatic mixed-function oxidase activity in mice treated with methylated benzenes and methylated naphthalenes. *Journal of Toxicology and Environmental Health* **2**, 1143-1146.

FLORIN I, RUTBERG L, CURVALL M and ENZELL C R (1980) Screening of tobacco smoke constituents for mutagenicity using the Ames' test. *Toxicology* **18**, 219-232.

GRIFFIN K A, JOHNSON C B, BREGER R K and FRANKLIN R B (1981) Pulmonary toxicity, hepatic, and extrahepatic metabolism of 2-methylnaphthalene in mice. *Toxicology and Applied Pharmacology* **61**, 185-196.

GRIFFIN K A, JOHNSON C B, BREGER R K and FRANKLIN R B (1982) Effect of inducers and inhibitors of cytochrome P-450-linked monooxygenases on the toxicity, *in vitro* metabolism and *in vivo* irreversible binding of 2-methylnaphthalene in mice. *Journal of Pharmacology and Experimental Therapeutics* **221**, 517-524.

GRIFFIN K A, JOHNSON C B, BREGER R K and FRANKLIN R B (1983) Pulmonary toxicity of 2-methylnaphthalene: Lack of a relationship between toxicity, dihydrodiol formation and irreversible binding to cellular macromolecules in DBA/2J mice. *Toxicology* **26**, 213-230.

GRIMES A J and YOUNG L (1956) The metabolism of 2-methylnaphthalene. *Biochemical Journal* **62**, 11p.

KADEN D A, HITES R A and THILLY W G (1979) Mutagenicity of soot and associated polycyclic aromatic hydrocarbons to *Salmonella typhimurium*. *Cancer Research* **39**, 4152-4159.

MALAMENT D S and SHKLAR G (1981) Inhibition of DMBA carcinogenesis of hamster buccal pouch by phenanthrene and dimethylnaphthalene. *Carcinogenesis* **2**, 723-729.

MELANCON M J, RICKERT D E and LECH J J (1982) Metabolism of 2-methylnaphthalene in the rat *in vivo*. *Drug Metabolism and Disposition* **10**, 128-133.

SCHMELTZ I, TOSK J and HOFFMANN D (1976) Formation and determination of naphthalenes in cigarette smoke. *Analytical Chemistry* **48**, 645-650.

SCHMELTZ I, TOSK J, HILFRICH J, HIROTA N, HOFFMANN D and WYNDER E L (1978) Bioassays of naphthalene and alkylnaphthalenes for co-carcinogenic activity. Relation to tobacco carcinogenesis. In: Jones P W and Freudenthal R I (eds) *Carcinogenesis, Polynuclear Aromatic Hydrocarbons* vol 3. New York, Raven Press, pp 47-60.

TESHIMA R, NAGAMATSU K, IKEBUCHI H, KIDO Y and TERAO T (1983) *In vivo* and *in vitro* metabolism of 2-methylnaphthalene in the guinea-pig. *Drug Metabolism and Disposition* **11**, 152-157.

WATER RESEARCH CENTRE (1981) Organic Micropollutants in Drinking Water. WRc Technical Report TR 159.

4. ACENAPHTHENE

4.1 Introduction

Acenaphthene (1,2-dihydroacenaphthylene, 1,8-ethylenenaphthalene, periethylenenaphthalene) is produced from coal-tar distillation, petroleum refinery and shale-oil processing. It is used in the manufacture of insecticides, fungicides, plastics and dyes. Acenaphthene is also a constituent of asphalt and tobacco smoke.

CAS Reg No:	83-32-9
Molecular weight:	154.2
Boiling point:	279°C
Solubility:	No data available
Evaporative half-life in water of depth 1 m:	No data available
Threshold odour concentration in water:	0.02–0.22 mg/l (Verschueren 1983)

4.2 Exposure

Acenaphthene was identified in only 2/14 treated water samples in the WRc survey (Water Research Centre 1981). A Japanese study detected acenaphthene at 200 ng/l in sewage influent, at 10 ng/l in sewage effluent and at 4 ng/l in tap water. It was also identified in sea water and sediment (Akiyama *et al* 1980). In the US, this compound has been detected in effluents from petrochemical, pesticide and wood preservative industries (United States Environmental Protection Agency 1980).

4.3 Toxicokinetics

There is little information on the mammalian metabolism of acenaphthene. Early work by Chang and Young (1943) suggested that cleavage of the aliphatic part of the acenaphthene molecule may be an important step in its metabolism. Naphthalene-1,8-dicarboxylic acid was identified in the urine of rats fed acenaphthene. Chang (1943) reported that 10% of a single oral dose of 200 mg of acenaphthene was eliminated in the faeces of rats, while 6% was eliminated in the same fashion in rats fed 1% acenaphthene in the diet.

4.4 Health effects

Oral LD50s of 10 g/kg in the rat and 2.1 g/kg in the mouse have been reported for acenaphthene (Knobloch *et al* 1969). Gerarde (1960) found that one mouse out of five died after intraperitoneal injection of 500 mg/kg/day of acenaphthene for 7 days. In another study, seven young rats given oral doses of 2 g/kg/day of acenaphthene in olive oil for 32 days showed loss of body weight and mild pathological changes in the liver and kidney (Knobloch *et al* 1969).

Rats exposed by inhalation to 12 mg/m^3 of acenaphthene, 4 hours/day, 6 days/week for 5 months developed toxic effects in the blood, lungs and 'glandular constituents' (Reshetyuk *et al* 1970).

In the earliest mutagenicity study, acenaphthene was found to be toxic to the Ames strains TA1535, TA1537, TA1538 and TA98 at the dose levels tested (200–2000 μg/plate) (Gibson *et al* 1978). More recent studies at non-toxic dose levels indicate that acenaphthene is non-mutagenic in the Ames test and in yeast (Nestmann *et al* 1980, Florin *et al* 1980, Gatehouse 1980, Nestmann and Lee 1983). Acenaphthene did give some evidence for mutagenicity in the presence of S-9 in a forward mutation assay in *Salmonella typhimurium* where resistance to 8-azaguanine was the genetic marker (Krishnan *et al* 1979).

No other toxicological data appear to be available for this compound.

4.5 Discussion

There are insufficient data for acenaphthene on which to base an assessment.

References

AKIYAMA T, KOGA M, SHINOHARA R, KIDO A and ETOH S (1980) Detection and identification of trace organic substances in the aquatic environment. *Journal of Uoeh* **2**, 285-300.

CHANG L H (1943) The fecal excretion of polycyclic hydrocarbons following their administration to the rat. *Journal of Biological Chemistry* **151**, 93-99.

CHANG L H and YOUNG L (1943) Metabolism of acenaphthene in the rat. *Journal of Biological Chemistry* **151**, 87-91.

FLORIN I, RUTBERG L, CURVALL M and ENZELL C R (1980) Screening of tobacco smoke constituents for mutagenicity using the Ames test. *Toxicology* **18**, 219-232.

GATEHOUSE D (1980) Mutagenicity of 1,2 ring-fused acenaphthenes against *S. typhimurium* TA1537 and TA1538: Structure–activity relationships. *Mutation Research* **78**, 121-135.
GERARDE H W (1960) Toxicology and biochemistry of aromatic hydrocarbons. Elsevier Monographs.
GIBSON T L, SMART V B and SMITH L L (1978) Non-enzymatic activation of polycyclic aromatic hydrocarbons as mutagens. *Mutation Research* **49**, 153-161.
KNOBLOCH K *et al* (1969) Acute and subacute toxicity of acenaphthene and acenaphthylene. *Medyayna Pracy* **20**, 210.
KRISHNAN S, KADEN D A, THILLY W G and HITES R A (1979) Cyanoarenes in soot: Synthesis and mutagenicity of cyanonaphthylenes. *Environmental Science and Technology* **13**, 1532-1534.
NESTMANN E R and LEE E G-H (1983) Mutagenicity of constituents of pulp and paper mill effluent in growing cells of *Saccharomyces cerevisiae*. *Mutation Research* **119**, 273-280.
NESTMANN E R, LEE E G-H, MATULA T I, DOUGLAS G R and MUELLER J C (1980) Mutagenicity of constituents identified in pulp and paper mill effluents using the *Salmonella*/microsome assay. *Mutation Research* **79**, 203-212.
RESHETYUK A L *et al* (1970) Toxicological evaluation of acenaphthene and acenaphthylene. *Gigiena Truda i Professional'nykh Zabolevanii* **14**, 46.
US ENVIRONMENTAL PROTECTION AGENCY (1980) Ambient water quality criteria for acenaphthene. US EPA, EPA-440/5-80-015.
VERSCHUEREN K (1983) *Handbook of environmental data on organic chemicals*. 2nd edn. New York, Van Nostrand Reinhold Company.
WATER RESEARCH CENTRE (1981) Organic micropollutants in drinking water. WRc Technical Report TR 159.

5. FLUORANTHENE

5.1 Introduction

Fluoranthene (idryl, 1,2-(1,8-naphthylene)benzene, benzo[*j*, *k*]fluorene) is a constituent of coal tar and a common environmental pollutant. There is no known commercial production or use of this compound.

CAS Reg No:	206-44-0
Molecular weight:	202.3
Boiling point:	250°C
Solubility:	265 μg/l at 25°C (Verschueren 1983)
Evaporative half-life in water:	No data available
Threshold odour concentration in water:	No data available

5.2 Exposure

5.2.1 Air

Fluoranthene concentrations in ambient air generally range from 0.1 to 20 $\mu g/m^3$ (Santodonato *et al* 1981). This compound has also been detected in cigarette smoke.

5.2.2 Food

A UK survey of fluoranthene in foodstuffs has indicated that, assuming a total daily food consumption of 1.46 kg, average intake of fluoranthene would be around 1 μg/day. Beverages were suggested to account for only 1% of this value (Dennis *et al* 1983).

5.2.3 Water

Fluoranthene has been identified in raw and treated water samples on many occasions (Sorrell *et al* 1980). In river waters, typical fluoranthene concentrations range from 40 to 300 ng/l, though water treatment appears to lower concentrations to below 12 ng/l (Water Research Centre 1981a). However, levels of 200-400 ng/l have been found in some drinking waters. In these cases, the source of fluoranthene is thought to be the coal-tar lining commonly applied to cast-iron mains (Water Research Centre 1981a).

In the WRc survey (Water Research Centre 1981b), fluoranthene was identified in only one of 14 drinking water samples tested.

5.3 Toxicokinetics

The only information available is from a study by La Voie *et al* (1982) in which the 2,3-dihydrodiol metabolite of fluoranthene was identified after incubation with rat liver microsomes.

5.4 Health effects

The limited toxicological data for fluoranthene have been reviewed by the US EPA (1978) and by the IARC (1983).

5.4.1 Acute and subacute toxicity

An oral LD50 of 2000 mg/kg has been reported for the rat. An LD50 of 3180 mg/kg by skin application in the rabbit and an intravenous LD50 of 100 mg/kg in the mouse have also been documented (Registry of Toxic Effects of Chemical Substances).

5.4.2 Chronic toxicity

No data appear to be available.

5.4.3 Genotoxicity

Both Gatehouse (1980) and Florin *et al* (1980) reported that fluoranthene was non-mutagenic in the Ames test using a plate incorporation method. In the same test system, however, La Voie *et al* (1982) found that fluoranthene was mutagenic to *Salmonella typhimurium* TA100 in the presence of S-9. The 2,3-dihydrodiol metabolite identified by this group was also found to be mutagenic. Fluoranthene has consistently given positive results for mutagenicity in bacterial assays in which the test organisms are incubated with the compound and a drug-metabolising enzyme system in a liquid medium. Two studies reported that fluoranthene was mutagenic to *Salmonella typhimurium* TA98 and TA100 in the fluctuation test (Mossanda *et al* 1979, Kinae *et al* 1979) while other studies in modified plate assays showed fluoranthene to be mutagenic to strains TA98 and TA100 (Bos *et al* 1987) and TA97,

TA98 and TA100 (Sakai *et al* 1985). Kaden *et al* 1979 also found that this compound was mutagenic in a forward mutation assay in *Salmonella typhimurium* TM677 where resistance to 8-azaguanine was the genetic marker. On an equimolar basis, fluoranthene exhibited greater mutagenic activity than benzo(*a*)pyrene in this assay.

Fluoranthene has also given positive results for mutagenicity in a human lymphoblastoid cell line (Thilly *et al* 1980).

Babson *et al* (1986) suggested that a major metabolic activation pathway of fluoranthene resulting in the production of mutagenic species involved the formation of the fluoranthene 2,3-diol, and the subsequent oxidation of this diol to fluoranthene 2,3-diol-1-10b-epoxide. However, Palitta *et al* (1986) showed that fluoranthene metabolism *in vivo* appeared to differ from that *in vitro* and did not produce sister chromatid exchanges in mouse bone marrow.

5.4.4 *Carcinogenicity*

Skin painting of mice, thrice weekly, for lifetime with a 0.1% solution of fluoranthene in acetone was not found to produce skin tumours (Wynder and Hoffmann 1959). In a later mouse study, thrice weekly skin treatment with a 1% solution of fluoranthene in acetone for 1 year also gave negative results (Hoffman *et al* 1972). Application of 10 doses of 0.1 mg of fluoranthene in acetone on alternate days to the shaved backs of 30 mice followed by thrice weekly painting with a 2.5% solution of croton oil for 20 weeks induced a single skin tumour in one mouse. A single skin tumour was also noted in a similarly treated vehicle control group (Hoffman *et al* 1972). A skin painting study in mice in which 50 mg of fluoranthene was applied in either decalin or a 1 : 1 mixture of decalin : *n*-dodecane for 82 weeks again did not produce tumours (Horton and Christian 1974).

Application of 40 μg of fluoranthene to the backs of mice, three times/week for 440 days did not produce skin tumours, but co-administration with 5 μg of benzo(*a*)-pyrene led to an enhancement of the number of skin tumours produced by benzo(*a*)pyrene alone. Fluoranthene also decreased the time to the first appearance of tumours (Van Duuren and Goldschmidt 1976). An earlier study also suggested co-carcinogenic activity for this compound (Hoffmann and Wynder 1963).

Some evidence for carcinogenicity of fluoranthene has been found in the mouse lung adenoma bioassay (Busby *et al* 1984). Newborn Swiss–Webster mice were given 1/7 of the total dose of fluoranthene by intraperitoneal injection on day 1, followed by 2/7 of the dose on day 8, and 4/7 of the dose on day 15. At 24 weeks of age the animals were sacrificed and the lungs examined for gross and microscopic evidence for tumours. A total dose of 3.5 mg/mouse of fluoranthene was found to elevate the total incidence and number of lung tumours. No increased tumour incidence was found with a total dose of 700 μg/mouse. The significance of this assay in relation to environmental exposure is unclear.

5.4.5 *Reproductive toxicity*

No data appear to be available.

5.5 Discussion

There are insufficient data for fluoranthene on which to base an assessment.

References

BABSON J R, RUSSO-RODRIGUEZ S E, WATTLEY R V, BERTSTEIN P L, RASTETTER W H, LIBER H L, ANDON B M, THILLY W G and WOGAN G N (1986) Microsomal activation of fluoranthene to mutagenic metabolites. *Toxicology and Applied Pharmacology* **85**, 355-366.

BOS R P, PRINSEN W J C, van ROOY J G M, JONGENEELEN F J, THEUWS J L G and HENDERSON P Th (1987) Fluoranthene, a volatile mutagenic compound present in creosote and coal tar. *Mutation Research* **187**, 119-125.

BUSBY W F Jr, GOLDMAN M E, NEWBERNE P M and WOGAN G N (1984) Tumorigenicity of fluoranthene in a newborn mouse lung adenoma bioassay. *Carcinogenesis* **5**, 1311-1316.

DENNIS M J, MASSEY R C, McWEENY D J, KNOWLES M E and WATSON D (1983) Analysis of polycyclic aromatic hydrocarbons in UK total diets. *Food and Chemical Toxicology* **21**, 569-574.

FLORIN I, RUTBERG L, CURVALL M and ENZELL C R (1980) Screening of tobacco smoke constituents for mutagenicity using the Ames test. *Toxicology* **18**, 219-232.

GATEHOUSE D (1980) Mutagenicity of 1,2 ring-fused acenaphthenes against *S. typhimurium* TA1537 and TA1538: Structure–activity relationships. *Mutation Research* **78**, 121-135.

HOFFMANN D and WYNDER E L (1963) Studies on gasoline engine exhaust. *Journal of the Air Pollution Control Association* **13**, 322-327.

HOFFMANN D, RATHKAMP F, NESNOW S and WYNDER E L (1972) Fluoranthenes: Quantitative determination in cigarette smoke, formation by pyrolysis, and tumor-initiating activity. *Journal of the National Cancer Institute* **49**, 1165-1175.

HORTON A W and CHRISTIAN G M (1974) Cocarcinogenic versus incomplete carcinogenic activity among aromatic hydrocarbons: Contrast between chrysene and benzo[*b*]triphenylene. *Journal of the National Cancer Institute* **53**, 1017-1020.

INTERNATIONAL AGENCY FOR RESEARCH ON CANCER (1983) IARC monographs on the evaluation of the carcinogenic risk of chemicals to humans, vol 32. Polynuclear aromatic compounds. Part 1. Chemical, environmental and experimental data. Lyon, France, IARC.

KADEN D A, HITES R A and THILLY W G (1979) Mutagenicity of soot and associated polycyclic aromatic hydrocarbons to *Salmonella typhimurium*. *Cancer Research* **39**, 4152-4159.

KINAE N, HASHIZUME T, MAKITA T, TOMITA I, KIMURA I and KANAMORI H (1979) Studies on the toxicity of pulp and paper mill effluents – I. Mutagenicity of the sediment samples derived from kraft paper mills. *Water Research* **15**, 17-24.

La VOIE E J, HECHT S S, BEDENKO V and HOFFMANN D (1982) Identification of the mutagenic metabolites of fluoranthene, 2-methylfluoranthene, and 3-methylfluoranthene. *Carcinogenesis* **3**, 841-846.

MOSSANDA K, PONCELET F, FOUASSIN A and MERCIER M (1979) Detection of mutagenic polycyclic aromatic hydrocarbons in African smoked fish. *Food and Cosmetics Toxicology* **17**, 141-143.

PALITTA F, COZZI R, FIORE M, PALOMBO F, POLCARO C, PEREX G and POSSAGNO E (1986) An *in vitro* and *in vivo* study on mutagenic activity of fluoranthene: comparison between cytogenetic studies and HPLC analysis. *Mutation Research* **174**, 125-130.

REGISTRY OF TOXIC EFFECTS OF CHEMICAL SUBSTANCES National Institute for Occupational Safety and Health, Cincinnati, Ohio.

SAKAI M, YOSHIDA D and MIZUSAKI S (1985) Mutagenicity of polycyclic aromatic hydrocarbons and quinones on *Salmonella typhimurium* TA97. *Mutation Research* **156**, 61-67.

SANTODONATO J, HOWARD P and BASU D (1981) Health and ecological assessment of polynuclear aromatic hydrocarbons. *Journal of Environmental Pathology and Toxicology* **5**, 108-109.

SORRELL R K, BRASS H J and REDING R (1980) A review of occurrences and treatment of polynuclear aromatic hydrocarbons in water. *Environment International* **4**, 245-254.

THILLY W G, DeLUCA J G, FURTH E E, HOPPE H, KADEN D A, KROLEWSKI J J, LIBER H L, SKOPEK T R, SLAPIKOFF S A, TIZARD R J and PENMAN B W (1980) Gene-locus mutation assays in diploid human lymphoblast lines. In: De Serres F J and Hollaender A (eds) *Chemical Mutagens. Principles and Methods for their Detection*, vol 6. New York, Plenum Press, pp 331-364.

US ENVIRONMENTAL PROTECTION AGENCY (1978) Ambient water quality criteria: Fluoranthene. US EPA, PB-292 433.

VAN DUUREN B L and GOLDSCHMIDT B M (1976) Carcinogenic and tumor-promoting agents in tobacco carcinogenesis. *Journal of the National Cancer Institute* **56**, 1237-1242.

VERSCHUEREN K (1983) *Handbook of environmental data on organic chemicals*. 2nd edn. New York, Van Nostrand Reinhold Company.

WATER RESEARCH CENTRE (1981a) A survey of polycyclic aromatic hydrocarbons levels in British waters. WRc Technical Report TR 158.

WATER RESEARCH CENTRE (1981b) Organic micropollutants in drinking water. WRc Technical Report TR 159.

WYNDER E L and HOFFMANN D (1959) A study of tobacco carcinogenesis VII. *Cancer* **12**, 1079-1086.

6. FLUORENE

6.1 Introduction

Fluorene (2,2′-methylenebiphenyl, *ortho*-biphenylenemethane, diphenylenemethane) is a constituent of coal tar. There is no known commercial production or use of this compound.

CAS Reg No:	86-73-7
Molecular weight:	166.2
Boiling point:	293°C

Solubility:	1.9 mg/l at 25°C (Verschueren 1983)
Evaporative half-life in water of depth 1 m:	No data available
Threshold odour concentration in water:	No data available

6.2 Exposure

This compound appears to be regularly present in drinking water samples, though at low ng/l levels (Akiyama *et a*l 1980, Benoit *et al* 1979). The WRc survey identified fluorene in raw water and in 2/14 samples of treated water (Water Research Centre 1981).

There are reports of the presence of fluorene in food and in cigarette smoke (Lo and Sandi 1978).

6.3 Toxicokinetics

Neish (1948) isolated two metabolites from the urine of rabbits dosed with fluorene; these were 2-hydroxyfluorene and its glucuronide conjugate. Incubation of fluorene with rat liver microsomes has been found to produce 1-hydroxyfluorene, 9-hydroxyfluorene and 9-ketofluorene (La Voie *et al* 1981a).

6.4 Health effects

There is very little information in the literature on the toxicology of fluorene.

6.4.1 Acute and subacute toxicity

No data appear to be available.

6.4.2 Chronic toxicity

Wilson *et al* (1947) fed groups of rats with diets containing 0.062–1.0% fluorene for 104 days. Depression of body weight gain, elevated liver weight and lowered spleen weight were found at the higher dose levels. No treatment-related effects were observed in groups of rats fed 0.125, 0.25 and 0.5% fluorene in the diet for 453 days.

6.4.3 Genotoxicity

Fluorene has been found to be non-mutagenic in bacterial systems (McCann *et al* 1975, Kaden *et al* 1979, La Voie *et al* 1981b, Hermann 1981, Mamber *et al* 1983).

Negative results for unscheduled DNA synthesis have been reported in primary cultures of rat hepatocytes (Probst *et al* 1981).

6.4.4 Carcinogenicity

A small study of female rats fed diets containing 0.05% fluorene for 18 months did not produce a significant increase in tumours compared to a control group (Morris *et al* 1960).

Fluorene also gave negative results for tumour initiation in Swiss Ha/ICR mice in which a 0.1% solution in acetone was applied to the skin ten times on alternate days.

After fluorene dosing, the animals were treated thrice weekly with 2.5 μg of the tumour promoter tetradecanoyl phorbol acetate in acetone for 20 weeks (La Voie *et al* 1980).

6.4.5 Reproductive toxicity

No data appear to be available.

6.5 Discussion

There are insufficient data for fluorene on which to base an assessment.

References

AKIYAMA T, KOGA M, SHINOHARA R, KIDO A and ETOH S (1980) Detection and identification of trace organic substances in the aquatic environment. *Journal of Uoeh* **2**, 285-300.

BENOIT F M, LEBEL G L and WILLIAMS D T (1979) Polycyclic aromatic hydrocarbons in Eastern Ontario drinking waters, 1978. *Bulletin of Environmental Contamination and Toxicology* **23**, 774-778.

HERMANN M (1981) Synergistic effects of individual polycyclic aromatic hydrocarbons on the mutagenicity of their mixtures. *Mutation Research* **90**, 399-409.

KADEN D A, HITES R A and THILLY W G (1979) Mutagenicity of soot and associated polycyclic aromatic hydrocarbons to *Salmonella typhimurium*. *Cancer Research* **39**, 4152-4159.

La VOIE E, TULLEY L, BEDENKO V and HOFFMANN D (1980) Mutagenicity, tumor initiating activity, and metabolism of tricyclic polynuclear aromatic hydrocarbons. In: Bjorseth A and Dennis A J (eds) *Polynuclear aromatic hydrocarbons. Chemistry and biological effects*. Columbus, Ohio, Batelle Press, pp 1041-1057.

La VOIE E J, THULLEY-FREILER L, BEDENKO V, GIRACH Z and HOFFMANN D (1981a) Comparative studies on the tumor-initiating activity and metabolism of methylfluorenes and methylbenzofluorenes. In: Cooke M and Dennis A J (eds) *Polynuclear aromatic hydrocarbons: Chemical analysis and biological fate*. 5th Int Symposium. Columbus, Ohio, Batelle Press, pp 417-427.

La VOIE E J, TULLEY L, BEDENKO V and HOFFMANN D (1981b) Mutagenicity of methylated fluorenes and benzofluorenes. *Mutation Research* **91**, 167-176.

LO M-T and SANDI E (1978) Polycyclic aromatic hydrocarbons (polynuclears) in foods. *Residue Reviews* **69**, 35.

MAMBER S W, BRYSON V and KATZ S E (1983) The *Escherichia coli* WP2/WP100 rec assay for detection of potential chemical carcinogens. *Mutation Research* **119**, 135-144.

McCANN J, CHOI E, YAMASAKI E and AMES B N (1975) Detection of carcinogens as mutagens in the *Salmonella*/microsome test: Assay of 300 chemicals. *Proceedings of the National Academy of Science* **72**, 5135-5139.

MORRIS H P, VELAT C A, WAGNER B P, DAHLGARD M and RAY F E (1960) Studies of carcinogenicity in the rat of derivatives of aromatic amines related to *N*-2-fluorenyl- acetamide. *Journal of the National Cancer Institute* **24**, 149 180.

NEISH W J P (1948) Metabolism of fluorene in the rabbit. *Biochemical Journal* **43**, 533-537.
PROBST G S, McMAHON R E, HILL L E, THOMPSON C Z, EPP J K and NEAL S B (1981) Chemically-induced unscheduled DNA synthesis in primary rat hepatocyte cultures. A comparison with bacterial mutagenicity using 218 compounds. *Environmental Mutagenesis* **3**, 11-32.
VERSCHUEREN K (1983) *Handbook of environmental data on organic chemicals.* 2nd edn. New York, Van Nostrand Reinhold Company.
WATER RESEARCH CENTRE (1981) Organic micropollutants in drinking water. WRc Technical Report TR 159.
WILSON R H, De EDS F and COX A J Jr (1947) The carcinogenic activity of 2-acetaminofluorene. *Cancer Research* **7**, 453-458.

7. THE METHYL FLUORENES

Three unspecified methylfluorene isomers were detected in the WRc survey, though they were found to occur somewhat infrequently (Water Research Centre 1981). Akiyama *et al* (1980) have identified a methylfluorene isomer in Japanese drinking water.

The only other information which could be found for these compounds is a study of their mutagenic potential in the Ames test (La Voie *et al* 1981). All the compounds tested (1-, 2-, 3-, 4- and 9-methylfluorene) proved non-mutagenic in *Salmonella typhimurium* TA98 and TA100 in the absence of metabolic activation. In the presence of S-9, the compounds were again negative, with the exception of 9-methylfluorene, which was mutagenic to both TA98 and TA100.

9-Methylfluorene was negative in the Swiss Ha/ICR mice tumour initiation test (La Voie *et al* 1980).

References

AKIYAMA T, KOGA M, SHINOHARA R, KIDO A and ETOH S (1980) Detection and identification of trace organic substances in the aquatic environment. *Journal of Uoeh* **2**, 285-300.
La VOIE E, TULLEY L, BEDENKO V and HOFFMANN D (1980) Mutagenicity, tumor initiating activity, and metabolism of tricyclic polynuclear aromatic hydrocarbons. In: Bjorseth A and Dennis A J (eds) *Polynuclear aromatic hydrocarbons. Chemistry and biological effects.* Columbus, Ohio, Batelle Press, pp 1041-1057.
La VOIE E J, TULLEY L, BEDENKO V and HOFFMANN D (1981) Mutagenicity of methylated fluorenes and benzofluorenes. *Mutation Research* **91**, 167-176.
WATER RESEARCH CENTRE (1981) Organic micropollutants in drinking water. WRc Technical Report TR 159.

8. PHENANTHRENE

8.1 Introduction

Phenanthrene is a constituent of coal tar and can be isolated from several types of crude petroleum. There is no known commercial production or use of this compound.

CAS Reg No:	85-01-8
Molecular weight:	178.2
Boiling point:	340°C
Solubility:	1.6 mg/l at 15°C (Verschueren 1983)
Evaporative half-life in water of depth 1 m:	No data available
Threshold odour concentration in water:	1 mg/l (Verschueren 1983)

8.2 Exposure

Little information exists on the environmental occurrence of phenanthrene. In the WRc survey, this compound was identified in raw water and in 7/14 samples of treated water (Water Research Centre 1981). Phenanthrene (in combination with anthracene) has also been detected in a range of Japanese waters (Akiyama *et al* 1980) and in Canadian drinking water (Benoit *et al* 1979).

Phenanthrene has been identified in some foods and in cigarette smoke (Lo and Sandi 1978).

8.3 Toxicokinetics

In mammals, this PAH is rapidly metabolised by the liver and excreted primarily in the urine. Boyland and Wolf (1950) suggested that epoxides were intermediates of phenanthrene metabolism when they identified 9,10-dihydroxy-9,10-dihydrophenanthrene and 1,2-dihydroxy-1,2-dihydrophenanthrene in the urine of rats and rabbits. Boyland and Sims (1965) later demonstrated that 9,10-epoxy-9,10-dihydrophenanthrene was converted by rats to the dihyroxydihydrophenanthrene. Other studies have also identified 3,4-dihydroxy-3,4-dihydrophenanthrene, a series of monohydroxylated and dihydroxylated compounds and their corresponding sulphate, glucuronide, glutathione and glycine conjugates as urinary metabolites of phenanthrene (Sims 1962, Boyland and Sims 1962a, b). It appears that in the rat and rabbit the major metabolites are derived from the 9,10- and 1,2-epoxides, with only small quantities of the 3,4-epoxide being formed. *In vitro* metabolic studies using rat liver microsomes correlate well with the findings *in vivo* (Sims 1970, Chaturapit and Holder 1978).

8.4 Health effects

There are very little data on the toxicology of this compound. Phenanthrene is known to be a human skin photosensitiser and mild allergen (Sandmeyer 1981).

8.4.1 Acute and subacute toxicity

An oral LD50 of 700 mg/kg and an intravenous LD50 of 56 mg/kg have been reported for this compound in the mouse (Registry of Toxic Effects of Chemical Substances).

Male Sprague–Dawley rats treated with a single intra-peritoneal injection of

150 mg/kg phenanthrene in DMSO showed a significant elevation of serum aspartate aminotransferase and gamma-glutamyl transpeptidase after 24 hours, but levels had returned to normal after 72 hours (Yoshikawa *et al* 1985).

8.4.2 Chronic toxicity

No data appear to be available.

8.4.3 Genotoxicity

Although most bacterial studies have indicated that phenanthrene is non-mutagenic (McCann *et al* 1975, Kaden *et al* 1979, Rosenkranz and Poirier 1979, Florin *et al* 1980, La Voie *et al* 1981), some positive results have been obtained under specialised conditions (Bucker *et al* 1979, Oesch *et al* 1981). Bucker *et al* (1979) found that phenanthrene was non-mutagenic to *Salmonella typhimurium* TA98, TA100, TA1535, TA1537 and TA1538 in the presence of mouse liver microsomes and an NADPH-generating system. However, when the compound was tested in the presence of an epoxide hydrolase inhibitor (1,1,1-trichloropropene-2,3-oxide) a dose-related mutagenic response was seen in TA1537 and a weaker response in TA98. A later study by the same group found similar results using rat liver S-9, and also showed that phenanthrene is mutagenic to TA100 when larger than normal quantities of rat liver S-9 are employed. Addition of reduced glutathione tended to lower activity, whereas the presence of adenosine-3′-phosphate-5′-sulphate phosphate (PAPS) enhanced activity nearly three fold (Oesch *et al* 1981).

Phenanthrene has not been found to mutate (Huberman and Sachs 1976) or transform mammalian cells (Kakunaga 1973, Mondal *et al* 1976, Pienta *et al* 1977) and is at best a very weak inducer of sister chromatid exchanges (Roszinsky-Kocher *et al* 1979, Abe and Sasaki 1977, Bayer and Bauknecht 1977, Popescu *et al* 1977). It has also been reported not to induce unscheduled DNA synthesis in primary cultures of rat hepatocytes (Probst *et al* 1981), or chromosome aberrations in a Chinese hamster lung cell line (Matsuoka *et al* 1979).

8.4.4 Carcinogenicity

There is some evidence that phenanthrene may be a weak initiating agent in mouse skin. Scribner (1973) applied phenanthrene (10 μmol in benzene) to the shaved backs of 8-week-old female CD-1 mice. One week later the animals began twice-weekly treatment with 5 μmol of the tumour promoter 12-*O*-tetradecanoyl-phorbol-13- acetate (TPA) for a period of 35 weeks. Although this treatment protocol was found to induce skin papillomas, interpretation must be cautious in view of the use of benzene as the solvent. Wood *et al* (1979) gave a single application of 10 μmol of phenanthrene in acetone to a group of 30 CD-1 mice. The animals were then treated twice weekly with 16 nmol of TPA in acetone for 35 weeks. Skin papillomas were seen in 5/30 mice of the test group and in 2/30 mice of a vehicle control group. A study by Salaman and Roe (1956) gave equivocal results for tumour initiation in mouse skin. The mice were given 10 applications of 0.3 ml of an 18% solution of phenanthrene in acetone (3 treatments per week) followed by prolonged treatment with croton oil as a promoter.

Short-term subcutaneous or intramuscular dosing studies followed by prolonged observation have failed to provide evidence for tumourigenicity of phenanthrene (Steiner 1955, Roe 1962, Grant and Roe 1963, Buening *et al* 1979).

Phenanthrene has been reported to inhibit the induction of mouse skin tumours by benzo(*a*)pyrene, 1,2,5,6-dibenzanthracene and 7,12-dimethylbenz(*a*)anthracene (Crabtree 1946, Huh and McCarter 1960), and to inhibit the development of 7,12-dimethylbenz(*a*)anthracene-induced hamster buccal pouch carcinomas (Malament and Shklar 1981).

8.4.5 Reproductive toxicity
No data appear to be available.

8.5 Discussion
Phenanthrene is a quite common organic micropollutant in drinking water. Its metabolism in the rabbit and rat have been well studied. The major metabolites are derived from the 9,10- and 1,2-epoxides.

Very little toxicological information is available on phenanthrene, though it is mutagenic in bacterial systems under specialised conditions. Genotoxicity tests in higher test systems have generally proved negative. Equivocal results for tumour initiation have been obtained with skin painting studies in mice.

There are insufficient data for this compound on which to base an assessment.

References

ABE S and SASAKI M (1977) Chromosome aberrations and sister chromatid exchanges in Chinese hamster cells exposed to various chemicals. *Journal of the National Cancer Institute* **58**, 1635-1640.

AKIYAMA T, KOGA M, SHINOHARA R, KIDO A and ETOH S (1980) Detection and identification of trace organic substances in the aquatic environment. *Journal of Uoeh* **2**, 285-300.

BAYER U and BAUKNECHT T (1977) The dose-dependence of sister-chromatid exchanges induced by 3 hydrocarbons, in the *in vivo* bone marrow test with Chinese hamsters. *Experientia* **33**, 25.

BENOIT F M, LEBEL G L and WILLIAMS D T (1979) Polycyclic aromatic hydrocarbons in Eastern Ontario drinking waters, 1978. *Bulletin of Environmental Contamination and Toxicology* **23**, 774-778.

BOYLAND E and SIMS P (1962a) The metabolism of phenanthrene in rabbits and rats: Mercapturic acids and related compounds. *Biochemical Journal* **84**, 564-570.

BOYLAND E and SIMS P (1962b) The metabolism of phenanthrene in rabbits and rats: Dihydrodihydroxy compounds and related glucosiduronic acids. *Biochemical Journal* **84**, 571-582.

BOYLAND E and SIMS P (1965) The metabolism of 9,10-epoxy-9,10-dihydrophenanthrene in rats. *Biochemical Journal* **95**, 788-792.

BOYLAND E and WOLF G (1950) Conversion of phenanthrene into dihydroxydihydrophenanthrenes. *Biochemical Journal* **47**, 64-69.

BUCKER M, GLATT H R, KLATT K L, AVNIR D, ITTAH Y, BLUM J and OESCH F (1979) Mutagenicity of phenanthrene and phenanthrene K-region derivatives. *Mutation Research* **66**, 337-348.

BUENING M K, LEVIN W, KARLE J M, YAGI H, JERINA D M and CONNEY A H (1979) Tumorigenicity of bay-region epoxides and other derivatives of chrysene and phenanthrene in newborn mice. *Cancer Research* **39**, 5063-5068.

CHATURAPIT S and HOLDER G M (1978) Studies on the hepatic microsomal metabolism of [^{14}C]phenanthrene. *Biochemical Pharmacology* **27**, 1865-1871.

CRABTREE H G (1946) Some effects of aromatic hydrocarbons on sulfur metabolism of tumor induction in mice. *Cancer Research* **6**, 553-559.

FLORIN I, RUTBERG L, CURVALL M and ENZELL C R (1980) Screening of tobacco smoke constituents for mutagenicity using the Ames test. *Toxicology* **18**, 219-232.

GRANT G and ROE F J C (1963) The effect of phenanthrene on tumour induction by 3,4-benzopyrene administered to newly born mice. *British Journal of Cancer* **17**, 261-265.

HUBERMAN E and SACHS L (1976) Mutability of different genetic loci in mammalian cells by metabolically activated carcinogenic polycyclic hydrocarbons. *Proceedings of the National Academy of Science* **73**, 188-192.

HUH T Y and McCARTER J A (1960) Phenanthrene as an anti-initiating agent. *British Journal of Cancer* **14**, 591-595.

KADEN D A, HITES R A and THILLY W G (1979) Mutagenicity of soot and associated polycyclic aromatic hydrocarbons to *Salmonella typhimurium*. *Cancer Research* **39**, 4152-4159.

KAKUNAGA T (1973) A quantitative system for assay of malignant transformation by chemical carcinogens using a clone derived from Balb/3T3. *International Journal of Cancer* **12**, 463-473.

La VOIE E J, TULLEY-FREILER L, BEDENKO V and HOFFMANN D (1981) Mutagenicity, tumor-initiating activity, and metabolism of methylphenanthrenes. *Cancer Research* **41**, 3441-3447.

LO M-T and SANDI E (1978) Polycyclic aromatic hydrocarbons (polynuclears) in foods. *Residue Reviews* **69**, 35.

MALAMENT D S and SHKLAR G (1981) Inhibition of DMBA carcinogenesis of hamster buccal pouch by phenanthrene and dimethylnaphthalene. *Carcinogenesis* **2**, 723-729.

MATSUOKA A, HAYASHI M and ISHIDATE M Jr (1979) Chromosomal aberration tests on 29 chemicals combined with S9 mix *in vitro*. *Mutation Research* **66**, 277-290.

McCANN J, CHOI E, YAMASAKI E and AMES B N (1975) Detection of carcinogens as mutagens in the *Salmonella*/microsome test: Assay of 300 chemicals. *Proceedings of the National Academy of Science* **72**, 5135-5139.

MONDAL S, BRANKOW D W and HEIDELBERGER C (1976) Two-stage chemical oncogenesis in cultures of C3H/10T1/2 cells. *Cancer Research* **36**, 2254-2260.

OESCH F, BUCKER M and GLATT H R (1981) Activation of phenanthrene to mutagenic metabolites and evidence for at least two different activation pathways. *Mutation Research* **81**, 1-10.

PIENTA R J, POILEY J A and LEBHERZ W B III (1977) Morphological transformation of early passage golden Syrian hamster embryo cells derived from cryopreserved primary cultures as a reliable *in vitro* bioassay for identifying diverse carcinogens. *International Journal of Cancer* **19**, 642-655.

POPESCU N C, TURNBULL D and DiPAOLO J A (1977) Sister chromatid exchange and chromosome aberration analysis with the use of several carcinogens and non-carcinogens. *Journal of the National Cancer Institute* **59**, 289-292.

PROBST G S, McMAHON R E, HILL L E, THOMPSON C Z, EPP J K and NEAL S B (1981) Chemically-induced unscheduled DNA synthesis in primary rat hepatocyte cultures: A comparison with bacterial mutagenicity using 218 compounds. *Environmental Mutagenesis* **1**, 11-32.

REGISTRY OF TOXIC EFFECTS OF CHEMICAL SUBSTANCES National Institute for Occupational Safety and Health, Cincinnati, Ohio.

ROE F J C (1962) Effect of phenanthrene on tumour-initiation by 3,4-benzopyrene. *British Journal of Cancer* **16**, 503-506.

ROSENKRANZ H S and POIRIER L A (1979) Evaluation of the mutagenicity and DNA-modifying activity of carcinogens and noncarcinogens in microbial systems. *Journal of the National Cancer Institute* **62**, 873-892.

ROSZINSKY-KOCHER G, BASLER A and ROHRBORN G (1979) Mutagenicity of polycyclic hydrocarbons. V. Induction of sister-chromatid exchanges *in vivo*. *Mutation Research* **66**, 65-67.

SALAMAN M H and ROE F J C (1956) Further tests for tumour-initiating activity: *N,N*-di-(2-chloroethyl)-p-aminophenyl-butyric acid (CB1348) as an initiator of skin tumour formation in the mouse. *British Journal of Cancer* **10**, 363-378.

SANDMEYER E E (1981) Aromatic hydrocarbons. In: Clayton G D and Clayton F E (eds) *Patty's industrial hygiene and toxicology*, 3rd revised edition, vol 2B, p 3355.

SCRIBNER J D (1973) Tumor initiation by apparently noncarcinogenic polycyclic aromatic hydrocarbons. *Journal of the National Cancer Institute* **50**, 1717-1719.

SIMS P (1962) The metabolism of phenanthrene in rabbits and rats: Phenols and sulphuric esters. *Biochemical Journal* **84**, 558-563.

SIMS P (1970) Qualitative and quantitative studies on the metabolism of a series of aromatic hydrocarbons by rat-liver preparations. *Biochemical Pharmacology* **19**, 795-818.

STEINER P E (1955) Carcinogenicity of multiple chemicals simultaneously administered. *Cancer Research* **15**, 632-635.

VERSCHUEREN K (1983) *Handbook of environmental data on organic chemicals*. 2nd edn. New York, Van Nostrand Reinhold Company.

WATER RESEARCH CENTRE (1981) Organic micropollutants in drinking water. WRc Technical Report TR 159.

WOOD A W, CHANG R L, LEVIN W, RYAN D E, THOMAS P E, MAH H D, KARLE J M, YAGI H, JERINA D M and CONNEY A H (1979) Mutagenicity and tumorigenicity of phenanthrene and chrysene epoxides and diol epoxides. *Cancer Research* **39**, 4069-4077.

YOSHIKAWA T, RUHR L P, FLORY W, GIAMALUA D, CHURCH D F and PRYOR W A (1985) Toxicity of polycyclic aromatic hydrocarbons.1 1. Effect of phenanthrene, pyrene and their ozonised products on blood chemistry in rats. *Toxicology and Applied Pharmacology* **79**, 218-226.

9. THE METHYL PHENANTHRENES

Three methylphenanthrene isomers were identified in the WRc survey (Water Research Centre 1981). All three were found in a single sample of drinking water. Methylphenanthrene isomers have also been reported in Japanese and Canadian drinking water (Akiyama *et al* 1980, Benoit *et al* 1979).

La Voie *et al* (1981) found that of all the possible methylphenanthrene isomers, 1-methylphenanthrene and 9-methylphenanthrene were the only ones mutagenic in the Ames test. Activity was observed only in strain TA100 in the presence of metabolic activation. These workers then used the Ames test as a bioassay to study the metabolism of these compounds and their potential mutagenic metabolites. It is apparent that oxidation at the 9,10-position is a deactivating metabolic reaction, as when this step is inhibited, for example by inserting a methyl group in the 1- or 9-position, phenanthrene becomes mutagenic. Further, in the case of the non-mutagenic methylphenanthrenes, the major metabolites derive from the 9,10-epoxide. HPLC analysis and mutagenicity testing of the metabolites of 1-methylphenanthrene and 9-methylphenanthrene suggest that the 3,4- or 5,6-dihydrodiols are the proximate mutagens.

Both 1-methylphenanthrene and 2-methylphenanthrene have been found to be mutagenic in a forward mutation assay with *Salmonella typhimurium* TM677 in the presence of metabolic activation (Kaden *et al* 1979). 1-Methylphenanthrene has also been reported to mutate diploid human (AHH-1) lymphoblasts (Crespi *et al* 1982) and to induce unscheduled DNA synthesis in primary cultures of rat hepatocytes (Tong *et al* 1981). Gibson *et al* (1978) reported that both 1- and 2-methylphenanthrene were negative in the Ames test to TA98, TA1535, TA1537 and TA1538. However, Sakai *et al* (1985) found 1-methylphenanthrene to be mutagenic to stains TA98, TA100 and TA97 with metabolic activation.

Ten applications of 0.1% acetone solutions of all five possible methylphenanthrene isomers to the shaved backs of mice followed by TPA treatment for 20 weeks was not found to produce skin tumours (La Voie *et al* 1981).

References

AKIYAMA T, KOGA M, SHINOHARA R, KIDO A and ETOH S (1980) Detection and identification of trace organic substances in the aquatic environment. *Journal of Uoeh* **2**, 285-300.

BENOIT F M, LEBEL G L and WILLIAMS D T (1979) Polycyclic aromatic hydrocarbons in Eastern Ontario drinking waters, 1978. *Bulletin of Environmental Contamination and Toxicology* **23**, 774-778.

CRESPI C L, MARLETTA M A and THILLY W G (1982) Development and application of a mutation assay in diploid human lymphoblasts competent in xenobiotic metabolism. *Environmental Mutagenesis* **4**, 304.

GIBSON T L, SMART V B and SMITH L L (1978) Non-enzymatic activation of polycyclic aromatic hydrocarbons as mutagens. *Mutation Research* **49**, 153-161.

KADEN D A, HITES R A and THILLY W G (1979) Mutagenicity of soot and associated polycyclic aromatic hydrocarbons to *Salmonella typhimurium*. *Cancer Research* **39**, 4152-4159.

La VOIE E J, TULLEY-FREILER L, BEDENKO V and HOFFMANN D (1981)

Mutagenicity, tumor-initiating activity, and metabolism of methylphenanthrenes. *Cancer Research* **41**, 3441-3447.

SAKAI M, YOSHIDA D AND MIZUSAKI S (1985) Mutagenicity of polycyclic aromatic hydrocarbons and quinones on *Salmonella typhimurium* TA97. *Mutation Research* **156**, 61-67.

TONG C, LASPIA M F, TELANG S and WILLIAMS G M (1981) The use of adult rat liver cultures in the detection of the genotoxicity of various polycyclic aromatic hydrocarbons. *Environmental Mutagenesis* **1**, 477-487.

WATER RESEARCH CENTRE (1981) Organic micropollutants in drinking water. WRc Technical Report TR 159.

11

Phthalate esters

1. INTRODUCTION

Phthalates, esters of 1,2-benzenedicarboxylic acid, are important industrial chemicals used to impart flexibility in plastic products. Di-(2-ethylhexyl)phthalate, the most important plasticiser, is also used as a dielectric fluid and a hydraulic fluid. Phthalate esters are usually prepared from the reaction of phthalic anhydride with the appropriate alcohols.

2. EXPOSURE

Phthalate esters have been detected in water samples throughout the world. Typically, they are found at low μg/l levels in both river water and drinking water (Commission of the European Communities 1984).

A range of phthalate esters have been detected by WRc in drinking water in the UK (Water Research Centre 1981, 1982).

Butyl benzyl phthalate
Di-*n*-butyl phthalate
Dibutyl phthalate isomers (four)
Diethyl phthalate
Di-isobutyl phthalate
Dimethyl phthalate
Dioctyl phthalate isomers (three)
Dipropyl phthalate isomers (two)

The most frequently identified compounds were di-*n*-butyl phthalate, di-isobutyl phthalate and diethyl phthalate.

Significant quantities of phthalate esters are found in food due to migration from packaging materials (Tomita *et al* 1977). Phthalate esters have also been identified in the atmosphere (Thomas 1973, Giam *et al* 1978). Di-(2-ethylhexyl)phthalate leaches

from the plastics in dialysis machines and with its metabolites has been identified in the blood of dialysis patients (Pollack *et al* 1985).
Although the overall exposure to phthalates is not clear, food is likely to represent the major source.

3. TOXICOKINETICS

3.1 Absorption

In most species, phthalates are readily absorbed from the gastrointestinal tract as the monoesters (White *et al* 1980, Lake *et al* 1977). Early studies demonstrated that bacterial activity was not very important for hydrolysis of the diesters, and it was therefore suggested that intestinal hydrolases played the most important role (White *et al* 1980, Rowland *et al* 1977, Kaneshima *et al* 1978a). However, a recent study by White *et al* (1983) found that inhibition of rat intestinal mucosal esterases *in vivo* also failed to change the rate of absorption of di-*n*-butyl phthalate. It was suggested that pancreatic esterases released in the intestine were responsible for hydrolysis of the ester.

It has recently been reported (Rhodes *et al* 1983) that less than 2% of an oral dose of di-(2-ethylhexyl)phthalate was absorbed by marmosets.

An *in vitro* study using both rat and human epidermis found that phthalate esters were only slowly absorbed (Dugard *et al* 1983).

3.2 Distribution

In Wistar rats maintained on diets containing 1000 ppm of di-(2-ethylhexyl)phthalate for 35 days, the greatest quantities of the ester were found in the liver and fat. At the end of the treatment period, the half-life of di-(2-ethylhexyl)phthalate was estimated to be about 1–2 days in the liver and 3–5 days in fat (Daniel and Bratt 1974). Following long-term intravenous infusion of di-(2-ethylhexyl)phthalate in a monkey, low levels of the ester were reported to be still detectable in the liver, testes, heart and fat 14 months after the last treatment (Jacobson *et al* 1977).

There is little information available on the distribution of the other phthalates, though di-*n*-butyl phthalate did not appear to accumulate in rats fed the ester at 0.1% in the diet for 4 or 12 weeks (Williams and Blanchfield 1975).

3.3 Metabolism

The first step in the metabolism of phthalate esters, hydrolysis of one of the ester linkages, occurs in the intestine. This step is generally thought to be essential for absorption (White *et al* 1980, Lake *et al* 1977, Rowland *et al* 1977, Kaneshima *et al* 1978b, White *et al* 1983).

In most species, the principal metabolites of phthalate esters are glucuronide conjugates of their monoesters (Tanaka *et al* 1978, Kaneshima *et al* 1978a, Lake *et al* 1976, Albro *et al* 1981, Peck *et al* 1978, Albro *et al* 1982). However, the rat does not appear to conjugate mono-(2-ethylhexyl)phthalate with glucuronide. The major metabolites of this compound in the rat result from ω and ω-1 oxidation of the alkyl groups (Albro *et al* 1982, Kluwe 1982, Albro *et al* 1973). Phthalates with small alkyl groups are metabolised to phthalic acid to a much greater extent than dibutyl or di-(2-ethylhexyl)phthalate (Albro *et al* 1973, Albro and Moore 1974).

3.4 Excretion

The urine is the principal route of excretion for phthalate esters in mammals. The most common metabolites are the monoesters and their glucuronide conjugates. Phthalic acid and side-chain metabolites may also be present (Williams and Blanchfield 1975, Tanaka *et al* 1978, Kaneshima *et al* 1978a, Lake *et al* 1976, Albro *et al* 1973, Albro and Moore 1974, Albro *et al* 1981, 1982, Peck *et al* 1978, Kluwe 1982, Ikeda *et al* 1980).

Following oral doses of dibutyl phthalate in the rat, around 90% was excreted in the urine within 48 hours (Williams and Blanchfield 1975, Tanaka *et al* 1978, Kaneshima *et al* 1978a). Although there was significant biliary excretion, only a small percentage of the dose appeared in the faeces. Therefore, entero-hepatic recirculation is probably important for phthalate esters.

4. HEALTH EFFECTS

4.1 Acute and subacute toxicity

Phthalate esters are of low acute toxicity in experimental animals. Oral LD50s reported for the rat (Shibko and Blumenthal 1973, Registry of Toxic Effects of Chemical Substances) are:

Butyl benzyl phthalate	2–18 g/kg
Dimethyl phthalate	6.8 g/kg
Diethyl phthalate	8.6–31 g/kg
Di-*n*-butyl phthalate	8–16 g/kg
Di-isobutyl phthalate	15–20 g/kg
Di-(2-ethylhexyl)phthalate	31 g/kg

The two most commonly reported target organs for phthalate ester-induced toxicity are the testes and liver. Although several phthalates have been shown to have marked effects on these organs at high doses, there is relatively little information on their effects at lower doses.

Severe damage to the testes was found in Sprague–Dawley rats given oral doses of 2 g/kg/day of di-*n*-butyl phthalate for 4 days (Cater *et al* 1977). No testicular damage was reported in rats given 1.4 g/kg/day of dimethyl phthalate, 1.6 g/kg/day of diethyl phthalate, 1.8 g/kg/day of dipropyl phthalate or 2.8 g/kg/day of di-*n*-octyl phthalate for the same period (Foster *et al* 1980). Dibutyl phthalate, di-isobutyl phthalate and di-(2-ethylhexyl)phthalate induced a lowering of testes weight, an increase in liver weight and severe testicular damage in Wistar rats fed the esters at 2% in the diet for 7 days. In identical experiments, dimethyl phthalate, diethyl phthalate and di-*n*-octyl phthalate had no effect on testes weight or pathology but did increase liver weight (Oishi and Hiraga 1980). Oral doses of 800 mg/kg/day of either mono-*n*-butyl-, mono-iso-butyl-, mono-*sec*-butyl but not mono-*tert*-butyl phthalate for 6 days produced marked testicular atrophy in Sprague–Dawley rats (Foster *et al* 1981). F-344 rats fed diets containing 0–10% of butyl benzyl phthalate for 14 days exhibited depression of body weight gain at 2.5%, testicular degeneration at 5% and thymic atrophy at 10%. No gross or histopathological effects were found in mice fed diets containing 0–2.5% of butyl benzyl phthalate for 14 days (United States National Toxicology Program 1981). Histological changes in the testes have been reported in dd-Y mice given 50 or 100 mg/kg/day of di-*n*-butyl phthalate by gavage for 30 days (Sajicki *et al* 1980).

In the rat, there appears to be an age-related sensitivity to the testicular toxicity of di-(2-ethylhexyl)phthalate (Gray and Butterworth 1980, Sjoberg *et al* 1982, 1985).

It is well documented that subacute administration of high doses of di-(2-ethylhexyl)phthalate (1–2 g/kg/day) can produce hepatomegaly, hepatic peroxisome proliferation and induction of peroxisomal enzymes in the rat (Lake *et al* 1976, Reddy *et al* 1976). Di-(2-ethylhexyl)phthalate also has marked effects on lipid metabolism, including inhibition of cholesterolgenesis and elevated fatty acid oxidation, in the liver and other tissues (Bell 1982). Oral doses of 2 g/kg/day of di-(2-ethylhexyl)phthalate for 14 days induced hepatomegaly, hepatic peroxisome proliferation and testicular atrophy in rats but not in marmosets (Rhodes *et al* 1983, Jackh *et al* 1984).

Phthalate esters with unbranched side-chains do not have similar effects on the liver as di-(2-ethylhexyl)phthalate. Oral doses of 1 g/kg/day of di-*n*-octyl phthalate for 14 days induced hepatomegaly but not hepatic peroxisome proliferation in Sprague–Dawley rats (Lake *et al* 1984). Wistar rats maintained on diets containing 2% of either di-*n*-octyl phthalate or di-*n*-hexyl phthalate for up to 21 days did not exhibit similar changes in the liver to those rats fed di-(2-ethylhexyl)phthalate. However, these esters induced a loss of glycogen in the liver at 3 days, accumulation of fat droplets around the central veins was evident after 10 days, while a loss of glucose-6-phosphatase activity accompanied by centrilobular necrosis was apparent by the end of the experiment (Mann *et al* 1985).

Di-(2-ethylhexyl)phthalate has also been shown to induce hepatic mixed function oxidase activity in the rat (Lake *et al* 1974, Aitio and Parkki 1978, Agarwal *et al* 1982).

4.2 Chronic toxicity

In an early study of dimethyl phthalate, no effects were seen in rats maintained on diets containing 2% of the compound for 2 years. Growth retardation was evident in rats fed diets containing 4% or 8% of dimethyl phthalate. Chronic nephritis was also apparent at the 8% dietary level (Lehman 1955).

Groups of 15 male and 15 female CD rats fed diets containing 0, 0.2, 1.0 or 5% of diethyl phthalate for 16 weeks exhibited a reduction in body weight gain and food intake in both sexes at the high dose and in females at the 1.0% dose level. Elevated liver weight/body weight ratio was found in females of all treatment groups but only at the top dose in male rats. All the treated females also exhibited significant increases in the relative weight of the stomach and small intestine. Increased relative kidney weights were seen in both sexes receiving 5% diethyl phthalate. There were no apparent changes in histopathology or in restricted examination of kidney function, serum enzymes or haematology (Brown 1978).

Groups of 10 male Sprague–Dawley rats fed diets containing 0, 0.01, 0.05 or 0.25% of di-*n*-butyl phthalate for 1 year did not exhibit changes in growth, gross pathology or histopathology of a limited numbers of tissues (Smith 1953). No histological changes in the liver, kidney or spleen were found in groups of 20 male and 20 female Wistar rats maintained for 1 year on diets containing 0.125% of di-*n*-butyl phthalate (Nikonorow *et al* 1973).

Carpenter *et al* (1953) observed increased liver and kidney weights but no changes in histology in groups of 32 male and 32 female Sherman rats maintained on diets containing 0.4% of di-(2-ethylhexyl)phthalate for 1 year. No effects were reported at 0.04% and 0.13% of diet. Similar results were found in the offspring from these rats which had also been fed di-(2-ethylhexyl)phthalate at 0.4% in the diet for 1 year. In a 90-day study, growth retardation was reported in groups of 5 male Wistar rats fed di-(2-ethylhexyl)phthalate in the diet at doses equivalent to 0.4, 0.9 and 1.9 g/kg body weight/day. Testicular atrophy was also noted in animals of the two higher dose groups. No effects were found in rats given 0.2 g/kg body weight/day (Shaffer *et al* 1945). In another study, groups of 15 male and 15 female CD rats were fed diets containing 0, 0.2, 1.0 or 2.0% of di-(2-ethylhexyl)phthalate for 17 weeks. At the top two dose levels there was reduced food intake and growth, an elevated liver weight/body weight ratio, lowered haemoglobin in males and lowered packed cell volume in both males and females, and a reduction in testes weight. Histological changes were found in the testes at all dose levels, but there were no effects in the liver. Increased relative kidney weights were also noted at 1.0% and 2.0%, and kidney function was adversely affected in females of the top dose group (Gray *et al* 1977). Histological changes in the testes were reported in F-344 rats fed diets containing 1.2% of di-(2-ethylhexyl)phthalate for 2 years, but not in those on a 0.6% diet. Pituitary changes were also seen in the high-dose males (United States National Toxicology Program 1982). Degeneration of the seminiferous tubules of the testes has been reported in B6C3F1 mice receiving a 0.6% di-(2-ethylhexyl)phthalate diet for 103 weeks but not with a 0.3% diet (United States National Toxicology Program 1982). Ferrets fed di-(2-ethylhexyl)phthalate at 1% in the diet for 14 months exhibited depression of body weight, elevated liver weight, morphological and biochemical changes in the liver, and testicular damage (Lake *et al* 1976). Elevated liver weight was found in female but not male guinea-pigs fed diets containing 0.04% and 0.13% of di-(2-ethylhexyl)phthalate for 1 year. No histological changes were found in either the liver, kidney, lung, spleen or testes (Carpenter *et al* 1953).

Depression of body weight gain and testicular degeneration were reported in rats maintained on diets containing 2.5% of butyl benzyl phthalate for 90 days (United States National Toxicology Program 1981). No changes in gross pathology or histopathology were found in B6C3F1 mice maintained on diets containing 0–2.5% butyl benzyl phthalate for 90 days (United States National Toxicology Program 1981). It has been reported (in an abstract) that dogs fed diets containing 1, 2 or 5% of butyl benzyl phthalate for 90 days exhibited no changes in gross pathology, histopathology, haematology or urinary parameters. Retarded growth was observed in animals receiving the highest dose level (Hammond 1981).

4.3 Genotoxicity

In general, phthalate esters appear to be at best only weakly mutagenic in bacterial assays. Seed (1982) reported that dimethyl phthalate, diethyl phthalate and di-*n*-butyl phthalate were weakly mutagenic to *Salmonella typhimurium* TA100 in liquid suspension assays where resistance to 8-azaguanine was the genetic marker. Dimethyl phthalate and diethyl phthalate were active both in the presence and absence of S-9, while di-*n*-butyl phthalate was active only in the absence S-9. A number of other phthalate esters gave negative results in this assay. Seed (1982) also reported that dimethyl phthalate was weakly mutagenic to *Salmonella typhimurium* TA100 in the histidine reversion assay. Kozumbo *et al* (1982) found that dimethyl phthalate and diethyl phthalate were weakly mutagenic in the Ames test to *Salmonella typhimurium* TA100 only in the absence of S-9. Tomita *et al* (1982) reported that di-(2-ethylhexyl)phthalate was weakly mutagenic in the Ames test to *Salmonella typhimurium* TA100 in the presence of S-9. The majority of studies, however, have failed to find mutagenic activity for phthalate esters in bacterial test systems (Zeiger *et al* 1982, Yoshikawa *et al* 1983, Simmon *et al* 1977).

Except in the case of di-(2-ethylhexyl)phthalate, there is much less information available on the genotoxicity of phthalate esters in higher test systems. The evidence for genotoxic activity of di-(2-ethylhexyl)phthalate is very weak. A wide range of *in vitro* and *in vivo* studies have given negative results for this compound (Rushbrook *et al* 1982, Hodgson *et al* 1982, Ishidate and Odashima 1977, Phillips *et al* 1982, Kirby *et al* 1983, Putman *et al* 1983, Butterworth *et al* 1984, Kornbrust *et al* 1984), though some indications of genetic damage were found in a mouse dominant lethal test (Singh *et al* 1974) and in Syrian hamster embryonic cells (Tomita *et al* 1982). Abe and Sasaki (1977) reported that dibutyl phthalate and di-(2-ethylhexyl)phthalate were able to induce sister chromatid exchanges in Chinese hamster cells *in vitro*.

4.4 Carcinogenicity

Only limited studies have been carried out on di-*n*-butyl phthalate. In an early study (Lefaux 1964), no carcinogenic activity for this compound was found in rats fed diets containing 0.01% for five generations or 0.03% and 0.05% for three generations. Tumours in two female rats and one male rat were reported in a study of two groups of 36 rats given either 0.5 or 1.0 ml/kg of a 50% solution of di-*n*-butyl phthalate in olive oil, by gavage, twice weekly for 1 year. No tumours were reported in two control groups receiving olive oil alone (Bornmann *et al* 1956).

Di-(2-ethylhexyl)phthalate has been tested as part of the United States National Toxicology Program (1982). Groups of 50 male and 50 female F-344 rats were fed diets containing 0, 6000 or 12 000 ppm for 103 weeks while groups of 50 male and 50 female B6C3F1 mice received diets containing 0, 3000 and 6000 ppm for the same length of time. A significant increase in hepatocellular carcinomas was found in treated female rats and male and female mice. An increased incidence of either hepatocellular carcinomas or neoplastic nodules was observed in high-dose male rats. An overall elevated tumour incidence was evident in high-dose female rats, high-dose male mice, and low- and high-dose female mice. Earlier studies of di-(2-ethylhexyl)phthalate did not give any evidence for carcinogenic potential, though the methods are now considered to be deficient (Carpenter *et al* 1953, Harris *et al* 1956).

In a United States National Toxicology Program study (1981), groups of 50 male and 50 female F-344 rats were fed diets containing 0, 0.6 or 1.2% of butyl benzyl phthalate for 28 weeks (males) and 103 weeks (females). An elevated incidence of myelomonocytic leukaemia was found in high-dose females. No evaluation of carcinogenicity could be made for the male rats as there were a large number of early deaths which resulted in termination of the study at 28 weeks. Groups of 50 male and 50 female B6C3F1 mice maintained on diets containing 0, 0.6 or 1.2% of butyl benzyl phthalate for 105–106 weeks did not exhibit any evidence of an increased tumour incidence (United States National Toxicology Program 1981).

4.5 Reproductive toxicity

Intraperitoneal injection of either 0.5, 1.0 or 2.0 ml/kg of dimethyl phthalate on days 3, 6 and 9 of gestation in Sprague–Dawley rats had no effect on the number of successful implants or the number of weaned offspring per litter (Peters and Cook 1973). An elevated incidence of skeletal abnormalities and a reduction in mean foetal weight were found in Sprague–Dawley rats given 0.338, 0.675 or 1.125 ml/kg of dimethyl phthalate by intraperitoneal injection on days 5, 10 and 15 of gestation. Similar results were found with diethyl phthalate at 0.506, 1.012 and 1.686 ml/kg (Singh *et al* 1972). Dimethyl phthalate showed no developmental toxicity in CD-1 mice when given orally at a dose estimated to be just below the threshold of lethal toxicity (Plasterer *et al* 1985).

Diethyl phthalate was tested for reproductive toxicity in CD-1 mice at doses of 0.0, 0.25, 1.25 or 2.5% in the diet over two generations. There were no effects in the F_0 generation but in the F_1 generation reduced litter size and reduced sperm concentrations were observed at the 2.5% dose. However, reduced body weight and increased liver weight was also observed in these animals (Reel 1984).

A reduction in placental weight, but no skeletal abnormalities, was found in Wistar rats given either 120 or 600 mg/kg/day of di-*n*-butyl phthalate by gavage from day 0 to 21 of gestation. An increase in the number of resorptions and a reduction in foetal body weight were also noted at the higher dose level (Nikonorow *et al* 1973). Piekacz (1971) also reported a significant decrease in mean foetal weight and treatment-related changes in placental weight in rats given daily doses of di-*n*-butyl phthalate at 5% of the acute LD50 by gavage for 3 months prior to and 21 days after conception. These effects were not observed at a dose of 1% of the LD50. Aldyreva *et al* (1975) reported increased embryonic loss in rats given 250 mg/kg of di-*n*-butyl phthalate by gavage on either day 5 or 6 of gestation. A marked reduction in placental weight was found in rats dosed on day 9 of gestation. Subcutaneous oedema, haemorrhages and kidney damage were also noted in the foetuses. In another study, an elevated incidence of skeletal abnormalities, a reduction in mean foetal weight but no increase in gross abnormalities was found in Sprague–Dawley rats given 0.305, 0.610 and 1.017 ml/kg of di-*n*-butyl phthalate by intraperitoneal injection on days 5, 10 and 15 of gestation. A significant increase in the number of resorptions was only observed at the highest dose level. Similar results were found with di-isobutyl phthalate (Singh *et al* 1972). No adverse effects on reproduction were observed in an early multigeneration study in which five generations of rats were maintained on diets containing 0.01% di-*n*-butyl phthalate or of three generations receiving diets containing 0.03% or 0.05% di-*n*-butyl phthalate (Lefaux 1964). ICR-JCL mice fed diets containing 0.05, 0.2, 0.4 and 1.0% of di-*n*-butyl phthalate throughout pregnancy exhibited a dose-related reduction in mean foetal body weight. A marked increase in resorptions and dead foetuses was found at the high dose. There was some evidence for effects on skeletal development (Shiota *et al* 1980).

Di-(2-ethylhexyl)phthalate and di-*n*-octyl phthalate have been reported to lower average foetal weight and induce gross abnormalities in Spague–Dawley rats given doses of 10 ml/kg by intraperitoneal injection on days 5, 10 and 15 of gestation. At 5 ml/kg, abnormalities were still found with di-*n*-octyl phthalate but not for di-(2-ethylhexyl)phthalate. A significant increase in resorptions was also noted at the higher dose of di-(2-ethylhexyl)phthalate but not with di-*n*-octyl phthalate. No skeletal abnormalities were produced by either phthalate ester (Singh *et al* 1972). No effects on reproduction were seen in groups of 20 female Wistar rats given 0.34 or 1.7 g/kg/day of di-(2-ethylhexyl)phthalate by gavage for 3 months prior to pregnancy. In groups of 10 rats given these same doses on days 0–21 of gestation, a significant reduction in foetal weight and increased numbers of resorptions occurred at both doses and a significant reduction in placental weight was found at 1.7 g/kg (Nikonorow *et al* 1973). Daily doses of either 1% or 5% of the LD50 of di-*n*-octyl phthalate by gavage for 3 months prior to and throughout the 21-day gestation period produced a statistically significant reduction in mean foetal weight, but no observable effect on skeletal ossification (Piekacz 1971). Gross and skeletal abnormalities were reported in ddy-Slc mice given single oral doses of 2.5 or 7.5 ml/kg of di-(2-ethylhexyl)phthalate on days 7 or 8 of gestation. Both treatments also produced a marked reduction in the number of living embryos (Yagi *et al* 1980). In another study, there was some evidence for changes in skeletal development and an increased incidence of malformed foetuses in ICR-JCL mice fed diets containing 0.1 or 0.2% of di-(2-ethylhexyl)phthalate throughout gestation. At higher dietary concentrations of 0.4% and 1.0%, there were no surviving foetuses (Shiota *et al* 1980).

5. DISCUSSION

Phthalate esters are ubiquitous environmental pollutants. The concentrations of these compounds in surface waters, however, are generally very low and hence food, particularly those products which are packaged with plastic materials, is likely to represent the major source of exposure.

Although phthalates are generally well absorbed as the monoesters from the gastrointestinal tract of most species, this would not appear to be the case for the marmoset. The significance of this for man awaits further study. In experimental animals, the metabolism and elimination of phthalate esters is relatively rapid. The most important route of metabolism in most species is conjugation with glucuronic acid. However, the rat does not seem to be able to do this efficiently, and hence in this species a wider range of side-chain metabolites is seen.

Phthalate esters are of very low acute toxicity, but several compounds have marked subacute effects on the liver and testes of rodents at high doses. Subacute and chronic toxicity studies have shown that the branched-chain phthalate esters are more potent in this respect than the esters with unbranched side-chains. There is evidence that the hepatic and testicular effects of di-(2-ethylhexyl)phthalate in rodents are not produced in the marmoset. Dibutyl phthalate, dimethyl phthalate and diethyl phthalate have been assessed for safety by the American College of Toxicology Panel on Cosmetic Ingredients (1985) who concluded that these compounds were safe for topical application in cosmetics.

The genotoxicity of di-(2-ethylhexyl)phthalate has been studied extensively, but there is less information available on the other compounds. Studies in bacterial systems indicate that phthalate esters are non-mutagenic or at best very weakly mutagenic. Data in higher test systems are largely confined to di-(2-ethylhexyl)-phthalate, though the evidence would indicate a similar lack of activity as found in bacteria.

Carcinogenicity bioassays of di-(2-ethylhexyl)phthalate and butyl benzyl phthalate have been carried out as part of the United States National Toxicology Program (1981, 1982). Di-(2-ethylhexyl)phthalate was unequivocally found to induce liver tumours in rats and mice. Butyl benzyl phthalate gave negative results in mice, but there was some evidence for an increased incidence of myelomonocytic leukaemia in female rats. Of the remaining esters, di-*n*-butyl phthalate gave no evidence for carcinogenicity in an early multigeneration study, but the other compounds have not been tested.

Currently, there is much debate as to the mechanism of carcinogenicity of di-(2-ethylhexyl)phthalate in rodents. It appears that di-(2-ethylhexyl)phthalate may be a non-genetic carcinogen, its ability to produce tumours instead relating to proliferation of peroxisomes. There is evidence that compounds which induce peroxisome proliferation in the liver of rodents do not have the same activity in man, and therefore the hepatocarcinogenicity seen in rodents may not be indicative of a carcinogenic hazard to man.

There is some evidence that di-(2-ethylhexyl)phthalate and di-*n*-octyl phthalate are teratogenic in rodents at very high dose levels. Other phthalate esters have been shown to be foetotoxic at high doses. Effects include lowered foetal weight, increased numbers of resorptions and in some cases an increase in skeletal abnormalities.

The low concentrations of phthalate esters observed in drinking water seem unlikely to represent a hazard to human health. To confirm this, however, futher toxicological information, particularly at lower doses, is essential.

REFERENCES

ABE S and SASAKI M (1977) Chromosome aberrations and sister chromatid exchanges in Chinese hamster cells exposed to various chemicals. *Journal of the National Cancer Institute,* **58**, 1635-1640.

AGARWAL D K, AGARWAL S and SETH P K (1982) Effect of di-(2-ethylhexyl)phthalate on drug metabolism, lipid peroxidation, and sulfhydryl content of rat liver. *Drug Metabolism and Disposition* **10**, 77–80.

AITIO A and PARKKI M (1978) Effect of phthalate esters on drug metabolizing enzyme activities in rat liver. *Archives Internationales de Pharmacodynamie et de Therapie* **235**, 187–195.

ALBRO P W and MOORE B (1974) Identification of the metabolites of simple phthalate diesters in rat urine. *Journal of Chromatography* **94**, 209–218.

ALBRO P W, THOMAS R and FISHBEIN L (1973) Metabolism of diethylhexyl phthalate by rats. Isolation and characterization of the urinary metabolites. *Journal of Chromatography* **76**, 321–330.

ALBRO P W, HASS J R, PECK C C, ODAM D G, CORBETT J T, BAILEY F J, BLATT H E and BARRETT B B (1981) Identification of the metabolites of di-(2-ethylhexyl) phthalate in urine from the African Green monkey. *Drug Metabolism and Disposition* **9**, 223–225.

ALBRO P W, CORBETT J T, SCHROEDER J L, JORDAN S and MATTHEWS H B (1982) Pharmacokinetics, interactions with macromolecules and species differences in metabolism of DEHP. *Environmental Health Perspectives* **45**, 19–25.

ALDYREVA M N, KLIMOVA T S, IZYNMOVA A S and TIMOFEEVSKAYA L A (1975) Effect of phthalate plasticizers on the reproductive function of rats. *Gigiena Truda i Professional'nykh Zabolevanii* **12**, 25–29.

AMERICAN COLLEGE OF TOXICOLOGY PANEL ON COSMETICS INGREDIENTS (1985) Final report on the safety assessment of dibutyl phthalate, dimethyl phthalate, and diethyl phthalate. *Journal of the American College of Toxicology* **4**, 267–303.

BELL F P (1982) Effects of phthalate esters on lipid metabolism in various tissues, cells and organelles in mammals. *Environmental Health Perspectives* **45**, 41–50.

BORNMANN G, LOESER A, MIKULICZ K and RITTER K (1956) Behaviour of the organism as influenced by various plasticizers. *Zeitschrift fur Lebensmittel-Untersuchung und Forschung* **103**, 413–424.

BROWN D, BUTTERWORTH K R, GAUNT I F, GRASSO P and GANGOLLI S D (1978) Short-term oral toxicity study of diethyl phthalate in the rat. *Food and Cosmetics Toxicology* **16**, 415–422.

BUTTERWORTH B E, BERMUDEZ E, SMITH-OLIVER T, EARLE L, CATTLEY R, MARTIN J, POPP J A, STROM S, JIRTLE R and MICHALOPOULOS G (1984) Lack of genotoxic activity of di(2-ethylhexyl)phthalate (DEHP) in rat and human hepatocytes. *Carcinogenesis* **5**, 1329–1335.

CARPENTER C P, WEIL C S and SMYTH H F Jr (1953) Chronic oral toxicity of di(2-ethylhexyl) phthalate for rats, guinea pigs, and dogs. *Journal of Industrial Hygiene and Occupational Medicine* **8**, 219–226.

CATER B R, COOK M W, GANGOLLI S D and GRASSO P (1977) Studies on dibutyl phthalate-induced testicular atrophy in the rat: effect on zinc metabolism. *Toxicology and Applied Pharmacology* **41**, 609–618.

COMMISSION OF THE EUROPEAN COMMUNITIES (1984) An inventory of organic pollutants which have been identified in various surface waters, effluent discharges, aquatic animals and plants, and bottom sediments. Eurocop-Cost, Project 64B, 4th Edition.

DANIEL J W and BRATT H (1974) The absorption, metabolism and tissue distribution of di(2-ethylhexyl)phthalate in rats. *Toxicology* **2**, 51–65.

DUGARD P H, SCOTT R C, RAMSEY J D and RHODES C (1983) Percutaneous absorption of phthalate esters: *in vitro* experiments on human and rat epidermal membranes. *Toxicology Letters* **18** (Suppl 1), 63.

FOSTER P M D, THOMAS L V, COOK M W and GANGOLLI S D (1980) Study of the testicular effects and changes in zinc excretion produced by some *n*-alkyl phthalates in the rat. *Toxicology and Applied Pharmacology* **54**, 392–398.

FOSTER P M D, LAKE B G, THOMAS L V, COOK M W and GANGOLLI S D (1981) Studies on the testicular effects and zinc excretion produced by various isomers of monobutyl-*o*-phthalate in the rat. *Chemicobiological Interactions* **34**, 233–238.

GIAM C S, CHAN H S, NEFF G S and ATLAS E L (1978) Phthalate ester plasticizers: a new class of marine pollutant. *Science* **199**, 419–421.

GRAY T J B and BUTTERWORTH K R (1980) Testicular atrophy produced by phthalate esters. *Archives of Toxicology* Suppl 4, 452–455.

GRAY T J B, BUTTERWORTH K R, GAUNT I F, GRASSO P and GANGOLLI S D (1977) Short-term toxicity study of di-(2-ethylhexyl) phthalate in rats. *Food and Cosmetics Toxicology* **15**, 389–399.

HAMMOND B G M (1981) Toxicology of butyl benzyl phthalate. *Toxicologist* **1**, 114.

HARRIS R S, HODGE H C, MAYNARD E A and BLANCHET H J Jr (1956) Chronic oral toxicity of 2-ethylhexyl phthalate in rats and dogs. *AMA Archives of Industrial Health* **13**, 259–264.

HODGSON J R, MYHR B C, McKEON M and BRUSICK D J (1982) Evaluation of di-(2-ethylhexyl)phthalate and its major metabolites in the primary rat hepatocyte unscheduled DNA synthesis assay. *Environmental Mutagenesis* **4**, 388.

IKEDA G J, SAPIENZA P P, COUVILLION J L, FARBER T M and van LOON E J (1980) Comparative distribution, excretion and metabolism of di-(2-ethylhexyl)phthalate in rats, dogs and miniature pigs. *Food and Cosmetics Toxicology* **16**, 637–642.

ISHIDATE M Jr and ODASHIMA S (1977) Chromosome tests with 134 compounds on Chinese hamster cells *in vitro* – a screening for chemical carcinogens. *Mutation Research* **48**, 337–354.

JACKH R, RHODES C, GRASSO P and CARTER J T (1984) Genotoxicity studies on di-(2-ethylhexyl) phthalate and adipate and toxicity studies on di-(2-ethylhexyl) phthalate in the rat and marmoset. *Food and Chemical Toxicology* **22**, 151–155.

JACOBSON M S, KEVY S V and GRAND R J (1977) Effects of a plasticizer leached from polyvinyl chloride on the subhuman primate: a consequence of chronic transfusion therapy. *Journal of Laboratory and Clinical Medicine* **89**, 1066–1079.

KANESHIMA H, YAMAGUCHI T, OKUI T and NAITOH M (1978a) Studies on the effects of phthalate esters on the biological system (part 2) – *in vitro* metabolism and biliary excretion of phthalate esters in rats. *Bulletin of Environmental Contamination and Toxicology* **19**, 502–509.

KANESHIMA H, YAMAGUCHI T and ITOH K (1978b) Studies on the effects of phthalate esters on the biological system: (Part 3). The *in vitro* metabolism of dibutyl phthalate in the small intestine of rats. *Bulletin of Environmental Contamination and Toxicology* **20**, 725–728.

KIRBY P E, PIZZARELLO R F, LAWLOR T E, HAWORTH S R and HODG-

SON J R (1983) Evaluation of di-(2-ethylhexyl)phthalate and its major metabolites in the Ames test and L5178Y mouse lymphoma mutagenicity assay. *Environmental Mutagenesis* **5**, 657–663.

KLUWE W M (1982) Overview of phthalate ester pharmacokinetics in mammalian species. *Environmental Health Perspectives* **45**, 31–10.

KORNBRUST D J, BARFKNECHT T R, INGRAM P and SHELBURNE J D (1984) Effect of di(2-ethylhexyl)phthalate on DNA repair and lipid peroxidation in rat hepatocytes and on metabolic cooperation in Chinese hamster V-79 cells. *Journal of Toxicology and Environmental Health* **13**, 99–116.

KOZUMBO W J, KROLL R and RUBIN R J (1982) Assessment of the mutagenicity of phthalate esters. *Environmental Health Perspectives* **45**, 103–109.

LAKE B G, GANGOLLI S D, WRIGHT M G, GRASSO P and LLOYD A G (1974) Studies on the effects of the oral administration of di-(2-ethylhexyl)-phthalate on some hepatic enzymes in the rat. *Biochemical Society Transactions* **2**, 322–325.

LAKE B G, GANGOLLI S D, GRASSO P and LLOYD A G (1975) Studies on the hepatic effects of orally administered di-(2-ethylhexyl)phthalate in the rat. *Toxicology and Applied Pharmacology* **32**, 355–367.

LAKE B G, BRANTOM P G, GANGOLLI S D, BUTTERWORTH K R and GRASSO P (1976) Studies on the effects of orally administered di-(2-ethylhexyl)phthalate in the ferret. *Toxicology* **6**, 341–356.

LAKE B G, PHILLIPS J C, LINNELL J C and GANGOLLI S D (1977) The *in vitro* hydrolysis of some phthalate diesters by hepatic and intestinal preparations from various species. *Toxicology and Applied Pharmacology* **39**, 239–248.

LAKE B G, RIJCKEN W R P, GRAY T J B, FOSTER J R and GANGOLLI S D (1984) Comparative studies of the hepatic effects of di- and mono-*n*-octyl phthalates, di-(2-ethylhexyl) phthalate and clofibrate in the rat. *Acta Pharmacologica et Toxicologica* **54**, 167–176.

LEFAUX R (1964) Chimie et toxicologie des matieres plastiques. Compagnie Francaise d'Editions, Paris.

LEHMAN A J (1955) Insect repellents. *Association of Food and Drug Officers of the United States Quarterly Bulletin* **19**, 87.

MANN A H, PRICE S C, MITCHELL F E, GRASSO P, HINTON R H and BRIDGES J W (1985) Comparison of the short-term effects of di(2-ethylhexyl) phthalate, di(*n*-hexyl) phthalate, and di(*n*-octyl) phthalate in rats. *Toxicology and Applied Pharmacology* **77**, 116–132.

NIKONOROW M , MAZUR H and PIEKACZ H (1973) Effect of orally administered plasticizers and polyvinyl chloride stabilizers in the rat. *Toxicology and Applied Pharmacology* **26**, 253–259.

OISHI S and HIRAGA K (1980) Testicular atrophy induced by phthalic acid esters: effect on testosterone and zinc concentrations. *Toxicology and Applied Pharmacology* **53**, 35–41.

PECK C C, ALBRO P W, HASS J R, ODOM D G, BARRETT B B and BAILEY F J (1978) Metabolism and excretion of the plasticizer di-2-ethylhexyl-phthalate in man. *Clinical Research* **26**, 101A.

PETERS J W and COOK R M (1973) Effect of phthalate esters on reproduction in rats. *Environmental Health Perspectives* **3**, 91–94.

PHILLIPS B J, JAMES T E B and GANGOLLI S D (1982) Genotoxicity studies of di-(2-ethylhexyl)phthalate and its metabolites in CHO cells. *Mutation Research* **102**, 297–304.
PIEKACZ H (1971) Effect of dioctyl- and dibutylphthalates on the organism of rats after oral administration in prolonged experiment. II Subacute and chronic toxicity. *Roczniki-Panstwowego Zakladu Higieny* **22**, 295–307.
PLASTERER M R, BRADSHAW W S, BOOTH G M and CARTER M W (1985) Developmental toxicity of nine selected compounds following prenatal exposure in the mouse: naphthalene, ρ-nitrophenol, sodium selenite, dimethyl phthalate, ethylenethiourea, and four glycol ether derivatives. *Journal of Toxicology and Environmental Health* **15**, 25–38.
POLLACK G M, BUCHANAN J F, SLAUGHTER R L, KOHLI R K and SHEN D D (1985) Circulating concentrations of di(2-ethylhexyl) phthalate and its de-esterified phthalic acid products following plasticizer exposure in patients receiving hemodialysis. *Toxicology and Applied Pharmacology* **79**, 257–267.
PUTMAN D L, MOORE W A, SCHECHTMAN L M and HODGSON J R (1983) Cytogenetic evaluation of di-(2-ethylhexyl)phthalate and its major metabolites in Fischer 344 rats. *Environmental Mutagenesis* **5**, 227–231.
REDDY J K, MOODY D E, AZARNOFF D L and RAO M S (1976) Di-(2-ethylhexyl)phthalate: an industrial plasticizer induces hypolipidemia and enhances hepatic catalase and carnitine acetyltransferase activities in rats and mice. *Life Sciences* **18**, 941–946.
REEL J R (1984) Diethyl phthalate: reproduction and fertility assessment in CD-1 mice when administered in the feed. National Toxicology Program, Research Triangle Park, NTP-84-262, PB 85–118636.
REGISTRY OF TOXIC EFFECTS OF CHEMICAL SUBSTANCES National Institute for Occupational Safety and Health, Cincinnati, Ohio.
RHODES C, ELCOMBE C R, BATTEN P L, BRATT H, JACKSON S J, PRATT I S and ORTON T C (1983) Comparative toxicity of di-(2-ethylhexyl)phthalate (DEHP) in rats and marmosets. *Toxicology Letters* **18** (Suppl 1), 63.
ROWLAND I R, COTTRELL R C and PHILLIPS J C (1977) Hydrolysis of phthalate esters by the gastro-intestinal contents of the rat. *Food and Cosmetics Toxicology* **15**, 17–21.
RUSHBROOK C J, JORGENSON T A and HODGSON J R (1982) Dominant lethal study of di-(2-ethylhexyl)phthalate and its major metabolites in ICR/SIM mice. *Environmental Mutagenesis* **4**, 387.
SAJIKI J, FUKUDA Y and YAMAGIWA J (1980) Pathological observations of the mouse intoxicated with phthalic acid ester. *Journal of Pharmacobiodynamics* **3**, s–14.
SEED J L (1982) Mutagenic activity of phthalate esters in bacterial liquid suspension assays. *Environmental Health Perspectives* **45**, 111–114.
SHAFFER C B, CARPENTER C P and SMYTH H F Jr (1945) Acute and subacute toxicity of di(2-ethylhexyl) phthalate with note upon its metabolism. *Journal of Industrial Hygiene and Toxicology* **27**, 130–135.
SHIBKO S I and BLUMENTHAL H (1973) Toxicology of phthalic acid esters used in food-packaging material. *Environmental Health Perspectives* **3**, 131–137.
SHIOTA K, CHOU M J and NISHIMURA H (1980) Embryotoxic effects of di-2-

ethylhexyl phthalate (DEHP) and di-*n*-butyl phthalate (DBP) in mice. *Environmental Research* **22**, 245–253.

SIMMON V F, KAUHANEN K and TARDIFF R G (1977) Mutagenic activity of chemicals identified in drinking water. In: *Progress in genetic toxicology,* ed. by D Scott, B A Bridges and F H Sobels. Elsevier/North Holland, pp 249–258.

SINGH A R, LAWRENCE W H and AUTIAN J (1972) Teratogenicity of phthalate esters in rats. *Journal of Pharmaceutical Sciences* **61**, 51–55.

SINGH A R, LAWRENCE W H and AUTIAN J (1974) Mutagenic and antifertility sensitivities of mice to di-(2-ethylhexyl) phthalate (DEHP) and dimethoxyethyl phthalate (DMEP). *Toxicology and Applied Pharmacology* **29**, 35–46.

SJOBERG P, PLOEN L, BONDESSON U and LINDQUIST N G (1982) Testicular toxicity of di-(2-ethylhexyl)phthalate in rats of different ages. *Teratology* **26**, 20A.

SJOBERG P, BONDESSON U, KJELLEN L, LINDQUIST N-G, MONTIN G, PLOEN L (1985) Kinetics of di-(2-ethylhexyl)phthalate in immature and mature rats and effects on testis. *Acta Pharmacologica et Toxicologica* **56**, 30–37.

SMITH C C (1953) Toxicity of butyl stearate, dibutyl sebacate, dibutyl phthalate, and methoxyethyl oleate. *Archives of Industrial Hygiene and Occupational Medicine* **7**, 310–318.

TANAKA A, MATSUMOTO A and YAMAHA T (1978) Biochemical studies on phthalic esters. 3. Metabolism of dibutyl phthalate (DBP) in animals. *Toxicology* **9**, 109–123.

THOMAS G H (1973) Quantitative determination and confirmation of identity of trace amounts of dialkyl phthalates in environmental samples. *Environmental Health Perspectives* **3**, 23–28.

TOMITA I, NAKAMURA Y and YAGI Y (1977) Phthalic acid esters in various foodstuffs and biological materials. *Ecotoxicology and Environmental Safety* **1**, 275–287.

TOMITA I, NAKAMURA Y, AOKI N and INUI N (1982) Mutagenic/carcinogenic potential of DEHP and MEHP. *Environmental Health Perspectives* **45**, 119–125.

UNITED STATES NATIONAL TOXICOLOGY PROGRAM (1981) Bioassay of butyl benzyl phthalate for possible carcinogenicity. NIH Publication No. 80–1769.

UNITED STATES NATIONAL TOXICOLOGY PROGRAM (1982) Carcinogenesis bioassay of di-(2-ethylhexyl)phthalate in F344 rats and B6C3F1 mice (feed study). NIH Publication No. 82–1773.

WATER RESEARCH CENTRE (1981) Organic micropollutants in drinking water. WRc Technical Report TR 159.

WATER RESEARCH CENTRE (1982) Frequency of occurrence data for compounds identified by GC–MS in XAD-2 samples taken for mutagenic testing survey. WRc Unpublished Report.

WHITE R D, CARTER D E, EARNEST D and MUELLER J (1980) Absorption and metabolism of three phthalate diesters by the rat small intestine. *Food and Cosmetics Toxicology* **18**, 383–386.

WHITE R D, EARNEST D L and CARTER D E (1983) The effect of intestinal esterase inhibition on the *in vivo* absorption and toxicity of di-*n*-butyl phthalate.

Food and Chemical Toxicology **21**, 99–101.
WILLIAMS D T and BLANCHFIELD B J (1975) The retention, distribution, excretion and metabolism of dibutyl phthalate-7-^{14}C in the rat. *Journal of Agricultural and Food Chemistry* **23**, 854–858.
YAGI Y, NAKAMURA Y, TOMITA I, TSUCHIKAWA K and SHIMOI N (1980) Teratogenic potential of di- and mono-(2-ethylhexyl)phthalate in mice. *Journal of Environmental Pathology and Toxicology* **4**, 533–544.
YOSHIKAWA K, TANAKA A, YAMAHA T and KURATA H (1983) Mutagenicity study of nine monoalkyl phthalates and a dialkyl phthalate using *Salmonella typhimurium* and *Escherichia coli*. *Food and Chemical Toxicology* **21**, 221–223.
ZEIGER E, HAWORTH S, SPECK W and MORTELMANS K (1982) Phthalate ester testing in the National Toxicology Program's Environmental Mutagenesis Test Development Program. *Environmental Health Perspectives* **45**, 99–101.

12

The aldehydes

1. THE ALDEHYDES

1.1 Introduction

Aldehydes are an important class of industrial chemicals. Formaldehyde is the most widely used member of the group, though higher aldehydes are used as fragrances in soap, detergents, creams, lotions and perfumes, and for flavouring food. Many of the higher aldehydes occur naturally in essential oils.

The study of the health effects of aldehydes has largely been centred on the lower members of the group, formaldehyde, acrolein and acetaldehyde in particular. Of the aldehydes identified in drinking water by WRc, only benzaldehyde has been studied to any significant extent. The toxicology of this compound is the subject of a separate review.

1.2 Exposure

1.2.1 Air

There is no evidence to suggest that aldehydes are present at significant levels in ambient air, although aldehydes have been detected in tobacco smoke and vehicle exhaust fumes (Kuwata *et al* 1979).

1.2.2 Food

There is little information available on the occurrence of higher aldehydes in food. However, several are constituents of essential oils. It is likely that food represents the most important source of exposure to these compounds.

1.2.3 Water

Benzaldehyde was the only member of this group to be regularly detected in the WRc survey (Water Research Centre 1981). The other aldehydes identified were:

Propanal
Hexanal
3-Methylhexanal

2-Methylheptanal
Phthalaldehyde
Terephthalaldehyde

A similar range of aldehydes has also been identified in the drinking water of Cincinnati, Ohio (Coleman *et al* 1980).

1.3 Toxicokinetics

Although no information appears to be available on the metabolism of these aldehydes *per se*, the biotransformation of aldehydes generally is well known. Both the aliphatic and aromatic hydrocarbons are rapidly metabolised in the liver. The aliphatic aldehydes are oxidised to the corresponding acids which are substrates for fatty acid oxidation. Aromatic aldehydes are also converted to their corresponding acids, though the subsequent step is conjugation with glycine, glucuronic acid or sulphate. A small amount of glutathione conjugation may also occur.

These pathways are very efficient in metabolising aldehydes and even relatively high doses appear to be handled quite readily.

1.4 Health effects

1.4.1 Acute and subacute toxicity

The limited information available indicates that the higher aldehydes are of relatively low acute toxicity in experimental animals.

Acute oral LD50s in the rat of 4.9 g/kg and 1.4 g/kg have been reported for *n*-hexanal and propanal respectively (Brabec 1981, Smyth *et al* 1951).

A depression in body weight gain was noted in a group of four male F-344 rats fed diets containing 2% hexanal for 3 weeks. This treatment resulted in only a minimal induction of hepatic peroxisomal proliferation, but hepatic catalase and carnitine acetyltransferase activities were significantly elevated (Moody and Reddy 1978). In a similar experiment (Moody and Reddy 1982), hexanal was also shown to significantly lower serum cholesterol and triglyceride levels.

No toxic effects were found in four male and four female rats exposed by inhalation to 90 ppm of propanal, 6 hours/day, 5 days/week for 4 weeks. Depression of body weight gain and histopathological changes in the liver were noted in rats exposed by inhalation to 1300 ppm of propanal, 6 hours/day for 6 days (Gage 1970).

Phthalaldehyde has been shown to inhibit rabbit pulmonary and hepatic microsomal cytochrome P-450 *in vitro* (Patel 1979).

A 1% solution of hexanal in petrolatum gave no evidence for sensitisation in a maximisation test in 25 volunteers (Opdyke 1973).

1.4.2 Chronic toxicity

No information appears to be available.

1.4.3 Genotoxicity

A whole range of higher aldehydes including hexanal and propanal were not found to be mutagenic in the Ames test to *Salmonella typhimurium* TA98, TA100, TA1535 and TA1537 (Florin *et al* 1980). Both phthalaldehyde and propanal have also given negative results for mutagenicity in preincubation experiments with *S. typhimurium* TA98 and TA100 (Sasaki and Endo 1978).

Propanal has been reported to be weakly mutagenic to *Drosophila* (Rapoport 1948).

1.4.4 Carcinogenicity
No information appears to be available.

1.4.5 Reproductive toxicity
No information appears to be available.

1.5 Discussion
With the exception of benzaldehyde, all the other aldehydes were only infrequently identified in drinking water. As many of the higher aldehydes are used as fragrances and flavours and are constituents of essential oils, food is likely to be the most important source of exposure to these compounds.

The health effects of the higher aldehydes have been poorly studied. However, they appear to be of relatively low acute and subacute toxicity and are non-mutagenic in the Ames test. There is no information available on chronic toxicity, carcinogenicity or reproductive toxicity.

References
BRABEC M J (1981) Aldehydes and Acetals. In: *Patty's Industrial Hygiene and Toxicology* Third Revised Edition, ed by G D Clayton and F E Clayton Vol 2A, John Wiley and Sons, pp 2629–2669.

COLEMAN W E, MELTON R G, KOPFLER F C, BARONE K A, AURAND T A and JELLISON M G (1980) Identification of organic compounds in a mutagenic extract of a surface drinking water by a computerized gas chromatography/mass spectrometry system (GC/MS/COM). *Environmental Science and Technology* **14,** 576-588.

FLORIN I, RUTBERG L, CURVALL M and ENZELL C R (1980) Screening of tobacco smoke constituents for mutagenicity using the Ames test. *Toxicology* **18,** 219-232.

GAGE J C (1970) The subacute inhalation toxicity of 109 industrial chemicals. *British Journal of Industrial Medicine* **27,** 1-18.

KUWATA K, UEBORI M and YAMASAKI Y (1979) Determination of aliphatic and aromatic aldehydes in polluted airs as their 2,4-dinitrophenylhydrazones by high performance liquid chromatography. *Journal of Chromatographic Science* **17,** 264-268.

MOODY D E and REDDY J K (1978) Hepatic peroxisome (microbody) proliferation in rats fed plasticizers and related compounds. *Toxicology and Applied Pharmacology* **45,** 497-504.

MOODY D E and REDDY J K (1982) Serum triglyceride and cholesterol contents in male rats receiving diets containing plasticizers and analogues of the ester 2-ethylhexanol. *Toxicology Letters* **10,** 379-383.

OPDYKE D L J (1973) Fragrance raw materials monographs. Aldehyde C-6. *Food and Cosmetics Toxicology* **11,** 111.
PATEL J M (1979) The destruction of pulmonary and hepatic cytochrome P-450 by phthalaldehyde. *Toxicology and Applied Pharmacology* **48,** 337-342.
RAPOPORT I A (1948) Mutations under the influence of unsaturated aldehydes. *Doklady Akademia Nauk SSSR* **61,** 713-715.
SASAKI Y and ENDO R (1978) Mutagenicity of aldehydes in *Salmonella. Mutation Research* **54,** 251-252.
SMYTH H F Jr, CARPENTER C P and WEIL C S (1951) Range-finding toxicity data: List 4. *Archives of Industrial Health and Occupational Medicine* **4,** 119-122.
WATER RESEARCH CENTRE (1981) Organic micropollutants in drinking water. WRc Technical Report TR 159.

2. BENZALDEHYDE

2.1 Introduction

Benzaldehyde is used as a flavouring agent, as a solvent, and as an intermediate in the manufacture of dyes, perfumes, cinnamic and mandelic acids. This compound is approved by the US Food and Drug Administration for use in food. Benzaldehyde can be prepared by the oxidation of toluene or by a catalysed reaction between benzyl chloride and lime.

CAS Reg. No:	100-52-7
Molecular weight:	106.1
Boiling point:	179.0°C
Solubility:	3300 mg/l at 25°C (Verschueren 1983)
Threshold odour concentration in water:	0.2–4.3 μg/l (Verschueren 1983)

2.2 Exposure

2.2.1 Air

Benzaldehyde has been identified in the atmosphere in the US (Bertsch *et al* 1974, Holzer *et al* 1977). It has also been detected in vehicle exhaust fumes at levels ranging from <0.1 to 13.5 ppm (Verschueren 1983, Kuwata *et al* 1979) and in tobacco smoke at 5.3–10.6 μg/cigarette (Kuwata *et al* 1979).

2.2.2 Food

This compound is used as a flavouring agent in some foods and medicines and occurs naturally in many other foodstuffs (Flavor and Extract Manufacturers' Association of the United States 1978). Occurrence in food appears to be the major source of exposure to this compound.

2.2.3 Water

Benzaldehyde was identified in 10/14 drinking water samples in the WRc survey (Water Research Centre 1981). It has also been detected in US drinking water (Coleman *et al* 1980) and in Japanese river water and drinking water (Akiyama *et al* 1980).

2.3 Toxicokinetics

In rats, exposure by inhalation led to rapid absorption of benzaldehyde. The peak residue concentrations in the blood, kidney, heart and brain occurred shortly after exposure, while those for the poorly perfused tissues such as skin, muscle, and fat were somewhat later. Most of the dose was eliminated in the urine as hippuric acid. The biological half-life of benzaldehyde in the blood was approximately 10 minutes (Kutzman *et al* 1980).

About 90% of an oral dose of 1000 mg of benzaldehyde was excreted in the urine of rabbits within 24 hours. Almost all of this was present as hippuric acid (Bray *et al* 1951).

Benzaldehyde has also been shown to be rapidly eliminated in the urine as hippuric acid following subcutaneous injection in both rats and rabbits (Stekol 1939).

The mechanism of biotransformation of benzaldehyde to hippuric acid is well known. The first step is oxidation to benzoic acid in the cytosol by aldehyde dehydrogenase. Benzoic acid is then conjugated with glycine in the mitochondrion to form hippuric acid, which is rapidly eliminated in the urine. This pathway is very efficient in metabolising benzaldehyde even at very high dose levels.

2.4 Health effects

2.4.1 Acute and subacute toxicity

The symptoms of acute toxicity in experimental animals are tremors, weakness, intestinal irritation and narcosis. At necropsy, there are no particular gross pathological changes. The acute oral LD50 of benzaldehyde in the rat has been reported to range from 1.3 to 2.85 g/kg. Acute oral LD50s of 2.02 g/kg and 1 g/kg have also been reported for the mouse and guinea-pig respectively (Jenner *et al* 1964, Sporn *et al* 1967, Peresedov 1974).

In a subacute study, groups of five male and five female F344 rats were treated by gavage with 0, 100, 200, 400, 800 or 1600 mg/kg body weight/day, 5 days/week for a total of 12 treatments. All the animals given 1600 mg/kg died after the second daily treatment. There were also some deaths at 800 mg/kg. The only other effects observed in this study were evident in the survivors at the 800 mg/kg dose level. These were depressed body weight gain, tremors, hyperexcitability, and inactivity. In groups of five male and five female B6C3F1 mice similarly treated with 0, 200, 400, 800, 1600 or 3200 mg/kg body weight, all the animals at the top two doses died during the dosing period. There were no clinical signs of toxicity, gross pathological changes or effects on body weight at the lower dose levels, though one mouse at 800 mg/kg died during treatment (Kluwe *et al* 1983).

A slight depression of body weight gain and a lowering of liver weight (in terms of percentage of original body weight) were noted in a group of three rats maintained on a diet of 1% benzaldehyde for 14 days (Hruban *et al* 1966).

2.4.2 *Chronic toxicity*

In a 90-day study, groups of 10 male and 10 female F344 rats were treated by gavage with 0, 50, 100, 200, 400 or 800 mg/kg body weight/day while groups of ten male and ten female B6C3F1 mice were similarly dosed with 0, 75, 150, 300, 600 or 1200 mg/kg body weight/day. Deaths of male and female rats and male mice occurred at the highest dose levels. Hyperexcitability, tremors and also periods of inactivity were observed in rats receiving the high dose but not in mice. Body weight gain was depressed in surviving male rats receiving 800 mg/kg, in female mice receiving 1200 mg/kg and in male mice receiving 600 mg/kg. Surviving male rats given 800 mg/kg also exhibited a marked reduction in thymus and testes weights while slightly elevated liver, kidney, thymus and heart weights were noted in surviving female rats at this dose level. Effects observed in both male and female rats at the highest dose level were renal tubular necrosis, necrotic lesions in the brain cerebellum and hippocampus, and mild epithelial hyperplasia and hyperkeratosis of the forestomach. The only pathological change found in mice was renal tubular necrosis in males at 1200 mg/kg. No toxic effects were seen in rats given 400 mg/kg or less, in male mice given 300 mg/kg or less or in female mice given 600–1200 mg/kg (Kluwe *et al* 1983).

There were no effects on growth, haematology or macroscopic and microscopic pathology in groups of five male and five female Osborne-Mendel rats fed diets containing either 0.1% benzaldehyde for 27–28 weeeks or 1% benzaldehyde for 16 weeks (Hagan *et al* 1967).

Rats given oral doses of 10 mg of benzaldehyde in oil on alternate days for 12 weeks did not show any changes in growth rate, liver weight, adrenal weight, hepatic nitrogen and lipid content, or adrenal ascorbic acid content. No effects on hepatic succinate dehydrogenase, aldolase or aspartic transaminase activities were found in rats given oral doses of 10 mg of benzaldehyde in oil on alternate days for 8 weeks (Sporn *et al* 1967).

A number of haematological changes were noted in rats exposed by inhalation to 26 mg/m3 of benzaldehyde, 5 days/week for 4 months. These effects were not apparent in rats exposed to a concentration of 6 mg/m3 (Peresedov 1974).

In a Japanese study, a group of 102 cancer patients were given daily doses of 10 mg/kg of beta-cyclodextrin benzaldehyde inclusion compound (approximately 0.83 mg/kg of benzaldehyde) by oral or rectal administration for periods ranging from 2 weeks to 2 years. Benzaldehyde treatment did not produce any changes in haematology or clinical chemistry (Kochi *et al* 1980).

2.4.3 *Genotoxicity*

Benzaldehyde gave negative results in the Ames test with *Salmonella typhimurium* TA98, TA100, TA1535 and TA1537, either in the presence or absence of metabolic activation, at doses ranging from 10 to 1000 μg/plate (Haworth *et al* 1983). The absence of mutagenic activity for benzaldehyde in the Ames test has also been reported by other groups (Sasaki and Endo 1978, Florin *et al* 1980, Rapson *et al* 1980, Kasamaki *et al* 1982).

A weak induction of chromosomal aberrations was found in Chinese hamster cells *in vitro* at a benzaldehyde concentration of 2.5 nM (Kasamaki 1982).

2.4.4 Carcinogenicity
No information appears to be available at present, though a US National Toxicology Program carcinogenicity bioassy is in progress.

2.4.5 Antitumour activity
Takeuchi *et al* (1978) implanted Swiss mice with a solid type of Ehrlich carcinoma. The mice were then given daily injections of 10 mg/kg/day of benzaldehyde for 9 days. Benzaldehyde treatment was found to inhibit tumour growth by 56% compared to an untreated control group. In a similar study, six CF-1 male mice were implanted with one million Ehrlich ascites cells. They were then given daily intraperitoneal injections of 1 mg/kg of benzaldehyde for 6 or 7 days. Benzaldehyde inhibited Ehrlich tumour growth by some 69% compared to controls (Hall *et al* 1978). No tumour growth was observed in mice implanted with transformed C3H/He mouse embryo cells which had been cultured in the presence of benzaldehyde. Tumours were found in mice implanted with cells which had not been cultured in the presence of benzaldehyde (Nambata *et al* 1980, Miyakawa *et al* 1979).

Benzaldehyde has also been shown to inhibit the growth of transformed cells *in vitro* (Nambata *et al* 1980, Miyakawa *et al* 1979).

The mechanism by which benzaldehyde inhibits the growth of transformed cells is not clear. However, an *in vitro* study has shown that benzaldehyde increases cell cycle duration primarily by a reduction in protein synthesis. It had only a small effect on protein degradation (Pettersen *et al* 1983).

2.4.6 Reproductive toxicity
Female breeding rats were given oral doses of 2 mg of benzaldehyde in oil on alternate days for 32 weeks. The number of offspring born, their weights after 1 and 3 weeks, and mortality of offspring were all reported to be within normal limits. The number of gestating animals was lower in the treated group compared to the control group (Sporn *et al* 1967).

2.5 Discussion
Benzaldehyde is widely used in the food industry as a flavouring agent. Although benzaldehyde was regularly identified in drinking water in the WRc survey, exposure from water would appear to be insignificant in comparison to exposure from food.

Benzaldehyde is likely to be rapidly absorbed by all routes and distributed primarily to the well-perfused tissues. Metabolism of benzaldehyde to hippuric acid is also very rapid. Excretion occurs almost exclusively via the kidneys.

Acute and chronic studies have shown that benzaldehyde is of very low toxicity. In a 90-day study, there were no effects in rats given daily oral doses of 400 mg/kg or in mice at 300 mg/kg. At higher dose levels in rats, the principal target organs were the brain, kidney and stomach. The only target organ in the mouse appeared to be the kidney. Benzaldehyde is not mutagenic in the Ames test but one study gave some evidence for cytogenetic effects in mammalian cells. No information appears to be available on carcinogenicity and there is only one limited study concerning reproductive effects. There is some evidence that benzaldehyde has antitumour activity by inhibiting cell growth.

The information available suggests that low levels of benzaldehyde in drinking water would be very unlikely to constitute a risk to human health.

References

AKIYAMA T, KOGA M, SHINOHARA R, KIDO A and ETOH S (1980) Detection and identification of trace organic substances in the aquatic environment. *Journal of Uoeh* **2,** 285-300.

BERTSCH W, CHANG R C and ZLATKIS A (1974) The determination of organic volatiles in air pollution studies: Characterization of profiles. *Journal of Chromatographic Science* **12,** 175-182.

BRAY H G, THORPE W V and WHITE K (1951) Kinetic studies of the metabolism of foreign organic compounds. 1. The formation of benzoic acid from benzamide, toluene, benzyl alcohol and benzaldehyde and its conjugation with glycine and glucuronic acid in the rabbit. *Biochemical Journal* **48,** 88-96.

COLEMAN W E, MELTON R G, KOPFLER F C, BARONE K A, AURAND T A and JELLISON M G (1980) Identification of organic compounds in a mutagenic extract of a surface drinking water by a computerized gas chromatography/mass spectrometry system (GC/MS/COM). *Environmental Science and Technology* **14,** 576-588.

FLAVOR AND EXTRACT MANUFACTURERS' ASSOCIATION OF THE UNITED STATES (1978) Scientific literature review of benzyl alcohol, benzaldehyde, benzoic acid and related substances in flavor usage. Vol. 1. Introduction and summary tables of data, bibliography. Food and Drug Administration, Washington, DC, NTIS PB-291 106.

FLORIN I, RUTBERG L, CURVALL M and ENZELL C R (1980) Screening of tobacco smoke constituents for mutagenicity using the Ames' test. *Toxicology* **18,** 219-232.

HAGAN E C, HANSEN W H, FITZHUGH O G, JENNER P M, JONES W I, TAYLOR J M, LONG E L, NELSON A A and BROUWER J B (1967) Food flavourings and compounds of related structure. 2. Subacute and chronic toxicity. *Food and Cosmetics Toxicology* **5,** 141-157.

HALL I H, SAJADI Z and LOEFFLER L J (1978) Antineoplastic agents III: Effects of dibromoethyl and vinyl esters of *N*-Benzyloxycarbonyl-L-phenylalanine on Ehrlich ascites tumour cell metabolism. *Journal of Pharmaceutical Sciences* **67,** 1726-1731.

HAWORTH S, LAWLOR T, MORTELMANS K, SPECK W and ZEIGER E (1983) *Salmonella* mutagenicity test results for 250 chemicals. *Environmental Mutagenesis* **5,** Suppl 1, 3-142.

HOLZER G, SHANFIELD H, ZLATKIS A, BERTSCH W, JUAREZ P, MAYFIELD H and LIEBICH H M (1977) Collection and analysis of trace organic emissions from natural sources. *Journal of Chromatography* **142,** 755-764.

HRUBAN Z, SWIFT H and SLESERS A (1966) Ultrastructural alterations of hepatic microbodies. *Laboratory Investigation* **15,** 1884-1901.

JENNER P M, HAGAN E C, TAYLOR J M, COOK E L and FITZHUGH O G (1964) Food flavourings and compounds of related structure. 1. Acute oral toxicity. *Food and Cosmetics Toxicology* **2,** 327-343.

KASAMAKI A, TAKAHASHI H, TSUMARA N, NIWA J, FUJITA T and URASAWA S (1982) Genotoxicity of flavoring agents. *Mutation Research* **105,** 387-392.

KLUWE W M, MONTGOMERY C A, GILES H D and PREJEAN J D (1983) Encephalopathy in rats and nephropathy in rats and mice after subchronic oral exposure to benzaldehyde. *Food and Chemical Toxicology* **21,** 245-250.

KOCHI M, TAKEUCHI S, MIZUTANI T, MOCHIZUKI,K, MATSUMOTO Y and SAITO Y (1980) Antitumour activity of benzaldehyde. Cancer Treatment Reports 64, 21-23.

KUTZMAN R S, MEYER G-J and WOLF A P (1980) Biodistribution and excretion of [^{11}C]benzaldehyde by the rat after two-minute inhalation exposures. *Xenobiotica* **10,** 281-288.

KUWATA K, UEBORI M and YAMASAKI Y (1979) Determination of aliphatic and aromatic aldehydes in polluted airs as their 2,4-dinitrophenylhydrazones by high performance liquid chromatography. *Journal of Chromatographic Science* **17,** 264-268.

MIYAKAWA T, ZUNDEL J-L and SAKAGUCHI K (1979) Selective inhibitory effect of benzaldehyde on the growth of simian virus 40-transformed cells. *Biochemical and Biophysical Research Communications* **87,** 1024-1030.

NAMBATA T, TERADA N, MIZUTANI T and TAKEUCHI S (1980) Effect of benzaldehyde on mouse embryo cells *in vitro. Gann* **71,** 572-573.

PERESEDOV V P (1974) Substantiation of the maximum permissible concentration of benzaldehyde in the air of a working zone. *Gigiena Truda i Professional-'nykh Zabolevanii* **11,** 40-41.

PETTERSEN E O, RONNING O W, NOME O and OFTEBRO R (1983) Effects of benzaldehyde on protein metabolism of human cells cultivated *in vitro. European Journal of Cancer and Clinical Oncology* **19,** 935-940.

RAPSON H W, NAZAR M A and BUTSKY V V (1980) Mutagenicity produced by aqueous chlorination of organic compounds. *Bulletin of Environmental Contamination and Toxicology* **24,** 590-596.

SASAKI Y and ENDO R (1978) Mutagenicity of aldehydes in *Salmonella. Mutation Research* **54,** 251-252.

SPORN A, DINU I and STANCIU V (1967) Investigations on the toxicity of benzaldehyde. *Igiena* **16,** 23-24.

STEKOL J A (1939) Studies on the mercapturic acid synthesis in animals. XI. The detoxification of benzyl chloride, benzyl alcohol, benzaldehyde and S-Benzylhomocysteine in the rabbit and rat. *Journal of Biological Chemistry* **128,** 199-205.

TAKEUCHI S, KOCHI M, SAKAGUCHI K, NAKAGAWA K and MIZUTANI T (1978) Benzaldehyde as a carcinostatic principle in figs. *Agricultural and Biological Chemistry* **42,** 1449-1451.

VERSCHUEREN K (1983) *Handbook of environmental data on organic chemicals.* Second edition. Van Nostrand Reinhold Company, New York.

WATER RESEARCH CENTRE (1981) Organic micropollutants in drinking water. WRc Technical Report TR 159.

13

The aliphatic hydrocarbons

1. INTRODUCTION

Aliphatic hydrocarbons are the major constituents of many petroleum-type mixtures and appear to be widely distributed in the environment.

In two surveys of UK drinking water, a group of 68 aliphatic alkanes and alkenes were detected by gas chromatography–mass spectrometry. Several of the compounds were identified frequently (Water Research Centre 1981, 1982):

Decane
Decane isomers (12)
Dodecane isomers (three)
Eicosane
Heptadecane
Heptane isomers (two)
Hexadecane
Hexane isomers (three)
Nonadecane
Nonane
Nonane isomers (seven)
Octadecane
Octane
Pentadecane
Tetradecane
Tridecane
Tridecane isomers (three)
Undecane
Undecane isomers (four)

Decadiene isomer
Decene isomers (four)
Dodec-1-ene
Heptadecene
Heptene isomers (four)
Hexadec-1-ene
Hexadiene isomers (two)
Hexene isomers (three)
Nonene
Octadecene
Octene isomer
Tetradecene
Undec-1-ene

A similar range of compounds has also been detected in the atmosphere.

Aliphatic hydrocarbons are lipophilic and therefore readily absorbed by all routes. On absorption, they are rapidly metabolised by oxidative enzymes and are then either excreted in the urine as glucuronide or glutathione conjugates or catabolised to carbon dioxide by conventional biochemical pathways.

Except in the case of *n*-hexane, toxicological information on individual compounds of this group is sparse. Moreover almost all the available data concern inhalation, reflecting the primary concern with these compounds, ie occupational exposure to hydrocarbon vapours. However, what information is available suggests that the aliphatic hydrocarbons are of relatively low acute and chronic toxicity.

n-Hexane, although the subject of much study because of its neurotoxicity, would not appear to present a hazard at the very low concentrations encountered in drinking water. Several of the C_{10}–C_{20} alkanes have been shown to be tumour promoters in mouse skin and the importance of chemicals like these in complex mixtures requires clarification.

Long-term inhalation studies conducted in the US have shown that complex mixtures of hydrocarbons have nephrotoxic potential in rats and mice (Bruner 1984, Busey and Cockrell 1984, Kitchen 1984, MacFarland 1984, MacNaughton and Uddin 1984). This phenomenon appears to be related to the alkane and alkene constituents but not to the aromatic fraction of the mixture (Halder *et al* 1984).

Early pathological changes observed in the kidneys of male rats following inhalation of unleaded gasoline (major components C_4–C_{12} paraffins) or synthetic jet fuels included (a) accumulation of hyaline droplets in cells of the proximal convoluted tubule, (b) focal degeneration of cells throughout the proximal convoluted tubule, (c) proximal tubular regeneration, (d) granular casts and dilated tubular lamina at the junction area between the proximal convoluted tubule and the descending limb of the loop of Henle, (e) mineralisation of tubules in the medulla. At the end of the studies, a significant increase in hyperplasias, dysplasias, adenomas and carcinomas was found in the kidney of male rats. Exacerbation of nephropathy routinely observed in old male rats has also been reported (MacFarland 1984).

Although epidemiological studies have failed to link exposure to hydrocarbons with cancer of the kidney (Higginson *et al* 1984, Raabe 1984, Wen *et al* 1984) there are several reports suggesting that hydrocarbons are nephrotoxic in man. However, the most commonly reported pathological effect, immune complex-type glomerulonephritis (Phillips 1984), was not observed in the experiments with rats and mice.

Despite the relatively limited toxicological information available on the aliphatic hydrocarbons identified by WRc, these compounds do not appear to warrant concern as micropollutants in drinking water.

References

BRUNER R H (1984) Pathologic findings in laboratory animals exposed to hydrocarbon fuels of military interest. In: *Advances in Modern Environmental Toxicology Vol 7 Renal Effects of Petroleum Hydrocarbons,* ed by M A Mehlman, G P Hemstreet III, J J Thorpe and N K Weaver. Princeton Scientific Publishers Inc, New Jersey, pp 133-140.

BUSEY W M and COCKRELL B Y (1984) Non-neoplastic exposure-related renal lesions in rats following inhalation of unleaded gasoline vapours. In *Advances in Modern Environmental Toxicology Vol 7 Renal Effects of Petroleum Hydrocar-*

bons, ed by M A Mehlman, G P Hemstreet III, J J Thorpe and N K Weaver. Princeton Scientific Publishers Inc, New Jersey, pp 57-64.

HALDER C A, WARNE T M and HATOUM N S (1984) Renal toxicity of gasoline and related naphthas in male rats. In: *Advances in Modern Environmental Toxicology Vol 7 Renal Effects of Petroleum Hydrocarbons,* ed by M A Mehlman, G P Hemstreet III, J J Thorpe and N K Weaver. Princeton Scientific Publishers Inc, New Jersey, pp 73-88.

HIGGINSON J, MUIR C S and BUFFLER P A (1984) The epidemiology of renal carcinoma in humans with a note on the effect of exposure to gasoline. In: *Advances in Modern Environmental Toxicology Vol 7 Renal Effects of Petroleum Hydrocarbons,* ed by M A Mehlman, G P Hemstreet III, J J Thorpe and N K Weaver. Princeton Scientific Publishers Inc, New Jersey, pp 203-226.

KITCHEN D N (1984) Neoplastic renal effects of unleaded gasoline in Fischer 344 rats. In: *Advances in Modern Environmental Toxicology Vol 7 Renal Effects of Petroleum Hydrocarbons,* ed by M A Mehlman, G P Hemstreet III, J J Thorpe and N K Weaver. Princeton Scientific Publishers Inc, New Jersey, pp 65-71.

MacFARLAND H N (1984) Xenobiotic-induced kidney lesions: Hydrocarbons. The 90-day and 2 year gasoline studies. In: *Advances in Modern Environmental Toxicology Vol 7 Renal Effects of Petroleum Hydrocarbons,* ed by M A Mehlman, G P Hemstreet III, J J Thorpe and N K Weaver. Princeton Scientific Publishers Inc, New Jersey, pp 51-56.

MacNAUGHTON M G and UDDIN D E (1984) Toxicology of mixed distillate and high-energy synthetic fuels. In: *Advances in Modern Environmental Toxicology Vol 7 Renal Effects of Petroleum Hydrocarbons,* ed by M A Mehlman, G P Hemstreet III, J J Thorpe and N K Weaver. Princeton Scientific Publishers Inc, New Jersey, pp 121-132.

PHILLIPS S C (1984) A review of the human kidney effects of hydrocarbon exposure. In: *Advances in Modern Environmental Toxicology Vol 7 Renal Effects of Petroleum Hydrocarbons,* ed by M A Mehlman, G P Hemstreet III, J J Thorpe and N K Weaver. Princeton Scientific Publishers Inc, New Jersey, pp 185-202.

RAABE G K (1984) Kidney cancer epidemiology in petroleum-related studies. In: *Advances in Modern Environmental Toxicology Vol 7 Renal Effects of Petroleum Hydrocarbons,* ed by M A Mehlman, G P Hemstreet III, J J Thorpe and N K Weaver. Princeton Scientific Publishers Inc, New Jersey, pp 259-271.

WATER RESEARCH CENTRE (1981) Organic micropollutants in drinking water. WRc Technical Report TR 159.

WATER RESEARCH CENTRE (1982) Frequency of occurrence data for compounds identified by GC–MS in XAD-2 samples taken for mutagenic testing survey. WRc Unpublished Report.

WEN C P, TSAI S P, MOFFITT K B, BONDY M and GIBSON R L (1984) Epidemiologic studies of the role of gasoline (hydrocarbon) exposure in kidney cancer risk. In: *Advances in Modern Environmental Toxicology Vol 7 Renal Effects of Petroleum Hydrocarbons,* ed by M A Mehlman, G P Hemstreet III, J J Thorpe and N K Weaver. Princeton Scientific Publishers Inc, New Jersey, pp 245-257.

2. HEXANE

2.1 Introduction

Hexane (C_6H_{14}) is normally one component of a mixture of alkanes used as fuel, as a solvent, thinner, degreasing agent and lubricant. The *n*-hexane isomer has a solubility in water of 9.5 mg/l at 20 oC (Verschueren 1983).

2.2 Exposure

Three unspecified hexane isomers were detected in drinking water in the WRc survey. The isomers occurred in 8/14, 5/14 and 3/14 samples respectively (Water Research Centre 1981).

Hexane isomers have also been identified in the atmosphere (Bertsch *et al* 1974, Holzer *et al* 1977, Ioffe *et al* 1977).

2.3 Toxicokinetics

The metabolism of *n*-hexane in mammals following exposure by inhalation has been studied extensively but there is very little information on metabolism after exposure by other routes.

In rats exposed to *n*-hexane by inhalation, the hydrocarbon is rapidly absorbed and distributed throughout the body. However, hexane is rapidly metabolised and hence has only a short biological half-life. The urine is the most important route of excretion for this compound.

The principal metabolites of hexane are similar in most mammalian species. Initially, hexane is converted to hexa*n*-2-ol, though smaller quantities of hexan-1-ol and hexan-3-ol can also be formed. Secondary metabolites derived from hexan-2-ol include 2,5-hexanedione, 2,5-dimethylfuran, methyl-*n*-butyl ketone and g-valero-lactone (Couri *et al* 1978, Perbellini *et al* 1980, Baker and Rickert 1981, Perbellini *et al* 1982).

Rats exposed by inhalation to 2-methylpentane were reported to excrete only 2-methylpentan-2-ol in the urine while rats exposed to 3-methylpentane excreted both 3-methylpentan-2-ol and 3-methylpentan-3-ol (Frontali *et al* 1981).

2.4 Health effects

2.4.1 Acute and subacute toxicity

In a study of the acute toxicity of hexane in Sprague–Dawley rats, oral LD50s of 15.8 g/kg, 32.3 g/kg and 28.7 g/kg were reported for 14-day-old animals, young adults and older adults respectively (Kimura *et al* 1971).

Other than a moderate accumulation of lipid, no evidence for liver cell injury was found in guinea-pigs given a single dose of 1000 mg/kg of hexane by intraperitoneal injection. After a dose of 500 mg/kg, there was only slight accumulation of lipid (Divincenzo and Krasavage 1974).

In a subacute study, rats were given doses of 660 mg/kg/day of *n*-hexane by intraperitoneal injection for either 2 days, 7 days, or twice weekly for 45 days. Hepatic necrosis was evident only in the group treated for 45 days. A decrease in serum albumin, total protein, cholesterol, acetylcholinesterase and carboxylesterase activities was found in animals treated for 7 days and 45 days but not at 2 days.

Elevated activity of serum alkaline phosphatase was found in the same groups, though serum FDP aldolase activity was enhanced in all three treatment groups (Goel *et al* 1982).

New Zealand rabbits exposed by inhalation to 3000 ppm of *n*-hexane, 8 hours/day for 8 days, exhibited toxicity in the lung characterised by centriacinar emphysema and micro-haemorrhages (Lungarella *et al* 1980).

2.4.2 Chronic toxicity

It is well documented that the major chronic effect of exposure to *n*-hexane in experimental animals and man is neurotoxicity. The nerve lesion is characterised by giant axonal swelling associated with the accumulation of neurofilaments. The biochemical mechanism of *n*-hexane neurotoxicity is unclear, although a γ-diketone metabolite, 2,5-hexanedione, appears to be important.

In a study of *n*-hexane, 2-methylpentane and 3-methylpentane, groups of five to seven male Wistar rats were given oral doses of 0.4 ml/day for 4 weeks, 0.6 ml/day for the next two weeks and 1.2 ml/day for the last 2 weeks of the treatment period. The hexane-treated rats showed a marked impairment of tail nerve conduction velocity. Significant impairment was also produced by the other two alkanes though they were less effective than *n*-hexane (Ono *et al* 1981). No clinical evidence (eg severe hindlimb weakness) or histological evidence of neuropathy was found in groups of five male Charles River rats treated by gavage with either 570 or 1140 mg/kg body weight/day of *n*-hexane, 5 days/week over a period of 90 days. At a dose of 4000 mg/kg body weight/day, 3/5 rats exhibited clinical evidence of neuropathy while 4/5 exhibited histological evidence of neuropathy. Testicular atrophy was also evident in this treatment group (Krasavage *et al* 1980).

Wistar rats exposed to 3000 ppm of *n*-hexane 12 hours/day, 7 days/week for 16 weeks, exhibited depression of body weight gain and compromised motor nerve conduction velocity, distal latency and mixed nerve conduction velocities of the tail nerve. Microscopic examination revealed damage to the peripheral nerve fibres and muscle fibres, and denervated neuromuscular junctions (Takeuchi *et al* 1981). In a study of male Sprague–Dawley rats exposed by inhalation to 500, 1500 or 5000 ppm of *n*-hexane, 1500 ppm of 2-methylpentane or 1500 ppm of 3-methylpentane for up to 14 weeks, histological evidence of neuropathy was found only in the group exposed to 5000 ppm of hexane (Frontali *et al* 1981). In the same study, rats exposed to hexane for 30 weeks exhibited neuropathy at a concentration of 2500 ppm but not at 500 ppm. However, Schaumburg and Spencer (1976) reported peripheral neuropathy in rats exposed to 400–600 ppm for 45–69 days.

A group of 12 male New Zealand rabbits were exposed by inhalation to 3000 ppm of *n*-hexane, 8 hours/day, 5 days/week for 24 weeks. After a further 120 days in clean air, the animals were sacrificed and the lungs examined by light and transmission electron microscopy. Pathological changes included enlargement of air spaces of the respiratory bronchioles and alveolar ducts, scattered foci of pulmonary fibrosis and focal proliferation of the non-ciliated bronchiolar epithelial cells. No clinical evidence of neuropathy or changes in body weight gain were reported in this study (Lungarella *et al* 1984).

In man, *n*-hexane neuropathy has been most commonly reported following occupational exposure. However, solvent abuse has also resulted in cases of hexane neurotoxicity.

2.4.3 Genotoxicity

Hexane was not found to be mutagenic in the Ames test to *Salmonella typhimurium* TA92, TA1535, TA100, TA1537, TA94 and TA98, either in the presence or absence of metabolic activation, at doses up to 10 mg/plate (Ishidate *et al* 1984). A negative result for mutagenicity has also been reported in mammalian cells (V79 Chinese hamster cells) *in vitro,* in which resistance to ouabain was the genetic marker (Lankas *et al* 1978).

Although there was no evidence for chromosome aberrations, an increased percentage of polyploid cells was found when a Chinese hamster fibroblast cell line was incubated with hexane (0.5 mg/ml) for 48 hours (Ishidate *et al* 1984).

2.4.4 Carcinogenicity

Hexane gave no evidence for tumour promotion when 20 μl of a solution in cyclohexane (20 g/100 ml) was applied to the initiated skin of Swiss mice, thrice weekly for 60 weeks (Sice 1966).

2.4.5 Reproductive toxicity

No teratogenic effects were found in the offspring of female CD-1 mice given either 260, 660, 1320 or 2200 mg/kg/day of *n*-hexane by gavage on days 6–15 of gestation. Maternal toxicity was observed at the high dose level. In the same study, pregnant mice were given 2170, 2830, 7920 or 9900 mg/kg/day by gavage (in three doses) on days 6–15 of gestation. There was no evidence of malformations in the offspring though average foetal body weights were lower than controls at the top two dose levels. With the exception of the low dose all the other treatments produced marked maternal toxicity (Marks *et al* 1980).

Pregnant F-344 rats were exposed by inhalation to 1000 ppm of *n*-hexane on days 8–12, 12–16 or 8–16 of gestation. There was no evidence of embryotoxic or teratogenic effects, but the postnatal growth of pups born from dams exposed on days 8–16 of gestation was significantly decreased compared to controls for up to 3 weeks after birth. Seven weeks after birth the litter weights had returned to normal (Bus *et al* 1979). In another study, no signs of neuropathy, or differences in litter size, sex ratio, age at eye opening or growth rate were found in Sprague–Dawley rats exposed by inhalation to either 0, 100, 2000 or 10 000 ppm of *n*-hexane, 7 hours/day for 15 days prior to conception and through to the 18th day of gestation (Howell and Cooper 1981).

2.5 Discussion

Isomers of hexane were frequently detected in UK drinking water in a WRc survey. Hexane has also been detected in the atmosphere.

The *n*-isomer of hexane is the alkane which has been most comprehensively studied with respect to its toxicity. Neuropathy has been reported in workers occupationally exposed to *n*-hexane and in glue sniffers inhaling products containing hexane. Studies in experimental animals have also demonstrated the neurotoxicity of this compound though there is relatively little information available on long-term effects at low doses particularly by the oral route of exposure. There is good evidence that 2,5-hexanedione is the neurotoxic metabolite of hexane.

The limited studies available indicate that *n*-hexane is non-genotoxic in bacteria or mammalian cells and is of very low reproductive toxicity in rats and mice. A full carcinogenicity study on hexane does not appear to have been carried out.

References

BAKER T S and RICKERT D E (1981) Dose-dependent uptake, distribution and elimination of inhaled *n*-hexane in the Fischer-344 rat. *Toxicology and Applied Pharmacology* **61,** 414-422.

BERTSCH W, CHANG R C and ZLATKIS A (1974) The determination of organic volatiles in air pollution studies: characterisation of profiles. *Journal of Chromatographic Science* **12,** 175-182.

BUS J S, WHITE E L, TYL R W and BARROW C S (1979) Perinatal toxicity and metabolism of *n*-hexane in Fischer-344 rats after inhalation exposure during gestation. *Toxicology and Applied Pharmacology* **51,** 295-302.

COURI D, ABDEL-RAHMAN M S and HETLAND L B (1978) Biotransformation of *n*-hexane and methyl *n*-butyl ketone in guinea pigs and mice. *American Industrial Hygiene Association Journal* **39,** 295-300.

DIVINCENZO G D and KRASAVAGE W J (1974) Serum ornithine carbamyl transferase as a liver response test for exposure to organic solvents. *American Industrial Hygiene Association Journal* **35,** 21-29.

FRONTALI N, AMANTINI M C, SPAGNOLO A, GUARCINI A M, SALTARI M C, BRUGNONE F and PERBELLINI L (1981) Experimental neurotoxicity and urinary metabolites of the C_5–C_7 aliphatic hydrocarbons used as glue solvents in shoe manufacture. *Clinical Toxicology* **18,** 1357-1367.

GOEL S K, RAO G S and PANDYA K P (1982) Toxicity of *n*-hexane and *n*-heptane: Some biochemical changes in liver and serum. *Toxicology Letters* **14,** 169-174.

HOLZER G, SHANFIELD H, ZLATKIS A, BERTSCH W, JUAREZ P, MAYFIELD H and LIEBICH H M (1977) Collection and analysis of trace organic emissions from natural sources. *Journal of Chromatography* **142,** 755-764.

HOWELL W E and COOPER G P (1981) Neurophysiological evaluation of prenatal *n*-hexane toxicity. *Toxicologist* **1,** 152.

IOFFE B V, ISIDOROV V A and ZENKEVICH I G (1977) Gas chromatographic–mass spectrometric determination of volatile organic compounds in an urban atmosphere. *Journal of Chromatography* **142,** 787-795.

ISHIDATE M Jr, SOFUNI T, YOSHIKAWA K, HAYASHI M, NOHMI T, SAWADA M and MATSUOKA A (1984) Primary mutagenicity screening of food additives currently used in Japan. *Food and Chemical Toxicology* **22,** 623-636.

KIMURA E T, EBERT D M and DODGE P W (1971) Acute toxicity and limits of solvent residue for sixteen organic solvents. *Toxicology and Applied Pharmacology* **19,** 699-704.

KRASAVAGE W J, O'DONOGHUE J L, DiVINCENZO G D and TERHAAR C

J (1980) The relative neurotoxicity of methyl-*n*-butyl ketone, *n*-hexane and their metabolites. *Toxicology and Applied Pharmacology* **52,** 433-441.

LANKAS G R, BAXTER C S and CHRISTIAN R T (1978) Effect of alkane tumor-promoting agents on chemically induced mutagenesis in cultured V79 Chinese hamster cells. *Journal of Toxicology and Environmental Health* **4,** 37-41.

LUNGARELLA G, FONZI L and CENTINI F (1980) Respiratory tract lesions induced in rabbits by short-term exposure to *n*-hexane. *Research Communications in Chemical Pathology and Pharmacology* **29,** 129-139.

LUNGARELLA G, BARNI-COMPARINI I and FONZI L (1984) Pulmonary changes induced in rabbits by long-term exposure to *n*-hexane. *Archives of Toxicology* **55,** 224-228.

MARKS T A, FISHER P W and STAPLES R E (1980) Influence of *n*-hexane on embryo and fetal development in mice. *Drug and Chemical Toxicology* **3,** 393-406.

ONO Y, TAKEUCHI Y and HISANAGA N (1981) A comparative study on the toxicity of *n*-hexane and its isomers on the peripheral nerve. *International Archives of Occupational and Environmental Health* **48,** 289-294.

PERBELLINI L, BRUGNONE F and PAVAN I (1980) Identification of the metabolites of *n*-hexane, cyclohexane and their isomers in men's urine. *Toxicology and Applied Pharmacology* **53,** 220-229.

PERBELLINI L, AMANTINI M C, BRUGNONE F and FRONTALI N (1982) Urinary excretion of *n*-hexane metabolites. A comparative study in rat, rabbit and monkey. *Archives of Toxicology* **50,** 203-215.

SCHAUMBURG H H and SPENCER P S (1976) Degeneration in central and peripheral nervous systems produced by pure *n*-hexane: An experimental study. *Brain* **99,** 182-192.

SICE J (1966) Tumor-promoting activity of *n*-alkanes and 1-alkanols. *Toxicology and Applied Pharmacology* **9,** 70-74.

TAKEUCHI Y, ONO Y, HISANAGA N, KITOH J and SUGIURA Y (1981) A comparative study of the toxicity of *n*-pentane, *n*-hexane and *n*-heptane to the peripheral nerve of the rat. *Clinical Toxicology* **18,** 1395-1402.

VERSCHUEREN K (1983) *Handbook of environmental data on organic chemicals,* 2nd edn. Van Nostrand Reinhold Company.

WATER RESEARCH CENTRE (1981) Organic micropollutants in drinking water. WRc Technical Report TR 159.

3. HEPTANE

3.1 Introduction

Heptane (C_7H_{16}) is used as a standard in testing the knock of gasoline engines. As a component of a complex mixture of hydrocarbons, it is also used as a fuel, solvent, thinner, degreasant, dry-cleaning agent and lubricant. The straight–chain isomer has a solubility in water of 3 mg/l at 20°C (Verschueren 1983).

3.2 Exposure

Two unspecified heptane isomers were detected in UK drinking water in the WRc survey. The isomers were identified in 7/14 and 2/14 samples respectively (Water

Research Centre 1981).

Heptane isomers have also been detected in the atmosphere (Grob and Grob 1971, Bertsch *et al* 1974, Holzer *et al* 1977, Ioffe *et al* 1977).

3.3 Toxicokinetics

There is relatively little information available on the metabolism of heptane.

Female Wistar rats exposed by inhalation to 2000 ppm of *n*-heptane, 6 hours/day, 5 days/week for 12 weeks, achieved a steady-state excretion of urinary metabolites after the second day. The major metabolites were found to be sulphate and glucuronide conjugates of heptan-2-ol, 6-hydroxyheptan-2-one and heptan-3-ol. Other minor metabolites included 2,5- and 2,6-heptanedione (Bahima *et al* 1984).

An earlier *in vitro* study using rat liver microsomes also showed that *n*-heptane could be converted to a wide range of oxidised metabolites (Frommer *et al* 1972).

3.4 Health effects

3.4.1 Acute and subacute toxicity

There appears to be no record in the literature of an oral LD50 value for heptane. An intravenous LD50 for *n*-heptane of 222 mg/kg has been reported in the mouse (Jeppsson 1975).

Rats dosed by intraperitoneal injection with 1.0 ml/kg (680 mg/kg) of *n*-heptane, daily, for 2 or 7 days, or twice weekly for 45 days exhibited microscopic changes in the liver only in those animals treated for 45 days. A significant decrease in serum protein, albumin, cholesterol and acetylcholinesterase and carboxylesterase activities was found after 7 and 45 days. A significant increase in serum alkaline phosphatase activity was also found after 7 and 45 days though serum FDP aldolase activity was elevated in all three groups (Goel *et al* 1982).

Heptane induced anaesthesia in mice exposed by inhalation to 16 000 ppm for 5 minutes. At a concentration of 48 000 ppm, three of four mice died (Swann *et al* 1974).

There was no evidence of neuropathy in male Wistar rats exposed by inhalation to 100, 500 or 1500 ppm of *n*-heptane, 6 hours/day, 5 days/week for 2 weeks. An increase in brain acid proteinase activity was evident during the second week but this was abolished 2 weeks after cessation of exposure (Savolainen and Pfaffli 1980).

3.4.2 Chronic toxicity

The studies available at present indicate that heptane does not induce neuropathy in experimental animals. It has been suggested that this is due to the formation of only small quantities of γ-diketone metabolites with heptane (Bahima *et al* 1984).

Groups of six to nine male Sprague–Dawley rats exposed by inhalation to 1500 ppm of *n*-heptane, 9 hours/day, 5 days/week for up to 30 weeks, did not show any changes in body weight gain or histology of peripheral nerves (Frontali *et al* 1981). Similarly, Takeuchi *et al* (1981) reported no electrophysiological or histological changes in the peripheral nerves of groups of seven male Wistar rats exposed by inhalation to 3000 ppm, 12 hours/day, 7 days/week for up to 16 weeks. In this study, depression of body weight gain was reported after 8 weeks but not at any other period. In the most recent study, no clinical evidence of neuropathy was observed in female Wistar rats exposed by inhalation to 2000 ppm of *n*-heptane, 6 hours/day, 5 days/week for 12 weeks (Bahima *et al* 1984).

Very little evidence of neurotoxicity was found in a group of 18 tyre workers exposed to solvent fumes containing more than 95% *n*-heptane for periods ranging from 1 to 9 years (Crespi *et al* 1979).

3.4.3 Genotoxicity
No information appears to be available.

3.4.4 Carcinogenicity
No information appears to be available.

3.4.5 Reproductive toxicity
No information appears to be available.

3.5 Discussion
There is relatively little toxicological information available on heptane and none at all by the oral route. However, heptane does not appear to possess the neurotoxic properties of hexane and would appear unlikely to present a risk to human health at the very low concentrations encountered in drinking water.

References

BAHIMA J, CERT A and MENENDEZ-GALLEGO M (1984) Identification of volatile metabolites of inhaled *n*-heptane in rat urine. *Toxicology and Applied Pharmacology* **76,** 473-482.

BERTSCH W, CHANG R C and ZLATKIS A (1974) The determination of organic volatiles in air pollution studies: characterisation of profiles. *Journal of Chromatographic Science* **12,** 175-182.

CRESPI V, DI COSTANZO M, FERRARIO F and TREDICI G (1979) Electrophysiological findings in workers exposed to *n*-heptane fumes. *Journal of Neurology* **222,** 135-138.

FROMMER U, ULLRICH V, STAUDINGER H and ORRENIUS S (1972) The monooxygenation of *n*-heptane by rat liver microsomes. *Biochimica et Biophysica Acta* **280,** 487-494.

FRONTALI N, AMANTINI M C, SPAGNOLO A, GUARCINI A M, SALTARI M C, BRUGNONE F and PERBELLINI L (1981) Experimental neurotoxicity and urinary metabolites of the C_5–C_7 aliphatic hydrocarbons used as glue solvents in shoe manufacture. *Clinical Toxicology* **18,** 1357-1367.

GOEL S K, RAO G S and PANDYA K P (1982) Toxicity of *n*-hexane and *n*-heptane: Some biochemical changes in liver and serum. *Toxicology Letters* **14,** 169-174.

GROB K and GROB G (1971) Gas-liquid chromatographic-mass spectrometric investigation of C_6-C_{20} organic compounds in an urban atmosphere. An application of ultra trace analysis on capillary columns. *Journal of Chromatography* **62,** 1.

HOLZER G, SHANFIELD H, ZLATKIS A, BERTSCH W, JUAREZ P, MAY-

FIELD H and LIEBICH H M (1977) Collection and analysis of trace organic emissions from natural sources. *Journal of Chromatography* **142,** 755-764.

IOFFE B V, ISIDOROV V A and ZENKEVICH I G (1977) Gas chromatographic–mass spectrometric determination of volatile organic compounds in an urban atmosphere. *Journal of Chromatography* **142,** 787-795.

JEPPSSON R (1975) Parabolic relationship between lipophilicity and biological activity of aliphatic hydrocarbons, ethers and ketones after intravenous injections of emulsion formulations into mice. *Acta Pharmacologica et Toxicologica* **37,** 56-64.

SAVOLAINEN H and PFAFFLI P (1980) Neurochemical effects on rats of *n*-heptane inhalation exposure. *Archives of Environmental Contamination and Toxicology* **9,** 727-732.

SWANN H E Jr, KWON B K, HOGAN G K and SNELLINGS W M (1974) Acute inhalation toxicology of volatile hydrocarbons. *American Industrial Hygiene Association Journal* **35,** 511-518.

TAKEUCHI Y, ONO Y, HISANAGA N, KITOH J and SUGIURA Y (1981) A comparative study of the toxicity of *n*-pentane, *n*-hexane and *n*-heptane to the peripheral nerve of the rat. *Clinical Toxicology* **18,** 1395-1402.

VERSCHUEREN K (1983) *Handbook of environmental data on organic chemicals.* 2nd edn. Van Nostrand Reinhold Company.

WATER RESEARCH CENTRE (1981) Organic micropollutants in drinking water. WRc Technical Report TR 159.

4. OCTANE

4.1 Introduction

Octane (C_8H_{18}) is widely used in organic synthesis, in the rubber industry, paper processing industry and as a solvent. The *n*-octane isomer has a solubility in water of 0.7 mg/l at 20°C (Verschueren 1983). The solubility of the other isomers decreases with increasing branching of the carbon chain.

4.2 Exposure

Octane was detected in 4/14 drinking water samples in the WRc survey (Water Research Centre 1981).

Thorburn and Colenutt (1979) reported an average octane concentration of 14.6 ppb in the atmosphere near the M1 at Luton and an average concentration of 5.6 ppb in a relatively rural area at Freshwater (IOW). Isomers of octane have also been identified in the atmosphere in other studies (Grob and Grob 1971, Bertsch *et al* 1974, Raymond and Guiochon 1974, Holzer *et al* 1977, Ioffe *et al* 1977).

4.3 Toxicokinetics

There is very limited information available on the toxicokinetics of octane.

Holmberg *et al* (1977) found higher concentrations of octane in the liver, brain and kidney compared to the blood in mice exposed to this compound for short periods by inhalation. The organ/blood ratio was found to increase with increasing concentration, the ratio being 30 times greater at 10 000 ppm than 100 ppm.

Rats exposed by inhalation to about 100 ppm of radiolabelled *n*-octane for 24 hours, and followed for up to 7 days, converted 60–70% of the total radioactivity used to metabolites. About 44% of the material metabolised was found in the urine, 21% in the faeces and 36% as carbon dioxide. A significant amount of radiolabelled material remained in the liver and kidneys (Brown and Salmon 1984).

4.4 Health effects

4.4.1 Acute and subacute toxicity

In the rat, intraperitoneal injection of 1.0 ml/kg/day (700 mg/kg) of *n*-octane for 2 or 7 days was found to lower hepatic mixed function oxidase activity. Depression of body weight gain and an increase in relative liver weight were only reported after treatment for 7 days (Khan and Pandya 1980, Khan *et al* 1980). A number of other biochemical changes have been reported in identical studies including elevated activity of alkaline phosphatase in the liver, spleen and bone marrow (Pandya and Khan 1982), lowered serum protein, albumin, cholesterol, acetylcholinesterase and carboxylesterase activities and an increase in the activity of serum FDP aldolase (Khan and Pandya 1985).

Iso-octane was not found to induce anaesthesia in mice exposed by inhalation to up to 8000 ppm for 5 minutes. At 16 000 ppm, 1/4 mice died and at 32 000 ppm 4/4 mice died (Swann *et al* 1974).

4.4.2 Chronic toxicity

No information appears to be available.

4.4.3 Genotoxicity

No information appears to be available.

4.4.4 Carcinogenicity

Octane gave no evidence for tumour-promoting activity when 20 μl of a solution in cyclohexane (20 g/100 ml) was applied thrice weekly to the initiated skin of female Swiss mice for 60 weeks (Sice 1966). However, twice weekly application of 60 μl of a solution in cyclohexane (75% v/v) to the initiated skin of male C3H mice for up to 50 weeks was found to produce an increase in the number of skin tumours compared to a solvent control group (Horton *et al* 1981).

4.4.5 Reproductive toxicity

No information appears to be available.

4.5 Discussion

There is insufficient toxicological information available for octane on which to base an assessment.

References

BERTSCH W, CHANG R C and ZLATKIS A (1974) The determination of organic volatiles in air pollution studies: characterisation of profiles. *Journal of Chromatographic Science* **12,** 175-182.

BROWN D C and SALMON A G (1984) The metabolism of *n*-octane, a component of white spirit. Poster presented at the British Toxicology Society Conference, University of Newcastle, 20/21 Sept 1984.

GROB K and GROB G (1971) Gas–liquid chromatographic–mass spectrometric investigation of C_6-C_{20} organic compounds in an urban atmosphere. An application of ultra trace analysis on capillary columns. *Journal of Chromatography* **62,** 1.

HOLMBERG B, JAKOBSON I and SIGVARDSSON K (1977) A study on the distribution of methylchloroform and *n*-octane in the mouse during and after inhalation. *Scandinavian Journal of Work Environment and Health* **3,** 43-52.

HOLZER G, SHANFIELD H, ZLATKIS A, BERTSCH W, JUAREZ P, MAYFIELD H and LIEBICH H M (1977) Collection and analysis of trace organic emissions from natural sources. *Journal of Chromatography* **142,** 755-764.

HORTON A W, BOLEWICZ L C, BARSTAD A W and BUTTS C K (1981) Comparison of the promoting activity of pristane and *n*-alkanes in skin carcinogenesis with their physical effects on micellar models of biological membranes. *Biochimica et Biophysica Acta* **648,** 107-112.

IOFFE B V, ISIDOROV V A and ZENKEVICH I G (1977) Gas chromatographic–mass spectrometric determination of volatile organic compounds in an urban atmosphere. *Journal of Chromatography* **142,** 787-795.

KHAN S and PANDYA K P (1980) Biochemical studies on the toxicity of *n*-octane and *n*-nonane. *Environmental Research* **22,** 271-276.

KHAN S and PANDYA K P (1985) Hepatotoxicity in albino rats exposed to *n*-octane and *n*-nonane. *Journal of Applied Toxicology* **5,** 64-68.

KHAN S, MUKHTAR H and PANDYA K P (1980) *n*-Octane and *n*-nonane induced alterations in xenobiotic metabolising enzyme activities and lipid peroxidation of rat liver. *Toxicology* **16,** 239-245.

PANDYA K P and KHAN S (1982) Effect of *n*-octane and *n*-nonane administration on alkaline phosphatase activity in tissues of female rats. *Biochemical Pharmacology* **31,** 201-203.

RAYMOND A and GUIOCHON G (1974) Gas chromatographic analysis of C_8–C_{18} hydrocarbons in Paris air. *Environmental Science & Technology* **8,** 143-148.

SICE J (1966) Tumor-promoting activity of *n*-alkanes and 1-alkanols. *Toxicology and Applied Pharmacology* **9,** 70-74.

SWANN H E Jr, KWON B K, HOGAN G K and SNELLINGS W M (1974) Acute inhalation toxicology of volatile hydrocarbons. *American Industrial Hygiene Association Journal* **35,** 511-518.

THORBURN S and COLENUTT B A (1979) A gas chromatographic comparison of volatile organic compounds in urban and rural atmospheres. *International Journal of Environmental Studies* **13,** 265-271.

VERSCHUEREN K (1983) *Handbook of environmental data on organic chemicals*,

2nd edn. Van Nostrand Reinhold Company.
WATER RESEARCH CENTRE (1981) Organic micropollutants in drinking water. WRc Technical Report TR 159.

5. NONANE

5.1 Introduction

Nonane (C_9H_{20}) is used in the manufacture of paraffin products and in the rubber and paper processing industries. The *n*-nonane isomer has a solubility of 0.07 mg/l at 20°C (Verschueren 1983). The solubility of the other isomers decreases with increasing branching of the carbon chain.

5.2 Exposure

n-Nonane was identified in 10/14 drinking water samples. Seven other unspecified nonane isomers were also detected in the survey, the most common occurring in up to 6/14 samples (Water Research Centre 1981).

Thorburn and Colenutt (1979) detected nonane in the atmosphere at levels of 13.4 ppb near the M1 at Luton and 3.6 ppb at Freshwater (IOW). Other studies have also detected nonane isomers in the atmosphere (Grob and Grob 1971, Bertsch *et al* 1974, Raymond and Guiochon 1974, Ioffe *et al* 1977).

5.3 Toxicokinetics

No information appears to be available.

5.4 Health effects

5.4.1 Acute and subacute toxicity

An intravenous LD50 for nonane of 219 mg/kg has been reported in the mouse (Jeppsson 1975).

Rats dosed by intraperitoneal injection with 1.0 ml/kg/day (720 mg/kg) of *n*-nonane for 2 or 7 days exhibited a reduction in hepatic mixed function oxidase activity. At 7 days, depression of body weight gain and an increase in relative liver weight were also noted (Khan and Pandya 1980, Khan *et al* 1980). In identical studies, a number of other biochemical changes were reported including elevated activity of alkaline phosphatase in the liver, spleen and bone marrow (Pandya and Khan 1982), lowered serum protein, albumin, cholesterol, acetylcholinesterase and carboxylesterase activities, and an increase in serum FDP aldolase activity (Khan and Pandya 1985).

An LD50 of 3200 ppm was reported for rats exposed to *n*-nonane vapour for 4 hours and then held for 14 days. Rats exposed to 1500 ppm, 6 hours/day for 7 days, exhibited slight irritation of the eyes and extremities, mild tremors and some uncoordination (Carpenter *et al* 1978).

5.4.2 Chronic toxicity

Carpenter *et al* (1978) exposed groups of 25 male Harlan–Wistar rats to 0, 360, 590 or 1600 ppm of *n*-nonane vapour for up to 13 weeks. Only rats exposed to 1600 ppm exhibited depression of body weight gain. No treatment-related changes in histopathology, haematology, clinical chemistry or urine analyses were found.

5.4.3 Genotoxicity

No information appears to be available.

5.4.4 Carcinogenicity

No information appears to be available.

5.4.5 Reproductive toxicity

No information appears to be available.

5.5 Discussion

There is insufficient information available for nonane on which to base an assessment.

References

BERTSCH W, CHANG R C and ZLATKIS A (1974) The determination of organic volatiles in air pollution studies: characterisation of profiles. *Journal of Chromatographic Science* **12,** 175-182.

CARPENTER C P, GEARY D L Jr, MYERS R C, NACHREINER D J, SULLIVAN L J and KING J M (1978) Petroleum hydrocarbon toxicity studies. *17.* Animal response to *n*-nonane vapor. *Toxicology and Applied Pharmacology* **44,** 53-61.

GROB K and GROB G (1971) Gas–liquid chromatographic–mass spectrometric investigation of C_6–C_{20} organic compounds in an urban atmosphere. An application of ultra trace analysis on capillary columns. *Journal of Chromatography* **62,** 1.

IOFFE B V, ISIDOROV V A and ZENKEVICH I G (1977) Gas chromatographic–mass spectrometric determination of volatile organic compounds in an urban atmosphere. *Journal of Chromatography* **142,** 787-795.

JEPPSSON R (1975) Parabolic relationship between lipophilicity and biological activity of aliphatic hydrocarbons, ethers and ketones after intravenous injections of emulsion formulations into mice. *Acta Pharmacologica et Toxicologica* **37,** 56-64.

KHAN S and PANDYA K P (1980) Biochemical studies on the toxicity of *n*-octane and *n*-nonane. *Environmental Research* **22,** 271-276.

KHAN S and PANDYA K P (1985) Hepatotoxicity in albino rats exposed to *n*-octane and *n*-nonane. *Journal of Applied Toxicology* **5**, 64-68.

KHAN S, MUKHTAR H and PANDYA K P (1980) *n*-Octane and *n*-nonane induced alterations in xenobiotic metabolising enzyme activities and lipid peroxidation of rat liver. *Toxicology* **16,** 239-245.

PANDYA K P and KHAN S (1982) Effect of *n*-octane and *n*-nonane administration

on alkaline phosphatase activity in tissues of female rats. *Biochemical Pharmacology* **31,** 201-203.
RAYMOND A and GUIOCHON G (1974) Gas chromatographic analysis of C_8–C_{18} hydrocarbons in Paris air. *Environmental Science & Technology* **8,** 143-148.
THORBURN S and COLENUTT B A (1979) A gas chromatographic comparison of volatile organic compounds in urban and rural atmospheres. *International Journal of Environmental Studies* **13,** 265-271.
VERSCHUEREN K (1983) *Handbook of environmental data on organic chemicals*, 2nd edn. Van Nostrand Reinhold Company.
WATER RESEARCH CENTRE (1981) Organic micropollutants in drinking water. WRc Technical Report TR 159.

6. C_{10} TO C_{20} ALKANES

6.1 Introduction

The higher alkanes, as a complex mixture, are used as fuels, solvents, thinners, degreasants, dry-cleaning agents and lubricants. These compounds tend to be less water-soluble than the lower alkanes. The *n*-isomer of decane has a solubility of 0.009 mg/l at 20°C (Verschueren 1983).

6.2 Exposure

Each of the alkanes from C_{10} through to C_{20} were found in at least two of the 14 samples examined in the WRc survey, decane being found in all 14 samples, undecane in 12/14 and dodecane in 11/14 (Water Research Centre 1981). In a Japanese study, most of the *n*-alkanes from C_{11} through to C_{29} were identified in tap water (Akiyama *et al* 1980).

Thorburn and Colenutt (1979) found levels of C_{10}–C_{14} alkanes ranging from 2.5 to 14.9 ppb in the atmosphere near the M1 at Luton. Slightly lower levels were present in the atmosphere at Freshwater (IOW). Higher alkanes have also been detected in the atmosphere in other studies (Grob and Grob 1971, Bertsch *et al* 1974, Raymond and Guiochon 1974, Holzer *et al* 1977, Ioffe *et al* 1977).

6.3 Toxicokinetics

Early studies demonstrated that a large proportion of an oral dose of *n*-hexadecane was absorbed by rats (El Mahdi and Channon 1933) and cats (Channon and Devine 1934), and that much of the dose was oxidised to fatty acids (Stetten 1943). Albro and Fishbein (1970) found an inverse linear relationship between percentage retention of oral doses of higher alkanes in rats and alkane chain length.

Following oral doses of radiolabelled hexadecane and octadecane in rats, up to 12% of the label was recovered in hepatic lipids. Hexadecane and octadecane were converted mainly to the C_{16} and C_{18} fatty acids respectively (McCarthy 1964).

In male Wistar rats given single doses of either 5 or 1000 mg/kg body-weight of radiolabelled *n*-heptadecane in the diet, about 55% of the radiolabel was eliminated as carbon dioxide within 6 hours. For six days following exposure, only very small quantities of label were found in the urine and faeces. At the end of this period between 25% and 37% of the radiolabel remained in the animal tissues, probably incorporated into lipids (Tulliez and Bories 1977). The rate of oxidation of *n*-heptadecane *in vitro* was much greater with hepatic microsomes from chicken than those from rat or rabbit (Perdu-Durand and Tulliez 1985).

In two Jersey cows, most of an oral dose of octadecane was excreted in the faeces (Bartley *et al* 1971).

6.4 Health effects

6.4.1 Acute and subacute toxicity

Intravenous LD50s in the mouse of 517, 1163 and 3505 mg/kg have been reported for *n*-undecane, *n*-tridecane and *n*-pentadecane respectively (Jeppsson 1975).

The effects of several of the C_6–C_{20} *n*-alkanes on the skin of miniature swine was studied by 48-hour closed patch tests (Motoyoshi *et al* 1979). The most irritant members of the group, *n*-octane and *n*-decane, caused severe blister formation and surface necrosis. With the exception of *n*-eicosane, all the alkanes tested were irritant to some degree. In more detailed studies with *n*-hexadecane, this alkane was found to be severely irritant to the skin of rabbits, guinea-pigs, rats and human volunteers (Motoyoshi *et al* 1979). Komatsu *et al* (1979) have also found that decane was irritant to rabbit skin, inducing a marked reduction in the biosynthesis of lipids, RNA and DNA during the first 3 days after application.

6.4.2 Chronic toxicity

Rats exposed by inhalation to 540 ppm of *n*-decane for 18 hours/day, 7 days/week for 57 days, exhibited a significant increase in body weight gain and a reduction in total white blood cell count. No histopathological changes were reported (Nau *et al* 1966).

6.4.3 Genotoxicity

n-Eicosane was not mutagenic in the Ames test to *Salmonella typhimurium* TA1535, TA1537, TA100 and TA98, in either the presence or absence of metabolic activation, at a dose level of up to 15 μmol/plate (Florin *et al* 1980).

Linear alkanes of even chain length C_{10} to C_{16} were not found to be mutagenic in V79 Chinese hamster cells where resistance to ouabain was the genetic marker (Lankas *et al* 1978).

6.4.4 Carcinogenicity

The only information available for the higher alkanes is on their carcinogenicity and tumour-promoting activity in mouse skin. Although none of the C_{10}–C_{20} alkanes have given any evidence for carcinogenic potential in this system, several have been shown to have marked tumour-promoting potential (Horton *et al* 1957, Saffiotti and Shubik 1963, Sice 1966, Horton and Christian 1974, Horton *et al* 1976, Van Duuren and Goldschmidt 1976, Horton *et al* 1981).

6.4.5 Reproductive toxicity

No information appears to be available.

6.5 Discussion

In a WRc survey, a large range of C_{10}–C_{20} paraffins were detected in UK drinking water. Such paraffins are the major constituents of many petroleum-type mixtures which are used as fuel. Hence the atmosphere is likely to represent another important source of exposure to these compounds.

Information on their metabolism is relatively limited, though it would appear that they are readily absorbed from the gastrointestinal tract and incorporated mainly into lipids.

Toxicological data on these compounds are very sparse. The information available suggests that they are of low acute toxicity and do not appear to have genotoxic potential. However, these compounds are irritant to the skin at high dose levels and have been shown to have tumour-promoting activity in the mouse skin system.

Although these compounds in themselves would not appear to present a risk to health at low concentrations in drinking water, their influence on the toxicity of other organics in drinking water requires study.

References

AKIYAMA T, KOGA M, SHINOHARA R, KIDO A and ETOH S (1980) Detection and identification of trace organic substances in the aquatic environment. *Journal of Uoeh* **2,** 285-300.

ALBRO P W and FISHBEIN L (1970) Absorption of aliphatic hydrocarbons by rats. *Biochimica et Biophysica Acta* **219,** 437-446.

BARTLEY E E, HELMER L G and MEYER R M (1971) Metabolism of ^{14}C-labeled octadecane by cattle. *Journal of Animal Science* **33,** 1351-1355.

BERTSCH W, CHANG R C and ZLATKIS A (1974) The determination of organic volatiles in air pollution studies: characterisation of profiles. *Journal of Chromatographic Science* **12,** 175-182.

CHANNON H J and DEVINE J (1934) The absorption of *n*-hexadecane from the alimentary tract of the cat. *Biochemical Journal* **28,** 467-471.

EL MAHDI M A H and CHANNON H J (1933) The absorption of *n*-hexadecane from the alimentary tract of the rat. *Biochemical Journal* **27,** 1487-1494.

FLORIN I, RUTBERG L, CURVALL M and ENZELL C R (1980) Screening of tobacco smoke constituents for mutagenicity using the Ames test. *Toxicology* **18,** 219-232.

GROB K and GROB G (1971) Gas–liquid chromatographic–mass spectrometric investigation of C_6–C_{20} organic compounds in an urban atmosphere. An application of ultra trace analysis on capillary columns. *Journal of Chromatography* **62,** 1-13.

HOLZER G, SHANFIELD H, ZLATKIS A, BERTSCH W, JUAREZ P, MAYFIELD H and LIEBICH H M (1977) Collection and analysis of trace organic emissions from natural sources. *Journal of Chromatography* **142,** 755-764.

HORTON A W and CHRISTIAN G M (1974) Cocarcinogenic versus incomplete carcinogenic activity among aromatic hydrocarbons: contrast between chrysene and benzo[*b*]triphenylene. *Journal of the National Cancer Institute* **53,** 1017-1020.

HORTON A W, DENMAN D T and TROSSET R P (1957) Carcinogenesis of the skin. 2. The accelerating properties of aliphatic and related hydrocarbons. *Cancer Research* **17,** 758-766.

HORTON A W, ESHLEMAN D N, SCHUFF A R and PERMAN W H (1976) Correlation of cocarcinogenic activity among *n*-alkanes with their physical

effects on phospholipid micelles. *Journal of the National Cancer Institute* **56,** 387-391.
HORTON A W, BOLEWICZ L C, BARSTAD A W and BUTTS C K (1981) Comparison of the promoting activity of pristane and *n*-alkanes in skin carcinogenesis with their physical effects on micellar models of biological membranes. *Biochimica et Biophysica Acta* **648,** 107-112.
IOFFE B V, ISIDOROV V A and ZENKEVICH I G (1977) Gas chromatographic–mass spectrometric determination of volatile organic compounds in an urban atmosphere. *Journal of Chromatography* **142,** 787-795.
JEPPSSON R (1975) Parabolic relationship between lipophilicity and biological activity of aliphatic hydrocarbons, ethers and ketones after intravenous injections of emulsion formulations into mice. *Acta Pharmacologica et Toxicologica* **37,** 56-64.
KOMATSU H, ASABA K and SUZUKI M (1979) Some biochemical effects of isopropyl myristate and squalene on rabbit skin. *Journal of the Society of Cosmetic Chemists* **30,** 263-278.
LANKAS G R, BAXTER C S and CHRISTIAN R T (1978) Effect of alkane tumor-promoting agents on chemically induced mutagenesis in cultured V79 Chinese hamster cells. *Journal of Toxicology and Environmental Health* **4,** 37-41.
McCARTHY R D (1964) Mammalian metabolism of straight-chain saturated hydrocarbons. *Biochimica et Biophysica Acta* **84,** 74-79.
MOTOYOSHI K, TOYOSHIMA Y, SATO M and YOSHIMURA M (1979) Comparative studies on the irritancy of oils and synthetic perfumes to the skin of rabbit, guinea pig, rat, miniature swine and man. *Cosmetics & Toiletries* **94,** 41-48.
NAU C A, NEAL J and THORNTON M (1966) C_9–C_{12} fractions obtained from petroleum distillates. An evaluation of their potential toxicity. *Archives of Environmental Health* **12,** 382-393.
PERDU-DURAND E F and TULLIEZ J E (1985) Hydrocarbon hydroxylation system in liver microsomes from four animal species. *Food and Chemical Toxicology* **23,** 363-366.
RAYMOND A and GUIOCHON G (1974) Gas chromatographic analysis of C_8–C_{18} hydrocarbons in Paris air. *Environmental Science & Technology* **8,** 143-148.
SAFFIOTTI U and SHUBIK P (1963) Studies on promoting action in skin carcinogenesis. National Cancer Institute Monograph No. 10, 489-507.
SICE J (1966) Tumor-promoting activity of *n*-alkanes and 1-alkanols. *Toxicology and Applied Pharmacology* **9,** 70-74.
STETTEN D Jr (1943) Metabolism of a paraffin. *Journal of Biological Chemistry* **147,** 327-332.
THORBURN S and COLENUTT B A (1979) A gas chromatographic comparison of volatile organic compounds in urban and rural atmospheres. *International Journal of Environmental Studies* **13,** 265-271.
TULLIEZ J E and BORIES G F (1977) Metabolism of a *n*-paraffin, heptadecane, in rats. *Lipids* **13,** 110-115.
VAN DUUREN B L and GOLDSCHMIDT B M (1976) Carcinogenic and tumor-promoting agents in tobacco carcinogenesis. *Journal of the National Cancer*

Institute **56,** 1237-1242.
VERSCHUEREN K (1983) *Handbook of environmental data on organic chemicals,* 2nd edn. Van Nostrand Reinhold Company.
WATER RESEARCH CENTRE (1981) Organic micropollutants in drinking water. WRc Technical Report TR 159.

7. THE ALKENES

7.1 Introduction

Alkenes (olefins) do not occur frequently in crude oils but are a feature of refined petroleum products, being produced either by petroleum cracking or pyrolysis of paraffins. They are used as raw materials for polymers, petrochemicals and detergents.

The alkenes are generally more chemically reactive than the alkanes because of the double bond. They also appear to be of slightly greater acute toxicity than the alkanes, probably for the same reason.

7.2 Exposure

A large number of alkenes were identified in a survey of treated waters by WRc (Table 1 of that survey). Two of three hexene isomers were the only compounds frequently detected in the survey (Water Research Centre 1981). There are relatively few other reports on the occurrence of alkenes in drinking water.

The lower alkenes are found in small quantities in ambient air.

7.3 Toxicokinetics

Although there is little published information on the metabolism of the alkenes, one would expect them to be readily absorbed by the gastrointestinal tract followed by rapid metabolism in the liver. Biotransformation probably occurs through one of two pathways: oxidation at the double bond followed by conjugation, and by ω or ω-1 oxidation with subsequent incorporation into unsaturated fatty acid metabolism.

7.4 Health effects

In general, the alkenes are of low acute toxicity in experimental animals. Within the group, chain branching and di-unsaturation tend to increase their toxicity (Sandmeyer 1981). At very high doses, the lower molecular weight members are weak anaesthetics while the higher members are narcotics.

The only toxicological information found for a specific alkene of this group is an intravenous LD50 in the mouse of 100 mg/kg for 5-decene (Registry of Toxic Effects of Chemical Substances).

Three of ten alkenes were shown to inhibit hepatic cytochrome P-450 activity in the rat. The three active compounds, 4-ethyl-1-hexene, 1-heptene and 3-methyl-1-octene, also led to the formation of identical, abnormal, hepatic pigments. It would appear that some alkenes may act as suicide substrates for cytochrome P-450 by alkylating the porphyrin group of the P-450 molecule. When these molecules are broken down and the iron scavenged, abnormal porphyrins are found in the bile (Ortiz de Montellano and Mico 1980).

In a study of Sprague–Dawley rats exposed by inhalation to 215–2049 ppm of polymerization naphtha (alkenes comprise about 92% of the mixture) 6 hours/day, 5 days/week for 15 exposures in 21 days, evidence of kidney damage was found only in males (Halder *et al* 1984). The changes reported in the kidney were similar to those found with unleaded gasoline and synthetic jet fuels described in the overview (Section 1).

7.5 Discussion

There is very little information available on the health effects of alkenes. Despite this, the very low levels of these compounds in drinking water and their rapid metabolism suggests that they probably do not present a significant risk to human health.

References

HALDER C A, WARNE T M and HATOUM N S (1984) Renal toxicity of gasoline and related naphthas in male rats. In: *Advances in Modern Environmental Toxicology Vol 7 Renal Effects of Petroleum Hydrocarbons* ed by M A Mehlman, G P Hemstreet III, J J Thorpe and N K Weaver. Princeton Scientific Publishers Inc, New Jersey, pp 73-88.

ORTIZ DE MONTELLANO P R and MICO B A (1980) Destruction of cytochrome P-450 by ethylene and other olefins. *Molecular Pharmacology* **18,** 128–135.

REGISTRY OF TOXIC EFFECTS OF CHEMICAL SUBSTANCES National Institute for Occupational Safety & Health, Cincinnati, Ohio.

SANDMEYER E E (1981) Aliphatic Hydrocarbons. In: *Patty's Industrial Hygiene and Toxicology* ed by G D Clayton and F E Clayton, 3rd Revised Edition, Volume 2B, John Wiley & Sons, New York pp 3175–3220.

WATER RESEARCH CENTRE (1981) Organic micropollutants in drinking water. WRc Technical Report TR 159.

14

The esters

1. INTRODUCTION

Esters are an important class of industrial chemicals. They are used as additives in the automotive and aircraft industry. They are also used as perfumes and flavourings in the soap and food processing industries. Other applications include use in lacquers, solvents, pharmaceuticals, plastics and resins.

The monocarboxylic acid esters occur frequently in natural products, particularly in fruits, to which they lend their pleasant odour and taste.

2. EXPOSURE

2.1 Air

Methylmethacrylate may be released to ambient air during the drying of acrylic-based paints (Schultz and Gunther 1972).

Vinyl acetate has been detected at levels of 5–10 ppm in the air of factories producing polyvinyl acetate, with maximum levels as high as 300 ppm (Deese and Joiner 1969).

There appear to be no data available on the occurrence of other esters in the atmosphere.

2.2 Food

The majority of esters identified in a survey of 14 drinking waters by WRc (1981) are found naturally in fruits or are used as added flavourings in food (Furia and Bellanca 1971, Food Additives and Contaminants Committee 1978). Food would therefore appear to be the major source of exposure to these compounds.

2.3 Water

Some 38 esters, including 14 phthalates, were identified in UK drinking water by WRc (1981 and 1982). The phthalate esters identified were reviewed previously (Chapter 11). The other esters identified are the subject of this report and are as follows:

Acetyl tri-*n*-butyl citrate
Amyl acetate
Butyl acetate
Dibutyl adipate isomers (two)
Dimethylmethylbenzoate isomer
Ethyl acetate
Ethyl propionate
Methyl benzoate
Methyl butanoate
Methyl iso-butanoate
Methyl laurate
Methyl methacrylate
Methyl-(2-methyl) butanoate
Methyl-(3-methyl) butanoate
Methyl-(2-methyl) propionate
Methyl myristate
Methyl oleate
Methyl palmitate
Methyl pentadecanoate
Methyl pentanoate
Methyl sorbate
Phenyl acetate
Vinyl acetate

The most frequently identified compounds were methyl butanoate, methyl-(2-methyl) butanoate, methyl benzoate, methyl iso-butanoate and methyl palmitate, occurring in from five to nine of 14 samples.

A number of these esters have also been identified in US drinking water (Coleman *et al* 1980).

3. TOXICOKINETICS

Acetate esters are readily absorbed from the gastrointestinal tract and through the lungs (Von Oettingen 1960).

Little information on *in vivo* metabolism of esters is available, but it is probable that esters are hydrolysed by esterases. The products of hydrolysis may be further catabolised by β-oxidation and enter normal intermediary metabolic pathways, or may be excreted by the kidney following conjugation.

The inhalation of vinyl acetate in rats leads to the accumulation of acetaldehyde in the blood (Simon *et al* 1985). The most probable pathway for this is hydrolysis of vinyl acetate to vinyl alcohol followed by oxidation to acetaldehyde.

In rats, most of a single intravenous dose of methyl methacrylate (5.7 mg/kg body weight) was expired as carbon dioxide in 10 days. Similar results were also found following administration of the same dose by oral gavage (Bratt and Hathway 1977).

In vitro studies on the metabolism of esters have shown that all esters investigated were hydrolysed to produce the corresponding acids and alcohols (Gallaher and

Loomis 1975, Longland *et al* 1977, Levey and Ocken 1969, Blickens and Diluzio 1965).

Yoshida *et al* (1970) showed that chicks may utilise methyl esters of fatty acids (carbon chain length 10–14) as sources of energy.

Since the toxic effects of acetaldehyde are similar to those observed after administration of vinyl acetate, namely impaired condition reflex activity and altered brain metabolism in rats (Davis and Walsh 1970, Cohen and Collins 1970), it is possible that this metabolite is responsible for vinyl acetate toxicity.

4. HEALTH EFFECTS

4.1 Acute and subacute toxicity

There are acute toxicity data for about half the compounds in this group. Oral LD50s ranging from 1.4 g/kg to 14.3 g/kg have been reported in the rat (Smyth 1969, Opdyke 1979, Sandmeyer and Kirwin 1981).

Saba and Di-Luzio (1968) have shown that a single dose of methyl palmitate (2 g/kg body weight) given intravenously in rats resulted in reticuloendothelial phagocytic depression, due to hepatic and splenic macrophage impairment. Similar immunologic depressant effects were observed in rats given an intravenous dose (17.5 mg/kg) of methyl pentadecanoate (Di-Luzio and Blickens 1966).

The acetate esters have been shown to cause CNS depression and slight eye and skin irritation in man at concentrations of 3300–14 000 ppm in air (Fassett 1963). The main effects of inhalation of butyl acetate in cats (20 ppm for 6 hours/day, for 6 days) were haematological changes and weight loss (Fassett 1963). Yoshida *et al* (1971) showed that rats were able to utilise butyl acetate and amyl acetate fed as 5% of the available energy in the diet, and that this did not result in any weight loss.

Symptoms of narcosis may be produced in rabbits by sublethal doses of methyl butanoate, butyl acetate and ethyl propionate (Fassett 1963, Munch 1972).

Vinyl acetate caused eye and nose irritation and depression of body weight gain in rats after exposure to 2000 ppm at 6 hours/day for 15 days (Gage 1970). Exposure to 630 ppm or 250 ppm for the same duration also resulted in depression of body weight gain, but all organs were normal at autopsy.

Daily exposure of workers to methyl methacrylate has resulted in contact sensitisation in some cases (Rycroft 1977, Hopkins 1985).

4.2 Chronic toxicity

There appears to be very little information on chronic toxicity of these esters.

Methyl benzoate administered (by an unspecified route) at 0.005 mg/kg and 2.5 mg/kg respectively for 6 months resulted in reticulocytosis, eosinophilia, monocytosis and an increase in phagocytic activity in rats (Bekker 1969). In a Russian study, high doses of methyl benzoate were stated to result in damage to the CNS, but no further details of the study were available (Kravetts-Bekker and Ivanova 1970).

Studies in which rats were exposed to methyl methacrylate (2 g/l in drinking water for 2 years) showed no significant alteration in haematologic values or concentrations of proteins and reducing substances. Female rats showed elevated kidney organ to body weight ratios, but no histopathological changes were noted. Administration of 100–1500 ppm methyl methacrylate (equivalent to 2.5–3.75 mg/kg body weight, assuming 1 mg/kg body weight of dry diet is equal to 40 ppm) in the diet of dogs also suggested that this compound does not possess any marked toxic potential following long-term exposure (Borzelleca *et al* 1964).

Studies of workers chronically exposed to small concentrations of esters are problematic, since the esters usually exist in a mixture of solvents. Nonetheless, workers exposed to solvents containing butyl acetate have shown behavioural changes and loss of coordination. Chronic exposure of workers to plasticisers including butyl adipate has been associated with polyneuritis and sensory impairment (Milkov *et al* 1969). The only toxic effects experienced by workers inhaling vinyl acetate were skin, nose and throat irritation (Deese and Joiner 1969).

4.3 Genotoxicity

Extracts of river water and industrial effluents containing methyl penta-decanoate, methyl oleate and methyl laurate were tested for mutagenicity using Ames tests (Somani *et al* 1980, Pereira *et al* 1982). Positive results were shown only with extracts containing methyl oleate or methyl pentadecanoate. However, these compounds were present in unspecified concentrations as trace constituents of a complex mixture, and therefore no conclusions can be drawn on the mutagenicity of these compounds.

Conflicting mutagenicity results have been obtained with methyl methacrylate using the Ames test. Negative results were found with the conventional Ames test (Ames *et al* 1975), using five strains of *Salmonella typhimurium*, with or without activation by induced rat liver S-9 mix. However, if the extracts were incubated with the bacteria and S-9 for 1 hour before mixing with agar and pouring onto plates, there was evidence of mutagenicity (Poss *et al* 1979).

Methyl laurate was a weak inducer of methylazoxymethanol mutagenicity (point mutation at the ouabain locus) in cultured V79 Chinese hamster cells (Wey and Baxter 1979).

Vinyl acetate has given negative results for mutagenicity in the Ames test (Bartsch *et al* 1979, Lijinsky and Andrews 1980). However, this compound has been shown to induce structural chromosome changes and sister chromatid exchanges in human lymphocyte cultures *in vitro* (He and Lambert 1985, Jantunen *et al* 1986). Vinyl acetate has also induced sister chromatid exchanges in CHO cells either with or without S-9 activation (Maki-Paakkanen *et al* 1984, Norppa *et al* 1985). Acetaldehyde, a metabolite of vinyl acetate, is thought to be responsible for the cytogenetic effects of this compound, as it also induces chromosome damage and sister chromatid exchanges in cultured human lymphocytes and CHO cells (He and Lambert 1985, Jansson 1982, Obe *et al* 1986).

Maki-Paakkanen and Norppa (1987) studied the effect of vinyl acetate on the induction of micronuclei in mice *in vivo* and in cultured human lymphocytes *in vitro*. Male mice were given a single intraperitoneal injection (250, 500, 1000 or 2000 mg/kg body weight) of vinyl acetate. After 30 hours the animals were killed, and peripheral erythrocytes were examined for micronuclei. The incidence of micronucleated polychromatic erythrocytes was significantly increased at the two highest doses. However, 1000 and 2000 mg/kg proved to be lethal doses, killing 6 and 8 out of 14 rats per group respectively. The human lymphocyte cultures were treated with 0.125,

0.25, 0.5, 1.0 and 2.0 mM vinyl acetate, in acetone. The incidence of micronuclei was significantly increased at the 0.5 and 1.0 mM dose levels, although no dose response was observed. No increase in micronuclei was observed at a dose of 2.0 mM, probably because toxicity reduced cell proliferation.

In a study by Zimmerman *et al* (1985), the ability of ethyl acetate to induce aneuploidy in *Saccharomyces cerevisiae* was demonstrated. It was shown that the ester could induce chromosome malsegregation, but did not induce mitotic recombination or point mutation in the yeast test system. It was suggested that this was because ethyl acetate acted on tubulin to affect spindle formation during mitosis.

4.4 Carcinogenicity

Rats receiving vinyl acetate in drinking water at a level of 2500 mg/l for life showed a higher incidence of some tumours over controls (Lijinsky and Reuber 1983). Out of 20 female rats, 5 developed carcinomas of the uterus and 6 developed adenoma or carcinoma of the thyroid at this dose. Only one of 20 male rats receiving the 2500 mg/l developed carcinoma of the thyroid. Rats dosed with 1000 mg/l vinyl acetate did not show any excess tumours over controls. It has been suggested that vinyl acetate forms epoxyethyl acetate, which is structurally similar to the ultimate epoxide carcinogens of vinyl chloride and vinyl carbamate. However, unlike these structural analogues, vinyl acetate was not found to induce pre-neoplastic enzyme-altered foci in rat liver (Laib and Bolt 1986). Therefore the mechanism by which vinyl acetate could act as a potential carcinogen is unclear.

Methyl oleate was at best weakly tumourigenic in a skin painting study in mice (Arffman and Glavind 1977). Out of 35 mice treated with 0.5 ml of a 20% v/v acetone solution three times a week for one year, 29 survived at 18 months. Induction of skin papillomas was observed in only one of these animals. No tumours were observed in 25 control animals. Methyl oleate also exhibited promoter activity when painted on the skin or injected subcutaneously, but not by oral administration. A single application of the initiator DMBA (50 μg) given to 30 mice was followed by application of methyl oleate as previously described. Of 5 mice surviving at 12 months, 2 and 3 mice were reported to have developed skin carcinomas and sarcomas respectively. Control mice (20) were treated with DMBA alone, and out of 11 surviving at 12 months, development of a sarcoma was observed in only one mouse.

4.5 Reproductive toxicity

Three groups of pregnant rats were dosed (methyl methacrylate) by intraperitoneal injection with 0.1, 0.2 and 0.4 g/kg body weight on each of days 5, 10 and 15 of gestation. Significantly decreased foetal body weights were observed in all three groups, but no skeletal effects were induced (Autian 1975, Singh *et al* 1972).

Pregnant rats given intraperitoneal injections of di-*n*-butyl adipate in the dose range 0.16–1.68 g/kg on the 5th, 6th and 16th day of gestation showed no adverse effects at the lower doses. Doses of 0.50–1.68 g/kg all produced a low incidence of gross abnormalities, including various non-malignant tumours of the blood vessels, twisted hindlegs and compacted head and neck, whilst a low incidence of skeletal abnormalities was observed at the highest dose level only. Foetal weight was reduced at 1.01 g/kg and above (Singh *et al* 1973).

5. DISCUSSION

As most of the esters identified in drinking water by WRc are widely used in the food processing industry, it is unlikely that water represents a significant source of exposure.

Esters are readily absorbed, but are rapidly hydrolysed before undergoing further oxidative metabolism or conjugation and excretion.

Acute studies suggest the esters to be of very low oral toxicity. Information on chronic toxicity is scarce, but the main concerns are haematological effects and effects on the CNS, the latter possibly being the result of 'alcohol intoxication' produced by ester hydrolysis (Tambo 1973).

Little information concerning the genotoxic and carcinogenic activity of the esters exists, and limited evidence available suggests the esters are generally not toxic to the reproductive system. Vinyl acetate, butyl adipate and methyl methacrylate were found to be only weakly embryotoxic.

Although there is only a limited amount of information available, it would appear very unlikely that low levels of these esters in drinking water constitute a risk to human health.

REFERENCES

AMES B N, MCCANN J and YAMASAKI E (1975) Methods for detecting carcinogens and mutagens with the Salmonella/mammalian-microsome mutagenicity test. *Mutation Research* **31**, 347-364.

ARFFMAN E and GLAVIND J (1977) Carcinogenicity in mice of some fatty acid esters. 1. Skin application. *Acta Pathologica et Microbiologica Scandinavica* Section A Pathology, 82A, 127.

AUTIAN J (1975) Structure–toxicity relationships of acrylic monomers. *Environmental Health Perspectives* **11**, 141-152.

BARTSCH H C, MALLEVEILLE A, BARBIN A and PLANCHE G (1979) Mutagenic and alkylating metabolites of halo-ethylenes, chlorobutadienes and dichlorobutenes produced by rodent or human liver tissues. Evidence for oxirane formation by P450-linked microsomal mono-oxygenases. *Archives of Toxicology* **41**, 249-277.

BEKKER A K (1969) Faktory Vneshnei Sredy i ikh Znachenie dlia Zdorov'ia Naseleniia 25 (Chem Abstr 72:64876j).

BLICKENS D A and DI-LUZIO N R (1965) Metabolism of methyl palmitate, aphagocytic and immunologic depressant, and its influence on tissue lipids. *Journal of the Reticuloendothelial Society* **2**, 60-74.

BORZELLECA J F, LARSON P S, HENNIGAR G R, HUF E G, CRAWFORD E M and BLACKWELL SMITH R Jr (1964) Studies on the chronic oral toxicity of monomeric ethyl acrylate and methacrylate. *Toxicology and Applied Pharmacology* **6**, 29-36.

BRATT H and HATHWAY D E (1977) Fate of methyl methacrylate in rats. *British Journal of Cancer* **36**, 114-119.

COHEN G and COLLINS M (1970) Alkaloids, from catecholamines in adrenal tissue: possible role for alcoholism. *Science* **167**, 1749-1751.

COLEMAN W E, MELTON R G, KOPFLER F C, BARONE K A, AURAND T A and JELLISON M G (1980) Identification of organic compounds in a mutagenic extract of a surface drinking water by computerised gas chromatography/mass spectrometry system (GC/MS/COM). *Environmental Science and Technology* **14**, 576-588.

DAVIS V E and WALSH M J (1970) Alcohol, amine and alkalis: A possible biochemical basis for alcohol addiction. *Science* **167**, 1005-1007.

DEESE D E and JOINER R E (1969) Vinyl acetate: A study of chronic human exposure. *American Industrial Hygiene Association Journal* **31**, 449-457.

DI-LUZIO N R and BLICKENS D A (1966) Influence of intravenously administered lipids on reticuloendothelial function. *Research Journal of the Reticuloendothelial Society* **3**, 250-270.

FASSETT D W (1963) Esters. In: *Patty's Industrial hygiene and toxicology*, edited by G D Clayton and F E Clayton, 2nd Edition, Vol 2, 1851. Interscience Publishers, New York.

FOOD ADDITIVES and CONTAMINANTS COMMITTEE (1978) Report on the review of flavourings in food. FACC/REP/25 London HMSO.

FURIA T E and BELLANCA N (1971) *Ferraroli's handbook of flavour ingredients.* Chemical Rubber Company, Cleveland, Ohio p 502.

GAGE J C (1970) The subacute inhalation toxicity of 109 industrial chemicals. *British Journal of Industrial Medicine* **27**, 1-18.

GALLAHER E and LOOMIS T (1975) Metabolism of ethyl acetate in the rat: hydrolysis to ethyl alcohol *in vitro* and *in vivo*. *Toxicology and Applied Pharmacology* **34**, 309-313.

HE S M and LAMBERT B (1985) Induction and persistence of SCE-inducing damage in human lymphocytes exposed to vinyl acetate and acetaldehyde *in vitro*. *Mutation Research* **158**, 201-208.

HOPKINS J (1985) Di(meth)acrylates–a sensitive question. *Food and Chemical Toxicology* **23**, 713-717.

INTERNATIONAL AGENCY FOR RESEARCH ON CANCER. Some monomers, plastics and synthetic elastomers, and acrolein. IARC Monographs on the evaluation of the carcinogenic risk of chemicals to humans. Volume **19**, pp. 187-211 and 341-366.

JANSSON T (1982) The frequency of sister chromatid exchanges in human lymphocytes treated with ethanol and acetaldehyde. *Hereditas* **97**, 301-303.

JANTUNEN K, MAKI-PAAKKANEN J and NORPPA H (1986) Induction of chromosome aberrations by styrene and vinyl acetate in cultured human lymphocytes: dependence on erythrocytes. *Mutation Research* **159**, 109-116.

KRAVETTS-BEKKER A A and IVANOVA O P (1970) Faktory Vneshnei Sredy i ikh Znachenie dlia Zdorov'ia Naseleniia **2**, 125. (Cited in OPDYKE 1974).

LAIB R J and BOLT H B (1986) Vinyl acetate, a structural analogue of vinyl carbamate, fails to induce enzyme-altered foci in rat liver. *Carcinogenesis* **7**, 841-843.

LEVEY M and OCKEN P R (1969) Purification and properties of pig liver esterase. *Archives of Biochemistry and Biophysics* **135**, 259-264.

LIJINSKY W and ANDREWS A W (1980) Mutagenicity of vinyl compounds in *Salmonella typhimurium*. *Teratogenicity, Carcinogenicity and Mutagenicity* **1**,

259-267.
LIJINSKY W and REUBER M D (1983) Chronic toxicity studies of vinyl acetate in Fischer rats. *Toxicology and Applied Pharmacology* **68**, 43-53.
LONGLAND R C, SHILLING W H and GANGOLLI S W (1977) The hydrolysis of flavouring esters by artificial gastrointestinal juices and rat tissue preparations. *Toxicology* **8**, 197-204.
MAKI-PAAKKANEN J and NORPPA H (1987) Induction of micronuclei by vinyl acetate in mouse bone marrow cells and cultured human lymphocytes. *Mutation Research* **190**, 41-45.
MAKI-PAAKKANEN J, TURSI F, NORPPA H, JARVENTAUS H and SORSA M (1984) Vinyl acetate is a potent inducer of chromosome damage in cultured mammalian cells. *Mutation Research* **130**, 249.
MILKOV L E, ALDYREVA M V, POPOVA T B, LOPUKHOVA K A, MAKARENKO Y L, MALYAR L M and SHAKHOVA T K (1969). Health status of workers exposed to phthalate plasticisers in the manufacture of artificial leather and films based on PVC resins. *Environmental Health Perspectives* **3**, 175-178.
MUNCH J C (1972). Aliphatic alcohols and alkyl esters. Narcotic and lethal potencies to tadpoles and to rabbits. *Industrial Medicine and Surgery* **41**, 31-33.
NORPPA H, TURSI F, PFAFFLI P, MAKI-PAAKKANEN J and JARVENTAUS H (1985) Chromosome damage induced by vinyl acetate through *in vitro* formation of acetaldehyde in human lymphocytes and Chinese hamster ovary cell. *Cancer Research* **45**, 4816-4821.
OBE G, JONAS R and SCHMIDT S (1986) Metabolism of ethanol *in vitro* produces a compound which induces sister chromatid exchanges in human peripheral lymphocytes *in vitro*: Acetaldehyde not ethanol is mutagenic. *Mutation Research* **174**, 47-51.
OPDYKE D L J (1974) Fragrance raw materials monographs: Methyl benzoate. *Food and Cosmetics Toxicology* **12**, 937-938.
OPDYKE D L J (1979) Fragrance raw materials monographs: Butyl acetate. *Food and Cosmetics Toxicology* **17**, 515-519.
PEREIRA W E, ROSTAD C E, TAYLOR H E, KLEIN J M (1982) Characterisation of organic contaminants in environmental samples associated with Mount St. Helens (Washington USA) 1980 volcanic eruption. *Environmental Science and Technology* **16**, 387.
PEROCCO P, BOLOGNESI S and ALBERGHINI W (1983) Toxic activity of seventeen industrial solvents and halogenated compounds on human lymphocytes cultured *in vitro*. *Toxicology Letters* **16**, 69-75.
POSS R, THILLY W G and KADEN D A (1979) Methyl methacrylate is a mutagen for *Salmonella typhimurium*. *Journal of Bone and Joint Surgery of America* **61**, 1203-1207.
RAJE R, AHMED S and WEISBROTH S (1985) Methyl methacrylate: tissue distribution and pulmonary damage in rats following acute inhalation. *Research Communications in Chemical Pathology and Pharmacology* **50**, 151-154.
RYCROFT R J G (1977) Contact dermatitis from acrylic compounds. *British Journal of Dermatology* **96**, 685-686.
SABA T M and DI-LUZIO N R (1968) Evaluation of humoral and cellular mechanisms of reticuloendothelial depression. *Life Science* **7**, 337-348.

SCHULZ H and GUNTHER R (1972) Paint processing and prevention of air pollution–investigation concerning organic substances from paint binders appearing in the drying air during paint drying in continuous ovens. *Staub-Reinhaltung der Luft* **32**, 1-11.

SIMON P, FILSER J G and BOLT H M (1985) Metabolism and pharmacokinetics of vinyl acetate. *Archives of Toxicology* **57**, 191-195.

SINGH A R, LAWRENCE W H and AUTIAN J (1972) Embryo-fetal toxicity and teratogenic effects of a group of methacrylate esters in rats. *Toxicology and Applied Pharmacology* **22**, 314-315.

SINGH A R, LAWRENCE W H and AUTIAN J (1973) Embryonic foetal toxicity and teratogenic effects of adipic acid esters in rats. *Journal of Pharmacological Science* **62**, 1596-1600.

SOMANI S M, TEECE R G and SCHAEFFER D J (1980) Identification of co-carcinogens and promoters in industrial discharges into and in the Illinois River. *Journal of Toxicology and Environmental Health* **6**, 315-331.

STENBACK F and SHUBIK P (1974) Lack of toxicity and carcinogenicity of some commonly used cutaneous agents. *Toxicology and Applied Pharmacology* **30**, 7-13.

TAMBO S (1973) Nichidai Igaku Zasshi 32, 349. Cited in Opdyke D L J (1979) Fragrance raw materials monographs: butylacetate. *Food and Cosmetics Toxicology* **17**, 515-519.

TREON J F, SIGMAN H, WRIGHT H and KITZMILLER K V (1949) The toxicity of methyl and ethyl acrylate. *Journal of Industrial Hygiene and Toxicology* **31**, 317-326.

VON OETTINGEN W F (1960) The aliphatic acids and their esters: toxicity and potential dangers. *AMA Archives of Industrial Health* **21**, 28-65.

WATER RESEARCH CENTRE (1981) Organic micropollutants in drinking water. WRc Technical Report TR 159

WATER RESEARCH CENTRE (1982) Frequency of occurrence for compounds identified by GC–MS in XAD-2 samples taken for mutagenic testing survey. WRc unpublished report.

WEY H E and BAXTER C (1979) Enhancement of chemically-induced mutagenesis in cultured V79 Chinese Hamster cells by certain fatty acid esters. *Toxicology and Applied Pharmacology* **48**, A134.

YOSHIDA M, MORIMOTO H and ODA R (1970) Availability of energy in esters of aliphatic acids and alcohols by growing chicks. *Agricultural and Biological Chemistry* **34**, 1668-1675.

YOSHIDA M, IKUMO H and SUZUKI O (1971) Evaluation of available energy of aliphatic chemicals by rats. An application of energy to mono-gastric animal. *Agricultural and Biological Chemistry* **35**, 1208-1215.

ZIMMERMAN F K, MAYER V W, SCHEEL I and RESNICK M A (1985) Acetone, methyl ethyl ketone, ethyl acetate, acetonitrile and other polar aprotic solvents are strong inducers of aneuploidy in *Saccharomyces cerevisiae*. *Mutation Research* **149**, 339-351.

15

The alicyclic hydrocarbons

1. INTRODUCTION

Six alicyclic hydrocarbons were identified in drinking water by WRc. Both cyclohexane and limonene were identified in 5/14 samples, but methylcyclopentane, menth-2-ene and two cyclohexadiene isomers have been detected less frequently.

There is very little information available on the occurrence of these compounds in the environment.

Toxicological information is also very limited. There is some information available for cyclohexane and limonene, but none at all for the remaining compounds.

2. CYCLOHEXANE

2.1 Introduction

Cyclohexane is widely used in industry as a solvent, paint and varnish remover, and in the manufacture of nylon. Cyclohexane can be prepared from benzene, cyclopentane or by the fractionation of crude oil.

CAS Reg. No:	110-82-7
Molecular weight:	84.2
Boiling point:	81°C
Solubility:	55 mg/l at 20°C (Verschueren 1983)
Threshold odour concentration in water:	0.02 mg/l (Verschueren 1983)

2.2 Exposure

In the WRc survey (Water Research Centre 1981) cyclohexane was detected in 5/14 drinking water samples tested. This compound has also been identified in Dutch and Czechoslovakian drinking water (Commission of the European Communities 1984).

Cyclohexane has been detected in the atmosphere in the US (Holzer *et al* 1977) and Russia (Ioffe *et al* 1977), but there appears to be no information on its occurrence in food.

2.3 Toxicokinetics

Following an oral dose of between 350 and 400 mg/kg of cyclohexane in rabbits, approximately 50% of the dose was excreted in the urine and 40% in the expired air within 2 days. At lower doses, however, excretion was almost exclusively via the urine. In the urine, the principal metabolites were glucuronide conjugates of cyclohexanol and *trans*-cyclohexane-1,2-diol. The expired air contained mostly unchanged cyclohexane (Elliott *et al* 1959).

Cyclohexanol has been identified in the urine of shoe factory workers exposed to cyclohexane (Perbellini and Brugnone 1980, Perbellini *et al* 1980).

2.4 Health effects

2.4.1 Acute and subacute toxicity

This compound appears to be of very low acute toxicity in experimental animals. The acute oral LD50 of cyclohexane in the rat has been reported to be 29.8 g/kg (Registry of Toxic Effects of Chemical Substances); Kimura *et al* (1971) investigated the acute toxicity of cyclohexane in groups of male Sprague–Dawley rats of different ages. The oral LD50 was found to be about 6 g/kg in 14-day old rats, 30 g/kg in young adult rats, and 13 g/kg in older adults. An intraperitoneal LD50 in the mouse of 1.3 g/kg has also been reported (Registry of Toxic Effects of Chemical Substances).

Treon *et al* (1943a) found that the minimum lethal oral dose of cyclohexane in rabbits was between 5.5 and 6.0 g/kg. The rabbits exhibited loss of body weight, elevated respiratory rate, severe diarrhoea and lethargy. At autopsy there was widespread vascular damage and collapse, extensive hepatocellular degeneration and glomerulonephritis.

A dose-dependent increase in solvent concentration was found in the perirenal fat and brain of Wistar rats exposed by inhalation to 300, 1000 or 2000 ppm of cyclohexane, 6 hours/day, 5 days/week for 2 weeks. Although there were no changes in brain RNA, glutathione or glutathione peroxidase, brain azoreductase activity was slightly inhibited (Savolainen and Pfaffli 1980).

2.4.2 Chronic toxicity

The only long-term studies which appear to be available are inhalation studies in the rat, rabbit and monkey.

Groups of six to nine male Sprague–Dawley rats were exposed for up to 30 weeks to 1500 ppm (9 hours/day, 5 days/week) or 2500 ppm (10 hours/day, 6 days/week) of cyclohexane. There were no effects on body weight, and histological examination of nerve tissue did not reveal any evidence for neuropathy (Frontali *et al* 1981).

No signs of toxicity were evident in rabbits exposed to 434 ppm, 6 or 8 hours/day, 5 days/week for 10 or 26 weeks. Slight pathological changes in the liver and kidney were found in rabbits exposed to 786 ppm for 10 weeks, while deaths occurred at concentrations of 7445 ppm and higher (Treon *et al* 1943b).

There were no signs of illness or changes in gross or microscopic pathology in a rhesus monkey exposed to 1243 ppm of cyclohexane for 10 weeks (Treon *et al* 1943b).

2.4.3 Genotoxicity

Cyclohexane was not found to be mutagenic in the Ames test to *Salmonella typhimurium* TA100, TA98, TA1535, and TA1537, in either the presence or absence of metabolic activation (McCann *et al* 1975).

2.4.4 Carcinogenicity

The only information which appears to be available is a study of the tumour-promoting activity of cyclohexane. The skin of 35 male C3H mice was given a single treatment of 60 μl of a 0.3% solution of 7,12-dimethylbenz[*a*]anthracene in benzene. After a 2-week interval the mice were treated with about 47 mg (60 μl) of cyclohexane twice weekly for up to 50 weeks. There was no significant increase in tumour incidence compared to a control group (Horton *et al* 1981).

2.4.5 Reproductive toxicity

No information appears to be available.

2.5 Discussion

This compound has been identified in water and air, but there appears to be no information on occurrence in food. It is readily metabolised in the rabbit to *trans*-cyclohexane-1,2-diol and cyclohexanol. Excretion is largely via the urine, particularly at low doses.

Cyclohexane is of low acute toxicity, but there is only very limited information available on chronic toxicity, mutagenicity, carcinogenicity and reproductive toxicity.

There is insufficient information available for cyclohexane on which to base an assessment of the risk to human health.

References

COMMISSION OF THE EUROPEAN COMMUNITIES (1984) An inventory of organic pollutants which have been identified in various surface waters, effluent discharges, aquatic animals and plants, and bottom sediments. Eurocop-Cost, Project 64B, 4th Edition.

ELLIOTT T H, PARKE D V and WILLIAMS R T (1959) The metabolism of cyclo[^{14}C]hexane and its derivatives. *Biochemical Journal* **72,** 193-200.

FRONTALI N, AMANTINI M C, SPAGNOLO A, GUARCINI A M, SALTARI M C, BRUGNONE F and PERBELLINI L (1981) Experimental neurotoxicity and urinary metabolites of the C5–C7 aliphatic hydrocarbons used as glue solvents in shoe manufacture. *Clinical Toxicology* **18,** 1357-1367.

HOLZER G, SHANFIELD H, ZLATKIS A, BERTSCH W, JUAREZ P, MAY-

FIELD H and LIEBICH H M (1977) Collection and analysis of trace organic emissions from natural sources. *Journal of Chromatography* **142,** 755-764.

HORTON A W, BOLEWICZ L C, BARSTAD A W and BUTTS C K (1981) Comparison of the promoting activity of pristane and *n*-alkanes in skin carcinogenesis with their physical effects on micellar models of biological membranes. *Biochimica et Biophysica Acta* **648,** 107-112.

IOFFE B V, ISIDOROV V A and ZENKEVICH I G (1977) Gas chromatographic–mass spectrometric determination of volatile organic compounds in an urban atmosphere. *Journal of Chromatography* **142,** 787-795.

KIMURA E T, EBERT D M and DODGE P W (1971) Acute toxicity and limits of solvent residue for sixteen organic solvents. *Toxicology and Applied Pharmacology* **19,** 699-704.

McCANN J, CHOI E, YAMASAKI E and AMES B N (1975) Detection of carcinogens as mutagens in the *Salmonella*/microsome test: assay of 300 chemicals. *Proceedings of the National Academy of Sciences USA: Biological Sciences* **72,** 5135-5139.

PERBELLINI L and BRUGNONE F (1980) Lung uptake and metabolism of cyclohexane in shoe factory workers. *International Archives of Occupational and Environmental Health* **45,** 261-269.

PERBELLINI L, BRUGNONE F and PAVAN I (1980) Identification of the metabolites of *n*-hexane, cyclohexane, and their isomers in men's urine. *Toxicology and Applied Pharmacology* **53,** 220-229.

REGISTRY OF TOXIC EFFECTS OF CHEMICAL SUBSTANCES National Institute for Occupational Safety & Health, Cincinnati, Ohio.

SAVOLAINEN H and PFAFFLI P (1980) Burden and dose-related neurochemical effects of intermittent cyclohexane vapour inhalation in rats. *Toxicology Letters* **7,** 17-22.

TREON J F, CRUTCHFIELD W E Jr and KITZMILLER K V (1943a) The physiological response of animals to cyclohexane, methylcyclohexane, and certain derivatives of these compounds. 1. Oral administration and cutaneous application. *Journal of Industrial Hygiene and Toxicology* **25,** 199-214.

TREON J F, CRUTCHFIELD W E Jr and KITZMILLER K V (1943b) The physiological response of animals to cyclohexane, methylcyclohexane, and certain derivatives of these compounds. 2. Inhalation. *Journal of Industrial Hygiene and Toxicology* **25,** 323-347.

VERSCHUEREN K (1983) *Handbook of environmental data on organic chemicals.* Second Edition. Van Nostrand Reinhold Company, New York.

WATER RESEARCH CENTRE (1981) Organic micropollutants in drinking water. WRC Technical Report TR 159.

3. LIMONENE

3.1 Introduction

Limonene (*p*-mentha-1,8-diene) is a monoterpene which occurs widely in plant oils. It is used as a flavouring agent in soaps, cosmetics and other consumer goods, as a solvent, a wetting and dispersing agent, aerosol stabiliser and in medicine in the treatment of cholesterol gallstones.

CAS Reg. No:	138-86-3
Molecular weight:	36.2
Boiling point:	178.0°C
Solubility:	No data available
Threshold odour concentration in water:	0.01 mg/l (Zoeteman 1984)

3.2 Exposure

In the WRc survey (Water Research Centre 1981), limonene was identified in 5/14 drinking water samples tested. No other data on occurrence in water appear to be available.

This compound has been detected in the atmosphere in the US (Bertsch *et al* 1974, Holzer *et al* 1977) and Russia (Ioffe *et al* 1977). However, limonene is a constituent of a wide range of essential oils, and therefore food is likely to represent the major source of exposure to this compound.

3.3 Toxicokinetics

In rats, an oral dose of limonene was rapidly absorbed by the gastrointestinal tract, with maximum concentrations found in the blood and tissues within 2 hours. Limonene was distributed primarily to the liver and kidney. Within 48 hours, about 60% of the dose had been excreted in the urine, 5% in the faeces and 2% in the expired air. A complex range of metabolites were detected in the urine. In bile duct cannulated rats, about 25% of the dose was excreted in the bile within 24 hours, indicating that limonene undergoes enterohepatic recirculation (Igimi *et al* 1974).

The metabolism of limonene in the rabbit appears to be very similar to that in the rat. Following an oral dose of limonene in three male rabbits, about 72% of the dose was excreted in the urine and 7% in the faeces within 72 hours. A complex range of metabolites were again detected in the urine, of which six were isolated. All were found to be products of side-chain oxidation (Kodama *et al* 1974).

The urine also appears to be the major route of excretion for limonene in the hamster, guinea-pig, dog and man (Kodama *et al* 1976). The major metabolites present in the urine tend to be specific for each species (Kodama *et al* 1976).

Three minor metabolites resulting from oxidation of the ring double bond have also been identified in dog and rat urine (Kodama *et al* 1976). Formation of the ring epoxide and side-chain epoxide following the incubation of limonene with rat liver microsomes have been reported (Watabe *et al* 1980, 1981).

3.4 Health effects

3.4.1 Acute and subacute toxicity

Limonene appears to be of low acute toxicity in experimental animals. Acute oral LD50s of 4.4–5.1 g/kg and 5.6–6.6 g/kg have been reported for the rat and mouse respectively (Tsuji *et al* 1975a).

Groups of ten male and ten female Sprague–Dawley rats were given daily oral doses of 277, 554, 1385, or 2770 mg/kg of limonene for one month. Lowered food consumption and body weight were noted in the high-dose animals. There were no changes in organ weights, haematology, urinalysis or clinical chemistry. The only histopathological changes observed were the presence of granular casts in the kidneys of male rats (Tsuji *et al* 1975a). Groups of young adult male Fischer-344 rats given oral doses of 75, 150 or 300 mg/kg *d*-limonene for up to 27 days showed renal toxicity considered to be the sequelae of hyaline droplet formation (Kanerva *et al* 1987).

Wistar rats given daily oral doses of 400 mg/kg for 30 days exhibited elevated liver weight, elevated hepatic phospholipid content, cytochrome P-450, aminopyrine demethylase and aniline hydroxylase activities, while hepatic and serum cholesterol were lowered. These effects were not found in rats given daily oral doses of 400 mg/kg for 2, 3 or 15 days (Ariyoshi *et al* 1975).

3.4.2 Chronic toxicity

Groups of nine to ten male and female Sprague–Dawley rats were given daily oral doses of 0, 277, 544, or 1385 mg/kg of limonene in a 1% Tween 80 solution for 6 months. A slight depression in body weight gain was observed in the high-dose animals. Significantly increased relative organ weights were found for the liver, kidney, thyroid, lung and adrenals. Relative liver and kidney weights were slightly elevated even at the lowest dose level. There were no changes in haematology, urinalysis or clinical chemistry. The only histopathological change observed was the presence of granular casts in the kidney of males at 544 and 1385 mg/kg (Tsuji *et al* 1975b).

Daily oral doses 0, 0.4, 1.2, and 3.6 ml/kg (about 0.33, 1.01, and 3.03 g/kg) of limonene were given to groups of three beagle dogs for 6 months. Nausea, vomiting and soft faeces were common in the initial stages of the study. Lowered body weights were found in males at 3.6 ml/kg and females at 1.2 and 3.6 ml/kg. At the high dose, slightly lowered haemoglobin, haematocrit and red blood cells were found in females, while lowered blood sugar and cholesterol were noted in both sexes. Protein casts were present in the kidneys of almost all treated animals. No other histopathological changes were reported (Tsuji *et al* 1975c).

Limonene administered by oral gavage at 150–2400 mg/kg/day in a subchronic (91 day) study induced renal alterations in male rats at all dose levels but not in female rats, or male or female mice (Kanerva and Alden 1987).

An investigation of the immunotoxicological effects of limonene in mice indicated an ability to modulate immume responses (Evans *et al* 1987).

3.4.3 Genotoxicity

Limonene was not found to be mutagenic in the Ames test to *Salmonella typhimurium* TA98, TA100, TA1535, and TA1537, in either the presence or absence of metabolic activation, at doses ranging from 0.3 to 3333 μg/plate (Haworth *et al* 1983). Similar results have been reported by other groups (Watabe *et al* 1980, 1981, Florin *et al* 1980). Watabe *et al* reported that the 1,2- and 8,9-epoxide metabolites of limonene were also non-mutagenic in the Ames test.

No evidence for mutagenic activity of limonene was found in the mammalian spot test. In this study, female C57BL/6JHan mice were bred with a specific male strain, and the pregnant animals were dosed with 215 mg/kg/day of limonene by intraperitoneal injection on days 9–11 of gestation. Mutagenic activity was measured by the frequency of expression of recessive hair colour genes in the offspring (Fahrig 1982).

3.4.4 Carcinogenicity

Limonene was not found to increase the incidence of lung tumours in strain A mice dosed with 4.8 or 24 g/kg of limonene in 0.1 ml of tricaprylin by intraperitoneal injection thrice weekly for 8 weeks (Stoner *et al* 1973). It was shown not to be a promoter of mouse skin tumours after initiation with DMBA (Elegbede *et al* 1986a).

Limonene has been reported to partially inhibit the carcinogenicity of benzo(*a*)-pyrene and benzo(*rst*)pentaphene in the mouse (Van Duuren and Goldschmidt 1976, Homburger *et al* 1971), and 7,12-dimethylbenz[*a*]anthracene in the rat (Elegbede *et al* 1984). Limonene also slightly inhibited the growth of implanted Walker tumours in the rat (Hendry *et al* 1951). Limonene increased the rate of regression of DMBA-induced mammary tumours in rat (Elegbede *et al* 1986b).

3.4.5 Reproductive toxicity

Daily oral doses of 0, 591, or 2869 mg/kg of limonene on days 9–15 of gestation were not found to be teratogenic in Wistar rats. At the highest dose level there was evidence for delayed maturation of foetuses, but there was also marked maternal toxicity, including a high incidence of mortality. No embryotoxic effects or maternal toxicity was found at 591 mg/kg (Tsuji *et al* 1975d).

Retarded ossification and an increased incidence of lumbar rib and fused rib were found in the pups of ICR mice given daily oral doses of 2363 mg/kg of limonene on days 7–12 of gestation. However, depressed body–weight gain was observed in the dams at this dose level. These effects were not found in pregnant mice given 591 mg/kg (Kodama *et al* 1977a).

Limonene was not found to be teratogenic in rabbits given daily oral doses of 0, 250, 500 or 1000 mg/kg on days 6–18 of gestation. Marked maternal toxicity was observed at the high dose level (Kodama *et al* 1977b).

3.5 Discussion

Limonene was identified in 5/14 drinking water samples tested in the WRc survey. It has also been identified in the atmosphere, but its occurrence in essential oils is likely to be the most important source of exposure to this compound. Limonene is rapidly absorbed by the gastrointestinal tract and distributed largely to the liver and kidney. A complex range of metabolites are found in the urine.

Limonene appears to be of low acute and chronic toxicity in rats and dogs. The most common effect observed was the presence of protein casts in the kidney. Limonene has given negative results in the Ames test and mammalian spot test. It has not been tested in a long-term carcinogenicity bioassay. Limonene is able to retard foetal development only at dose levels which also cause maternal toxicity.

References

ARIYOSHI T, ARAKAKI M, IDEGUCHI K, ISHIZUKA Y, NODA K and IDE H (1975) Studies on the metabolism of *d*-limonene (*p*-mentha-1,8-diene). 3. Effects of *d*-limonene on the lipids and drug-metabolising enzymes in rat livers. *Xenobiotica* **5,** 33-38.

BERTSCH W, CHANG R C and ZLATKIS A (1974) The determination of organic volatiles in air pollution studies: characterisation of profiles. *Journal of Chromatographic Science* **12,** 175-182.

ELEGBEDE J A, ELSON C E, QURESHI A, TANNER M A and GOULD M N (1984) Inhibition of DMBA-induced mammary cancer by the monoterpene *d*-limonene. *Carcinogenesis* **5,** 661-664.
ELEGBEDE J A, MALTZMANN T H, VERMA A K, TANNER M A, ELSON C E and GOULD M N (1986a) Mouse skin tumour promoting activity of orange peel oil and *d*-limonene: a re-evaluation. *Carcinogenesis* **7,** 2074-2049.
ELEGBEDE J A, ELSON C E, TANNER M A, QURESHI A and GOULD M N (1986b) Regression of rat primary mammary tumours following dietary *d*-limonene. *Journal of the National Cancer Institute* **76,** 323-325.
EVANS D L, MILLER D M, JACOBSEN K L and BUSH P B (1987) Modulation of immune responses in mice by *d*-limonene. *Journal of Toxicology and Environmental Health* **20,** 51-66.
FAHRIG R (1982) Effects of food additives in the mammalian spot test. In: *Progress in Clinical and Biological Research* **109.** Mutagens in our Environment, edited by R R Liss, Inc, New York pp 339–348.
FLORIN I, RUTBERG L, CURVALL M and ENZELL C R (1980) Screening of tobacco smoke constituents for mutagenicity using the Ames test. *Toxicology* **18,** 219-232.
HAWORTH S, LAWLOR T, MORTELMANS K, SPECK W and ZEIGER E (1983) *Salmonella* mutagenicity test results for 250 chemicals. *Environmental Mutagenesis* **5,** 3-142.
HENDRY J A, HOMER R F, ROSE F L and WALPOLE A L (1951) Cytotoxic agents: 2. Bis-epoxides and related compounds. *British Journal of Pharmacology* **6,** 235-255.
HOLZER G, SHANFIELD H, ZLATKIS A, BERTSCH W, JUAREZ P, MAYFIELD H and LIEBICH H M (1977) Collection and analysis of trace organic emissions from natural sources. *Journal of Chromatography* **142,** 755-764.
HOMBURGER F, TREGER A and BOGER E (1971) Inhibition of murine subcutaneous and intravenous benzo(*rst*)pentaphene carcinogenesis by sweet orange oils and *d*-limonene. *Oncology* **25,** 1-10.
IGIMI H, NISHIMURA M, KODAMA R and IDE H (1974) Studies on the metabolism of *d*-limonene (*p*-mentha-1,8-diene). 1. The absorption, distribution and excretion of *d*-limonene in rats. *Xenobiotica* **4,** 77-84.
IOFFE B V, ISIDOROV V A and ZENKEVICH I G (1977) Gas chromatographic–mass spectrometric determination of volatile organic compounds in an urban atmosphere. *Journal of Chromatography* **142,** 787-795.
KANERVA R L and ALDEN C L (1987) Review of kidney sections from a subchronic d-limonene oral dosing study conducted by the National Cancer Institute. *Food and Chemical Toxicology* **25,** 355-358.
KANERVA R L, RIDDER G M, LEFEVER F R and ALDEN C L (1987) Comparison of short-term renal effects due to oral administration of decalin or *d*-limonene in young adult male Fischer-344 rats. *Food and Chemical Toxicology* **25,** 345-353.
KODAMA R, NODA K and IDE H (1974) Studies on the metabolism of *d*-limonene (*p*-mentha-1,8-diene). 2. The metabolic fate of *d*-limonene in rabbits. *Xenobiotica* **4,** 85-95.
KODAMA R, YANO T, FURUKAWA K, NODA K and IDE H (1976) Studies on

the metabolism of *d*-limonene (*p*-mentha-1,8-diene). 4. Isolation and characterisation of new metabolites and species differences in metabolism. *Xenobiotica* **6,** 377-389.

KODAMA R, OKUBO A, ARAKI E, NODA K, IDE H and IKEDA T (1977a) Studies on *d*-limonene as a gallstone solubiliser. 7. Effects on development of mouse fetuses and offsprings. *Oyo Yakuri* **13,** 863-873.

KODAMA R, OKUBO A, SATO K, ARAKI E, NODA K, HIROYUKI I and IKEDA T (1977b) Studies on *d*-limonene as a gallstone solubiliser. 9. Effects on development of rabbit fetuses and offsprings. *Oyo Yakuri* **13,** 885-898.

STONER G D, SHIMKIN M B, KNIAZEFF A J, WEISBURGER J H, WEISBURGER E K and GORI G B (1973) Test for carcinogenicity of food additives and chemotherapeutic agents by the pulmonary tumor response in strain A mice. *Cancer Research* **33,** 3069-3085.

TSUJI M, FUJISAKI Y, ARIKAWA Y, MASUDA S, KINOSHITA S, OKUBO A, NODA K, IDE H and IWANAGA Y (1975a) Studies on *d*-limonene, as gallstone solubiliser. 2. Acute and subacute toxicities. *Oyo Yakuri* **9,** 387-401.

TSUJI M, FUJISAKI Y, ARIKAWA Y, MASUDA S, KINOSHITA S, OKUBO A, NODA K, IDE H and IWANAGA Y (1975b) Studies on *d*-limonene as a gallstone solubiliser. 3. Chronic toxicity in rats. *Oyo Yakuri* **9,** 403-412.

TSUJI M, FUJISAKI Y, ARIKAWA Y, MASUDA S, TANAKA T, SATO K, NODA K, IDE H and KIKUCHI M (1975c) Studies on *d*-limonene as a gallstone solubiliser. 4. Chronic toxicity in dogs. *Oyo Yakuri* **9,** 775-808.

TSUJI M, FUJISAKI Y, OKUBO A, ARIKAWA Y, NODA K, IDE H and IKEDA T (1975d) Studies on *d*-limonene as a gallstone solubiliser. 5. Effects on development of rat fetuses and offsprings. *Oyo Yakuri* **10,** 179-186.

VAN DUUREN B L and GOLDSCHMIDT B M (1976) Carcinogenic and tumour-promoting agents in tobacco carcinogenesis. *Journal of the National Cancer Institute* **56,** 1237-1242.

WATABE T, HIRATSUKA A, ISOBE M and OZAWA N (1980) Metabolism of *d*-limonene by hepatic microsomes to non-mutagenic epoxides toward *Salmonella typhimurium. Biochemical Pharmacology* **29,** 1068-1071.

WATABE T, HIRATSUKA A, OZAWA N and ISOBE M (1981) A comparative study on the metabolism of *d*-limonene and 4-vinylcyclohex-1-ene by hepatic microsomes. *Xenobiotica* **11,** 333-344.

WATER RESEARCH CENTRE (1981) Organic micropollutants in drinking water. WRC Technical Report TR 159.

ZOETEMAN B C J (1984) Threshold odour concentrations in water of chemical substances. RID-Mededeling 74-3.

16

The alicyclic/aromatic hydrocarbons

1. INTRODUCTION

Indan (indane, 2,3-dihydroindene) is derived from coal tar. The information available on this compound is extremely limited.

Indene (indonaphthene) is used as a starting material for the synthesis of plastics, elastomers, polyester fibres, plasticizers, drugs, and in the production of coumarone-indene resins. It is also used in paint, coating, and tile manufacturing. Indene is a constituent of asphalt and naphtha.

	INDAN	INDENE
CAS Reg No:	496-11-7	95-13-6
Molecular weight:	118.2	116.2
Boiling point:	178°C	182°C
Threshold odour concentration in water:	No data available	0.001 mg/l (Verschueren 1983)

2. EXPOSURE

Indan and indene were the only alicyclic/aromatic hydrocarbons to be detected in UK drinking water by WRc (Water Research Centre 1981, 1982). In the first survey (Water Research Centre 1981), indan was detected in 5/14 samples but indene was not identified. In the second survey (Water Research Centre 1982), indan and indene were detected in 2/14 and 1/14 samples respectively.

There is very little other information available on the occurrence of these compounds in the environment, though indan has been detected in potable water previously (Commission of the European Communities 1984), and both indan and indene were identified in the atmospheres of Paris (Raymond and Guiochon 1974) and Leningrad (Ioffe *et al* 1977).

3. TOXICOKINETICS

A group of four rabbits were given 200 mg/kg body weight of indene by stomach tube on two consecutive days. From the urine collected over 3 days, about 25% of the dose was identified as indan-2-one and 5% of the dose as *cis*- and *trans*-indane-1,2-diol. These metabolites were also identified in the urine of rabbits dosed with indene by subcutaneous injection (Brooks and Young 1956).

In rats (body weight 200–250 g), about 5% of a dose of 250 mg of indene given by stomach tube was identified in the urine as indan-2-one. Indane-1,2-diol was also identified (Brooks and Young 1956).

No information appears to be available for indan.

4. HEALTH EFFECTS

4.1 Acute and subacute toxicity

Of ten male rats given single oral doses of 5 ml/kg of indan in olive oil, seven died soon after treatment (Gerarde 1960).

In an identical study with indene, all ten rats died after single oral doses of 5 ml/kg. Macroscopic changes found at autopsy were a generalised vasodilation, hyperaemia and haemorrhage of the gastrointestinal tract, and pulmonary oedema and haemorrhage. Histological examination revealed hepatotoxicity and the presence of haemoglobin crystals in the pulmonary capillaries (Gerarde 1960).

Although oral doses of 3 ml/day of indan for three days had no effect, 5 ml/day of indene for 5 days was reported to increase bile flow in dogs (Smith and Whipple 1930).

In rats, 3/4 animals died following subcutaneous injection of 1 ml of indene but there was no mortality after doses of 0.05, 0.2 or 0.5 ml. Fatty liver was noted in animals receiving 0.5 ml and 1 ml but not at the lower dose levels (Cameron and Doniger 1939).

In a similar study in mice, mortality was observed at all dose levels (0.05–0.5 ml). Fatty liver was found in mice receiving 0.1 and 0.2 ml, while both fatty liver and hepatic necrosis were observed at 0.5 ml (Cameron and Doniger 1939).

Mortality was also reported in rats and guinea-pigs given intraperitoneal injections of indene ranging from 0.05 to 0.25 ml and 0.01 to 0.25 ml respectively. Fatty liver was noted in both rats and guinea-pigs, while hepatic necrosis was found only in guinea-pigs (Cameron and Doniger 1939).

Application of indene to the shaven and unshaven skin of rats (one to eight treatments of 0.1 ml) and guinea-pigs (three treatments of 0.5 ml) did not produce local or systemic effects (Cameron and Doniger 1939).

No deaths were recorded in groups of 5–20 Wistar rats exposed by inhalation to between 800 and 900 ppm of indene for periods ranging from 4 to 45 hours. Hepatotoxic effects were noted in all groups of rats, the severity increasing with increasing exposure time. Effects on the spleen and kidney were also noted in rats exposed for 45 hours. No signs of toxicity were evident in a group of 15 rats exposed to 400 ppm for 40 hours. Three of ten mice died after exposure to 400 ppm of indene for 12 hours. Moderate to severe changes were found in the liver (Cameron and Doniger 1939).

Direct aspiration of liquid indene into the lungs of a range of experimental animals has been reported to induce chemical pneumonitis, pulmonary oedema and haemorrhage (Gerarde 1960).

4.2 Chronic toxicity

No information appears to be available.

4.3 Genotoxicity

Indan and indene gave negative results in Ames spot tests with *Salmonella typhimurium* TA98, TA100, TA1535 and TA1537, both in the presence and absence of metabolic activation, at dose levels ranging from 0.03 to 30 μmol/plate (Florin *et al* 1980, Curvall *et al* 1982).

4.4 Carcinogenicity

No information appears to be available.

4.5 Reproductive toxicity

No information appears to be available.

5. DISCUSSION

There appears to be very little information available for indan and indene. There are limited studies on the metabolism of indene in the rat and rabbit, and some information on the acute toxicity of indene by several routes in rodents. Indene appears to be primarily a hepatotoxin at high doses. Both indan and indene were reported to be non-mutagenic in the Ames test.

Although the limited data available would suggest that these compounds have similar properties to the aromatic hydrocarbons and are therefore unlikely to present a risk to human health at the concentrations detected in drinking water, there appear to be no long-term toxicity studies on indan and indene with which to support this contention.

REFERENCES

BROOKS C J W and YOUNG L (1956) The metabolic conversion of indene into *cis*- and *trans*-indane-1:2-diol. *Biochemical Journal* **63**, 264-269.

CAMERON G R and DONIGER C R (1939) The toxicity of indene. *Journal of Pathology and Bacteriology* **49**, 529-533.

COMMISSION OF THE EUROPEAN COMMUNITIES (1984) An inventory of organic pollutants which have been identified in various surface waters, effluent discharges, aquatic animals and plants, and bottom sediments. Eurocop-Cost, Project 64B, 4th edn.

CURVALL M, FLORIN I and JANSSON T (1982) Mutagenicity of some indoles and related compounds in the Ames test. *Toxicology* **23**, 1-10.

FLORIN I, RUTBERG L, CURVALL M and ENZELL C R (1980) Screening of tobacco smoke constituents for mutagenicity using the Ames test. *Toxicology* **18**, 219-232.

GERARDE H W (1960) *Toxicology and biochemistry of aromatic hydrocarbons.* Amsterdam, Elsevier Publishing Company.

IOFFE B V, ISODOROV V A and ZENKEVICH I G (1977) Gas chromatographic–mass spectrometric determination of volatile organic compounds in an urban atmosphere. *Journal of Chromatography* **142**, 787-795.

RAYMOND A and GUIOCHON G (1974) Gas chromatographic analysis of C_8–C_{18} hydrocarbons in Paris air. *Environmental Science and Technology* **8**, 143-148.

SMITH H P and WHIPPLE G H (1930) Bile salt metabolism. VII. Indene, hydrindene and isatin. *Journal of Biological Chemistry* **89**, 719-725.

VERSCHUEREN K (1983) *Handbook of environmental data on organic chemicals.* 2nd edn. Van Nostrand Reinhold Company.

WATER RESEARCH CENTRE (1981) Organic micropollutants in drinking water. WRc Technical Report TR 159.

WATER RESEARCH CENTRE (1982, unpublished) Frequency of occurrence data for compounds identified by GC–MS in XAD-2 samples taken for mutagenic testing survey.

17

The ketones

1. ACETOPHENONE

Acetophenone is a colourless liquid, with a sweet almond-like smell, used in perfume manufacturing, and as a solvent for the synthesis of pharmaceuticals, rubber, chemicals, dyestuffs and corrosion inhibitors. It is also used in the manufacture of plasticisers, as a tobacco flavouring, and as an intermediate in the synthesis of pharmaceuticals.

$CH_3.CO.C_6H_5$	
CAS Reg No:	98-86-2
Molecular weight:	120.16
Molecular formula	C_8H_8O
Boiling point:	202.0 °C
Threshold odour concentration:	0.30 ppm

Synonyms: acetophenon, acetyl benzene, benzoyl methide, 1-phenylethanone, hypnone, methyl phenyl ketone.

1.1 Exposure

Acetophenone was identified in tap, sea and river water in the Kitakyushu area of Japan; the level in the tap water was 5.4 ng/l (Akiyama *et al* 1980). It was detected in raw Kanawha River water at levels of between 19 and 29 μg/l (Dostal *et al* 1965), and identified in the drinking water of Cincinnati, Ohio (Coleman *et al* 1980). WRc identified acetophenone in only one of 14 UK drinking water samples examined (Water Research Centre 1981), although in a later unpublished study it was found in four of the 14 samples examined.

Acetophenone has been identified in the atmosphere of Houston (Bertsch *et al* 1974) and Zurich (Grob and Grob 1971), as well as being found in gasoline exhaust at levels of between <0.1 and 0.4 ppm (Dostal *et al* 1965).

It has also been found in oils of castoreum and labdanum resin, buds of balsam poplar, and in the heavy oil fraction of coal tar (Dostal *et al* 1965, Opdyke 1973b).

1.2 Toxicokinetics

Williams (1959) suggested that acetophenone undergoes asymmetrical reduction to the carbinol, and then is further metabolised to benzoic and mandelic acids. Rabbits have been reported to excrete approximately 50% of a dose of acetophenone as methylphenylcarbinyl glucuronide, with about 20% as hippuric acid (Williams 1959). It has been suggested that acetophenone is converted to benzoic acid and methylphenylcarbinol in both dogs and rabbits, with only small amounts (less than 2%) of mandelic acid (Opdyke 1973b).

Chinchilla rabbits, of 3 kg body weight, were each given a single dose of 450 mg/kg acetophenone by stomach tube. Urine was collected for 24 hours and examined for metabolites. Of the dose, 47% was recovered as the glucuronide. This was mainly found conjugated with methylphenylcarbinol. Only 3% of the dose was recovered as the ethereal sulphate (Smith *et al* 1954).

A single dose of 100 mg/kg acetophenone given to each of eight male albino rats of 250 g body weight by intraperitoneal injection was eliminated as mandelic acid, benzoylformic acid, benzoic acid, hydroxyacetophenone and phenylgloxal in urine within 24 hours of dosing (Sullivan *et al* 1976). In addition to these metabolites $^{14}CO_2$ was exhaled by another group of rats which were intraperitoneally dosed with [methyl-^{14}C]acetophenone; 10% of the label was exhaled as carbon dioxide in the first 4 hours, and 30% in 13 hours (Sullivan *et al* 1976).

In a study of rabbits given [methyl-^{14}C]acetophenone by intraperitoneal injection, 10% of the label was exhaled as carbon dioxide in the first 4 hours, and 30% after 13 hours (Sullivan *et al* 1976).

Rabbits each given one intraperitoneal injection of 2000 mg acetophenone eliminated 48.8% of the dose via the urine as the glucuronide. No other parameters were measured (Thierfielder and Klenk 1924).

Rabbits subcutaneously dosed with acetophenone appeared to eliminate hippuric acid and methylphenylcarbinol glucuronic acid in their urine. Smaller amounts of mandelic acid, free acetophenone, and free methylphenylcarbinol were also identified. Of the dose, 35.7% had been reduced to the carbinol and conjugated with glucuronic acid before elimination, while 24.3% of the administered acetophenone had been oxidised to benzoic acid (Thierfielder and Daiber 1923).

Fifteen male rabbits, weighing 3.8–4.3 kg, were each administered 5360 mg (between 1250 and 1410 mg/kg) of acetophenone by intraperitoneal injection, and urine was collected for 48 hours. Approximately 0.1% of the dose was excreted unchanged. 1-Phenylethanol accounted for 3.6% of the dose, omega-, *para*, and *meta*-hydroxyacetophenone accounted for 0.75%, 0.4% and 0.1% of the dose respectively. A substantial portion of 1-phenylethanol, up to half the total amount, was extracted from the urine in the unconjugated form (Kiese and Lenk 1974).

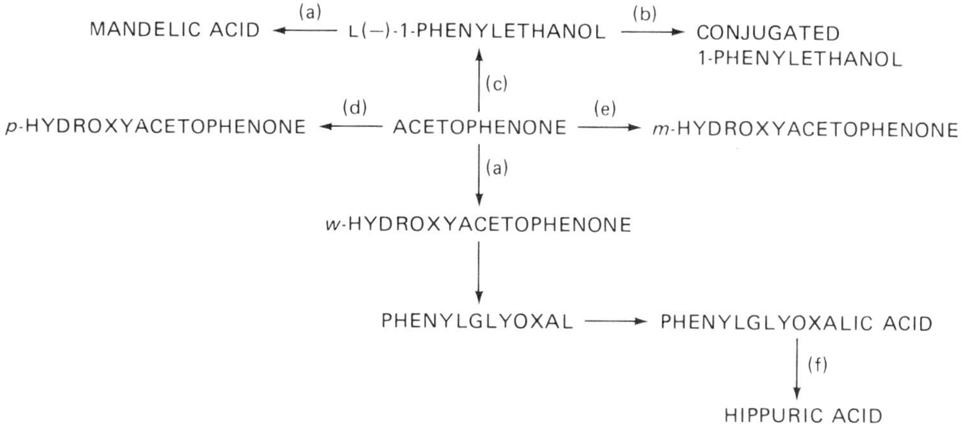

where: (a) = ω-oxidation
(b) = conjugation
(c) = reduction
(d) = *p*-hydroxylation
(e) = *m*-hydroxylation
(f) = decarboxylation conjugation

Acetophenone has been reported to be reduced by incubation with rat liver post-mitochondrial supernatant (Maylin and Anders 1969). The reduction of acetophenone was found by Culp and McMahon (1968) to be due to an NADPH-mediated enzyme, associated with the cytosol. The enzyme, referred to as aromatic A-K reductase, was initially isolated from rabbit kidney cortex tissue, and later from the kidney cortex of rats and hogs, as well as rabbit liver, but not from the heart, lung or smooth muscle. The reaction was found to be irreversible when tested with the alcohol analogue of acetophenone, 1-phenylethanol.

Leibman (1971) examined the *in vitro* metabolism of a number of ketones in complete cytosol and microsomal fractions of the liver, and found that acetophenone reduction took place almost exclusively in the cytosol. It was found that the reduction occurred primarily in the liver and kidney of rabbit. Slight activity was observed in both the heart and lungs, but not the brain. Enzymic reduction occurred in the presence of both NADPH and NADH in a ratio of 10 : 1 respectively, suggesting that a number of enzymes may be involved. This reaction was found to be reversible, with NADP and NAD utilised during the oxidation of 1-phenylethanol, which is further evidence for the involvement of more than one enzyme, since aromatic A-K reductase does not catalyse the oxidation of 1-phenylethanol to acetophenone (Leibman 1971).

1.3 Toxicity

Due to the low volatility of acetophenone, significant exposure by the pulmonary route is unlikely, ingestion being the far more likely route of exposure. The acute oral toxicity of acetophenone appears to be relatively low, although anaesthetic effects have been noted. The majority of the limited number of toxicological studies available relate to acute and subchronic toxicity. There is a distinct lack of chronic and human toxicity data. Krasavage *et al* (1982) and Opdyke (1973b) have reviewed the toxicity of acetophenone.

1.3.1 Acute toxicity

The oral LD50 of acetophenone in the rat has been determined to be 900 mg/kg in Sherman rats (Smyth and Carpenter 1948), and 3200 mg/kg in Osborne–Mendel rats (Jenner *et al* 1964). Another study gives the figure as 1.87 ml/kg (1930 mg/kg) in female rats of an unspecified strain (Smyth *et al* 1970). The intraperitoneal LD50 in mouse has been reported as 200 mg/kg and 1070 mg/kg (NIOSH 1978, Quevauviller 1946). Central nervous depression has been observed in mice receiving intraperitoneal doses of between 400 and 500 mg/kg (Quevauviller 1946).

All six rats exposed, by inhalation, to between 4400 and 5000 ppm of acetophenone survived an exposure period of 2 hours. When the exposure time was doubled to 4 hours, all six rats died. Death was attributed to anaesthesia. Congestion of the liver, lungs and kidneys was observed in these animals (US EPA 1976).

The dermal LD50 of acetophenone has been reported to be in excess of 20 ml/kg (20 600 mg/kg) for guinea-pigs (Smyth and Carpenter 1944). Slight erythema has been reported to occur when applied undiluted to the clipped belly of rabbits, and left uncovered. A 15% solution of acetophenone caused severe eye injury to rabbits (US EPA 1976). Another study, in which undiluted acetophenone (771 mg) was applied to the eyes of rabbits, revealed moderate irritation and transient corneal injury (Smyth and Carpenter 1948).

1.3.2 Subchronic and chronic toxicity

A slight degree of liver damage was reported in a group of 15 male rats, of between 60 and 70 g body weight, exposed to 1.43 ppm of acetophenone, by inhalation, for 70 days. Cholinesterase activity was monitored in five of the rats, and a number of changes, although not consistent ones, were noted. In three of the rats the cholinesterase activity decreased by 22%, and in one the activity increased by 45%. A distinct decrease in albumin/globulin ratio was observed in these rats, even though the total protein remained the same. Rats exposed by inhalation to 0.143 ppm displayed no apparent signs of toxicity. No deaths were recorded at either exposure level (Imasheva 1971).

Sherman rats orally dosed with between 1.0 and 102.0 mg/kg of acetophenone per day for a period of 30 days suffered no ill effects. Growth, appetite, and micropathology remained normal (Smyth and Carpenter 1948).

No mortalities occurred in groups of rats fed either 1.0, 6.0, or 25.0 mg/kg of acetophenone daily for 30 days. A significant increase in liver weight relative to total body weight was the only deviation from normal (US EPA 1976).

Three groups of ten male and ten female Osborne–Mendel rats were fed 1000, 2500 or 10 000 ppm of acetophenone daily for 17 weeks. On examination, no effects on growth, haematology or macroscopic pathology were observed (Hagan *et al* 1967).

1.3.3 Human toxicity

In the early part of this century, acetophenone was used to sedate and induce sleep in mental patients during treatment. The acetophenone was only of secondary importance as a sedative, and at therapeutic levels caused a burning sensation in the stomachs of some patients (US EPA 1976).

Acetophenone, tested at a concentration of 2% in petrolatum, caused no irritation of human skin during a 48-hour closed patch test. No sensitisation reactions occurred in these 25 volunteers (Opdyke 1973b, US EPA 1976).

1.4 Mutagenicity

Florin *et al* (1980) reported that acetophenone did not exhibit mutagenic activity in *Salmonella typhimurium* TA98, TA100, TA1535, and TA1537, when tested either with or without the presence of S-9 from arcolor-induced rats, at 3 μmol/plate.

In another study, acetophenone displayed no mutagenic activity in *Salmonella typhimurium* TA98, TA100, and TA1535 under the same conditions (Elliger *et al* 1984).

1.5 Teratogenicity and carcinogenicity

Application of 480 mg/kg of acetophenone daily to the skin of pregnant rats on days 10–15 of gestation caused no changes in gestation period, size of litter, weight of offspring, time for the appearance of teeth or hair, opening of eyes, or the appearance of reflexes (Lagno and Bakhtizina 1969).

No data concerning the carcinogenicity of this compound were found.

1.6 Discussion

Acetophenone has been reported to occur in a number of water sources up to levels of 29 μg/l. It was identified in both surveys of UK drinking water samples carried out by WRc.

Acetophenone appears to be metabolised to methylphenylcarbinol and benzoic acid. The benzoic acid is conjugated with glycine to form hippuric acid, which is eliminated largely in the urine. Minor metabolites also reported include *o*-, *m*-, *p*-hydroxyacetophenone and mandelic acid.

Limited studies indicate that acetophenone is of relatively low acute oral toxicity, the LD50 via this route being reported to be between 900 and 3200 mg/kg in rat. On the whole, toxicological data are sparse.

Acetophenone does not appear to be mutagenic, and one study involving the dermal application of acetophenone revealed no teratogenic effects. No carcinogenicity studies have been undertaken to date.

Insufficient information is available for a complete toxicological evaluation of this compound to be made.

2. 9,10-ANTHRAQUINONE

9,10-anthraquinone is found as yellowish-green crystals, which are reported to be insoluble in water, although no actual solubility data were found. It is used as an intermediate for dyes and organics, and as a bird repellent for seeds.

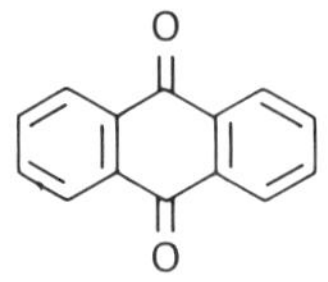

CAS Reg No:	84-65-1
Molecular weight:	208.22
Molecular formula:	$C_{14}H_8O_2$

Synonyms: Anthraquinone; anthracene, 9,10-dihydro-9,10-dioxo-; 9,10-anthracenedione; anthradione; corbit; hoelite; morkit; and 9,10-dioxoanthracene.

9,10-Anthraquinone has been detected in the tap water of the Kitakyushu area of Japan at a level of 5.2 ng/l (Akiyama *et al* 1980). It has been identified in 12 drinking water samples from Ontario at levels of between 0.1 and 2.1 ng/l (Benoit *et al* 1979), and in two raw water samples in Ontario at 0.9 and 4.7 ng/l (Benoit *et al* 1979). Anthraquinone was identified in the drinking water of Cincinnati, Ohio (Coleman *et al* 1980), and in 4/14 drinking water samples in an unpublished survey by WRc.

The intraperitoneal LD50 of 9,10-anthraquinone in rats has been reported to be 3500 mg/kg (Volodchenko *et al* 1971). Experimental animals chronically exposed to oral doses of anthraquinone were reported to show slight anaemia, poor blood coagulation, hepatitis and a slight impairment of nitrogen excretion by the kidneys. 9,10-Anthraquinone was the least toxic in comparison with 1,2-diamino- and 1,5-diamino-anthraquinone. Actual dose levels and exposure times were not specified in this Russian study (Volodchenko and Ladunskii 1972). It has been reported that mice are not affected by an oral dose of 5000 mg/kg (Worthing 1979).

Anthraquinone has been reported to be non-mutagenic in a number of studies. It did not exhibit any mutagenic activity in a variety of *Salmonella typhimurium* tester strains. Strains used have been TA1535, TA1538 (Anderson and Styles 1978, Brown, 1980), TA98, TA100, TA1535 (Brown 1980), TA2637 (Tikkanen *et al* 1983), and TM677 (kaden *et al* 1979), all with or without the presence of either phenobarbitol or Arcolor 1254 induced rat liver S-9. Liberman *et al* (1982) found that anthraquinone exhibited a weak mutagenic effect in *Salmonella typhimurium* TA 1537, TA 1538, and TA 98, in the absence of metabolic activation.

Anthraquinone also gave negative results in *in vitro* mammalian cell transformation assays with both Chang (human liver) and BHK-21 (baby Syrian hamster kidney) cells, with and without metabolic activation (Styles 1978).

Eighteen mice of each sex of two hybrid strains, B6C3F1 and B6AKF1, were given anthraquinone in the diet at a concentration of 1206 ppm for 18 months . No significant increase in the number of tumours occurred compared to the controls (Bionetics Research Lab Inc 1968, Innes *et al* 1969). Anthraquinone again caused no increase in the tumour incidence in mice of the same hybrid strains given daily subcutaneous injections of 1000 mg/kg for 18 months (Bionetics Research Lab Inc 1968).

3. BENZOPHENONE

Benzophenone is a solid at room temperature, and has a geranium-like odour. It is reported to be insoluble in water, although no actual figures were found. Benzophenone can be prepared by the Friedel-Crafts method by reacting benzene with benzoyl chloride, in the presence of aluminium chloride.

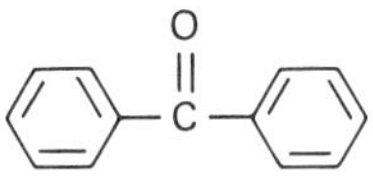

CAS Reg No:	119-61-9
Molecular weight:	182.21
Molecular formula:	$C_{13}H_{10}O$
Boiling point:	304.5 °C
Melting point:	48.5

Synonyms: diphenyl ketone, benzoylbenzene, diphenylmethanone

Benzophenone is widely used as a fixative for heavy perfumes, such as geranium, the new-mown hay, especially when used in soaps. It is also used in the manufacture of antihistamines, hypnotics, and insecticides.

3.1 Exposure

Benzophenone does not appear to occur naturally, although it is used as a fragrance in soap, detergent, perfume, creams and lotions. In the past, benzophenone has been used as a sun-protecting agent (Opdyke 1973). It was detected in Japanese tap water at 8.8. ng/l (Akiyama *et al* 1980), and identified in 1/14 drinking water samples in an unpublished survey by WRc. Benzophenone has been detected in the atmosphere of Alabama (Holzer *et al* 1977).

3.2 Absorption, distribution, metabolism and excretion

The main route for the metabolism of benzophenone is reduction of the keto group to yield benzhydrol, which is then conjugated with glucuronic acid (Williams 1959). Robinson (1958) found that between 46 and 61% of an oral dose of benzophenone was excreted as the glucuronide in rabbits' urine within 48 hours of dosing. No ethereal sulphates were found, and it seems likely that hydroxylation of the aromatic ring does not occur to any significant extent.

$$(C_6H_5)2.CO \rightarrow (C_6H_5)2CH.OH \rightarrow (C_6H_5)2CH.O.C_6H_9O_6$$

When incubated with the S-9 fraction of rabbit liver in the presence of an NADPH-generating system, benzophenone was reduced to the corresponding secondary alcohol, benzhydrol (Leibman 1971).

3.3 Toxicity

There appear to be very limited data on the toxicity of benzophenone. The oral LD50 has been reported to be in excess of 10 000 mg/kg in the rat (Opdyke 1973a), and 2895 mg/kg in male Swiss mice (Caprino *et al* 1976). In lethal doses, benzophenone has been reported to induce sedation, progressive depression of motor activity, unstable gait, tremors and respiratory impairment. No lesions or gross abnormalities of visceral organs were noted at autopsy (Caprino *et al* 1976). The dermal LD50 in rabbit was found to be 3535 mg/kg (Opdyke 1973a), while the intraperitoneal LD50 in mouse was 727 mg-kg (Caprino *et al* 1976).

No sensitisation reactions occurred in a maximisation test, when a 6% solution of benzophenone in petrolatum was tested in 25 human volunteers (Opdyke 1973a).

No significant increase in the number of tumours in mice was observed following the dermal application of benzophenone. Groups of 50 7-week-old female Swiss mice received 0.02 ml of either 50, 25, or 5% benzophenone in acetone, which was applied to a 1-inch square shaved area of dorsal skin twice daily for the lifespan of the animals. Tumours occurred in 28, 32, and 52% of the animals treated with 50, 25, and 5% of benzophenone, respectively. The number of tumours was not statistically significant when compared to untreated controls, in which a 42% tumour rate was observed (Stenbuck and Shubik 1974).

4. 2,6-DISUBSTITUTED *p*-BENZOQUINONES

2,6-Di-*tert*-butyl-*p*-benzoquinone was identified in five, and 2,6-dimethyl-*p*-benzoquinone in two, or 14 drinking water samples in an unpublished survey by WRc.

2,6-Di-*tert*-butyl-*p*-benzoquinone is a metabolite of the commonly used anti-oxidant butylated hydroxytoluene (BHT). The only toxicological information found was an intraperitoneal LD50 of 2270 mg/kg body weight in male ddY (Yamamoto *et al* 1980). No data were found on the toxicity of 2,6-dimethyl-*p*-benzoquinone.

5. 1-INDANONE

1-Inadanone (alpha-hydrindone) is a solid which is synthesised by an internal Friedel–Crafts reaction on beta-phenylpropionyl chloride.

Molecular weight:	132
Molecular formula:	C_9H_8O
Melting point:	42.0 °C

1-Indanone was identified in 1/14 drinking water samples by WRc. It has also been identified in sea and river water in the Kitakyushu area of Japan (Akiyama *et al* 1980).

1-Indanone was found to be non-mutagenic in *Salmonella typhimurium* TA98,

TA11, TA1535 and TA1537 with and without S-9 mix from aroclor-induced rats (Florin *et al* 1980).

No other data on the toxicity of 1-indanone were found.

6. 9-FLUORENONE

Fluorenone is a solid at room temperature, consisting of yellow rhombic or bipyrimidal crystals. It is prepared by the oxidation of fluorene with chromium trioxide in glacial acetic acid.

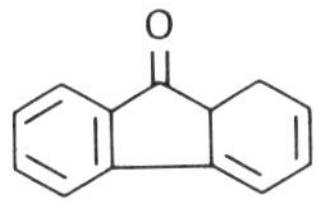

CAS Reg No:	486-25-9
Molecular weight:	180.21
Molecular formula:	$C_{13}H_8O$
Melting point:	84.0 °C
Boiling point:	341.5 °C

Synonyms: 9-H-fluoren-9-one; diphenylene ketone; 9-oxo-fluorene.

9-Fluorenone was identified in two of 14 drinking water samples in a survey by WRC (Water Research Centre 1981).

Subcutaneous injection of rabbits with 3 mmol of fluoreneone caused a decrease in hepatic aryl hydrocarbon hydroxyklase and epoxide hydrolase activities. Hepatic or intestinal NADPH cytochrome *c* reductase, hepatic cytochrome P-450 and ethoxyresorufin *O*-deethylase, hepatic and intestinal ethoxycoumarin *O*-deethylase, and glutathione *S*-transferase were unaffected (Hietanen and Vaniop 1982). Noradrenaline-induced oxidative metabolism of isolated fat cells from adult hamsters was inhibited by 54% when incubated with a 1.0 mM solution of 9-fluorenone (Pettersson *et al* 1980).

Only one long-term study appears to have been carried out. Albino rats were fed 9-fluorenone in the diet at concentrations of between 0.031 and 0.50% for 100–600 days. Concentrations of 0.125% and above caused a significant decrease in the rate of growth of the animals. The livers, kidneys and possibly testes were significantly heavier than in the controls. No increased incidence of tumours was apparent in this experiment or in another study of rats subjected to subcutaneous injection of 20 mg of 9-fluorenone for 6 months (Wilson *et al* 1947).

Fluorenone was non-mutagenic in *Salmonella typhimurium* TA98, TA100, TA1535, and TA1537, with and without S-9 from arcolor-induced rats, when tested at 30 μmole/plate. Precipitation of the fluorenone made the result obtained difficult to evaluate (Florin *et al* 1980).

7. ISOPHORONE

Isophorone is an unsaturated, cyclic ketone or aliphatic enone, which is found as a colourless liquid. It has a low volatility, and a sharp peppermint-like odour, and is chiefly employed as a solvent for the formulation of lacquers and other surface coatings. It is also used as an intermediate for alcohols, a raw material for 3,5-dimethyl-aniline, and in the manufacture of pesticides. Isophorone is produced commercially by passing acetone over calcium oxide, calcium carbide, or mixtures of these at 350°C and 1 atmosphere of pressure. The United States commercial production of isophorone was 28 million pounds in 1973.

$$OCCHC(CH_3)CH_2C(CH_3)_2CH_2$$

CAS Reg. No:	78-59-1
Molecular weight:	138.23
Molecular formula:	$C_9H_{14}O$
Boiling point:	215.2 °C
Solubility:	12 000 mg/l
Threshold odour concentration:	0.20

Synonyms: 3,5,5-trimethyl-2-cyclohexen-1-one, isoacetophorone, isoforon, 1,1,3-trimethyl-3-cyclohexene-5-one.

7.1 Exposure

7.1.1 Water

Isophorone was identified in one of 14 UK drinking water samples examined by WRc (Water Research Centre 1981). The US EPA detected isophorone at an average level of 2.3 μg/l in several finished drinking water samples taken from the New Orleans area (US EPA 1974). In a follow-up survey, isophorone was only identified in the finished drinking water of one of ten cities. It was identified only in Cincinnati, at a level of 0.02 μg/l, but this water was categorised as being contaminated with industrial discharge (US EPA 1975). Another study has also identified isophorone in the drinking water of the Cincinnati area of Ohio (Coleman *et al* 1980). In a nationwide survey of the US, isophorone occurred at concentrations up to 9.5 μg/l (US EPA 1975). It has also been detected in water from the Delaware River, near a highly industrialised region, at concentrations of less than 0.1 ppb (Sheldon and Hites 1978). Levels of between 25 and 90 ppb isophorone were detected in raw Kanawha River water (Dostal *et al* 1965). Isophorone has also been detected at 0.04 mg/l in wastewater from a tyre manufacturing plant (Jungclaus *et al* 1976), and in the effluents from latex and chemical plants in Alabama (Shackelford and Keith 1976).

7.1.2 Air and food

No data were found on the occurrence of isophorone in air or food.

7.2 Toxicokinetics

Truhaut *et al* (1970) identified dimethyl-5,5-cyclohexen-1-one- 3-carboxylic acid, and its glucuronide, in the urine of rabbits 24 hours after oral dosing with 1000 mg/kg isophorone. They later identified the same metabolite and its glucuronide in rat urine (Truhaut *et al* 1973).

In a further study by the same group, New Zealand rabbits, of 2.5 kg body weight, were dosed with 1000 mg/kg of isophorone by stomach tube. Their 24- and 48-hour urine, and expired air, was collected and examined for possible metabolites. Isophorone was partly eliminated unchanged in the expired air and urine. A number of metabolites found in the urine were characterised, including dimethyl-5,5-cyclohexen-1-one-3-carboxylic acid, which was probably formed by the methyloxidation of isophorone and the secondary alcohol, isophorol (trimethyl-3,5,5-cyclohexen-2-ol-1) which was probably formed by the reduction of the ketonic group, and eliminated as the glucuronide. Another metabolite, dihydroisophorone (trimethyl-3,5,5-cyclohexanone) was probably formed by the hydrogenation of the cyclohexene ring. *Cis*- and *trans*-trimethyl-3,5,5-cyclohexanol-1 were found in only small quantities (Dutertre-Catella *et al* 1978).

7.3 Toxicity

Reviews of the toxicity of isophorone have been published by the US EPA (1978) and Krasavage *et al* (1982).

7.3.1 Acute toxicity

Oral LD50s have been reported for isophorone of 2000 mg/kg and greater than 3200 mg/kg for mice (Bukhalovskii and Shugaev 1976, Krasavage *et al* 1982), and 2370 mg/kg, 1870 mg/kg, 2100 mg/kg, 2120 mg/kg and greater than 3200 mg/kg for rats (Union Carbide 1975, Smyth *et al* 1969a, Krasavage *et al* 1982). The intraperitoneal LD50 has been found to be 400 mg/kg for mice, and between 400 and 800 mg/kg for rats (Krasavage *et al* 1982)

Guinea-pigs and rats were exposed by inhalation to between 300 and 4600 ppm of isophorone for a maximum single exposure of up to 24 hours at the lower level and up to 8 hours at the higher exposure level, the other periods being between these two. A number of symptoms were exhibited by the majority of animals, including irritation of eyes and nose, followed by lacrimation, swelling of nose, instability, respiratory difficulty or irregularity, diarrhoea, and finally light narcosis. This was followed by death in a number of animals (Smyth and Seaton 1940). An increased heart rate was observed in those animals exposed for periods over 12 hours. Irritation of eyes and nose was observed immediately at all levels of 800 ppm and above, but did not occur during 24-hour exposures to 300 ppm. Although not observed in rats, opacity of the cornea or corneal necrosis was found in guinea-pigs after exposure to 840 ppm or more for periods of at least 4 hours. The only symptom appearing during continuous 24-hour exposure to 300 ppm of isophorone was an accelerated heart rate. Deaths were seen in groups of rats exposed to 1840 ppm or more for periods of 4 hours, and was attributed to respiratory paralysis. No guinea-pigs died at any of the exposure levels. Gross pathology included petechial and massive haemorrhages of the lungs, congestion of the stomach and liver, excess peritoneal fluid, and a discoloration of the kidneys and spleen. A temporary drop in red blood cell and haemoglobin levels was seen in the majority of animals. White blood cell levels appeared unchanged (Smyth and Seaton 1940).

Union Carbide (1975) reported that a single 8-hour exposure to approximately

600 ppm isophorone killed one of six rats exposed. In the same study it was found that the dermal LD50 in rabbit was 1390 mg/kg. It has also been reported to be 1500 mg/kg (Krasavage *et al* 1982). Isophorone has been reported to be only a weak irritant to the skin of rabbits, although it caused reversible irritation of the conjunctiva and corneal opacity. It has also been reported to be a moderate irritant to the eye of rabbit in a number of other studies (Carpenter and Smyth 1946, Truhaut *et al* 1972, Union Carbide 1963).

7.3.2 Subacute toxicity

Groups of ten male Wistar rats and ten guinea-pigs were exposed to isophorone vapours at concentrations of either 25, 50, 100, 200 or 500 ppm for 8 hours/day, 5 days/week, for 6 weeks. Exposure to 25 ppm of isophorone caused no ill effects. Deaths occurred at concentrations of 100 ppm and above, with a 45% mortality rate being seen in those receiving 500 ppm isophorone. These animals also displayed a loss of appetite, and so lost weight before death. The authors made no distinction between the results with guinea-pigs and with rats (Smyth *et al* 1942). Animals exposed to 500 ppm isophorone often developed chronic conjunctivitis and nasal irritation, although no corneal necrosis occurred. Lung irritation was observed, resulting in congestion, capillary leakage and desquamation of epithelium in these animals. Liver damage was observed in a small proportion of the animals, and was confined to congestion and slight cloudy swelling. The kidney pathology was seen to be abnormal in 66% of the animals exposed to concentrations of greater than 50 ppm, dilation of Bowman's capsule and cloudy swelling of convoluted tubular epithelium being most typical (Smyth *et al* 1942).

7.3.3 Subchronic toxicity

Four groups of 20 male and female CFE albino rats were fed 0, 750, 1500 or 3000 ppm isophorone in the diet, for 90 days. No significant differences were observed in body weights or food consumption of any of the groups at the end of the study, although the body weight of the 3000 ppm male group was significantly depressed for several weeks of the study before returning to normal. There was no significant difference between the treated and control group with regard to haematology, blood chemistry or urinalysis. No pathological lesions were observed when the animals were examined grossly or microscopically (US EPA 1972).

Four groups of one male and one female beagle were each fed either 0, 35, 75 or 150 mg/kg isophorone in the form of gelatin capsules daily for 90 days. Body weights, organ weights, and food consumption were within normal limits in all animals. All animals survived the 90-day treatment period, before being sacrificed and thoroughly examined. No abnormalities were observed in haematology, biochemical and urinalyses tests. All organs and tissues appeared normal on close examination (US EPA 1972).

7.3.4 Human toxicity

During experimental work on laboratory animals, humans have reported isophorone concentrations of 300 ppm and above to be irritant to eyes and nose. Conjunctivitis has been observed in those exposed to 300 ppm for a few minutes, but this was transient. As a result of this finding, groups of 11 or 12 human volunteers were exposed by inhalation to either 40, 85, 200 or 400 ppm of isophorone for a few minutes. All reported eye, nose and throat irritation. There were a few complaints of nausea, headache, dizziness, faintness, inebriation, and feelings of suffocation at concentrations of 200 and 400 ppm. At the lower two concentrations, symptoms of irritation and narcotic action appeared to decrease with time (Smyth and Seaton 1940).

Isophorone has been reported to cause irritation to the eyes, nose and throats of human volunteers when exposed by inhalation to 25 ppm isophorone for 15 minutes. The majority of subjects did not subject to the odour during an 8-hour exposure to 10 ppm (Silverman *et al* 1946). Workers exposed to between 5 and 8 ppm isophorone for an unspecified length of time complained of fatigue and malaise. No complaints were reported after exposure to between 1 and 4 ppm (NIOSH 1978).

A one-minute exposure to 200 ppm isophorone has been reported to be intolerable for humans, and only half of an unspecified number found 40 ppm tolerable. In the same study, no sensitisation reactions were noted in ten human volunteers tested (Union Carbide 1963).

7.4 Carcinogenicity

Isophorone in corn oil was administered to rats and mice by gavage 5 days/week for 103 weeks at doses of 0, 250 or 500 mg/kg body weight. Dosed male rats developed proliferative and non-proliferative lesions of the kidney. Carcinomas of the preputial gland were observed in high-dose male rats or mice but there was some indication of increased hepatocellular and mesenchymal neoplasms in high-dose male mice (Bucher *et al* 1986).

7.5 Mutagenicity and teratogenicity

No mutagenicity or teratogenicity data for isophorone were found.

7.6 Discussion

Isophorone is usually present in drinking water at low ug/l levels. WRc identified isophorone in only one of 14 UK drinking water samples examined.

Little is known about the toxicokinetics in isophorone, although a number of metabolites from rabbit urine have been isolated and characterised.

Isophorone appears to have a relatively low acute oral toxicity in experimental animals; the oral LD50 in rat has been reported to be within the 2000–3200 mg/kg range. The vapour of isophorone appears to be highly irritating to the eyes, nose and throat of both humans and experimental animals.

8. BUTAN-2-ONE

Butan-2-one is a colourless liquid used as a solvent or swelling agent for resins, as an intermediate in the manufacture of ketones and amines, as a flush-off paint stripper, for the extraction and production of wax from lube oil fractions of petroleum, and as a solvent in nitrocellulose coatings and vinyl films.

$CH_3.CO.CH_2.CH_3$

CAS Reg No:	78-93-3
Molecular weight:	72.12
Molecular formula:	C_4H_8O
Boiling point:	79.6 °C
Solubility in water:	353 000 mg/l

Synonyms: methyl ethyl ketone, MEK, methyl acetone.

8.1 Exposure

Water

Butan-2-one was identified in three of 14 UK drinking water samples examined by WRc (Water Research Centre 1981). It has also been detected in the tap water of Philadelphia, Seattle, Iowa, Miami, and Cincinnati by the US EPA (Keith 1976a), and in the tap water of the District of Columbia, USA (Eurocop-cost 1976).

Air

Butan-2-one has been identified in the urban air of Osaka, Japan (Kuwata *et al* 1979), in cigarette smoke at 500 ppm (Kuwata *et al* 1979, Verschueren 1977), and in gasoline exhaust at levels of between <0.1 and 1.0 ppm (Kuwata *et al* 1979, Verschueren 1983).

Food

It has been detected as an impurity, within the products of the dry-distillation of wood, and in the oil of black tea. It has also been found in coffee, cheese, bread, citrus oils and natural products such as grape and raspberry (Opdyke 1975c).

8.2 Absorption, distribution, metabolism, and excretion

Butan-2-one is readily absorbed by all routes of exposure; its metabolism appears to follow both oxidative and reductive pathways, the ketone undergoing ω-1 carbon atom oxidation to the corresponding hydroxyketone, which then undergoes reduction to the diol. The secondary alcohol, butan-2-ol, is formed by the reduction of the ketone, and is then eliminated in the urine as *O*-sulphates or *O*-glucuronides, or may enter the intermediary metabolism to be eliminated as carbon dioxide, or incorporated into tissues (Williams 1959).

Examination of the blood serum of male guinea-pigs for periods of up to 16 hours after intraperitoneal injection of 450 mg/kg showed that at least three metabolites had been formed. These metabolites were characterised as butan-2-ol, 3-hydroxybutan-2-one and 2,3-butanediol. The butan-2-one was found to have a serum half-life of 270 minutes, and serum clearance time of 12 hours, while the three metabolites were all cleared from the serum within 16 hours of dosing (DiVincenco *et al* 1976).

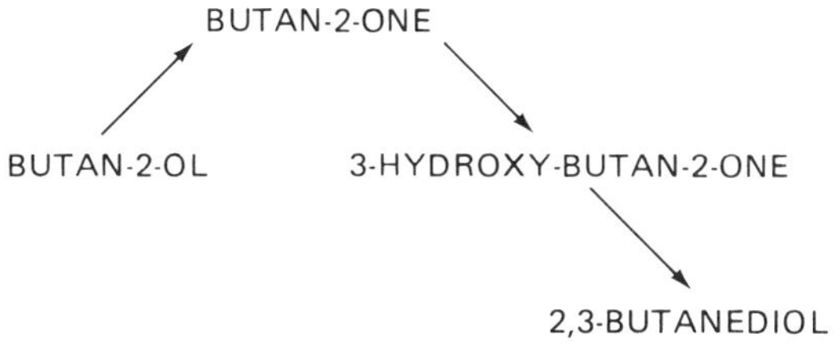

In dogs, approximately 30–33% of an oral dose of 300–500 mg/kg was eliminated unchanged in the expired air (Williams 1959). Humans exposed to 300 ppm of butan-2-one by inhalation for 2 hours were reported to eliminate 23 ppm unchanged in the expired air, with a smaller amount in the urine (Tadas *et al* 1972). Butan-2-one has been reported to be rapidly absorbed by hydrated and dehydrated skin of the human forearm. Rapid absorption was indicated by the appearance of unchanged butan-2-one in the expired air soon after dosing. The exposure lasted for 8 hours, a constant rate of absorption being reached in 2–5 hours. The rate was highest in the hydrated skin. Similar excretion of unchanged butan-2-one in expired air was observed following the ingestion of a 375 mg capsule of butan-2-one by volunteers (Munies 1965, Wurster and Munies 1965). Butan-2-one has been detected in the urine of normal, healthy adults (Tsao and Pfeiffer 1957, Zlatkis *et al* 1973). It has also been identified in the urine, milk and blood of cows fed unspecified concentrations of this ketone. The highest concentration was found in the urine (Loney *et al* 1963).

Leibman (1971) examined the *in vitro* metabolism of butan-2-one by complete cytosol and microsomal fractions of rat liver. It was found that butan-2-one reduction occurred almost exclusively in the cytosol, and that both NADPH and NADH could serve as reducing agents (Leibman 1971). These NADPH and NADH-dependent reductions may reflect the activity of a number of different cytosolic enzymes rather than NADH-dependent alcohol dehydrogenase and NADPH-dependent aromatic A-K reductase, which did not cause the reduction of this ketone in *in vitro* test systems (Merritt and Tomkins 1959, Culp and McMahon 1968).

8.3 Toxicity

Few data are available concerning the long-term oral toxicity of butan-2-one. It does appear to be of low toxicity by the oral route in short-term studies. It also appears to have a low inhalation toxicity, and although it has been widely reported not to be neurotoxic itself, it does appear to potentiate polyneuropathy caused by other solvents. It is also thought that it may potentiate the hepatoxicity of carbon tetrachloride.

8.3.1 Acute toxicity

Carpenter (1954) reported the oral LD50 of a 10% dispersion of butan-2-one in 1% Tergitol, in male Sherman rats, to be 3980 mg/kg, while the figure for female Carworth–Wistar rats was 5530 mg/kg (Smyth *et al* 1962). The effect of age on susceptibility to poisoning has been examined for butan-2-one using Sprague–Dawley rats of three age groups: 14 days old (16–50 g body weight), young adults

(80–160 g), and older adults (300–470 g). The oral LD50s for these groups were 2500, 2900 and 2700 mg/kg respectively (Kimura *et al* 1971).

In the study by Carpenter (1954) no deaths were recorded at an oral dose level of 3160 mg/kg, while a 100% mortality rate was recorded at 6300 mg-kg butan-2-one. At the higher dose levels, butan-2-one caused narcosis and central nervous depression. At the highest sublethal doses, narcosis was found to last for as long as 15 hours. With fatal doses, death usually occurred within 48 hours. Gross pathological findings included congestion or haemorrhage of the lungs, congestion of the liver and intestine, and discoloration of the liver, and spleen (Carpenter 1954).

Butan-2-one did not appear to be hepatoxic to male Sprague–Dawley rats (180–250 g body weight) receiving oral doses of 1.87 ml/kg (1510 mg/kg). Serum alanine aminotransaminase (ALT) and hepatic glucose-6-phosphatase activities did not differ significantly from controls when monitored for up to 16 hours, although the hepatic trigyceride content was significantly elevated (163%) 16 hours after treatment. Butan-2-one did appear to potentiate the hepatotoxic effect induced by carbon tetrachloride treatment. One group of rats were given an intraperitoneal injection of 0.1 ml/kg of carbon tetrachloride in corn oil 16 hours after an oral dose of 1.87 kl/kg butan-2-one. The rats were sacrificed 24 hours after carbon tetrachloride administration. Compared to animals receiving the injection of carbon tetrachloride alone, the serum ALT levels were increased by approximate 2000%, the hepatic glucose-6-phosphatase decreased by approximately 50%, and there was a 100% increase in liver tryglyceride content. Examination of the livers also revealed centrilobular fatty vacuolation and necrosis (Traiger and Bruckner 1975).

These authors also attempted to determine the effect of the sovent on the hepatic ultrastructure and microsomal drug-metabolising activity of the rat. Animals given an oral dose of 1.87 ml/kg (1510 mg/kg) butan-2-one were killed 16, 28, or 40 hours after dosing. At each of these times, an increased acetanilide hydroxylase activity of between 50 and 97% was found. Aminopyrine-*N*-demethylase activity was significantly increased in those sacrificed after 40 hours, the increase being less pronounced at 16 or 28 hours. Electron microscopic examination of the hepatocytes revealed an increase in the smooth endoplasmic reticulum content of the cells. These results suggest that the potentiation of carbon tetrachloride hepatotoxicity may be related, in part, to an induction of the mixed function oxidase system.

Guinea-pigs exposed by inhalation to 3300 ppm butan-2-one for 13.5 hours showed no signs of intoxication. Those subjected to 10 000 ppm suffered irritation of the eyes and nose within 4 minutes, and narcosis was noted after 4–5 hours. Guinea-pigs exposed to 33 000 ppm showed narcosis, and subsequently death. Exposure to 100 000 ppm for between 45 and 55 minutes did not cause death, although narcosis was observed after only 10 minutes (Krasavage *et al* 1982). Irritation of eyes and nose, lacrimation, incoordination, narcosis, respiratory distress and death have also been noted at 100 000 ppm. Corneal opacity has been reported to develop after 30 minutes in some cases (US EPA 1976).

No deaths were seen in guinea-pigs exposed by inhalation to 100 000 ppm for a few minutes (Patty *et al* 1935). Those exposed to lethal doses showed marked congestion of the internal organs, especially the liver and kidney, and to a lesser extent the brain. The lungs showed a degree of emphysema. Guinea-pigs surviving 100 000 ppm for 30 minutes developed corneal opacity, from which they recovered after 8 days or more (Patty *et al* 1935). Rats exposed to 2000 ppm of butan-2-one vapour for 2 hours have been reported to suffer no ill effects. At 4000 ppm, four of six rats died (Smyth 1956). Exposure to 8000 ppm for 8 hours was reported to result in the death of three of six rats, while 16000 ppm killed all six (Smyth *et al* 1962).

The inhalation LC50 of butan-2-one in male albino rats has been reported to be 11700 ppm. Narcosis occurred in the majority of survivors. No deaths were recorded in rats exposed to 7850 ppm for 4 hours, while at 18100 ppm a 100% mortality rate was found (La Belle and Brieger 1955).

Four lever-pressing, 90–120-day-old Holtzman, Sprague-Dawley rats were exposed by inhalation to 25 ppm butan-2-one during 6-hour experimental sessions. It was found that the response rate increased in all four animals, the highest increase being from 12.17 to 61.00 responses/minute. The response rate remained high for 11 days after the end of the exposure (Garcia *et al* 1978). Higher concentrations of between 500 and 3500 ppm have been reported to cause narcosis in chickens, cats, or rats (Abdel-Rahman *et al* 1976).

Groups of four male guinea-pigs received a single intraperitoneal injection of either 750, 1500 or 2000 mg/kg butan-2-one dissolved in corn oil. A moderate elevation in serum ornithine carbamyl transferase activity was observed in those animals dosed with 2000 mg-kg. At this dose level, one of the four animals died. Haematoxylin-and eosin-stained tissues showed no evidence of liver damage, although Oil Red O staining showed a slight accumulation of lipid at the two higher dose levels (DiVincenzo and Krasavage 1974). Intraperitoneal LD50s of 1.27 and 0.73 ml/kg (1023 and 588 mg/kg) have been reported for rats and guinea-pigs respectively (Krasavage *et al* 1982). The intraperitoneal LD50 of butan-2-one in mice has been reported to be 616 mg/kg (NIOSH 1978).

The acute dermal 14-day LD50 has been reported to be in excess of 5000 mg/kg (Moreno 1975), in excess of 8100 mg/kg (Smyth *et al* 1962), and 10200 mg/kg (Carpenter 1949) in rabbit. When applied full strength to intact or abraded rabbit skin for 24 hours under an occlusion butan-2-one was moderately irritating (Opdyke 1975c).

8.3.2 Subacute and chronic toxicity

Butan-2-one has been widely reported not to be neurotoxic itself (Opdyke 1975c, Krasavage *et al* 1982, Spencer and Schaumberg 1976, Saida *et al* 1975), although it does appear to potentiate polyneuropathy caused by some other solvents such as hexan-2-one (methyl *n*-butyl ketone) (Opdyke 1975c, Krasavage *et al* 1982, Saida *et al* 1975, Duckett *et al* 1974), nonan-5-one (di-*n*-butyl ketone) (Shifman *et al* 1981), heptan-3-one (ethyl *n*-butyl ketone) (O'Donoghue *et al* 1984), and *n*-hexane (Altenkirch *et al* 1978).

Saida *et al* (1975) did not observe any signs of neuropathy in rats exposed by inhalation to 1125 ppm for 5 months, although it did appear to potentiate the neurotoxic effect of hexan-2-one. Rats exposed to air containing butan-2-one and hexan-2-one vapours in a ratio of 1125 : 225 ppm, developed clinical signs (paralysis) of neuropathy after 25 days, whereas those inhaling 225 ppm of hexan-2-one alone exhibited neuropathy after 66 days (Saida *et al* 1975).

Rats exposed by inhalation to a mixture of 2000 ppm pf butan-2-one and 200 ppm of hexan-2-one for 8 hours/day, 5 days/week, for 6 weeks, developed muscular weakness of the limbs, and some deaths occurred. Histological examination of the sciatic nerves of these rats, and of rats exposed to 200 ppm of hexan-2-one, alone, showed axonal hypertrophy, beading and degeneration, associated with widespread perinodal and segmental breakdown of myelin representing the early changes of neuropathy (Duckett *et al* 1974).

Cats, of 2-3 kg body weight, receiving twice-daily subcutaneous injections of 150 mg/kg of butan-2-one, 5 days/week, over nearly 9 months, displayed no clinical or pathological evidence of neuropathy (Spencer and Schaumberg 1976). In a similar study (Krasavage *et al* 1982), beagle dogs also did not develop neuropathologic changes. Rats interperitoneally injected with between 100 and 200 mg/kg of butan-2-one, a 9 : 1 mixture of butan-2-one and hexan-2-one, or a 9 : 1 mixture of butan-2-one and 4-methyl-2-pentanone (methyl isobutyl ketone), respectively, for 35 weeks, showed no clinical or neuropathologic changes. It has been reported that rats inhaling either 2150 ppm of butan-2-one for 6 weeks, or 4740 ppm for 4 weeks, showed no signs of neurotoxicity (Krasavage *et al* 1982).

Typical distal axonopathy was observed in 300 g male rats given 2000 mg/kg heptan-3-one (ethyl *n*-butyl ketone) by gavage, daily, 5 days/week, for 14 weeks. Butan-2-one given by gavage at a dose level of 1500 mg/kg/day, 5 days/week for 14 weeks, potentiated heptan-3-one neurotoxicity, characterised by giant axonal swelling and neurofilamentous hyperplasia. Butan-2-one also appeared to increase the urinary excretion of two known neurotoxic gamma-diketones, 2,5-heptanedione, and 2,5,-hexanedione, when given by gavage with heptan-3-one. When rats were exposed to a combination of heptan-3-one (700 ppm) and butan-2-one (700 or 1400 ppm) by inhalation for up to 4 days, serum 2,5-heptanedione levels were increased approximately 2.5 times, although 2,5-hexanedione levels remained normal. No effect was seen at butan-2-one levels of 70 ppm (O'Donaghue *et al* 1984).

No signs of neuropathy were observed in a group of three Sprague–Dawley rats receiving 750 mg/kg butan-2-one in corn oil, by gavage, twice-weekly for up to 14 weeks. All three animals died, and were found to have aspiration pneumonia on necroscopy. A 17% decrease in body weight, compared to controls receiving 1 ml/kg corn oil, had been found after 4 weeks of treatment. Rats receiving nonan-5-one dissolved in corn oil at a daily dose of 150 mg/kg for 3 weeks, increased to 750 mg/kg for 8 weeks, and then 1500 mg/kg for 3 weeks developed typical neurotoxic symptoms, such as hind-limb paralysis, and muscular wasting. Giant axonal swellings filled with neurofilaments were observed on closer examination. Another group of rats receiving the same doses of nonan-5-one, in conjunction with twice-weekly doses of 750 mg/kg butan-2-one in corn oil, developed these symptoms after 11 rather than 14 weeks, indicating that butan-2-one had accelerated the onset of neuropathy caused by nonan-5-one (Shifman *et al* 1981).

The nervous system responses of male Wistar rats inhaling 10 000 ppm *n*-hexane, 1100 ppm butan-2-one/8900 ppm *n*-hexane, and 6000 ppm butan-2-one for 8 hours/day, 7 days/week, for up to 19 weeks, have been investigated. On examination, motor neuropathy of the dying back type with giant swelling of axons in the peripheral and central nervous system had developed in animals exposed to *n*-hexane and the *n*-hexane/butan-2-one mixture, but not in those exposed to butan-2-one alone. Severe potentiation of *n*-hexane neurotoxicity and accelerated onset of morphological and clinical signs were demonstrated in the animals exposed to the mixture. Animals exposed to the ketone alone did not develop any obvious motor impairment up to the 7th week, when all animals died without neurological symptoms. Pathological and histological examination revealed severe signs of bronchopneumonia in all of the animals (Altenkirch *et al* 1978).

Hetland *et al* (1976) and Couri *et al* (1977) reported that hepatic microsomal enzyme activities were significantly enhanced in young male Wistar rats exposed to either 750 ppm of butan-2-one or a mixture of 225 ppm hexan-2-one/750 ppm butan-2-one continuously or intermittently (7 hours/day) for 7 days. Exposure to hexan-2-one vapour alone (225 ppm) caused no effect. Hexobarbital sleeping times were significantly reduced following exposure to butan-2-one or to the mixture of butan-2-one and hexan-2-one, while hexan-2-one alone had no effect. Aniline hydroxylase, aminopyrine demethylase, neoprontosil reductase and *p*-nitrobenzoate reductase activities were significantly enhanced two- or threefold over the control values when the rats were continuously exposed to the mixture of butan-2-one and hexan-2-one. In the intermittent group, only *p*-aminophenol production was affected, the aniline hydroxylase activity being increased (Hetland *et al* 1976, Couri *et al* 1977).

Twenty-five rats and 15 guinea-pigs were exposed by inhalation to 235 ppm butan-2-one for 7 hours/day, 5 days/week, for 7 weeks. No deaths that could be attributed to the ketone occurred, and there were no signs of intoxication. There were no significant differences from the controls in growth, haematological or pathological parameters (La Bella and Brieger 1955).

Groups of 15 male and 15 female Sherman rats were exposed to either 125, 250, 500 or 1000 ppm butan-2-one for 30 days. Daily exposure times were not specified. No significant histopathological changes were seen in lung, liver or kidney. No statistically significant deviations from normal were seen in body, liver or kidney weights (Mellon Institute 1950).

Fischer-344 rats of both sexes were exposed to 1250, 2500, or 5000 ppm butan-2-one vapours for 6 hours/day, 5 days/week, for a period of 90 days. Clinical pathology, necropsy, and histopathology studies did not reveal any abnormalities or lesions attributable to butan-2-one exposure. A slight decrease in mean body weight was observed in the 5000 ppm dose group; these animals also had a slight, but significant, increase in liver weight, liver weight/body weight ratio, and liver weight/brain weight, at necropsy. A slight, but non-significant, increase in absolute liver weight was observed in the 1200 and 2500 ppm dose groups, but only in female rats. An increased serum alanine aminotransaminase (ALT) activity was observed in females exposed to 2500 ppm butan-2-one, while the activity was significantly decreased in those inhaling 5000 ppm. Female rats exposed to 5000 ppm also exhibited increased alkaline phosphatase, potassium and glucose levels (Clavender *et al* 1983).

Only mild desquamation was noted ion guinea-pigs having 2 ml butan-2-one, butan-2-one/4-methylpentan-2-one (9 : 1), or butan-2-one/methyl *n*-butyle ketone, dropped onto their backs, each day, for 31 weeks (Krasavage *et al* 1982).

8.3.3 Human toxicity

Smith and Meyers (1944) reported the findings of inhalation and dermal exposures of butan-2-one to workers in raincoat factories, where the ketone was used as a solvent. Concentrations of between 300 and 600 ppm butan-2-one were detected in the ambient air, and additional exposure occurred because the workers tended to wash their hands in the solvent. A number of the workers complained of dermititis and/or numbness of the fingers and arms. One worker also complained of numbness of the legs. They also found that exposure of the face and other bare skin to the vapour of butan-2-one is enough to cause dermatitis if proper ventilation is not employed. Other employees were exposed to a mixture of between 398 and 561 ppm butan-2-one, and between 330 and 495 ppm acetone. The effects noted included gastric complaints, headaches, and fainting in two women employed in brushing waterproofing materials, which were dissolved in the solvents, onto raincoats (Smith and Meyers 1944).

One worker in a plastics factory exposed to tetrahydrofuran-polyester glue and to butan-2-one, both by inhalation and dermal contact, developed a toxic polyneuritis involving paraesthesia of the fingers, loss of utility of the hand muscles and leucocytosis, which might have been due to butan-2-one or the mixture of the two chemicals (Viader *et al* 1975).

Exposure of humans by inhalation to between 90 and 270 ppm butan-2-one for 4 hours has been associated with a shortening in time estimates in males, and an increased variation in females in time-estimation tests of 5, 10, and 30 seconds (Nakaaki 1974). Exposure of humans to 100 ppm for between 3 and 5 minutes caused slight irritation of the nose and throat. Mild eye irritation was noted in some subjects at 200 ppm, and levels in excess of 300 ppm proved intolerable, eye, nose and throat irritation being seen (Nelson *et al* 1943). Occupational exposure to between an estimated 300 and 500 ppm butan-2-one concentration has been reported to cause headaches, irritation and nausea. Exposures to 700 ppm led to no permanent untoward effects. Momentary exposure to 33 000 ppm and 100 000 ppm produced intolerable irritation of the eyes, nose, and throat (Elkins 1959).

Cases of toxic distal neuropathy have been reported in workers of a plant producing plastic-coated and colour-printed fabrics. Of 1157 employees screened, 86 cases were verified. The neuropathy was attributed to exposure to methyl *n*-butyl ketone which was present in a solvent mixture with butan-2-one. In 194 employees described as suspect cases on the basis of electrodiagnostic studies, the results of haemotological studies appeared normal. However, an unusual pattern was reported for erythrocyte and plasma cholinesterase values in 96 of the employees with abnormal electrodiagnostic findings. Erythrocyte acetylcholinesterase (AChE) activities were found to be decreased by 33%, while plasma cholinesterase (butyrocholinesterase or BuChE) activities were increased by some 150%, compared to neurologically normal subjects. No relationship with the severity of the peripheral neuropathy was found. Average airborne concentrations behind the printing machines were 36 ppm methyl *n*-butyl ketone and 516 ppm butan-2-one. A possible synergistic effect with butan-2-one, tetrahydrofuran, trichloroethylene or phthalate plasticiser could not be ruled out. When a group of ten affected employees returned to work under conditions of reduced solvent exposure, values for erythrocyte AChE and serum BuChE did not differ significantly from values found in ten unaffected workers. No cases of toxic neuropathy were found in workers exposed to butan-2-one in another factory where methyl *n*-butyl ketone had never been used.

Damage to the horny layer of human forearm skin, often requiring complete regeneration, was noted on exposure to butan-2-one for periods of 1 hour/day for 6 days (Malten *et al* 1968). Butan-2-one has also been reported to cause defatting and partial hydration of the stratum corneum of hydrated human forearm skin without producing irritation or inflammation (Munies 1965, Wurster and Munies 1965). Dermatitis resulting from excessive occupational skin contact with butan-2-one is not uncommon (Rowe and Wolf 1963).

Butan-2-one tested at 20% in petrolatum produced no irritation after a 48-hour closed-patch test on humans, and no sensitisation reactions during a maximisation test in 24 volunteers (Opdyke 1975c).

8.4 Reproductive toxicity

Pregnant Sprague–Dawley rats, weighing approximately 250 g, were exposed by inhalation to either 1000 or 3000 ppm of butan-2-one for 7 hours/day on days 6–15 of gestation. Neither concentration caused maternal toxicity, but a degree of embryotoxicity and weak teratogenicity were observed. Butan-2-one concentrations of 3000 ppm causeed some retardation of foetal development (delayed ossification of sternebrae) and increased gross, skeletal and soft-tissue anomalies, including acaudia, imperforated anus and brachygnathia. There was no significant increase in gross, soft tissue, or specific skeletal abnormalities in litters of those rats exposed to 1000 ppm, although the total number of litters containing foetuses with anomalous skeletons was significantly increased compared to the controls (Schwetz *et al* 1974).

Groups of 25 pregnant Sprague–Dawley rats were exposed to either 400, 1000 or 3000 ppm of butan-2-one by inhalation for 7 hours/day on days 6–15 of gestation. A group of 35 pregnant rats acted as controls, being exposed to filtered room air only. A degree of maternal toxicity, as indicated by a decreased weight gain and increased water consumption, was observed in rats exposed to 3000 ppm of butan-2-one. Slight foetotoxicity was observed among litters of rats exposed to the highest level of butan-2-one, as evidenced by a significant increase in the incidence of extra lumbar ribs, and the occurrence of delayed ossification of cervical central, compared to the controls. No significant embryotoxic or teratogenic effects were seen in rats at any of the levels of exposure (Deacon *et al* 1981).

8.5 Mutagenicity and carcinogenicity

Butan-2-one was found to be non-mutagenic in *Salmonella typimurium* TA98, TA100, TA1535, and TA1537, with and without S-9 from arcolor-induced Sprague–Dawley rats. The Ames tests were carried out at a concentration of 3 μmol/plate (Florin *et al* 1980). No carcinogeniticity studies appear to have been carried out to date.

8.6. Discussion

Butan-2-one was identified in three of 14 UK drinking water samples examined by WRC. It has also been identified in the tap water of a number of US cities.

Butan-2-one is readily absorbed by all routes of exposure; its metabolism appears to follow both oxidative and reductive pathways, the ketone undergoing ω-1 carbon atom oxidation to the corresponding hydroxyketone which then undergoes reduc tion to the diol. The secondary alcohol, butan-2-ol, is formed by the reduction of the ketone, and is then eliminated in the urine as *O*-sulphates or *O*-glucuronides, or may enter intermediary metabolism to be eliminated as carbon dioxide, or incorporated into tissues.

Few data are available concerning the long-term oral toxicity of butan-2-one. Short-term studies suggest that this ketone is of low oral toxicity. The LD50 of butan-2-one in the rat has been reported to be between 2700 and 5530 mg/kg.

It also appears to have a low inhalation toxicity, and although it has been widely reported not to be neurotoxic itself, it does appear to potentiate polyneuropathy caused by other solvents. It is also thought that it may potentiate the hepatotoxicity of carbon tetrachloride, although it does not cause any hepatotoxic effects itself. These effects are believed to be due to induction of enzymes by the ketone.

Reproductive toxicity studies have proved rather inconclusive, slight foetotoxic and embryotoxic effects being reported. One study showed butan-2-one to be non-mutagenic. No carcinogenicity data appear to be available.

9. BUTAN-2,3-DIONE

Butan-2,3-dione is a yellowish-green liquid with a quinone odour, although the vapours smell rather more like carbon tetrachloride. It is made from methyl ethyl ketone (butan-2-one) by conversion to the nitroso compound and then decomposition to butan-2,3-dione by hydrolysis with HCl. It is widely used as a carrier of aromas, especially those in butter, vinegar, coffee, and numerous other foodstuffs.

	$CH_3COCOCH_3$
CAS Reg No:	431-03-8
Molecular formula:	$C_4H_6O_2$
Molecular weight:	86.09
Threshold odour concentration:	8.6 ppb (Pietrzak and Barylko-Pikielna 1976)

Synonyms: diacetyl, biacetyl, 2,3-diketobutane, 2,3-butanedione, dimethylgloxyal.

9.1 Exposure

Butan-2,3-dione is used as a food flavouring, especially in baked goods, sweets and ice cream. It is also found in milk, butter, wine, tea, coffee, honey, a number of vegetables, fruits, and natural oils (Opdyke 1979b, Colley *et al* 1969).

Butan-2,3-dione was identified in six of 14 UK drinking water samples examined by WRc (Water Research Centre 1981), although it was only detected in one of another 14 samples examined in a subsequent unpublished survey.

Very few data on exposure to butan-2,3-dione were found in the literature, although the likely maximum intake by man has been calculated to be approximately 10 mg/day, half of which may be through the ingestion of the flavouring in soft drinks (Colley *et al* 1969).

9.2 Toxicokinetics

No information concerning the toxicokinetics of butan-2,3-dione appears to be available.

9.3 Toxicity

Oral LD50s of butan-2,3-dione in rats have been reported as 1580 mg/kg (Jenner *et al* 1964) and 3000 mg/kg in females and 3400 mg/kg in males of the CFE strain (Colley *et al* 1969). At lethal doses, death followed soon after convulsions. At lower doses, salivation, vasodilation and reduced motor activity were observed. No macroscopic abnormalities were noted. Similar observations were made in rats following intraperitoneal injection with butan-2,3-dione. The LD50 by this route was 400 and 640 mg/kg in male and female CFE rats respectively (Colley *et al* 1969). The acute dermal LD50 in rabbit has been reported to be in excess of 5000 mg/kg (Opdyke 1979b).

When applied full strength to intact or abraded rabbit skin under an occlusion for a period of 24 hours, butan-2,3-dione was described as being moderately to markedly irritating (Opdyke 1979b). Testing at 2% in petrolatum produced no irritation after a 48-hour closed-patch test on human volunteers. No sensitisation reactions occurred in a maximisation test carried out on 29 volunteers, using a similar concentration and vehicle (Opdyke 1979b).

Rats were given butan-2,3-dione by oral intubation at doses of 10, 30, 90 or 540 mg/kg/day, for 90 days. No adverse effects were seen at the lower three dose levels. At 540 mg/kg/day, a decrease in body weight gain, an increase in water consumption, anaemia, an increased leucocyte count, and an increase in the relative weights of the liver, kidneys, adrenal and pituitary glands were observed. Stomach lesions showing necrosis, with infiltration by inflammatory cells, were seen at autopsy (Colley *et al* 1969).

A slight increase in the number of pulmonary tumours was observed in A/He mice intraperitoneally injected with doses of either 71.8 or 350.0 mg/kg thrice-weekly, for 8 weeks. The butan-2,3-dione was administered in 0.1 ml of water. Twenty-four weeks after the first injection the survivors were sacrificed and examined for tumours. The incidence of pulmonary tumours was 20% in untreated controls, 32% for vehicle controls (0.1 ml water), 40% in the group receiving 71.8 mg/kg butan-2,3-dione and 65% in the group receiving 350.0 mg/kg. This increase was significant compared to the controls; however, when the study was repeated, there was no significant increase in tumours in the treated animals (Stoner *et al* 1973).

Bjeldanes and Chew (1979) found that butan-2,3-dione was mutagenic in *Salmonella typhimurium* TA100 either with or without incubation with S-9 mix. No mutagenic activity was seen when the test was carried out using strain TA98. Butan-2,3-dione did not exhibit mutagenic activity in a test system using root tip meristems of *Vicia faba* (Loveless 1951).

10. MENTHONE

Three stereochemical isomers of menthone (2-isopropyl-5-methyl- *p*-menthan-3-one, or *p*-menthan-3-one), have been reported to occur naturally. These are *d*-menthone, *l*-menthone, and the racemate of the two, *dl*-menthone. Menthone is a bitter liquid, with a slight peppermint odour, which is prepared by the oxidation of menthol, or by partial hydrogenation of thymol.

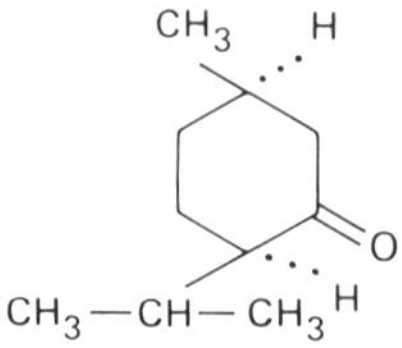

CH_3CHCH_3 H

CAS Reg No:	
dl-p-menthan-3-one	1074-95-9
d-p-menthan-3-one	89-80-5
l-p-menthan-3-one	491-07-5
Molecular weight:	154.28
Molecular formula:	$C_{10}H_{18}O$
Boiling point:	
dl-p-menthan-3-one	204.0 °C
d-p-menthan-3-one	210.5 °C
l-p-menthan-3-one	209.6 °C

Menthone is commonly used as a fragrance in cream, detergent, perfume and soap, as well as a flavouring in foodstuffs. WRc identified menthone in only one of a survey of 14 UK drinking water samples (Water Research Centre 1981).

l-Menthone is the isomer most commonly found in nature. It is a constituent of the essential oils of Russian and American peppermint, geranium, *Andropogon fragrans*, and a number of other plants (Opdyke 1976b).

Opdyke (1976b) reported that the urine of rabbits dosed with menthone contained a glucuronide which when treated with warm dilute sulphuric acid produced pulegone (*p*-menthen-3-one). He suggested that the substance isolated from the urine was ketomenthone, which was probably formed by the oxidation of menthone. In contrast to this, Williams (1940) reported the reduction of *l*-menthone to *d*-neomethylglucuronide in rabbit. Rabbits (2–3 g body weight) given 3000 mg *l*-menthone by stomach tube eliminated 30–40% of the dose in the urine as hydroxy derivatives conjugated with glucuronic acid. Of the dose, 10–15% was isolated as urinary *d*-neomenthylglucuronide, indicating that at least part of the menthone molecule is reduced at the carbonyl group.

The oral LD50 of menthone has been reported to be 2.18 ml/kg (1990 mg/kg) in the rat (Opdyke 1976b). The dermal LD50 of menthone in the rabbit has been reported to be in excess of 5000 mg/kg (Opdyke 1976b). When applied full strength to intact or abraded rabbit skin under an occlusion for 24 hours, only mild irritation was observed (Opdyke 1976b).

An 8% solution of menthone in petrolatum produced no irritation during a 48-hour closed-patch test in human volunteers, and produced no sensitisation reactions in 25 volunteers subjected to a maximisation test (Opdyke 1976b).

Groups of ten male and ten female rats were given 0, 200, 400 or 800 mg/kg body weight of menthone by gavage for 28 days. After 19 days the dose in the highest dose group of females was reduced to 400 mg/kg. There was a dose-dependent decrease in plasma creatinine and a dose-dependent increase in plasma alkaline phosphatase and bilirubin. Relative weights of liver and spleen were increased and cyst-like spaces were observed in the white matter of the cerebellum of the two highest dose groups (Madsen *et al* 1986).

Menthone showed a significant but weak mutagenic response in *Salmonella typhimurium* TA97. It was not mutagenic in TA1535, TA100 and TA98 and although a statistically significant increase in revertants was observed at the two lowest dose levels in TA1537 these did not constitute a doubling of the number of revertants over control values (Anderson and Jensen 1984).

Groups of 20 female A/He mice were given 20 intraperitoneal injections totalling either 4.75 or 1.90 g/kg/mouse over a period of 7 weeks. The menthone was dissolved in 0.1 ml tricaprylin, and administered thrice-weekly. Nineteen weeks after the first injection the animals were sacrificed. There was no significant increase in pulmonary tumours over control animals (Stoner *et al* 1973).

11. ISOMENTHONE

Isomenthone is a colourless, oily liquid, used as a fragrance in soaps, detergents, creams, lotions, and perfumes. WRc identified isomenthone in only one of a survey of 14 UK drinking water samples (Water Research Centre 1981).

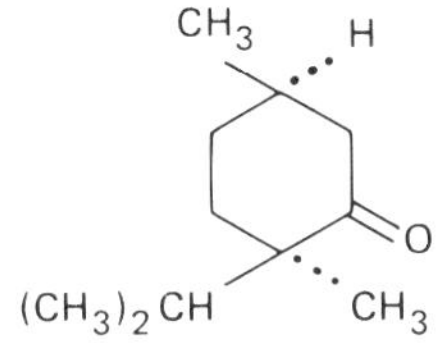

$(CH_3)_2CH$ CH_3

CAS Reg No:	491-07-6
Molecular weight:	154.28
Molecular formula:	$C_{10}H_{18}O$

Synonyms: (2)-*p*-menthan-3-one, 2-isopropyl-5-methyl-cyclohexanone, or 5-methyl-2-(1-methylethyl)-cyclohexanone.

Williams (1959, 1940) suggests that *d*-isomenthone undergoes reduction in the rabbit when given at a dose of 3000 mg via stomach tube, since *d*-isomenthylglucuronide has been identified in the urine. Another possible reduction product, *d*-neoisomenthol, was not detected.

Very few toxicological data appear to be available. Two unpublished papers were cited in a brief toxicological review of isomenthone (Opdyke 1976a).

The dermal LD50 of isomenthone in the rabbit has been reported to be in excess of 5000 mg/kg (Opdyke 1976a). When applied full strength to intact or abraded rabbit skin under an occlusion for 24 hours, only mild irritation occurred (Opdyke 1976a).

An 8% solution of isomenthone in petrolatum produced no irritation after a 48-hour closed-patch test in human volunteers, and produced no sensitisation reactions in 25 volunteers subjected to a maximisation test (Opdyke 1976a).

12. 6-METHYL-5-HEPTEN-2-ONE

6-methyl-5-hepten-2-one (methyl heptenone) is used to a limited extent as a fragrance. It was identified in one of a survey of 14 drinking water samples by WRc (Water Research Centre 1981). It has been reported to occur naturally in lemongrass and the essential oils from *Artemisia scoparia*, *Urtica dioica* and others (Opdyke 1975a).

$$_{3}HC\text{–}C(CH_3)\text{=}CH\text{–}CH_2\text{–}CH_2\text{–}CO\text{–}CH_3$$

CAS Reg No:	409-02-9
Molecular weight:	126.22
Molecular formula:	$C_8H_{14}O$

Very few toxicological data appear to be available on 6-methyl-5-hepten-2-one.

Oral LD50's of 6-methyl-5-hepten-2-one in rat have been reported to be 3500 mg/kg (NIOSH 1983) and 4100 mg/kg (Opdyke 1975a). The dermal LD50 was greater than 5000 mg/kg (Opdyke 1975a).

This compound has been reported to be a skin irritant in rabbit, when applied undiluted to intact or abraded skin and held there for 24 hours under an occlusion (Opdyke 1975a). 6-Methyl-5-hepten-2-one, when tested at 3% in petrolatum, produced no irritation during a 48-hour closed-patch test in humans. No sensitisation reactions occurred at this concentration in a maximisation test carried out on 25 human volunteers (Opdyke 1975a).

6-Methyl-5-hepten-2-one was non-mutagenic in *Salmonella typhimurium* TA98, TA100, TA1535, and TA1537, in the Ames test either with or without the presence of S-9 mix from arcolor-induced rats, when tested at 3 μmol/plate (Florin *et al* 1980).

13. 3-HYDROXY-2-BUTANONE

3-Hydroxy-2-butanone (acetoin) is a slightly yellow liquid, or crystalline solid, used in the preparation of flavours and essences.

$$CH_3\text{–}CH(OH)\text{–}CO\text{–}CH_3$$

CAS Reg No:	513-86-0
Molecular weight:	88.12
Molecular formula:	$C_4H_8O_2$

Synonyms: acetoin, acetylmethyl carbinol, 2,3-butanolone, dimethyl ketol, 2-butanol-3-one, 1-hydroxyethyl methyl ketone, gamma-hydroxy-beta-oxobutane.

13.1 Exposure

3-Hydroxy-2-butanone was identified in one of 14 drinking water samples examined by WRc (Water Research Centre 1981). It has been detected in a large number of foodstuffs, including corn, a variety of fruits, bread, chicken, fish, tomato, peas, and a number of alcoholic and non-alcoholic beverages (Opdyke 1979a). From data provided by seven of the leading flavouring manufacturers in the UK it has been estimated that the total daily intake of 3-hydroxy-2-butanone by humans is in the region of 0.5 mg/kg/day (Gaunt *et al* 1972).

13.2 Toxicokinetics

Between 5 and 25% of a dose of 3-hydroxy-2-butanone administered to a dog was reported to have been excreted as butane-2,3-diol in the first 24 hours after dosing. Small amounts of the unchanged compound were also detected in the urine (Westerfield and Berg 1943).

Sprague–Dawley rats dosed by intraperitoneal injection with ^{14}C-labelled 3-hydroxy-2-butanone were found to eliminate $^{14}CO_2$ in the expired air. The average 12-hour $^{14}CO_2$ production was found to be 15% of the injected dose, and the 18-hour figure was 22%. The conversion was up to 47.7% after 20 hours in a rat injected with 3-hydroxy-2-butanone intracardially (Gabriel *et al* 1972).

Decerebrated cats of between 2.5 and 4.0 kg body weight were intravenously injected with 750 mg 3-hydroxy-2-butanone. After 120 minutes the blood of these animals contained approximately 22% of the administered dose in the form of butane-2,3-diol, and approximately 5% as unchanged 3-hydroxy-2-butanone (Dawson and Hullin 1954a).

Carbon dioxide, acetoacetate, and acetate were found to be oxidation products of 3-hydroxy-2-butanone when incubated with a rabbit kidney tissue dispersion (Dawson and Hullin 1954b).

13.3 Toxicity

Both the acute oral LD50 in rats and the acute dermal LD50 in rabbits have been reported to be in excess of 5000 mg/kg (Moreno 1977). When applied full strength to the intact or abraded skin of rabbits for 24 hours under an occlusion, 3-hydroxy-2-butanone was moderately irritant. 3-hydroxy-2-butanone produced no irritation in humans during a 48-hour closed-patch test when tested at a concentration of 10% in petrolatum (Opdyke 1979a). No sensitisation reactions occurred due to a 10% solution of 3-hydroxy-2-butanone in a maximisation test on 31 human volunteers (Opdyke 1979a).

Subcutaneous injection of 2000 mg 3-hydroxy-2-butanone in rats, of 150 g body weight, resulted in death within 6 hours of dosing. Animals dosed with 500 mg by subcutaneous injection developed paralytic symptoms, but this was followed by rapid recovery. Intraperitoneal injection of 500 mg, or subcutaneous injection of 250 mg, had no adverse effects on the rats. No increase in liver glycogen occurred in fasted rats fed between 1500 and 2000 mg 3-hydroxy-2-butanone (Westerfield and Berg 1943).

CFE strain rats were given drinking water containing 0,750, 3000 or 12 000 mg/l of 3-hydroxy-2-butanone for a period of 13 weeks. No anomalies attributable to the treatment were seen at the 750 or 300 mg/l dose levels. Parameters monitored included body weight gain, haematology, serum chemistry, renal cell excretion, urinary concentration tests, organ weights and histopathology. The 12 000 mg/l dose level caused a decrease in the rate of body weight gain associated with a reduction in food and water consumption. The relative liver weight was increased, and a slight anaemia was observed. No animals died during this study (Gaunt *et al* 1972).

Groups of 20 female A/He mice were given 20 intraperitoneal injections totalling either 60 or 12 g/kg/mouse over a period of 7 weeks. The 3-hydroxy-2-butanone was dissolved in 0.1 ml water and administered thrice-weekly. Twenty-two weeks after the first injection the animals were sacrificed. There was no significant increase in pulmonary tumours over controls (Stoner *et al* 1973).

14. OCTANONE

Octanone is a colourless liquid with a pleasant fruity odour. A number of isomers exist, but toxicological information on most of them is not available. The only information found concerns the 2- and 3-isomers.

2-OCTANONE (methyl hexyl ketone)	CH_3–CO–$[CH_2]_5$–CH_3
CAS Reg No:	111-13-7
3-OCTANONE (amyl ethyl ketone)	CH_3–$[CH_2]_4$–CO–CH_2–CH_3
CAS Reg No:	106-68-3
Molecular weight:	128.24
Molecular formula:	$C_8H_{16}O$

14.1 Exposure

Very few data are available concerning exposure to any of the isomers of octanone. An uncharacterised isomer of octanone was identified in one of 14 UK drinking water samples examined by WRc (Water Research Centre 1981), and 3-octanone was found in a Cincinnati drinking water sample (Coleman *et al* 1980).

2-Octanone has been identified in small quantities in the essential oil of *Ruta montana* L., as well as in bananas and citrus fruits (Opdyke 1975b). 3-Octanone has been detected in lavender oil (Opdyke 1974).

14.2 Toxicity

The acute oral LD50 in rats and the acute dermal LD50 in rabbits have been reported to be in excess of 5000 mg/kg for 2- and 3-octanone (Opdyke 1974, 1975b). The oral LD50 of 2-octanone in mice has been reported to be 3100 mg/kg (Abbasov *et al* 1977), and 1600 mg/kg (Hall and Carlson 1976), and 9200 mg/kg in rats (Abbasov *et al* 1977). The intraperitoneal LD50 of 2-octanone was between 800 and 1600 mg/kg for both rats and mice, while a figure of 406 mg/kg of 3-octanone has been quoted for mice (Krasavage *et al* 1982).

Rats fed 20 mg/kg of 2-octanone daily for 16 days had reduced serum cholesterol, triglyceride and glycerol levels. Serum lipase activity was significantly elevated (Hall and Carlson 1976, Carlson *et al* 1975).

Rats exposed by inhalation to 8.9 mg/l of 2-octanone for 6 hours exhibited signs of mild eye irritation (Krasavage *et al* 1982). Guinea-pigs were seen to suffer from eye and nasal irritation immediately on exposure to 1300 ppm of 2-octanone. Muscular weakness followed, and persisted for some 10 hours, before the animals went into coma after approximately 12 hours. Guinea-pigs exposed by inhalation to 1300 ppm for 1 hour suffered from no serious disturbances (Rowe and Wolf 1963).

Application of unspecified amounts of 2- or 3-octanone to intact or abraded rabbit skin for 24 hours, under an occlusion, has been reported to cause some irritation, the 2-isomer being classified as slightly irritating, while the 3-isomer was classified as being moderately irritating (Opdyke 1974, 1975b). Guinea-pigs have been reported to lose weight over a 2-week period when 2-octanone was applied to their skin under an occlusion (Krasavage *et al* 1982). Both 2- and 3-octanone do not appear to cause sensitisation reactions in guinea-pigs (Sharp 1978).

No irritation was produced in 25 humans subjected to 48-hour closed-patch tests with either 3-octanone at 2% (Opdyke 1974) or 2-octanone at 4% in petrolatum (Opdyke 1975b). The same concentration caused no sensitisation reactions in a maximisation test (Opdyke 1974, 1975b).

14.3 Mutagenicity

2-Octanone has been reported to be non-mutagenic in a number of unspecified *Salmonella typhimurium* tester strains (McMahon *et al* 1979).

15. PENTAN-2-ONE

Pentan-2-one (methyl-*n*-propylketone, ethylacetone) is a colourless liquid with a limited usage, although it possesses very good solvent properties.

$$CH_3.CO.CH_2.CH_2.CH_3$$

CAS Reg No:	107-87-9
Molecular formula:	$C_5H_{10}O$
Molecular weight:	86.15
Boiling point:	102.2 °C
Solubility at 20 °C	43 000
Threshold odour concentration:	8.0 ppm

15.1 Exposure

Pentan-2-one has been identified in the tap water of Cincinnati, Philadelphia, Ottuma, and Miami by the US EPA (Coleman *et al* 1976); in Ottuma, Iowa the concentration was 0.1 μg/l (Keith 1976b). WRc identified pentan-2-one in four of 14 UK drinking water samples (Water Research Centre 1981).

It has been detected in white bread, soybeans, bananas, tobacco, and evaporated milk. It was found at levels of 0.98 ppm in Swiss cheese, at levels of between 0.007 and 0.026 ppm in milk, and 0.025 and 0.045 ppm in cream (US EPA 1976).

Pentan-2-one has been detected in the exhaust fumes of gasoline engines at levels of between <0.1 and 0.8 ppm (Verschueren 1977).

15.2 Toxicokinetics

Little information concerning the toxicokinetics of this compound is available. Percutaneous absorption has been reported to occur in guinea-pigs when 20 ml/kg of pentan-2-one was applied to their skin (Krasavage *et al* 1982). Absorption from the gastrointestinal tract appears to occur readily in dogs. Within 24 hours of oral dosing, one dog receiving a single dose of 358 mg/kg of pentan-2-one eliminated 21.2% of the ketone unchanged in the expired air; another dog receiving 381 mg/kg eliminated 27.1% of the dose in the same manner (Krasavage *et al* 1982, US EPA 1976). Neubreur (1901) reported that rabbits orally dosed with 1400 mg/kg of pentan-2-one, in two portions, eliminated a number of unidentified urinary metabolites of pentan-2-one in the glucuronide form. Pentan-2-one has been detected in normal human urine (Zlatkis *et al* 1973).

15.3 Toxicity

The oral LD50 of pentan-2-one has been reported to be 3730 ml/kg (3021 mg/kg) in the rat (Smyth *et al* 1962). One of six rats died after exposure by inhalation to 2000 ppm of pentan-2-one for a period of 4 hours, while at 4000 ppm all six rats died within the exposure period (Smyth *et al* 1962).

No poisonings of man have been reported, although inhalation of approximately 1500 ppm of pentan-2-one has been reported to cause irritation of the nasal passages and eyes of man (Yant *et al* 1936).

It has been reported that pentan-2-one caused narcosis, depression of cardiac and respiratory rates, and a loss of cranial nerve reflexes in guinea-pigs exposed to its vapours for an unspecified duration of time. Levels of between 25 000 and 40 000 ppm caused generalised vascular congestion (Specht *et al* 1940). Lethargy was observed in guinea-pigs inhaling between 30 000 and 50 000 ppm, but those inhaling between 15 000 and 20 000 ppm, for up to 8 hours, or 5000 ppm for 1 hour showed no abnormal clinical signs (Yant *et al* 1936). Four of ten female guinea-pigs exposed to 10 000 ppm for 9 hours died during exposure; the others died within 48 hours of the end of exposure. In these guinea-pigs, congestion and emphysema of the lungs and kidney along with distention of the renal tubules were the primary pathological effects. Slight congestion of the liver and adrenals was also reported (US EPA 1976).

Intraperitoneal injection of pentan-2-one at doses of between 250 and 500 mg/kg caused agitation and hypertesthesia in mice. When the dose was 2000 mg/kg, additional adverse effects included loss of balance, staggering, paresis, loss of sensitivity, and a 20% mortality rate. At 2500 mg/kg a 100% mortality rate was noted (Giroux *et al* 1954). Death has been reported to occur due to respiratory failure in rats intraperitoneally injected with 2530 mg/kg of pentan-2-one (Haggard *et al* 1945). The Eastman Kodak Co reported an intraperitoneal LD50 of 800 mg/kg in rats, and 1600 mg/kg in mice for pentan-2-one (Krasavage *et al* 1982).

Slight to moderate irritation was reported when pentan-2-one was placed in the conjunctival sacs of rabbits' eyes, or applied to the backs of guinea-pigs under an impervious cuff. Levels of up to 20 ml/kg of pentan-2-one have been reported to cause no clinical abnormalities when applied to the backs of guinea-pigs. When this procedure was repeated for 10 days, some slight erythema and oedema was observed (Krasavage *et al* 1982). Smyth *et al* (1962) reported the dermal LD50 in rats to be 8.0 ml/g.

In a study (Krasavage *et al* 1982) in which drinking water was used as the vehicle for dosing, rats received either 144 mg/kg/day for 10 months or 250 or 454 mg/kg/day for 13 months. No neuropathologic changes in the central or peripheral nervous systems were noted. Clinical signs, organ weights and histology were all normal. At the highest dose level the only abnormality was a 9% reduction in body weight gain compared to controls. In another experiment, rats exposed by inhalation to 305 ppm of pentan-2-one during two 16-hour and two 20-hour periods, four consecutive days/week, for 17 or 18 weeks, also showed no signs of neurologic damage. Histopathologic screening of a number of tissues showed no damage (Krasavage *et al* 1982).

16. PENTAN-3-ONE

Pentan-3-one is a colourless liquid with an acetone-like odour, commonly used as a solvent.

$CH_3.CH_2.CO.CH_2.CH_3$

CAS Reg No:	96-22-0
Molecular formula:	$C_5H_{10}O$
Molecular weight:	86.15
Boiling point:	101.5 °C
Solubility at 20 °C:	47 000 mg/l

Synonyms: *sym*-dimethylacetone, diethyl ketone, propione, ethyl ketone, methacetone, and dimethylacetone.

Pentan-3-one was identified in only one of the 14 drinking water samples examined by WRc (Water Research Centre 1981). No other exposure data are available.

Culp and McMahon (1968) isolated and purified an enzyme which caused some reduction of pentan-2-one, called aromatic A-K reductase, from the kidney cortex of rats and hogs as well as rabbit liver. Neubauer (1901) found that oral administration of 1030 mg/kg of pentan-3-one to rabbits caused an increase in the urinary excretion of glucuronic acid. Two dogs orally dosed with 332 and 109 mg/kg excreted 8.8 and 0% of the dose respectively unchanged in the expired air within 24 hours of administration (US EPA 1976).

The oral LD50 has been reported to be 2100 mg/kg (Windholz 1976), and 2140 mg/kg in the rat (NIOSH 1978). Death has been reported to occur due to respiratory failure in rats intraperitoneally injected with a single dose of 2790 mg/kg of pentan-3-one (Haggard *et al* 1945). Smyth *et al* (1954) reported that an inhalation exposure of 8000 ppm for 4 hours killed four of six Carworth–Wistar rats. The acute dermal 14-day LD50 in rabbit is 16 200 mg/kg (Smyth *et al* 1954). The intravenous LD50 has been reported to be 5.97 mmol/kg (514 mg/kg) in mice (Jeppsson 1975).

17. 3-METHYL-BUTAN-2-ONE

$$CH_3.CO.CH(CH_3).CH_3$$

CAS Reg No:	563-80-4
Molecular formula:	$C_5H_{10}O$
Molecular weight:	86.15

17.1 Exposure

The US EPA have identified 3-methyl-2-butanone (isopropyl methyl ketone) in the tap water of Cincinnati, Philadelphia, Ottuma (Iowa), Miami and Seattle (Eurocop-cost), while WRc found it in one of 14 UK drinking water samples tested (Water Research Centre 1981).

17.2 Metabolism

The metabolism of 3-methyl-butan-2-one has been reported to occur slowly, with between 38 and 54% of a 1000 mg/kg dose given to rats eliminated unchanged. Excretion occurred mainly via exhaled air (Haggard *et al* 1945). A portion of the dose has been reported to be excreted in the urine in the form of glucuronide conjugates (Williams 1959).

17.3 Toxicity

The oral LD50 of 3-methyl-2-butanone has been reported as 5.66 ml/kg (4.55 g/kg) in rats (Carpenter *et al* 1974), 3200 mg/kg in both male rats and mice (Krasavage *et al* 1982), and 4100 mg/kg in rats (Haggard *et al* 1945).

Death due to respiratory failure has been reported to occur in rats injected intraperitoneally with 2980 mg/kg of 3-methyl-2-butanone (Haggard *et al* 1945). The Eastman Kodak Co reported an intraperitoneal LD50 of 800 mg/kg for 3-methyl-butan-2-one in rats, and between 200 and 400 mg/kg in male mice (Krasavage *et al* 1982).

Oedema and necrosis were reported after 3-methyl-2-butanone was applied to the abdomen of guinea-pigs for 24 hours at levels of between 5 and 20 ml/kg. Two weeks after the treatment, residual eschars and scarring of the tissue was noted (Krasavage *et al* 1982). Rabbits having 3-methyl-2-butanone applied to their uncovered abdomens suffered only slight irritation. When applied undiluted to intact and abraded skin for a period of 24 hours, under an occlusive dressing, moderate irritation was observed (Krasavage *et al* 1982). Carpenter (1974) reported the dermal LD50 in rabbit to be 6.35 ml/kg.

None of 25 volunteers subjected to skin sensitisation tests, using a 10% solution of 3-methyl-2-butanone, showed symptoms of sensitisation or irritation (Krasavage *et al* 1982).

18. ACETONE

Acetone (2-propanone, dimethyl ketone, beta-ketopropane, pyroacetic ether, dimethylformaldehyde, dimethylketal, ketone propane) is a colourless liquid with a characteristic odour. It is used as a solvent for fats, oils, waxes, resins, rubber, plastics, lacquers, varnishes and rubber cements. It is also used in the manufacture of many organic chemicals, including acetic acid (ketene process), chloroform, methyl isobutyl ketone and some explosives.

Acetone occurs as a micropollutant in blood and urine.

CAS Reg No:	67-64-1
Molecular weight:	58.09
Boiling point:	56.50 °C

18.1 Exposure

WRc identified acetone in an initial survey of drinking water, but it was not found in a subsequent more detailed survey (Water Research Centre 1981). This compound has also been identified in Japanese tap water (Akiyama *et al* 1980).

Acetone was detected in rural air in Talladega National Forest, Alabama, USA (Holzer *et al* 1977) and in urban air in Leningrad (Ioffe *et al* 1977).

18.2 Metabolism

Acetone is a naturally occurring constituent of blood and urine. It is readily absorbed from the gastrointestinal tract and lungs. It has a high solubility in water, and is rapidly and widely distributed among the various tissues relative to their water content. Large doses of acetone are primarily eliminated unchanged in expired air, but smaller doses are largely metabolised and eliminated as carbon dioxide (Flory and Weir, 1978, 190, 203, 274). The level of acetone in rat blood was measured following intraperitoneal injection of a range of acetone concentrations (25–2000 mg/kg). At blood acetone concentrations above 1000 mg/l, 75% or more of the acetone was eliminated unchanged, but at blood acetone concentrations below this level metabolism played an increasingly important role. At blood acetone concentrations of 150 mg/l, only 40% or less was eliminated unchanged, and 60% or more was metabolised (Haggard *et al* 1944).

Fasting appears to increase the rate of acetone metabolism. In rats given 50, 100 or 300 mg/kg acetone, metabolism was respectively 17%, 26% or 30% higher respectively in fasted animals than controls (Haggard *et al* 1944).

The half-life of acetone in the blood of dogs and humans has been found to be approximately 3 hours (DiVincenzo *et al* 1973).

The pathways of acetone metabolism are primarily direct oxidation to a 3-carbon glycolytic intermediate ('pyruvate' formation) and secondly as acetate and formate formation (Mourkides *et al* 1959). Following administration of radiolabelled acetone in rats, radioactivity was found in glycogen, various amino acids and cholesterol (Mourkides *et al* 1959, Price and Rittenberg 1950).

It has been suggested that acetone is converted via acetol to 1,2-propanediol (Ruddick 1972).

18.3 Health effects

Acetone is of low acute toxicity in rats. LD50 values (Kimura *et al* 1971) in four age groups were:

Newborn	1.74 g/kg (1.34–3.00)
14-day-old	4.43 g/kg (3.08–6.33)
Young adults	7.20 g/kg (5.38–9.57)
Older adults	6.72 g/kg (6.16–7.36)

Smyth *et al* (1962) reported an oral LD50 for acetone of 8.46 g/kg for rats.

The growth rate of rats (compared to controls) was not reduced by daily 4-hour inhalation of acetone vapour for 10 days at concentrations of 3000 to 16000 ppm. Several rats after a single exposure to 12000 or 16000 ppm showed symptoms of ataxia. However, a tolerance rapidly developed, and this response was not seen on subsequent days. Conditioned avoidance behaviour, as studied by a modification of the pole-climb method, altered at concentrations of 6000 ppm and above, and was also associated with a developed tolerance in several rats (Goldberg *et al* 1964).

Male Sprague–Dawley rats were given a single intraperitoneal injection of acetone (3.5 g/kg) 30 minutes before sacrifice. Then the liver 9000×*g* supernatant fraction was investigated, and showed an increase in activity of aniline hydroxylation and phenacetin *O*-deethylation (Kitada *et al* 1978). Female Wistar rats were given acetone (60 mmol/kg, as a 50% solution in saline) by intraperitoneal injection. The animals were sacrificed at 0.5 and 48 hours after acetone administration, and hepatic microsomes prepared. Investigation of the drug-metabolising activity of the hepatic microsomes showed an increase in aniline *p*-hydroxylation and a short (2 hours) inhibition of aminopyrine *N*-demethylation (Clark and Powis 1974). Male Simonson rats were given 1% acetone in drinking water for 5 days. The 9000×*g* supernatant fraction from rat liver was studied, and an increase in aniline and *p*-nitroanisole metabolism was reported. Also in this study, acetone was added to a 9000×*g* supernatant preparation to see what kind of binding spectrum it would produce. It produced a type I binding spectrum similar to hexobarbital. This indicates that acetone can interact with cytochrome P450 and may be a substrate, inhibitor or both for the hepatic oxidative enzymes (Furner *et al* 1972).

Male hooded Wistar rats were injected intraperitoneally with 0.5 ml/kg body weight acetone twice-daily for 3 days. Aniline and *p*-nitroanisole metabolism were elevated in the liver of treated rats. However, the cytochrome P-450 content was decreased (Farquharson and Stock 1975).

Acetone causes inhibition of non-specific cholinesterase isolated from cat liver (Hagiwara 1960). Acetone has been shown to potentiate the effects of 1,1-dichlor-oethylene, resulting in increased serum alanine alpha-ketoglutarate transaminase activity (Jaegar *et al* 1975). It also potentiates acetonitrile acute toxicity (Freeman and Hayes 1985).

Acetone is reported to produce moderate corneal injury (Grade 5 on a scale of 1–10) in the rabbit eye (Carpenter and Smyth 1946). Rengstorff *et al* (1976) found that small multiple doses of acetone administered topically or intracutaneously onto the backs of guinea-pigs produced cataracts. Repetition of the experiment with rabbits by dropping 1 ml of acetone directly on an area of clipped dorsal thorax three times a week for 3 weeks failed to induce any cataracts in any of the ten experimental rabbits.

Topical application of acetone to human skin for 30 or 90 minutes produced cellular damage mainly in the stratum corneum and the stratum spinosum. Acetone induced marked intracellular oedema of keratinised cells, and vacuolation of spinous cells. Seventy-two hours after discontinuation of the solvent application, most of the normal ultrastructural pattern in the superficial layers had been restored, while the viable parts of the epidermis showed residual cell degeneration (Lupulescu *et al* 1973).

Nelson *et al* (1943) used a group of unacclimatised volunteers to assess the effects of acetone vapour upon the eyes, nose and throat. Acetone was found to produce slight irritation at 300 ppm but 500 ppm was tolerated by most subjects.

In groups of rats exposed by inhalation to 19 000 ppm acetone vapour for 3 hours/day, 5 days/week for 8 weeks there was no effect on lactic dehydrogenase activity, glutamic-pyruvic transaminase activity, blood urea nitrogen, liver triglyceride content, organ histopathology, lung fluid content or organ weights (Bruckner and Peterson 1978).

Cellulose acetate filter press workers chronically exposed by inhalation to an average of 1006 ppm acetone, 8 hours/day, were studied by Raleigh and McGee (1972). A few workers complained of eye, nose or throat irritation, and a few complained of having a headache or of feeling lightheaded. Generally these complaints occurred when the concentration of acetone in air was over 1000 ppm. There was no evidence of central nervous effects as determined by lack of disturbance in gait and finger-to-nose test. Psychomotor tests revealed no lessened ability to perform these tests before, during or after exposure.

A case of acute intoxication due to exposure to over 12 000 ppm acetone was reported by Ross (1973). The men exposed had symptoms ranging from eye and throat irritation, headaches and limb weakness to confusion, nausea, vomiting and unconciousness.

No data appear to be available on the chronic toxicity of acetone.

Acetone was non-mutagenic in the Ames test with *Salmonella typhimurium* TA1535, TA1537, TA1538, TA98 and TA100 in either the presence or absence of metabolic activation (De Flora 1981). Acetone is a strong inducer of aneuploidy in *Saccharomyces cerevisiae* diploid strain D61.M. However, acetone was shown not to induce recombination and point mutation (Zimmermann *et al* 1985).

Van Duuren *et al* (1971) applied acetone to the skin of mice three times a week for 1 year, and reported after this time that no tumours had occurred in any of the 60 control or 20 acetone-treated animals.

19. CYCLOHEXANONE

Cyclohexanone (ketohexamethylene, pimelic ketone, sextone, anone) is a colourless, oily liquid with an acetone-like odour. It is used as a solvent for cellulose acetate, nitrocellulose, various insecticides, natural resins, crude rubber, waxes and fats. It is also used in the occurred adipic acid for nylon. Cyclohexanone is sometimes used in the solvent for PVC cement and primers used in solvent-welded joints for water pipes.

CAS Reg No:	108-94-1
Molecular weight:	98.1
Boiling point:	115.6 °C

19.1 Exposure

Cyclohexanone was identified by WRc in one of an unpublished study of 14 water samples analysed by gas chromatography–mass spectrometry.

19.2 Metabolism

In rabbits, hexanone is reduced to cyclohexanol and then conjugated to glucuronic acid to give cyclohexyl glucuronide, which is excreted in the urine (Elliot *et al* 1959). Traces of hydroxycyclohexylmercapturic acid and *cis*-2-hydroxycyclohexyl-mercapturic acid as its methyl ester were detected in ethereal extracts of acidified urine from rats and rabbits dosed with cyclohexanone (James and Waring 1971). Another sulphur-containing compound was found, which was thought to be the sulphate ester of the 2-hydroxycyclohexylmercapturic acid. The production of these sulphur-containing metabolites caused a slight decrease in total glutathione.

19.3 Health effects

An oral LD50 value of 1.54 g/kg and a dermal LD50 value of 0.95 g/kg have been reported for cyclohexanone in the rat (Smyth *et al* 1969).

When cyclohexanone was given orally to young white rabbits, the minimum lethal dose was found to lie between 1.0 and 1.6 g/kg. The sequence of symptoms following oral administration of lethal doses was ataxia, lethargy, collapse, narcosis, loss of reflexes and death. The minimum lethal dose of cyclohexanone for rabbits by cutaneous application was between 10.2 and 23.0 g/kg (Treon *et al* 1943).

The maximum safe concentration for the prolonged exposure (50 periods of 6 hours each) of rabbits to cyclohexanone by inhalation is thought to be a little below 0.75 mg/l cyclohexanone in air (190 ppm), since this concentration is reported to produce only very minor degenerative changes in the liver and kidneys (Treon *et al* 1943).

Various concentrations of cyclohexanone were applied to the shaved backs of male rabbits, and covered with an occlusive patch for 24 hours to determine its irritancy. Topical application of 12.4% cyclohexanone produced very slight irritation, 24.8% and 49.5% caused slight and moderate irritation respectively, while undiluted (99+%) cyclohexanone produced marked irritation. Ophthalmic tests in rabbits showed that 2.5% cyclohexanone was not irritating, but concentrations of 5–40% showed a dose-dependent irritation ranging from slight to marked irritation (Gupta *et al* 1979).

Mice were given 10%, 20% or 50% of the intraperitoneal LD50 dose daily for three consecutive days and then given 50 mg/kg pentobarbital sodium 24 hours after the final cyclohexanone injection. There was no effect on the pentobarbital sleeping time at these concentrations of cyclohexanone, suggesting that cyclohexanone does not cause induction or inhibition of the oxidative microsomal enzymes (Gupta *et al* 1979).

A range of concentrations of cyclohexanone (0.002–0.01 mol/l) caused a decrease in force of cardiac muscle contraction in an isolated rabbit heart preparation (Gupta *et al* 1979).

When cyclohexanone was administered by intraperitoneal injection 5 days/week, at the end of one week the LD50 was between one third and one quarter of the acute LD50, whereas by the end of 10 weeks the LD50 was about one tenth of the acute LD50. The authors state that there is a cumulative toxic effect of cyclohexanone (Gupta *et al* 1979).

Embryonated chicken eggs were exposed at 0 or 96 hours incubation time for either 3, 6 or 12 hours respectively to cyclohexanone vapours. Embryos sacrificed at 13 days incubation showed no gross pathology. Newly hatched chicks were normal at first but gradually showed increasingly severe locomotor problems; either an inability to walk, due to spastic extension of their legs, or toes severely curled inward (Weller and Griggs 1975).

Cyclohexanone was not mutagenic in *Salmonella typhimurium* strains TA100, TA98, TA1535 and TA1537 in experiments at two different laboratories (Haworth *et al* 1983).

20. 2-HEXANONE

2-Hexanone (n-butylmethyl ketone, methyl *n*-butyl ketone (MnBK), propylacetone) is a clear liquid with an odour resembling acetone but more pungent. 2-Hexanone is better known by its synonym methyl *n*-butyl ketone (MBK). It is used as a solvent, especially in paints, and in the printing of plasticised fabrics.

CAS Reg No:	591-78-6
Molecular weight:	100.18
Boiling point:	128 °C

20.1 Exposure

A hexanone isomer was identified in one of 14 UK drinking water samples analysed by WRc (Water Research Centre 1981).

20.2 Metabolism

A study in guinea-pigs showed that 2-hexanone is hydroxylated to 5-hydroxy-2-hexanone, which is then either oxidised to 2,5-hexanedione, reduced to 2,5-hexanediol or converted to a small extent to 2,5-dimethyl-2,3-dihydrofuran. 2-Hexanone may be reduced to 2-hexanol which can be further metabolised to 2,5-hexanediol, 5-hydroxy-2-hexanone, and 2,5-hexanedione. Of the 2-hexanone metabolites, 5-hydroxy-2-hexanone, 2,5-hexanediol and 2-hexanol were all cleared from the blood in 6–8 hours, whereas 2,5-hexanedione was cleared in approximately 16 hours (DiVincenzo *et al* 1976).

Male Charles River CD rats dosed with radiolabelled 2-hexanone excreted radiolabelled carbon dioxide in the expired air and radiolabelled 2-hexanol, 5-hydroxy-2-hexanone, 2,5-hexanedione, norleucine, 2,5-dimethylfuran, gamma-valerolactone and urea in the urine. The 2-hexanone used was labelled in the C-1 position, and radioactive carbon dioxide accounted for the single largest proportion of excreted radioactivity. A likely route of radiolabelled carbon dioxide formation is by alpha-oxidation of 2-hexanone to alpha-ketohexanoic acid followed by decarboxylation to carbon dioxide (DiVincenzo *et al* 1977).

In humans, 2-hexanone is readily absorbed by the lungs, the gastrointestinal tract and the skin. About 75–92% of the hexanone vapour was absorbed when humans were exposed to 10 or 50 ppm for 7.5 hours or to 100 ppm for 4 hours. The major metabolite of 2-hexanone in man was carbon dioxide, with 2,5-hexanedione also being detected in the blood. 2-Hexanone is excreted relatively slowly in the expired air and the urine (approx 65% of an oral dose excreted in 8 days). This suggests that repeated daily exposures may lead to a build-up of neurotoxic metabolites, eg 2,5-hexanedione (DiVincenzo *et al* 1978).

20.3 Health effects

A rat acute oral LD50 of 2.59 g/kg for 2-hexanone has been reported (Smyth *et al* 1954). The oral LD50 in mice has been reported as 100 mg/kg, and the intraperitoneal LD50 for rats and guinea-pigs has been reported as 1142 and 1140 ml/kg respectively (Krasavage et al 1982).

Neurotoxic effects may develop in the periphery following exposure to 2-hexanone or its metabolite 2,5-hexandione over a period of weeks in experimental animals and man. Symptoms include clumsiness and lack of muscular coordination. Examination of the nerve fibres reveals accumulations of 10 nm filaments, identical in size and form to neurofilaments, within the axon. These accumulations cause enlargement of the proximal paranodes at the nodes of Ranvier, and later the whole internode swells irregularly, causing thinning of the myelin covering. Later, secondary masses are found, and degeneration is found in many fibres below these giant swellings (Cavanagh 1979).

Groups of male rats were administered equimolar doses (6.6 mmol/kg) of 2-hexanone and its metabolites by gavage 5 days/week for 90 days to determine their relative neurotoxicity. All test compounds produced both clinical and histologic evidence for neuropathy. The relative neurotoxicity of the test compounds in decreasing order of potency was: 2,5-hexanedione, 5-hydroxy-2-hexanone, 2,5-hexanediol, 2-hexanone and 2-hexanol. The neurotoxicity of each compound was found to be directly related to the degree of its metabolism to 2,5-hexanedione as determined by measuring the area under the serum concentration time curve of 2,5-hexanedione (Krasavage *et al* 1980).

Nine rats were exposed by inhalation for 8 hours/day, 5 days/week for 6 weeks to 200 ppm 2-hexanone. Eight other rats were exposed to a mixture of 200 ppm 2-hexanone and 2000 ppm methyl ethyl ketone for a similar period; three rats died during this experiment. All treated animals showed muscular weakness of all limbs, which in the case of the 2-hexanone-treated rats lasted a few hours after the experiment each night, and for the 2-hexanone/methyl ethyl ketone group lasted at least 24 hours. Histological examination of the sciatic nerves revealed axonal hypertrophy and segmental breakdown of myelin. These observations were interpreted as early changes of a neuropathy which is primarily axonal with secondary myelin breakdown (Duckett *et al* 1974). The enhancement of 2-hexanone neurotoxicity by combined exposure with methyl ethyl ketone was also demonstrated by Abdel-Rahman *et al* (1976).

Cats receiving twice-daily subcutaneous injections of 150 mg/kg undiluted commercial grade 2-hexanone (99.66% purity) 5 days/week for up to 8.5 months developed damage to the peripheral and central nervous system (Spencer and Schaumberg 1976).

Guinea-pigs were given drinking water containing 0.1% or 0.25% 2-hexanone, 0.1% or 0.5% 2-hexanol, 0.1% or 0.5% 2,5-hexanedione, and a control group received water for 24 weeks. Dynamic pupillometry indicated that 2-hexanone, 2,5-hexanedione and 2-hexanol caused a decreased pupillary response throughout the first 5 weeks, and by the 24th week all treatment groups showed a greatly impaired pupillary response (Abdel-Rahman *et al* 1978).

Groups of pregnant female Fischer 344 rats were exposed by inhalation to 500, 1000 and 2000 ppm 2-hexanone for 6 hours/day throughout gestation. Dose-related differences in maternal weight gain, in pup weight at birth, in the number of pups per litter and in postnatal growth of the offspring were seen. Behavioural tests suggested that young offspring of treated dams were more active than those of controls, and their geriatric counterparts less active than those of controls. No consistent age-related patterns were seen (Peters *et al* 1981).

21. 3-HEXANONE

CAS Reg No:	589-38-8
Molecular weight:	100.18
Boiling point:	124 °C

A hexanone isomer was identified in one of fourteen UK drinking water samples analysed by WRc (Water Research Centre 1981).

3-Hexanone (ethyl propyl ketone) was reported to have an oral LD50 value of 2.69 g/kg in rats and a dermal LD50 value of 2.54 g/kg in rabbits (Carpenter *et al* 1974).

No other toxicological data appear to be available.

22. CAMPHOR

Camphor (1,7,7-trimethylbicyclo[2.2.1]heptan-2-one, 2-bornanone, 2-camphanone, 2-keto-1,7,7-trimethylnorcamphane, gum camphor) consists of colourless or white crystalline masses. It has a penetrating, fragrant, aromatic odour and an aromatic, slightly bitter and cooling taste. Camphor is a by-product of the wood processing industry, although it is also produced on a commercial basis. It is used as an odorant/flavouring in household, pharmaceutical and industrial products, as a plasticiser, for cellulose esters and ethers, insect repellants, explosives, lacquers and varnishes, and as a preservative in the pharmaceutical and cosmetics industry.

CAS Reg No:	76-22-2
Molecular weight:	152.23
Boiling point:	204 °C

22.1 Exposure

Camphor was found in a raw water sample in a survey carried out by WRc (Water Research Centre 1981). Camphor was also identified in Japanese tap water (Akiyama *et al* 1980). It was found in Zurich tap water at 2 ng/l, in spring water at 2 ng/l, and in lake Zurich at 12 ng/l at the surface and 2 ng/l at a depth of 30 m (Grob and Grob 1974).

Naturally occurring camphor is found in the twigs, leaves and stem of the camphor tree of China and Japan. It is also the major constituent of pine oil (Verschueren 1983).

22.2 Metabolism

Camphor is easily absorbed through the mucous membranes and gastrointestinal tract in man (Aronow 1976). It is known to cross the human placenta, since it was identified in amniotic fluid, foetal blood, brain, liver and kidney 36 hours after the mother ingested 12 g of camphor (Riggs *et al* 1965).

Studies have shown that camphor is metabolised in dogs and rabbits to 3-hydroxycamphor, 5-endo-hydroxycamphor and 5-exo-hydroxycamphor, all of which are conjugated with glucuronic acid and excreted in the urine. The hydroxylation reactions were shown to occur in microsomes isolated from dog and rabbit liver, and were NADPH-dependent. *d*-Camphor is not detectably reduced by rat liver $9000 \times g$ supernatant fraction, while *l*-camphor undergoes a small amount of reduction to borneol, with an even smaller amount of isoborneol formed. In rabbit $9000 \times g$ supernatant fraction, *d*-camphor was strongly reduced to borneol whereas *l*-camphor reduction was much less than that for *d*-camphor, and produced three times more isoborneol than borneol (Liebman and Ortiz 1973).

22.3 Health effects

Both the acute oral LD50 in rats and the acute dermal LD50 in rabbits were reported to be greater than 5 g/kg (Moreno 1976). The acute oral LD50 for mice has been reported at 1.31 g/kg (Horikawa and Okada 1975).

The minimum lethal doses for synthetic and natural camphors administered subcutaneously as a 20% solution in olive oil were 1.7 g/kg and 2.2 g/kg respectively (Christensen and Lynch 1937). The minimum lethal dose for an intraperitoneal injection of camphor was found to be 3.5 ml of a 20% solution in olive oil/kg (Sampson and Fernandez 1939).

Intoxication from camphor has been frequently reported in the literature. Signs of camphor intoxication include nausea, vomiting and mental changes such as excitement, hallucinations and delirium (Phelan 1976).

Workmen exposed to 33–194 mg camphor/m^3 air for 8 hours/day, 5 days/week at a synthetic camphor packaging plant had inflammation of the nose and throat but no lymph adenopathy. No permanent changes were caused, and symptoms disappeared soon after leaving the camphor atmosphere (Gronka *et al* 1969).

23. FENCHONE

Fenchone (1,3,3-trimethylbicyclo[2.2.1]heptan-2-one, *d*-1,3,3-trimethyl-2-norbornanone, *d*-1,3,3-trimethyl-2-norcamphanone) is an oily liquid with a camphor-like odour. Fenchone occurs naturally in many essential oils, with the highest levels being found in fennel oil. It is used in perfumes and as a flavouring.

CAS Reg No:	1195-79-5
Molecular weight:	152.26
Molecular formula:	$C_{10}H_{16}O$
Melting point:	6.1 °C

23.1 Exposure
Fenchone was identified in one of 14 drinking water samples analysed by WRc in an unpublished survey.

23.2 Metabolism
The metabolism of *d*-fenchone to 4-hydroxyfenchone, 5-hydroxyfenchone and pi-apofenchone-3-carboxylic acid has been demonstrated. These metabolites are conjugated to glucuronic acid, and excreted in the urine (Reinhartz and Zanke 1936).

23.3 Health effects
The acute oral LD50 value for fenchone in the rat was reported as 6.16 g/kg. Toxic signs included depression, scrawny appearance, porphyrin-like deposit around the eyes and nose for a week after treatment. Time until death varied from 4 hours to 9 days (Jenner *et al* 1964). The acute dermal LD50 value in rabbits was reported as greater than 5 g/kg (Levenstein 1975).

Fenchone when applied full strength to intact or abraded rabbit skin for 24 hours under occlusion produced mild irritation (Levenstein 1975). When tested at 4% in petrolatum in a 48-hour closed-patch test on humans, fenchone produced no irritation. Fenchone did not produce sensitisation reactions when tested at 4% in petrolatum on 25 volunteers in a maximisation test (Klingman 1975).

The median convulsive dose for fenchone administered subcutaneously in sesame oil is reported as 1.13 g/kg in mice (Wenzel and Ross 1957). The hexobarbitone sleep time in mice was reduced by the subcutaneous administration of 500 mg/kg fenchone 5 minutes after an intraperitoneal injection of 100 mg/kg hexobarbital sodium. An intraperitoneal injection of 500 mg/kg fenchone, however, had no effect on pentobarbitone-depressed respiration in rats.

Inhalation of fenchone produces a dose-dependent increase in volume output of respiratory tract fluid, which reaches a peak at an amount that produces a just detectable scent to inhaled air. The increase seen was greater in the autumn months (Boyd and Sheppard 1971).

24. 4-METHYL-2-PENTANONE
4-Methyl-2-pentanone is a colourless liquid with a faint ketonic and camphor odour. It is used as a solvent for paints, varnishes, gums, resins and nitrocellulose. 4-Methyl-2-pentanone is also used in the manufacture of methylamylalcohol, in extraction processes and organic syntheses. 4-methylpentan-2-one is more commonly known as methyl isobutyl ketone (MiBK) or less commonly as isopropyl acetone.

CAS Reg No:	108-10-1
Molecular weight:	100.16
Boiling point:	118 °C
Odour threshold concentration:	0.10 ppm

24.1 Exposure
Methyl isobutyl ketone was identified in four of 14 UK drinking water samples examined by WRc (Water Research Centre 1981).

24.2 Metabolism
4-Methyl-2-pentanone is metabolised by hydroxylation at the ω-1 carbon to form 4-hydroxy-4-methyl-2-pentanone, and by reduction of the carbonyl group to give the secondary alcohol 4-methyl-2-pentanol. These two metabolites were identified in guinea-pig serum after intraperitoneal administration of 450 mg/kg body weight 4-methyl-2-pentanone. The major metabolite was 4-hydroxy-4-methyl-2-pentanone, whose clearance time was 16 hours. The half-life of 4-methyl-2-pentanone was 66 minutes, and its clearance time was 6 hours (DiVincenzo *et al* 1976).

4-Methyl-2-pentanone was found to be a volatile constituent in urine collected over a 24-hour period from unexposed men and women (Zlatkis and Liebich 1971).

24.3 Health effects
The acute oral rat LD50 value for 4-methyl-2-pentanone as a 20% emulsion in Tergitol 7 surfactant was reported as 2.08 g/kg (Smyth *et al* 1951).

When placed in the rabbit eye, 0.1 ml of undiluted 4-methyl-2-pentanone caused some irritation within 10 minutes. After 8 hours, inflammation and swelling were visible, and by 24 hours exudate was also present (Krasavage *et al* 1982).

Baboons exposed by inhalation to 50 ppm 4-methyl-2-pentanone for 24 hours a day for a 7-day period showed no significant effect upon accuracy of performance of a match-to-sample task, but did show a slowing of response time. When the exposure atmosphere was 100 ppm methyl ethyl ketone combined with 50 ppm 4-methyl-2-pentanone, no effect was seen on response time (Geller *et al* 1979).

Twelve subjects, of mixed sexes, were placed in a 1200 cubic foot gas cabinet and exposed to a given concentration of 4-methyl-2-pentanone for 15 minutes. Afterwards, each individual classified the effect of the vapour on the eyes, nose and throat as either not irritating, slightly irritating or very irritating. From this data a sensory limit of 100 ppm was indicated as the highest concentration that could be tolerated for an 8-hour period (Silverman *et al* 1946).

Six young adult rats were exposed by inhalation to 1500 ppm commercial grade 4-methyl-2-pentanone for 6 hours/day, 5 days/week for up to 5 months. These animals displayed a normal weight gain, slight narcosis during exposure, and no signs of neurological dysfunction after 5 months exposure. Areas of the central nervous system and the proximal parts of the peripheral nervous system were examined histologically, and showed no peculiarities. However, the most distal parts of the tibial and ulnar nerves showed many axons containing large numbers of dilated, glycogen-filled mitochondrial remnants, adaxonal Schwann cell invaginations and rare focal swellings. These minimal distal axonal changes may be due to the 3%

methyl *n*-butyl ketone which is a contaminant in commercial grade 4-methyl-2-pentanone (Spencer *et al* 1975). Cats receiving twice-daily subcutaneous injections of 150 mg/kg undiluted 4-methyl-2-pentanone or a 9 : 1 mixture of methyl ethyl ketone and 4-methyl-2-pentanone for 5 days/week for up to 8.5 months showed no detectable signs of nervous system damage (Spencer and Schaumberg 1976).

25. METHYLETHYLCYCLOHEXANONE ISOMER

Methylethylcyclohexanone isomer was identified in one of 14 drinking water samples in a survey by WRc (Water Research Centre 1981).

No data appear to be available for this compound.

26. 3-METHYL-2-PENTANONE

3-Methyl-2-pentanone was identified in four of 14 drinking water samples in a survey by WRc (Water Research Centre 1981).

No data appear to be available for this compound.

27. METHYLPROPYLCYCLOHEXANONE ISOMER

Methylpropylcyclohexanone isomer was identified in one of 14 drinking water samples in a survey by WRc (Water Research Centre 1981).

No data appear to be available for this compound.

28. REFERENCES

ABBASOV B M, ZEINALOBA K G and SAFAROVA I A (1977) Toxicology of some ketones. *Gigiena Truda i Professional'nykh Zabolevaniia* **11**, 145-8.

ABDEL-RAHMAN M S, HETLAND L B and COURI D (1976) Toxicity and metabolism of methyl *n*-butyl ketone. *Journal of the American Industrial Hygiene Association* **37**, 95-102.

ABDEL-RAHMAN M S, SALADIN J J, BOHMAN C E and COURI D (1978) The effect of 2-hexanone and 2-hexanone metabolites on pupillomotor activity and growth. *Journal of the American Industrial Hygiene Association* **39**, 94-99.

AKIYAMA T, KOGA M, SHINOHARA R, KIDO A and ETOH S (1980) Detection and identification of trace organic substances in the aquatic environment. *Journal of Uoeh* **2**, 285-300.

ALLEN N, MENDELL J R, BILLMAIER D J, FONTAINE R E and O'NEILL J (1975) Toxic polyneuropathy due to methyl *n*-butyl ketone. An industrial outbreak. *Archives of Neurology* **32**, 209-218.

ALTENKIRCH H, STOLTENBURG G and WAGNER H M (1978) Experimental studies on hydrocarbon neuropathies induced by methyl ethyl ketone (MEK). *Journal of Neurology* **219**, 159-170.

ANDERSON D and STYLES J A (1978) An evaluation of six short-term tests for detecting organic chemical carcinogens. Appendix 2. The bacterial mutation test. *British Journal of Cancer* **37**, 924-930.

ANDERSON P H and JENSEN N J (1984) Mutagenic investigation of peppermint oil in the Salmonella/mammalian-microsome test. *Mutation Research* **138**, 17-20.

ARONOW R (1976) Camphor poisoning. *Journal of the American Medical Association* **235**, 1260.

BENOIT F M, LEBEL G L and WILLIAMS D T (1979) Polycyclic aromatic hydrocarbon level in Eastern Ontario drinking waters. *Bulletin of Environmental Contamination and Toxicology* **23**, 774-778.

BERTSCH W, CHANG R C and ZLATKIS A (1974) The determination of organic volatiles in air pollution studies: characterization of profiles. *Journal of Chromatographic Science* **12**, 175–182.

BIONETICS RESEARCH LABS INC (1968) Evaluation of carcinogenic, teratogenic, and mutagenic activities of selected pesticides and industrial chemicals. Volume 1. Carcinogenic study. August 1968, US Department of Commerce, Maryland, NTIS PB-223 159, pp 276-277.

BJELDANES L F and CHEW H (1979) Mutagenicity of 1,2-dicarbonyl compounds: Maltol, kojic acid, diacetyl and related compounds. *Mutation Research* **67**, 367-371.

BOYD E M and SHEPPARD E P (1971) An autumn-enhanced mucotropic action of inhaled terpenes and related volatile agents. *Pharmacology* **6**, 65-80.

BROWN J P (1980) A review of the genetic effects of naturally occurring flavinoids, anthraquinones and related compounds. *Mutation Research* **75**, 243-277.

BRUCKNER J V and PETERSON R G (1978) Effect of repeated exposure of mice and rats to concentrated toluene and acetone vapors. *Toxicology and Applied Pharmacology* **45**, 359.

BUCHER J R, HUFF J and KLUWE W M (1986) Toxicology and carcinogenesis studies of isophorone in F344 rats and B6C3F1 mice. *Toxicology* **39**, 207-219.

BUKLAHOVSKI A A and SHUGAEV B B (1976) Toxicity and hygienic standardization of isophorone, dihydroisophorone, and dimethylphenylcarbinol. *Promyshlennost' Sinteticheskogo Kauchuka* p 4.

CAPRINO L, TOGNA G and MAZZEI M (1976) Toxicological studies of photosensitizer agents and photodegradable polyolefins. *European Journal of Toxicology* **9**, 99-103.

CARLSON G L, HALL I H and PIANTADOSI C (1975) Cycloalkanones. Part 7: hypocholesterolemic activity of aliphatic compounds related to 2,8-dibenzylcyclooctanone. *Journal of Medicinal Chemistry* **18**, 1024-1026.

CARPENTER C P (1949) Acute toxicity of methyl ethyl ketone. Report 12-59, Mellon Institute of Industrial Research. Cited in US Department of Commerce National Technical Information Service, PB-252 970. Investigations of selected potential environmental contaminants; ketonic solvents. Syracuse Research Corp, prepared for Environmental Protection Agency (May 1976).

CARPENTER C P (1954) Methyl propyl ketone, range finding tests on, Report 17-132, Mellon Institute of Industrial Research. Cited in US Department of Commerce National Technical Information Service, PB-252 970. Investigation of selected potential environmental contaminants; ketonic solvents. Syracuse Research Corp, prepared for Environmental Protection Agency (May 1976).

CARPENTER C P and SMYTH H F (1946) Chemical burns of the rabbit cornea. *American Journal of Ophthalmology* **29**, 1363-1372.

CARPENTER C P, WEIL C S and SMYTH H F Jr (1974) Range-finding toxicity data: List 8. *Toxicology and Applied Pharmacology* **28**, 313-319.

CAVANAGH J B (1979) The 'Dying Back' process. *Archives of Pathology and Laboratory Medicine* **103**, 659-664.

CHRISTENSEN B V and LYNCH H J (1937) A comparative study of the pharmacological actions of natural and synthetic camphor. *Journal of the American Pharmaceutical Association* **26**, 786-794.

CLARK H and POWIS G (1974) Effect of acetone administered *in vivo* upon hepatic microsomal drug metabolizing activity in the rat. *Biochemical Pharmacology* **23**, 1015-1019.

CLAVENDER F L, CASEY H W, SALEM H, SWENBERG J A and GRALLA E D (1983) A 90-day vapor inhalation toxicity study of methyl ethyl ketone. *Fundamental and Applied Toxicology* **3**, 264-270.

COLEMAN E W, LINGG R D, MELTON R G and KOPFLER F C (1976) The occurrence of volatile organics in five drinking water supplies using gas chromatography/mass spectrometry. In: *Identification and analysis of organic pollutants in water*, ed by L H Keith. Ann Arbor Science, Michigan.

COLEMAN W E, MELTON R G, KOPFLER F C, BARONE K A, AURAND T A and JELLISON M G (1980) Identification of organic compounds in a mutagenic extract of a surface drinking water by a computerized gas chromatography/mass spectrometry system(GC/MS/COM). *Environmental Science and Technology* **14**, 576-588.

COLLEY J, GAUNT I F, LANSDOWN A B G, GRASSO P and GANGOLLI S D (1969) Acute and short-term toxicity of diacetyl in rats. *Food and Cosmetics Toxicology* **7**, 571-580.

COURI D, HETLAND L B, ABDEL-RAHMAN M S and WEISS H (1977) The influence of inhaled ketone solvent vapours on hepatic microsomal biotransformation activities. *Toxicology and Applied Pharmacology* **41**, 285-289.

CULP H W and McMAHON R E (1968) Reductase for aromatic aldehydes and ketones. *Journal of Biological Chemistry* **243**, 848-852.

DAWSON J and HULLIN R P (1954a) Metabolism of acetoin. 1. The formation and utilization of acetoin and butane-2:3-diol in the decerebrated cat. *Biochemical Journal* **57**, 177-179.

DAWSON J and HULLIN R P (1954b) Metabolism of acetoin. 2. Metabolic conversions of acetoin, pyruvate and acetate by rabbit-kidney dispersions. *Biochemical Journal* **57**, 180.

DEACON N M, PILNY M D, JOHN J A, SCHWETZ B A, MURRAY F J, YAKEL H O and KUNA R A (1981) Embryo- and fetotoxicity of inhaled methyl ethyl ketone in rats. *Toxicology and Applied Pharmacology* **59**, 620-622.

DE FLORA S (1981) Study of 106 organic and inorganic compounds in the Salmonella/microsome test. *Carcinogenesis* **2**, 283-298.

DIVINCENZO G D and KRASAVAGE W J (1974) Serum ornithine carbamyl transferase as a liver response test for exposure to organic solvents. *American Industrial Hygiene Association Journal* **35**, 21-29.

DIVINCENZO G D, YANNO F J and ASTILL B D (1973) Exposure of man and dog to low concentrations of acetone vapour. *American Industrial Hygiene Association Journal* **34**, 329-336.

DIVINCENZO G D, KAPLAN C J and DEDINAS J (1976) Characterization of the metabolites of methyl *n*-butyl ketone, methyl iso-butyl ketone and methyl ethyl ketone in guinea pig serum and their clearance. *Toxicology and Applied Pharmacology* **36**, 511-522.

DIVINCENZO G D, HAMILTON M L, KAPLAN C J and DEDINAS J (1977) Metabolic fate and disposition of ^{14}C-labelled methyl *n*-butyl ketone in the rat. *Toxicology and Applied Pharmacology* **41**, 547-560.

DIVINCENZO G D, HAMILTON M L, KAPLAN C J, KRASAVAGE W J and O'DONOGHUE J L. (1978) Studies on the respiratory uptake and excretion and the skin absorption of methyl *n*-butyl ketone in humans and dogs. *Toxicology and Applied Pharmacology* **44**, 593-604.

DOSTAL K A, PIERSON R C, HAGER D G and ROBECK G G (1965) Carbon bed design criteria study at Nitro, W.Va. *Journal of the American Water Works Association,* 670-674.

DUCKETT S, WILLIAMS N and FRANCIS S (1974) Peripheral neuropathy associated with inhalation of methyl-*n*-butyl ketone. *Experientia* **30**, 1283-1284.

DUTERTRE-CATELLA H, PHU-LICH M N, QUAN D Q and TRUHAUT R (1978) Transformations metaboliques de la trimethyl-3,5,5,cyclo-hexene-2, one-1 (isophorone). *Toxicology Research Journal* **1**, 209-216.

ELKINS H B (1959) *The chemistry of industrial toxicology*. 2nd edn. Wiley, New York.

ELLIGER C A, HENIKA P R and MACGREGOR J T (1984) Mutagenicity of flavones, chromones and acetophenones in *Salmonella typhimurium*. New structure-activity relationships. *Mutation Research* **135**, 77-86.

ELLIOTT T H, PARKE D V and WILLIAMS R T (1959) Studies in detoxication. 79. The metabolism of cyclo[^{14}C]hexane and its derivatives. *Biochemical Journal* **72**, 193-200.

EUROCOP-COST (1976) An inventory of organic pollutants which have been identified in various surface waters, effluent discharges, aquatic animals and plants, and bottom sediments. Cost project-64B. Luxembourg, Commission of the European Communities, 1976.

FARQUHARSON T A and STOCK B H (1975) Modified response of hepatic microsomes from rats administered polar aprotic solvents. *Australian Journal of Pharmaceutical Sciences* **NS4**, 111-115.

FILSER J G, JUNG P and BOLT H M (1982) Increased acetone exhalation induced by metabolites of halogenated C1 and C2 compounds. *Archives of Toxicology* **49**, 107-116.

FLORIN I, RUTBERG L, CURVALL M and ENZELL C R (1980) Screening of tobacco smoke constituents for mutagenicity using the Ames Test. *Toxicology* **18**, 219-232.

FLORY D A and WEIR F W (1978) Development of reclaimed potable water quality criteria, Spectrix Corporation Report No, NAS9-15368.

FREEMAN J J and HAYES E P (1985) Acetone potentiation of acute acetonitrile toxicity in rats. *Journal of Toxicology and Environmental Health* **15**, 609-621.

FURNER R L, NEVILLE E D, TALARICO K S and FELLER D D (1972) A common modality of action of simulated space stresses on the oxidative metabolism of ethylmorphine, aniline and *p*-nitroanisole by male rat liver. *Toxicology and Applied Pharmacology* **21**, 569-581.

GABRIEL M A, JABARA H and AL-KHALIDI U A S (1971) Metabolism of acetoin in mammalian liver slices and extracts. Interconversion with butane-2,3-diol and biacetyl. *Biochemical Journal* **124**, 793-800.

GABRIEL M A, ILBAWI M and AL-KHALID U A S (1972) The oxidation of acetoin to CO_2 in intact animals and in liver mince preparation. *Comparative Biochemistry and Physiology* **41**, 493-502.

GARCIA C R, GELLER I and KAPLAN H L (1978) Effects of ketones on lever-pressing behavior of rats. *Proceedings of the Western Pharmacological Society* **21**, 433-438.

GAUNT I F, BRANTOM P G, KISS I D, GRASSO P and GANGOLLI S D (1972) Short-term toxicity of acetoin (acetylmethylcarbinol) in rats. *Food and Cosmetics Toxicology* **10**, 131-141.

GELLER I, GAUSE E, KAPLAN H and HARTMANN R J (1979) Effects of acetone, methyl ethyl ketone and methyl isobutyl ketone on a match-to-sample task in the baboon. *Pharmacology Biochemistry and Behaviour* **11**, 401-406.

GIROUX J, GRANGER R and MONNIER P (1954) Comparative study of 2-pentanone and 2-ethyl butanone in the mouse. *Travaux-Societe de Pharmoacie de Montpelier* **14**, 342-346.

GOLDBERG M E, JOHNSON H E, POZZANI U C and SMYTH H F Jr (1964) Effect of repeated inhalation of vapours of industrial solvents on animal behaviour. 1. Evaluation of nine solvent vapors on pole-climb performance in rats. *American Industrial Hygiene Association Journal* **25**, 369-375.

GROB K and GROB G (1971) Gas–liquid chromatographic–mass spectrometric investigation of C6–C20 organic compounds in an urban atmosphere. Application of ultratrace analysis on capillary columns. *Journal of Chromatography* **62**, 1-13.

GROB K and GROB G (1974) Organic substances in potable water and its precursor. Part 2. Applications in the area of Zurich. *Journal of Chromatography* **90**, 303-313.

GRONKA P, BOBKOSKIE R L, TOMCHICK G J and RAKOW A B (1969) Camphor exposures in a packaging plant. *American Industrial Hygiene Association Journal* **30**, 276-279.

GUPTA P K, LAWRENCE W H, TURNER J E and AUTIAN J (1979) Toxicological aspects of cyclohexanone. *Toxicology and Applied Pharmacology* **49**, 525-533.

HAGAN E C, HANSEN W H, FITZHUGH O G, JENNER P M, JONES W I, TAYLOR J M, LONG F, NELSON A A and BROUWER J B (1967) Food flavourings and compounds of related structure. 2. Subacute and chronic toxicity. *Food and Cosmetics Toxicology* **5**, 141.

HAGGARD H W, GREENBURG L A and McCULLOUGH TURNER J (1944) The physiological principles governing the action of acetone together with determination of toxicity. *Journal of Industrial Hygiene and Toxicology* **26**, 133-151.

HAGGARD H W, MILLER D P and GREENBERG L A (1945) The amyl alcohols and their ketones: their metabolic fates and comparative toxicities. *Journal of Industrial Hygiene and Toxicology* **27**, 1-14.

HAGIWARA Y (1960) Benzoylcholinesterase. Report 2: activation of nonspecific cholinesterase by polyhydric alcohols. *Japanese Journal of Pharmacology* **9**, 137-149.

HALL I H and CARLSON G L (1976) Cycloalkanones. Part 9. Comparison of analogs which inhibit cholesterol and fatty acid synthesis. *Journal of Medicinal Chemistry* **19**, 1257-61.

HAWORTH S, LAWLOR T, MORTELMANS K, SPECK W and SEIGER E (1983) Salmonella mutagenicity test results for 250 chemicals. *Environmental Mutagenous Supplement* **1**, 3-142.

HETLAND L B, COURI D and ABDEL-RAHMAN M S (1976) The influence of inhaled ketone solvent vapours on hepatic microsomal biotransformation activities. *Toxicology and Applied Pharmacology* **37**, 111.

HIETANEN E and VANIO H (1982) Effects of fluorenone and trifluorenone on the monooxygenase, epoxide hydrolase and glutathione *S*-transferse activities in rabbits. *Developments in Biochemistry* **23**, 777-780.

HOLZER G, SHANFIELD H, ZLATKIS A, BERTSCH W, JUAREZ P, MAYFIELD H and LIEBICH H M (1977) Collection and analysis of trace organic emmissions from natural sources. *Journal of Chromatography* **142**, 755-764.

HORIKAWA E and OKADA T (1975) Acute toxicity of phenol camphor. *Shika Gakuho* **75**, 934. (As reported in *Food and Cosmetics Toxicology* **13**, 665-671 1975.) Cited in Opdyke, D L J (1975). Fragrance raw materials monographs. Camphor USP.

IMASHEVA N B (1971) Threshold concentrations of acetophenone during short- and long-term inhalation. AICE Survey of USSR Air Pollution Literature, 8, 79-93.

INNES J R M , ULLAND B M, VALERO M G, PETRUCELLI L, FISHBEIN L, HART E R, PALLOTTA A J, BATES R R, FALK H L, GART J J, KLEIN M, MITCHELL I and PETERS J (1969) Bioassay of pesticides and industrial chemicals for tumourigenicity in mice: A preliminary note. *Journal of the National Cancer Institute* **42**, 1101-1114.

IOFFE B V, ISIDOROV V A and ZENKEVICH I G (1977) Gas chromatographic –mass spectometric determination of volatile organic compounds in an urban atmosphere. *Journal of Chromatography* **142**, 787–795.

JAEGAR R J, CONOLLY R B, REYNOLDS E S and MURPHYS D (1975) Biochemical toxicology of unsaturated halogenated monomers. *Environmental Health Perspectives* **11**, 121-128.

JAMES S P and WARING R H (1971) The metabolism of alicyclic ketones in the rabbit and rat. *Xenobiotica* **1**, 573-580.

JENNER P M, HAGAN E C, TAYLOR J M, COOK E L and FITZHUGH O G (1964) Food flavourings and compounds of related structure. 1. Acute oral toxicity. *Food and Cosmetics Toxicology* **2**, 327-343.

JEPPSSON R (1975) Parabolic relationship between lipophilicity and biological activity of aliphatic hydrocarbons, ethers and ketones after intravenous injections of emulsion formulations into mice. *Acta Pharmacologica et Toxicologica* **37**, 56-64.

JUNGCLAUS G A, GAMES L M and HITES R A (1976) Identification of trace organic compounds in tire manufacturing plant waste waters. *Analytical*

Chemistry **48**, 1894-1897.
KADEN D A, HITES R A and THILLY W G (1979) Mutagenicity of soot and associated polycyclic aromatic hydrocarbons to *Salmonella typhimurium*. *Cancer Research* **39**, 4152-4159.
KEITH L H (1976a) Identification of organic compounds in drinking water from thirteen US cities. Paper given at an informal colloquium, Voorburg, Holland 18th February.
KEITH L H (ed) (1976b) *The identification and analysis of organic pollutants in water*. Ann Arbor Science Publishers Inc.
KIESE M and LENK W (1974) Hydroxyacetophenones: urinary metabolites of ethylbenzene and acetophenone in the rabbit. *Xenobiotica* **4**, 337-343.
KIMURA E T, EBERT D M and DODGE P W (1971) Acute toxicity and limits of solvent residue for sixteen organic solvents. *Toxicology and Applied Pharmacology* **19**, 699-704.
KITADA M, KAMATAKI T and KITAGAWA H (1978) Enhancement *in vivo* of drug oxidations following administration of benzphetamine, acetone, metyrapone and dimethylsulphoxide. *Japanese Journal of Pharmacology* **28**, 213-221.
KRASAVAGE W J, O'DONOGHUE J L, DIVINCENZO G D and TERHAAR C J (1980) The relative neurotoxicity of methyl *n*-butyl ketone, *n*-hexane and their metabolites. *Toxicology and Applied Pharmacology* **52**, 433-441.
KRASAVAGE W J, O'DONOGHUE J L and DIVINCENZO G D (1982) Ketones. In: *Patty's Industrial Hygiene and Toxicology*, Vol 2C, 3rd edn, ed by F E Clayton and G D Clayton. Wiley–Interscience Publ, New York. pp 4709-4800.
KUWATA K, UEBORI M and YAMASAKI Y (1979) Determination of aliphatic and aromatic aldehydes in polluted airs as their 2,4-dinitrophenylhydrazones by high performance liquid chromatography. *Journal of Chromatographic Science* **17**, 264-268.
LA BELLE C W and BRIEGER H (1955) Vapour toxicity of a composite solvent and its principal components. *Archives of Industrial Health* **12**, 623-627.
LEIBMAN K C (1971) Reduction of ketones in liver cytosol. *Xenobiotica* **1**, 97-104.
LEIBMAN K C and ORTIZ E (1973) Mammalian metabolism of terpenoids. 1 Reduction and hydroxylation of camphor and related compounds. *Drug Metabolism and Disposition* **1**, 543-551.
LIBERMAN D F, FINK R C, SCHAEFER L, MULCAHY R J and STARK, A A (1982) Mutagenicity of anthraquinone and hydroxlated anthraquinones in the Ames/Salmonella microsome system. *Applied Environmental Microbiology* **43**, 1354-1359.
LONEY B E, BASSETTE R and WARD G M (1963) Some volatile components in milk, blood, and urine from cows fed silage, bromegrass, and hay and grain. *Journal of Dairy Science* **46**, 922.
LOVELESS A (1951) Qualitative aspects of the chemistry and biology of radiomimetic (mutagenic) substances. *Nature* **167**, 338-342.
LUPULESCU A P, BIRMINGHAM D J and PINKUS H (1973) An electron microscopic study of human epidermis after acetone and kerosene administration. *Journal of Investigative Dermatology* **60**, 33-45.
MADSEN C, WURTZEN G and CARTENSEN J (1986) Short-term toxicity study

in rats dosed with methone. *Toxicology Letters* **32**, 147-152.
MALTEN K E, SPRUIT D, BOEMAARS H G M and DE KEIZER M J M (1968) Horny layer injury by solvents. *Berufsdermatosen* **16**, 135.
MAYLIN G A and ANDERS M W (1969) Effect of phenobarbital treatment on the stereochemistry of ethyl benzene metabolism. *Pharmacologist* **11**, 251.
McMAHON R E, CLINE J C and THOMPSON C Z (1979) Assay of 855 test chemicals in ten tester strains using a modification of the Ames test for bacterial mutagens. *Cancer Research* **39**, 682-93.
MELLON INSTITUTE (1950) Methyl ethyl ketone. Report 14-33, unpublished. 1950. Courtesy of Union Carbide Corp. Cited in US Environmental Protection Agency (1976). Investigation of selected potential environmental contaminants; ketonic solvents. US Department of Commerce, Washington DC, NTIS PB-252 970.
MERCK INDEX (1976) *An encyclopedia of chemicals and drugs*. 10th Edition. Merck and Co, Inc, Rahway, NJ.
MERRITT A D and TOMKINS G M (1959) Reversible oxidation of cyclic secondary alcohols by liver alcohol dehydrogenase. *Journal of Biological Chemistry* **234**, 2778-2782.
MOURKIDES G A, HOBBS D C and KOEPPE R E (1959) The metabolism of acetone-2-C^{14} by intact rats. *Journal of Biological Chemistry* **234**, 27-30.
MUNIES R (1965) Investigation of some factors influencing the percutaneous absorption of methyl ethyl ketone. Dissertation, University of Wisconsin, 1965. (In: *Dissertation Abstracts*, 1966, **26**, 5384.)
MUNIES R and WURSTER D E (1965) Investigation of some factors influencing percutaneous absorption. 3. Methyl ethyl ketone. *Journal of Pharmaceutical Sciences* **54**, 1281.
NAKAAKI K (1974) An experimental study of the effect of exposure to organic solvent vapor in human subjects. *Journal of Science of Labour* **50**, 89.
NATIONAL CANCER INSTITUTE (1979) Chemicals on standard protocol. National Cancer Institute, Carcinogeniesis Testing Program.
NATIONAL INSTITUTE FOR OCCUPATIONAL SAFETY AND HEALTH Registry of toxic effects of chemical substances. US Dept Health, Education and Welfare. Cincinnati, Ohio.
NELSON K W, EGE J F Jr, ROSS M, WOODMAN L E and SILVERMAN L (1943) Sensory response to certain industrial solvent vapors. *Journal of Industrial Hygiene and Toxicology* **25**, 282-285.
NEUBAUER O (1901) Concerning the pairing of glucuronic acid with materials of the aliphatic series. *Archiv für Experimentelle Pathologie und Pharmakoligie* **46**, 133-154. Cited in Krasavage W J, O'Donoghue J L and Divincenzo G D (1982) *Patty's Industrial Hygiene and Toxicology*, Vol 2C, 3rd edn, edited by F E Clayton and G D Clayton). Wiley–Interscience Publ, New York. pp 4709-4800.
NIOSH (1978) Criteria for a recommended standard for occupational exposure to ketones. US Dept of Health, Education and Welfare, National Institute for Occupational Safety and Health DHEW (NIOSH). Publication No 78-173.
O'DONOGHUE J L, KRASAVAGE W J, DIVINCENZO G D and KATZ G V (1984) Further studies on ketone neurotoxicity and interactions. *Toxicology and*

Applied Pharmacology **72**, 201-209.
OPDYKE D L J (1973a) Fragrance raw materials monographs. Benzophenone. *Food and Cosmetics Toxicology* **11**, 873-874.
OPDYKE D L J (1973b) Fragrance raw materials monographs. Acetophenone. *Food and Cosmetics Toxicology* **11**, 99-100.
OPDYKE D L J (1974) Fragrance raw materials monographs. Ethyl amyl ketone. *Food and Cosmetics Toxicology* **12**, 715.
OPDYKE D L J (1975a) Fragrance raw materials monograph. Methyl heptenone. *Food and Cosmetics Toxicology* **13**, 859.
OPDYKE D L J (1975b) Fragrance raw materials monographs. Methyl hexyl ketone. *Food and Cosmetics Toxicology* **13**, 861.
OPDYKE D L J (1975c) Fragrance raw materials monographs. Methyl ethyl ketone. *Food and Cosmetics Toxicology* **15**, 627-632.
OPDYKE D L J (1976a) Fragrance raw materials monograph. Isomenthone. *Food and Cosmetics Toxicology* **14**, 315.
OPDYKE D L J (1976b) Fragrance raw materials monograph. Menthone Racemic. *Food and Cosmetics Toxicology* **14**, 475-476.
OPDYKE D L J (1979a) Fragrance raw material monographs. Acetoin. *Food Cosmetics Toxicology* **17**, 509-511.
OPDYKE D L J (1979b) Fragrance raw materials monographs. Diacetyl. *Food and Cosmetics Toxicology* **17** (suppl), 765-8.
PATTY F A, SCHRENK H H and YANT W P (1935) Butanone. United States Public Health Report 50, 1217.
PETERS M A, HUDSON P M and DIXON R L (1981) The effect totigestational exposure to methyl *n*-butyl ketone has on postnatal development and behaviour. *Ecotoxicology and Environmental Safety* **5**, 291-306.
PETTERSSON B, CURVALL M and ENZELL C R (1980) Effects of tobacco smoke compounds on the noradrenaline induced oxidative metabolism in isolated brown fat cells. *Toxicology* **18**, 1-15.
PHELAN W J (1976) Camphor poisoning: over the counter dangers. *Pediatrics* **57**, 428-431.
PIETRZAK E and BARYLKO-PIKIELNA N (1976) Determination of odor absolute threshold of some sulphur compounds. *Acta Alimentaria Polonica* **2**, 207.
PRICE D T and RITTENBERG D (1950) The metabolism of acetone. 1. Gross aspects of catabolism and excretion. *Journal of Biological Chemistry* **185**, 449-459.
QUEVAUVILLER A (1946) Toxicite, pouvoir hypnotique de l'acetephenone et des thienylacetones. Comptes Rendus des Seances de la Societe de Biologie et de ses filiales **140**, 367-369.
RALEIGH R L and McGEE W A (1972) Effects of short, high-conçentration exposures to acetone as determined by observation in the work area. *Journal of Occupational Medicine* **14**, 607-610.
REINHARTZ F and ZANKE W (1936) Der Abbau des Fenchons im tierischen Organismus. *Berichte-Deutache Chemiscke Gessellschaft* **69**, 2259. (As cited in *Food and Cosmetics Toxicology* **14**, 769-771, 1976).
RENGSTORFF R, PETRALI J and SIM V (1976) Attempt to induce cataracts in

rabbits by cutaneous application of acetone. *American Journal of Optometry and Physiological Optics* **53**, 41-42.

RIGGS J, HAMILTON R, HOMEL S and McCABE J (1965) Camphorated oil intoxication in pregnancy. *Obstetrics and Gynecology* **25**, 255-258.

ROBINSON D (1958) Studies in detoxification. 74. The metabolism of benzhydrol, benzophenone, and *p*-hydroxybenzophenone. *Biochemical Journal* **68**, 584-586.

ROSS D S (1973) Short communications. Acute acetone intoxication involving eight male workers. *Annals of Occupational Hygiene* **16**, 73-75.

ROWE V K and WOLF M A (1963) Ketones. In: *Patty's Industrial Hygiene and Toxicology,* 2nd edn, ed by F A Patty Volume 2. Interscience, New York.

RUDDICK J A (1972) Toxicology, metabolism and biochemistry of 1,2 propanediol. *Toxicology and Applied Pharmacology* **21**, 102-111.

SAIDA K, MENDELL J R and WEISS H S (1975) Peripheral nerve changes induced by methyl *n*-butyl ketone and potentiation by methyl ethyl ketone. *Journal of Neuropathology and Experimental Neurology* **35**, 207-225.

SAKAMI W and LASAYE J M (1950) Formation of formate and labile methyl groups from acetone in the intact rat. *Journal of Biological Chemistry* **187**, 369-378.

SAMPSON W L and FERNANDEZ L (1939) Experimental convulsions in the rat. *Journal of Pharmacology and Experimental Therapeutics* **65**, 275-280.

SCHWARTZ L (1898) Uber die Oxydation des Acetones und der homologer Ketone der Fett saurerethe. *Archiv für Experimentelle Pathologie und Pharmakologie* **40**, 168. Cited in Krasavage W J, O'Donoghue J L, Divencenzo G D (1982). *Patty's Industrial Hygiene and Toxicology*, Vol 2C, 3rd edn, ed by F E Clayton and G D Clayton). Wiley–Interscience Publ., New York. pp 4709-4800.

SCHWETZ B A, LEONG B K J and GEHRING P J (1974) Embryo- and fetotoxicity of inhaled carbon tetrachloride, 1,1-dichloroethane and methyl ethyl ketone in rats. *Toxicology and Applied Pharmacology* **28**, 452-464.

SHACKELFORD W M and KEITH L H (1976) Frequency of organic compounds identified in water. US EPA 600/4-76-062. U S EPA, Athens, GA, p 626.

SHARP D W (1978) The sensitization potential of some perfumed ingredients tested using a modified Draize procedure. *Toxicology* **9**, 261-271.

SHELDON L S and HITES R A (1978) Organic compounds in Delaware River. *Environmental Science and Technology* **12**, 1188.

SHIFMAN M A, GRAHAM D G, PRIEST J W and BOULDIN T W (1981) The neurotoxicity of 5-nonanone: preliminary report. *Toxicology Letters*, 283-288.

SILVERMAN L, SCHULTE H F and FIRST M W (1946) Further studies on sensory response to certain industrial solvent vapours. *Journal of Industrial Hygiene and Toxicology* **28**, 262-266.

SMITH A R and MEYERS M R (1944) *New York State Department of Labour Industrial Bulletin* **23**, 174-176.

SMITH J N, SMITHIES R A and WILLIAMS R T (1954) Studies in detoxification. 56. The metabolism of alkylbenzenes. Stereochemical aspects of the biological hydroxylation of ethylbenzene to methylphenylcarbinol. *Biochemistry* **56**, 320-324.

SMYTH H F (1956) Hygienic standards for daily inhalation. *American Industrial Hygiene Association Journal* **17**, 129-185.

SMYTH H F and CARPENTER C P (1944) The place of the range finding test in the industrial toxicology laboratory. *Journal of Industrial Hygiene and Toxicology* **26**, 269.

SMYTH H F and CARPENTER C P (1948) Further experience with the range finding test in the industrial toxicology laboratory. *Journal of Industrial Hygiene and Toxicology* **30**, 63-68.

SMYTH H F and SEATON J (1940) Acute response of guinea pigs and rats to inhalation of the vapors of isophorone. *Journal of Industrial Hygiene and Toxicology* **22**, 477-483.

SMYTH H F, SEATON J and FISCHER L (1942) Response of guinea pigs and rats to repeated inhalation of vapors of mesityl oxide and isophorone. *Journal of Industrial Hygiene and Toxicology* **24**, 46-50.

SMYTH H F, CARPENTER C P and WEIL C S (1951) Range-finding toxicity data: list 4. *American Medical Association Journal of Industrial Health and Occupational Medicine* **4**, 119-122.

SMYTH H F, CARPENTER C P, WEIL C S and POZZANI U C (1954) Range finding toxicity data: list 5. *Archives of Industrial Hygiene and Occupational Medicine* **10**, 61-68.

SMYTH H F, CARPENTER C P, WEIL C S, POZZANI U C and STRIEGEL J A (1962) Range-finding toxicity data: list 6. *American Industrial Hygiene Association Journal* **23**, 95-107.

SMYTH H F, CARPENTER C P, WEIL C S, POZZANI U C, STRIEGEL J A and NYCUM J S (1969a) Range-finding toxicity data: list 7. *American Industrial Hygiene Association Journal* **30**, 470-472.

SMYTH H F, WEIL C S, WEST J S and CARPENTER C P (1969b) An exploration of joint toxic action: twenty seven industrial chemicals intubated in rats in all possible pairs. *Toxicology and Applied Pharmacology* **14**, 340-347.

SMYTH H F, WEIL C S, WEST J S and CARPENTER C P (1970) An exploration of joint toxic action. 2. Equitoxic versus equivolume mixtures. *Toxicology and Applied Pharmacology* **17**, 498-503.

SPECHT H, MILLER J W, VALAER P J and SAYERS R R (1940) Acute response of guinea-pigs to the inhalation of ketone vapors. *National Institutes of Health Bulletin* **176**, Div Ind Hyg pp 1-66.

SPENCER P S and SCHAUMBERG H H (1976) Feline nervous system response to chronic intoxication with commercial grades of methyl *n*-butyl ketone, methyl isobutyl ketone and methyl ethyl ketone. *Toxicology and Applied Pharmacology* **37**, 301-311.

SPENCER P S, SCHAUMBERG H H, RALEIGH R L and TERHAAR C J (1975) Nervous system degeneration produced by the industrial solvent methyl *n*-butyl ketone. *Archives of Neurology* **32**, 219-222.

STENBACK F and SHUBIK P (1974) Lack of toxicity and carcinogenicity of some commonly used cutaneous agents. *Toxicology and Applied Pharmacology* **30**, 7-13.

STONER G D, SHIMKIN M B, KNIAZEFF A J, WEISBURGER J H, WEISBURGER E K and GORI G B (1973) Test for carcinogenicity of food additives and chemotherapeutic agents by the pulmonary tumor response in Strain A mice. *Cancer Research* **33**, 3069-3085.

STYLES J A (1978) An evaluation of six short-term tests for detecting organic chemical carcinogens. Appendix 2. Mammalian cell transformation *in vitro*. *British Journal of Cancer* **37**, 931-935.

SULLIVAN H R, MILLER W M and McMAHON R E (1976) Reaction pathways of *in vivo* stereoselective conversion of ethylbenzene to mandelic acid. *Xenobiotica* **6**, 49-54.

TADA O, NAKAAKI K and FUKABORI S (1972) An experimental study on acetone and methyl ethyl ketone concentrations in urine and expired air after exposure to those vapours. *Journal of Science of Labour* **48**, 305.

THIERFIELDER H and DAIBER K (1923) Zur Kenntnis des Verhaltens fettaromatischer Ketone im Tierkorper. *Zeitschrift für Physiologie* **130**, 380-396.

THIERFIELDER H and KLENK E (1924) Zur Kenntnis des Verhaltens des Acetophenons und Benzols im Tierkorper. *Zeitschrift für Physiologie* **141**, 13-28.

TIKKANEN L, MATSUSHIMA T and NATORI S (1983) Mutagenicity of anthraquinones in the Salmonella preincubation test. *Mutation Research* **116**, 297-304.

TRAIGER G J and BRUCKNER J V (1975) The participation of 2-butanone in 2-butanol-induced potentiation of carbon tetrachloride hepatotoxicity. *Journal of Pharmacology and Experimental Therapeutics* **196**, 493-500.

TRAIGER G J, BRUCKNER J V and COOKE P H (1975) Effect of 2-butanol and 2-butanone on rat hepatic ultrastructure and microsomal drug metabolising enzyme activity. *Toxicology and Applied Pharmacology* **33**, 132.

TREON J F, CRUTCHFIELD W E Jr and KITZMILLER K V (1943a) The physiological response of rabbits to cyclohexane, methylcyclohexane and certain derivatives of these compounds. 1. Oral administration and cutaneous application. *Journal of Industrial Hygiene and Toxicology* **25**, 199-214.

TREON J F, CRUTCHFIELD W E Jr and KITZMILLER K V (1943b) The physiological response to cyclohexane, methylcyclohexane and certain derivatives of these compounds. 2. Inhalation. *Journal of Industrial Hygiene and Toxicology* **25**, 323-347.

TRUHAUT R, DUTERTRE-CATELLA H and PHU-LICH M N (1970) Premiers resultats de l'etude du metabolisme chez le lapin d'un solvent industriel : l'isophorone. *Comptes Rendus de l'Academie des Sciences, Paris, Serie D* **271**, 1333-1336.

TRUHAUT R, DUTERTRE-CATELLA H and PHU-LICH M N (1972) Toxicity of an industrial solvent, isophorone. Irritating effect on the skin and mucous membranes. *Journal of European Toxicology* **5**, 31-37.

TRUHAUT R, DUTERTRE-CATELLA H and PHU-LICH M N (1973) Metabolic transformations of 3,5,5-trimethylcyclohexanone (dihydroisophorone). New metabolic pathway dismutation. *Comptes Rendus de l'Academie des Sciences, Paris, Serie D* **276**, 2223.

TSAO M V and PFEIFFER E L (1957) Isolation and identification of a new ketone body in normal urine. *Proceedings of the Society of Experimental Biology* **94**, 628.

UNION CARBIDE (1963) Toxicological studies–isophorone, summary data sheet. Union Carbide Corporation, Industrial Medicine and Toxicology Department, New York.

UNION CARBIDE (1975) Ketones technical booklet (F-41971A)/Union Carbide Corporation, Chemical and Plastics Division, New York.

UNITED STATES ENVIRONMENTAL PROTECTION AGENCY (1972) US Environmental Protection Agency, Pesticides Tolerance Division internal memo from W E Parkin (Toxicology Branch) to D M Baker (Pesticides Control Branch) regarding Pesticide Petition No 2F1224. May 11, 1972. Cited in United States Environmental Protection Agency (1978). Isophorone: Ambient Water quality criteria. EPA, Washington DC, NTIS PB-296 798.

UNITED STATES ENVIRONMENTAL PROTECTION AGENCY (1974) Draft analytical report: New Orleans area water supply study. Region 4, Surveillance and Analysis Division, Lower Mississippi River Facility.

UNITED STATES ENVIRONMENTAL PROTECTION AGENCY (1975) Preliminary assessment of suspected carcinogens in drinking water: report to Congress. US *Environmental Protection Agency*, Washington DC.

UNITED STATES ENVIRONMENTAL PROTECTION AGENCY (1976) Investigation of selected potential environmental contaminants; ketonic solvents. US Department of Commerce, Washington DC, NTIS PB-252 970.

UNITED STATES ENVIRONMENTAL PROTECTION AGENCY (1978) Isophorone: Ambient water quality criteria. EPA, Washington DC. NTIS PB-296 798.

VAN DUUREN B L, SIVAK A, KATZ C and MELCHIONNE S (1971) Cigarette smoke carcinogenesis: importance of tumour promoters. *Journal of the National Cancer Institute* **47**, 235-240.

VERSCHUEREN K (1983) *Handbook of environmental data on organic chemicals.* Second edition. Van Nostrand Reinhold Company.

VIADER F, LECHEVALIER B and MORIN P (1975) Polynevrite toxique chez un travailleur du plastique. Role possible du methyl-ethyl-cetone. *Nouvelle Presse Medicale* **4**, 1813.

VOLODCHENKO V A and LADUNSKII V V (1972) Comparative biological features of diaminoanthraquinone and anthraquinone isomers. *Gigiena Truda i Professional'nykh Zabolevaniia* **11**, 44-45. (In: *Chemical Abstracts* 1973, **78**, 53643d).

VOLODCHENKO V A, GUDZ Z A and TIMCHENKO A N (1971) Basis for setting the maximum permissible concentration of anthraquinone in the atmosphere of the working area. *Gigiena Truda i Professional'nykh Zabolevaniia* **15**, 58-9.

WATER RESEARCH CENTRE (1981) Organic micropollutant in drinking water. Technical Report TR159 Water Research Centre, Marlow.

WELLER E M and GRIGGS J H (1975) Hazards of embryonic exposure to chemical vapours. *Anatomical Record* **184**, 561.

WENZEL D G and ROSS C R (1957) Central stimulating properties of some terpenones. *Journal of the American Pharmaceutical Association* **46**, 77-82.

WESTERFIELD W W and BERG R L (1943) Observations on the metabolism of acetoin. *Journal of Biological Chemistry* **148**, 523-528.

WILLIAMS R T (1940) Studies in detoxication. 7. The biological reduction of *l*-menthone to *d*-neomenthol and *d*-isomenthone to *d*-isomenthol in the rabbit. The conjugation of *d*-neomenthol with glucuronic acid. *Biochemical Journal* **34**,

690-697.

WILLIAMS R T (1959) *Detoxification mechanisms. The metabolism and detoxification of drugs, toxic substances and other organic compounds*. 2nd edn. Chapman and Hall Ltd, London.

WILSON R H, DeEDS F and COX A J (1947) The carcinogenic activity of 2-acetaminofluorene. 4. Action of related compounds. *Cancer Research* **7**, 453-458.

WINDHOLZ M (ed) (1976) *The Merck Index*, 9th edn. New Jersey, Merck and Co.

WORTHING C R (ed) (1979) *The Pesticide Manual. A World Compendium*, 6th edn. The British Crop Protection Council, Croydon, p18.

WURSTER D E and MUNIES R (1965) Factors influencing percutaneous absorption. 2. Methyl ethyl ketone. *Journal of Pharmaceutical Sciences* **54**, 554.

YAMAMOTO K, TAJIMA K and MIZUTANI T (1980) The acute toxicity of butylated hydroxytoluene and its metabolites in mice. *Toxicology Letters* **6**, 173-175.

YANT W P, PATTY F A and SCHRENK H H (1936) Pentanone. *US Public Health Report* **51**, 392.

ZIMMERMANN F K, MAYER V W, SCHEEL I and RESNICK M A (1985) Acetone, methyl ethyl ketone, ethyl acetate, acetonitrile and other polar aprotic solvents are strong inducers of aneuploidy in *Saccharomyces cerevisiae. Mutation Research* **149**, 339-351.

ZLATKIS A and LIEBICH H M (1971) Profile of volatile metabolites in human urine. *Clinical Chemistry* **17**, 592-594.

ZLATKIS A, BERTSCH W, LICHTENSTEIN H A, TISHBEE A, SHUNBO F, LIEBICH H M, LOSCIA A M and FLEISCHER N (1973) Profile of volatile metabolites in urine by gas chromatography–mass spectrometry. *Analytical Chemistry* **45**, 763-767.

18

The ethers

1. INTRODUCTION

The ethers have a wide range of industrial applications, though they are particularly useful as solvents and fragrances.

Of the group of ethers detected in drinking water by WRc, dioxane is the only compound for which much toxicological information is available. Almost all the information described therefore relates to this compound.

2. EXPOSURE

In the WRc survey (Water Research Centre 1981), 1,1-diethoxyethane and ethoxy-propoxyethane were the most frequently detected compounds occurring in 6/14 and 4/14 drinking water samples respectively. The other compounds identified were:

Dibenzofuran
Diisopropyl ether
Dimethoxybutane isomer
Dioxane
Dimethyldioxane isomer
Diphenyl ether
Dipropoxymethane
Ethoxymethoxymethane
Ethyl isopropyl ether
Methyl tetrahydrofuran isomer

Ethers have also been detected in drinking water in the US (Coleman *et al* 1980) and Japan (Akiyama *et al* 1980), but there appears to be no information available on occurrence in food or air.

3. TOXICOKINETICS

In the rat, an intraperitoneal dose of dioxane was distributed primarily to the liver, kidney, spleen, lung, colon and skeletal muscle (Woo *et al* 1977a).

Young and Gehring (1975) have shown that dose has a very important bearing on the pharmacokinetics of dioxane. Rats given single oral doses of 10 mg/kg of dioxane eliminated about 0.4% of the dose in the expired air. However, rats given oral doses of 1000 mg/kg were found to eliminate about 25% of the dose in the expired air. Correspondingly, the percentage of dose excreted in the urine decreased with increasing dosage. The half-life of dioxane in plasma was also greater at the higher dose compared to the lower dose. This 'saturation' of the normal metabolic pattern at high doses has implications for the dose levels used in toxicological studies. High dose levels are unlikely to be representative of the pharmacokinetics, and hence the toxicity of dioxane, which would be found in low exposure situations similar to that for drinking water.

The major urinary metabolite of dioxane in the rat appears to be either 2-hydroxyethoxyacetic acid (Braun and Young 1977) or its lactone, *p*-dioxane-2-one (Woo *et al* 1977b, 1977c), the form depending on pH. The lactone is thought to be the chemical form present *in vivo* (Woo *et al* 1977c).

Rats pretreated with Aroclor 1254 to induce broad-spectrum hepatic mixed-function oxidases (MFO) or phenobarbitone to induce cytochrome P-450 exhibited enhanced metabolism of dioxane to *p*-dioxane-2-one. Only a slight induction of dioxane metabolism was found after pretreating with 3-methylcholanthrene, a compound which tends to induce cytochrome P-448. Both cobalt chloride, an inhibitor of hepatic MFO synthesis, and 2,4-dichloro-6-phenyl-phenoxy ethylamine, an inhibitor of MFO function, repressed the metabolic conversion of dioxane (Woo *et al* 1977d, 1978).

In four male volunteers exposed by inhalation to 50 ppm of dioxane for 6 hours, the half-life of elimination was found to be approximately 1 hour. Almost all of the dose was eliminated in the urine as 2-hydroxyethoxyacetic acid (Young *et al* 1977).

4. HEALTH EFFECTS

For ethers, it would appear that as the aliphatic chain length increases and the volatility decreases, their toxic potential tends to decrease. The reverse relationship is true for skin irritation.

The principal target organs for the toxicity of dioxane are the liver and kidney. In the liver, toxicity is normally associated with the centrilobular region. Toxicity to the tubular epithelium is the most common effect in the kidney.

4.1 Acute and subacute toxicity

Early case-histories of exposure to dioxane by inhalation or skin contact reported that the most common pathological changes were hepatic centrilobular necrosis, cortical necrosis and haemorrhage of the kidney, and oedema and demylenisation of nerve fibres in the brain (Barber 1934, Johnstone 1959).

Dioxane appears to be of low acute toxicity in experimental animals. The acute oral LD50 of dioxane in a variety of species ranges from 2 to 6 g/kg (Registry of Toxic Effects of Chemical Substances).

Intravenous injection of 10 mg of dioxane into male Sprague–Dawley rats was found to rapidly lower hepatic RNA polymerase A and RNA polymerase B activity. At 1 hour post-injection, RNA polymerase B activity had recovered to control levels, while RNA polymerase A had increased to 40% greater than control. A secondary decrease in RNA polymerase B activity was observed at 4 hours post-injection. This had recovered to control levels again by 24 hours post-injection (Kurl *et al* 1981).

Acute oral LD50s in the rat have also been reported for some of the other ethers (Registry of Toxic Effects of Chemical Substances):

Dioxane	5.2 g/kg
1,1-Diethoxyethane	4.6 g/kg
Di-isopropyl ether	8.5 g/kg
1,3-Dimethoxybutane	3.7 g/kg
Dimethyldioxane	3.0 g/kg
Diphenyl ether	3.4 g/kg

4.2 Chronic toxicity

In a study by Stott *et al* (1981), groups of male Sprague–Dawley rats were exposed to average daily doses of 0, 10 or 1000 mg/kg body weight of dioxane via their drinking water for 11 weeks. At the high dose, there were some pathological changes in the liver, an increase in the liver weight/body weight ratio, and a slight increase in hepatic DNA synthesis. No toxic effects were found in animals given 10 mg/kg body weight/day.

4.3 Genotoxicity

Dioxane has given negative results in the Ames test with *Salmonella typhimurium* TA98, TA100, TA1538, TA1535 or TA1537 at doses up to 103 mg/plate, either in the presence or absence of metabolic activation (Stott *et al* 1981, Haworth *et al* 1983).

Dioxane was not found to induce unscheduled DNA synthesis in primary cultures of rat hepatocytes (Stott *et al* 1981).

Exposure of rats to 10 or 1000 mg/kg body weight/day of dioxane via drinking water for 11 weeks did not result in any detectable alkylation of DNA and did not appear to induce hepatic DNA repair (Stott *et al* 1981).

Diphenyl ether has also given negative results in the Ames test (Haworth *et al* 1983, Florin *et al* 1980).

4.4 Carcinogenicity

The first indication of carcinogenic potential for dioxane in experimental animals was reported by Argus *et al* (1965). A group of 26 male Wistar rats were exposed to 10 g/l of dioxane in their drinking water for up to 455 days. Hepatocellular carcinomas were found in six of the treated animals. No tumours of this type were evident in the control group of nine animals. Extensive histological changes in the liver and kidney were present in most animals exposed to dioxane. In a further study (Argus *et al* 1973), groups of 30 male Charles River CD rats were exposed to 0, 7.5, 10, 14 or 18 g/l of dioxane in their drinking water for up to 13 months. In addition to marked changes in the structure of both the liver and kidney, a dose-dependent increase in the incidence of liver nodules and hepatomas was observed. Of the 120 rats exposed to dioxane in this study, six developed nasal carcinomas, an extremely rare event in rats (Hoch-Ligeti *et al* 1970).

Groups of 60 male and 60 female Sherman rats were exposed to 0, 0.1, 1.0 or 10 g/l of dioxane in their drinking water for up to 2 years (Kociba *et al* 1974). At the highest dose, corresponding to daily intakes of approximately 1000 mg/kg body weight for males and 1600 mg/kg body weight for females, there was reduced survival, and depression of body weight gain and water intake. A significant increase in hepatocellular carcinomas and nasal carcinomas was apparent in this group but not in any other group. Degenerative changes in the liver and kidney similar to those reported before were evident at both 1.0 and 10 g/l. The dioxane concentration in drinking water at which no toxic effects were observed corresponded to a dose of approximately 10 mg/kg body weight/day in males and 19 mg/kg body weight/day in females.

In a group of 23 male guinea-pigs receiving drinking water containing 5–20 g/l of dioxane for a 23-month period, two animals developed carcinoma of the gall bladder while three had hepatomas. No liver tumours were reported in ten control animals (Hoch-Ligeti and Argus 1970).

No evidence for the carcinogenicity of dioxane was found in groups of 50 male and 50 female B6C3F1 mice receiving drinking water containing 5 or 10 g/l of dioxane for 40–43 weeks (King *et al* 1973).

In the only inhalation study published to date, no significant increase in tumour incidence was observed in 288 male and 288 female Wistar rats exposed to 111 ppm of dioxane for 7 hours/day, 5 days/week for 2 years. There were also no apparent effects on haematology, clinical chemistry or histopathology (Torkelson *et al* 1974).

Thrice-weekly painting of dioxane (in acetone) on the dorsal skin of Swiss–Webster mice was not found to produce a significant excess of skin tumours. However, dioxane painting led to an increased incidence of skin tumours in mice pretreated with 50 μg of dimethylbenzanthracene (DMBA) compared to mice exposed to DMBA alone (King *et al* 1973).

4.5 Reproductive toxicity

Dioxane was evaluated for teratogenic potential in rats by oral gavage on days 6–15 of gestation at doses of 0–1.0 ml/kg/day (1.034 mg/kg). There were no adverse effects except embryotoxicity manifested by reduced foetal weight occurring only at the highest dose level (Giavini *et al* 1985).

5. DISCUSSION

The only ether of this group for which there is a significant amount of toxicological information is dioxane. Although this compound does cause injury to the liver and kidney at high doses, the most important toxicological finding is its carcinogenic activity in rats. The mechanism of carcinogenicity of dioxane is a matter of debate at present, though it would appear that cytotoxic rather than genetic events are essential for tumour formation. This is an important distinction, as current evidence indicates that there are no-effect levels for certain compounds which do not act by direct genetic mechanisms. It appears unlikely that exposure to very low doses of dioxane from drinking water would constitute a health hazard to man.

There is insufficient information available for the remaining compounds on which to base an assessment.

REFERENCES

AKIYAMA T, KOGA M, SHINOHARA R, KIDO A and ETOH S (1980) Detection and identification of trace organic substances in the aquatic environment. *Journal of Uoeh* **2,** 285-300.

ARGUS M F, ARCOS J C and HOCH-LIGETI C (1965) Studies on the carcinogenic activity of protein-denaturing agents: Hepatocarcinogenicity of dioxane. *Journal of the National Cancer Institute* **35,** 949-958.

ARGUS M F, SOHAL R S, BRYANT G M, HOCH-LIGETI C and ARCOS J C (1973) Dose–response and ultrastructural alterations in dioxane carcinogenesis. Influence of methylcholanthrene on acute toxicity. *European Journal of Cancer* **9,** 237-243.

BARBER H (1934) Haemorrhagic nephritis and necrosis of liver from dioxan poisoning. *Guy's Hospital Reports* **84,** 267-280.

BRAUN W H and YOUNG J D (1977) Identification of beta-hydroxyethoxyacetic acid as the major urinary metabolite of 1,4-dioxane in the rat. *Toxicology and Applied Pharmacology* **39,** 33-38.

COLEMAN W E, MELTON R G, KOPFLER F C, BARONE K A, AURAND T A and JELLISON M G (1980) Identification of organic compounds in a mutagenic extract of a surface drinking water by a computerized gas chromatography/mass spectrometry system (GC/MS/COM). *Environmental Science and Technology* **14,** 576-588.

FLORIN I, RUTBERG L, CURVALL M and ENZELL C R (1980) Screening of tobacco smoke constituents for mutagenicity using the Ames test. *Toxicology* **18,** 219-232.

GIAVINI E, VISMARA C and BROCCIA M L (1985) Teratogenesis study of dioxane in rats. *Toxicology Letters* **26,** 85-88.

HAWORTH S, LAWLOR T, MORTELMANS K, SPECK W and ZEIGER E (1983) *Salmonella mutagenicity* test results for 250 chemicals. *Environmental Mutagenesis* **5,** Suppl 1, 3-142.

HOCH-LIGETI C and ARGUS M F (1970) Effect of carcinogens on the lung of guinea-pigs. In: Nettesheim P, Hanna M G Jr and Deatherage J W (eds) *The morphology of experimental respiratory carcinogenesis, Gatlinburg, TN.* AEC Symposium Series No 21, US National Technical Information Service, pp 267-279.

HOCH-LIGETI C, ARGUS M F and ARCOS J C (1970) Induction of carcinomas in the nasal cavity of rats by dioxane. *British Journal of Cancer* **24,** 164-167.

JOHNSTONE R T (1959) Death due to dioxane? *AMA Archives of Industrial Health* **20,** 445-447.

KING M E, SHEFNER A M and BATES R R (1973) Carcinogenesis bioassay of chlorinated dibenzodioxins and related chemicals. *Environmental Health Perspectives* **5,** 163-170.

KOCIBA R J, McCOLLISTER S B, PARK C, TORKELSON T R and GEHRING P J (1974) 1,4-Dioxane. I. Results of a 2-year ingestion study in rats. *Toxicology and Applied Pharmacology* **30,** 275-286.

KURL R N, POELLINGER L, LUND J and GUSTAFSSON J-A (1981) Effects of dioxane on RNA synthesis in the rat liver. *Archives of Toxicology* **49,** 29-33.

REGISTRY OF TOXIC EFFECTS OF CHEMICAL SUBSTANCES National Institute for Occupational Safety and Health, Cincinnati, Ohio.

STOTT W T, QUAST J F and WATANABE P G (1981) Differentiation of the mechanisms of oncogenicity of 1,4-dioxane and 1,3-hexachlorobutadiene in the rat. *Toxicology and Applied Pharmacology* **60,** 287-300.

TORKELSON T R, LEONG B K J, KOCIBA R J, RICHTER W A and GEHRING P J (1974) 1,4-Dioxane. II. Results of a 2-year inhalation study in rats. *Toxicology and Applied Pharmacology* **30,** 287-298.

WATER RESEARCH CENTRE (1981) Organic micropollutants in drinking water. WRc Technical Report TR 159.

WOO Y-T, ARGUS M F and ARCOS J C (1977a) Tissue and subcellular distribution of ^{3}H-dioxane in the rat and apparent lack of microsome-catalyzed covalent binding in the target tissue. *Life Sciences* **21,** 1447-1456.

WOO Y-T, ARCOS J C, ARGUS M F, GRIFFIN G W and NISHIYAMA K (1977b) Metabolism *in vivo* of dioxane: Identification of *p*-dioxane-2-one as the major urinary metabolite. *Biochemical Pharmacology* **26,** 1535-1538.

WOO Y-T, ARCOS J C, ARGUS M F, GRIFFIN G W and NISHIYAMA K (1977c) Structural identification of *p*-dioxane-2-one as the major urinary metabolite of *p*-dioxane. *Naunyn-Schmiedeberg's Archives of Pharmacology* **299,** 283-287.

WOO Y-T, ARGUS M F and ARCOS J C (1977d) Metabolism *in vivo* of dioxane: Effect of inducers and inhibitors of hepatic mixed-function oxidases. *Biochemical Pharmacology* **25,** 1539-1542.

WOO Y-T, ARGUS M F and ARCOS J C (1978) Effect of mixed-function oxidase modifiers on metabolism and toxicity of the oncogen dioxane. *Cancer Research* **38,** 1621-1625.

YOUNG J D and GEHRING P J (1975) The dose-dependent fate of 1,4-dioxane in male rats. *Toxicology and Applied Pharmacology* **33,** 183.

YOUNG J D, BRAUN W H, RAMPY L W, CHENOWETH M B and BLAU G E (1977) Pharmacokinetics of 1,4-dioxane in humans. *Journal of Toxicology and Environmental Health* **3,** 507-520.

19

The miscellaneous oxygenated compounds

1. INTRODUCTION

This group is comprised largely of alcohols. Most of the information available is on phenol, 2-ethylhexanol and 2-phenylphenol and therefore these compounds have been reviewed individually.

All the compounds were identified only infrequently in the WRc survey and there appears to be relatively little other information on their occurrence in the environment.

2. PHENOL

2.1 Introduction

Phenol (carbolic acid, hydroxybenzene) is commercially produced by cumene oxidation and is used as an intermediate in the manufacture of a wide range of important chemicals including phenolic resins, bisphenol-A, caprolactam, alkylphenols and adipic acid. Although the use of phenol as a disinfectant has diminished considerably since the 19th century, it is still present in some mouth, throat and skin preparations.

CAS Reg No:	108-95-2
Molecular weight:	94
Boiling point:	182°C at 760 mm Hg
Solubility:	82 g/l at 15°C (Verschueren 1983)
Threshold odour concentration in water:	1.0–7.5 mg/l (Verschueren 1983)

2.2 Exposure

Phenol was identified in 5/14 treated water samples examined in the WRc survey (Water Research Centre 1981). The US EPA (1980) have reported the occurrence of this compound in some raw waters at low μg/l levels, but not in treated water. Phenol has been identified in both raw and treated water in Japan (Akiyama *et al* 1980).

There is little information on levels in air. Inhalation of phenol is primarily associated with occupational exposure.

Large quantities of phenolic compounds are present in food. It is thought that some may be broken down by microbiological action in the gastrointestinal tract to phenol itself. There are no accurate data for exposure to phenol by this route, and therefore the average daily intake is difficult to assess.

Exposure to phenol may also occur through the use of some mouthwashes or skin preparations.

2.3 Toxicokinetics

Phenol is readily absorbed by all routes. One study has reported that significant amounts (12% in 30 minutes) of 2.5–10 g/l solutions of phenol can be absorbed through the skin of the human forearm, although the rate of absorption at much lower concentrations is not clear (Baranowska-Dutkiewicz 1981).

An oral dose of phenol is rapidly distributed throughout the body, with the highest levels occurring in the liver, heart, kidneys, lungs, blood and muscle (Deichmann 1944).

In rabbits, 72% of an oral dose of 300 mg/kg of phenol was excreted in the urine within 24 hours, roughly half as free phenol and half as conjugated phenol. About 23% had been converted to other metabolites such as carbon dioxide, hydroquinone (1,4-dihydroxybenzene) and catechol (1,2-dihydroxybenzene). Trace amounts were found in the faeces, expired air and carcass (Deichmann 1944).

In a detailed study by Capel *et al* (1972), several species including man were found to excrete four major metabolites in the urine. These were the sulphate and glucuronide conjugates of phenol and hydroquinone. In the human studies, 90% of an oral dose was excreted in 24 hours, principally as the sulphate conjugate of phenol. Other species, notably the cat and pig, showed quite different metabolic patterns.

Incubation of phenol with rat liver microsomes has been shown to produce hydroquinone and catechol in the ratio of 20:1 (Sawahata and Neal 1983). In another study, sulphydryl conjugates of 1,4-benzoquinone were detected following the incubation of phenol with mouse liver microsomes (Lunte and Kissinger 1983).

2.4 Health effects

2.4.1 Acute and subacute toxicity

Phenol is of relatively low acute toxicity in experimental animals. Oral LD50s of 384 mg/kg and 270 mg/kg have been reported for the rat and mouse respectively (Registry of Toxic Effects of Chemical Substances). The cat, however, appears to be more sensitive than other species, presumably because of its inability to conjugate phenol with glucuronic acid. Toxic effects in animals produced by acute oral exposure to phenol include swelling, necrosis and haemorrhage of the mucous membranes of the throat and oesophagus, pulmonary damage, myocardial necrosis and liver changes. Death due to CNS depression is usually preceded by muscular twitching and convulsions (Deichmann and Keplinger 1981).

In an unpublished study by Dow Chemical Company, reported by the US EPA

(1980), a group of rats given oral doses of 100 mg/kg/day for 20 days developed changes in both the liver and kidney. No such effects were observed at doses of 10 or 50 mg/kg/day.

There is growing evidence that the metabolites responsible for the haematotoxicity of benzene are derived from phenol and are perhaps free-radicals and quinones. This poses the question, does exposure to phenol produce similar toxic effects in the bone marrow as exposure to benzene? Two recent studies in mice suggest that this is not the case (Bolcsak and Nerland 1983, Tunek *et al* 1981). Phenol was shown to have some haematotoxic potential, but its activity was much weaker than that of benzene. Clearly, if phenol metabolites are involved in the toxicity of benzene to the bone marrow, then the reactive metabolites are reaching the target sites after exposure to benzene but not after exposure to phenol. The reason for this difference is unclear.

In man, the acute toxicity of phenol is characterised by its action on higher centres. Ingestion of large amounts can cause a burning sensation in the mouth, abdominal pain, sweating, cyanosis, lowering of body temperature, decreased respiration, loss of reflex activity and death from respiratory failure.

Three major incidents of subacute phenol poisoning in humans have been reported following consumption of contaminated drinking water. However, in all three incidents there is some doubt as to the precise concentrations of phenol involved.

Following accidental spillage of a large quantity of phenol in Wisconsin, USA, symptoms of phenol poisoning such as burning of the mouth, mouth sores, diarrhoea and dark urine were reported in some individuals drinking contaminated well water. Epidemiological investigation of the incident found that 17/39 members of a high-dose group, 5/61 of a low-dose group and 2/58 of a control group exhibited two or more of the above symptoms during an 8-month period. The cases in the low-dose and control groups occurred randomly throughout the period whereas the cases in the high-dose group occurred during two particular months. The daily intake of phenol by these individuals was estimated to be about 10–240 mg/person/day. No attempt was made to estimate phenol exposure from skin contact with contaminated water (Baker *et al* 1978).

In another incident, employees and patients of a Georgia hospital developed some symptoms of phenol poisoning after a water tank, which was part of a solar heating system, had been lined with a phenolic resin which had not cured properly. GC–MS analysis of the water in the tank found a concentration of 0.35 mg/l of phenol. A number of other phenolic compounds were also identified. As the tank had been installed several months earlier it is likely that the employees and patients were exposed to much higher levels of phenol than 0.35 mg/l. When investigated the tank showed 'several large, rusted areas and considerable muddy sediment in the interior free space' (Trincher and Rissing 1983).

The most recent incident occurred in the UK in January 1984 and involved a considerable spill of phenol into the River Dee (Welsh Water and North West Water 1984, Jarvis *et al* 1985). Water for potable use is abstracted from the River Dee by the Chester Water Works Company, the Wrexham and East Denbighshire Water Company, Welsh Water and North West Water. During the incident, which lasted for about one week, large numbers of complaints were received of antiseptic taste and also some complaints of illness among the two million exposed population. A retrospective epidemiological study of 594 households in one of the exposed areas provided some evidence for symptoms of 'phenol poisoning' in consumers. There are, however, difficulties in attributing a particular concentration of phenol for the effects observed. Firstly, the highest phenol concentrations reported were lower than the value previously calculated from animal studies for protection of human health. Secondly, there is some evidence to suggest that the peak concentration of phenol in the river may have been missed and that phenol concentrations in supply were therefore probably underestimated. Thirdly, analytical evidence suggests that in areas supplied with water from treatment works disinfecting with chlorine, the finished water contained a complex mixture of chemicals with 2,4,6-trichlorophenol predominating. These difficulties make an asessment of the role of phenol in this incident extremely uncertain.

2.4.2 Chronic toxicity

Exposure of rats to phenol in their drinking water for five generations did not appear to have any visible effects at 100, 500 or 1000 mg/l. At higher doses, effects on reproduction and deaths of young animals were found (Heller and Pursell 1938). In another study, there were no apparent effects in rats exposed to 800, 1200 or 1600 mg/l of phenol in their drinking water for 12 months, though at 2000 and 2400 mg/l depression of body weight gain was observed (Deichmann and Oesper 1940). Histological examination of tissues was not carried out in either study.

In a study by the Dow Chemical Company (US EPA 1980), rats were given 135 oral doses of 50 or 100 mg/kg of phenol during a 6-month period. Slight changes in the kidney were observed at both doses, while slight liver damage was found only at the higher dose.

In a range-finding study by the National Cancer Institute (1980) groups of ten male and female F-344 rats and B6C3F1 mice were given drinking water containing 0.1, 0.3, 1.0, 3.0 or 10.0 g/l phenol for 90 days. Depression of body weight gain was observed in rats and mice at 10.0 g/l. No histopathological changes were found in any group.

Chronic poisoning effects reported in humans include vomiting, difficulty in swallowing, diarrhoea, anorexia, liver and kidney damage, headaches, fainting and other mental disturbances.

2.4.3 Genotoxicity

In the Ames *Salmonella*/microsome assay, several groups have reported negative results for phenol with a range of *Salmonella* strains and using a variety of different procedures, including the standard plate test (Epler *et al* 1979, Kinoshita *et al* 1981, Pool and Lin 1982), the plate test but with preincubation (Haworth *et al* 1983), in a suspension assay (Thompson and Melampy 1981) and in spot tests (Florin *et al* 1980). However, a single study by Wild *et al* (1980) found that phenol was weakly mutagenic to *Salmonella typhimurium* TA98 in the presence of S9. Phenol has been reported to be mutagenic to *E. coli* Sd-4 (Demerec *et al* 1951).

In mammalian cell cultures, positive results have been reported in three test systems. In each case, a metabolising enzyme system was required for activity. Phenol was found to mutate V79 Chinese hamster cells at a concentration of 250–500 μg/ml (Paschin and Bahitova 1982), increase sister chromatid exchange frequency in human lymphocytes at 282 μg/ml (Morimoto *et al* 1983), and inhibit DNA synthesis in HeLa cells at 188 μg/ml (Painter and Howard 1982).

Phenol did not significantly increase the incidence of chromosome aberrations in the bone marrow of Sprague–Dawley rats given single oral or intraperitoneal doses of phenol ranging from 80 to 500 mg/kg (Thompson and Gibson 1984). Phenol has also given negative results in an *in vivo* micronucleus assay and in the Basc *Drosophila* test (Wild *et al* 1980). An earlier report suggested that phenol was mutagenic in *Drosophila* after exposing isolated gonads *in vitro* and implanting them into host larvae (Hadorn and Niggli 1946).

A dose-related increase in chromosomal damage in spermatogonia and primary spermatocytes has been reported in a mouse multigeneration study. The animals were given 0.08, 0.8 or 8 mg/l of phenol in the drinking water for five generations (Bulsiewicz 1977).

2.4.4 Carcinogenicity

In a National Cancer Institute study (1980) groups of 50 male and female F-344 rats and B6C3F1 mice were given drinking water containing 2.5 or 5.0 g/l phenol for 103 weeks. A dose-related depresion of body weight gain was observed for both rats and mice. Both species also exhibited lowered water consumption. An increased incidence of leukaemia or lymphomas was found in male rats receiving the lower dose, but not in any other group.

Twice-weekly application of 2.5 mg of phenol in benzene to the shaved backs of mice for up to one year produced papillomas in 5/14 surviving animals. During the first 6 weeks of phenol treatment many animals exhibited skin wounds and hyperplasia. Almost all mice similarly exposed to phenol, though pretreated with a single dose of 75 μg of dimethylbenzanthracene (DMBA), developed papillomas. By 26 weeks, about 50% of these animals had also developed malignant tumours. Few tumours were found in DMBA-treated mice which had not been exposed to phenol. Further experiments showed that the promotion of DMBA carcinogenesis by phenol was dose-dependent (Boutwell and Bosch 1959). Similar results were reported in a study by Salaman and Glendenning (1957). Phenol has been found to partially inhibit benzo[*a*]pyrene skin carcinogenesis when given simultaneously (Van Duuren *et al* 1973, Van Duuren and Goldschmidt 1976).

2.4.5 Reproductive toxicity

Phenol did not exhibit any evidence of teratogenic potential in Sprague–Dawley rats given 20, 63 or 200 mg/kg body weight by intraperitoneal injection on days 9–11 or 12–14 of gestation. A reduction in foetal body weight was found at the highest dose for days 12–14 but not for days 9–11 (Minor and Becker 1971). Although the multigeneration study of Heller and Pursell (1938) was not specifically designed for teratogenicity, no evidence of such an effect was observed.

2.5 Discussion

In view of the presence of phenolics in food, it is probable that under normal circumstances waterborne phenol would represent only a small fraction of total intake.

Phenol is readily absorbed by all routes, though it is rapidly conjugated with either sulphate or glucuronic acid, followed by elimination in the urine. Small quantities of oxidative metabolites such as catechol, hydroquinone and benzoquinones can be formed. Such metabolites have been suggested to be involved in the haematotoxicity of benzene, though phenol does appear to have much weaker activity than benzene in this respect.

Although there are many reports in the literature of human poisoning with phenol, these are largely concerned with severe toxicity experienced after very high doses and do not readily aid an assessment of possible health effects at lower levels. The three major incidents of phenol poisoning through drinking water all suffer from uncertainty concerning the precise phenol concentrations involved.

Acute and chronic animal studies indicate that phenol is of relatively low toxicity. This compound does not appear to be mutagenic in the Ames test, but has given positive results in some higher test systems. Phenol gave inconclusive results in an NCI carcinogenicity study in which rats and mice were exposed through drinking water.

Based on a 6-month toxicity study in rats by the Dow Chemical Company and incorporating an uncertainty factor of 500, the US EPA calculated a maximum permissible concentration of 3.5 mg/l for phenol.

It appears unlikely that very low concentrations of phenol in drinking water would present a risk to human health.

References

AKIYAMA T, KOGA M, SHINOHARA R, KIDO A and ETOH S (1980) Detection and identification of trace organic substances in the aquatic environment. *Journal of Uoeh* **2,** 285-300.

BAKER E L, BERTOZZI P E, FIELD P H, BASTEYNS B J and SKINNER H G (1978) Phenol poisoning due to contaminated drinking water. *Archives of Environmental Health* **33,** 89-94.

BARANOWSKA-DUTKIEWICZ B (1981) Skin absorption of phenol from aqueous solutions in men. *International Archives of Occupational and Environmental Health* **49,** 99-104.

BOLCSAK L E and NERLAND D E (1983) Inhibition of erythropoiesis by benzene and benzene metabolites. *Toxicology and Applied Pharmacology* **69,** 363-368.

BOUTWELL R K and BOSCH D K (1959) The tumor-promoting action of phenol and related compounds for mouse skin. *Cancer Research* **19,** 413-424.

BULSIEWICZ H (1977) The influence of phenol on chromosomes in mice (*Mus musculus*) in the process of spermatogenesis. *Folia Morphologica (Warsaw)* **36,** 13-22.

CAPEL I D, FRENCH M R, MILLBURN P, SMITH R L and WILLIAMS R T (1972) The fate of [^{14}C]-phenol in various species. *Xenobiotica* **2,** 25-34.

DEICHMANN W B (1944) Phenol studies. 5 The distribution, detoxification and excretion of phenol in the mammalian body. *Archives of Biochemistry* **3,** 345.

DEICHMANN W B and KEPLINGER M L (1981) Phenols and phenolic Compounds. In *Patty's Industrial Hygiene and Toxicology* ed by G D Clayton and F E Clayton, 3rd Revised Edition, Vol 2A. John Wiley & Sons Inc. pp 2567-2627.

DEICHMANN W and OESPER P (1940) Ingestion of phenol — effects on the albino rat. *Industrial Medicine* **9,** 296.

DEMEREC M, BERTANI G and FLINT J (1951) A survey of chemicals for mutagenic activity in *E. coli. American Naturalist* **85,** 119-136.

EPLER J L, RAO T K and GUERIN M R (1979) Evaluation of feasibility of mutagenic testing of shale oil products and effluents. *Enviromental Health Perspectives* **30,** 179-184.

FLORIN I, RUTBERG L, CURVALL M and ENZELL C R (1980) Screening of tobacco smoke constituents for mutagenicity using the Ames test. *Toxicology* **18,** 219-232.

HADORN E and NIGGLI H (1946) Mutations in *Drosophila* after chemical treatment of gonads *in vitro. Nature* **157,** 162-163.

HAWORTH S, LAWLOR T, MORTELMANS K, SPECK W and ZEIGER E (1983) *Salmonella* mutagenicity test results for 250 chemicals. *Environmental Mutagenesis* **5,** Supl 1, 3-142.

HELLER V G and PURSELL L (1938) Phenol-contaminated waters and their physiological action. *Journal of Pharmacology and Experimental Therapeutics* **63,** 99.

JARVIS S N, STRAUBE R C, WILLIAMS A L J and BARTLETT C L R (1985) Illness associated with contamination of drinking water supplies with phenol. *British Medical Journal* **290,** 1800-1802.

KINOSHITA T, SANTELLA R, PULKRABEK P and JEFFREY A M (1981) Benzene oxide: genetic toxicity. *Mutation Research* **91,** 99-102.

LUNTE S M and KISSINGER P T (1983) Detection and identification of sulfydryl conjugates of *p*-benzoquinone in microsomal incubations of benzene and phenol. *Chemicobiological Interactions* **47,** 195-212.

MINOR J L and BECKER B A (1971) A comparison of the teratogenic properties of sodium salicylate, sodium benzoate and phenol. *Toxicology and Applied Pharmacology* **19,** 373.

MORIMOTO K, WOLFF S and KOIZUMI A (1983) Induction of sister-chromatid exchanges in human lymphocytes by microsomal activation of benzene metabolites. *Mutation Research* **119,** 335-360.

NATIONAL CANCER INSTITUTE (1980) Bioassay of phenol for possible carcinogenicity. NTIS PB80-217946

PAINTER R B and HOWARD R (1982) The HeLa DNA-synthesis inhibition test as a rapid screen for mutagenic carcinogens. *Mutation Research* **92,** 427-437.

PASCHIN Y V and BAHITOVA L M (1982) Mutagenicity of benzo[*a*]pyrene and the antioxidant phenol at the HGPRT locus of V79 Chinese hamster cells. *Mutation Research* **104,** 389-393.

POOL B L and LIN P Z (1982) Mutagenicity testing in the *Salmonella typhimurium* assay of phenolic compounds and phenolic fractions obtained from smokehouse smoke condensates. *Food and Chemical Toxicology* **20,** 383-391.

REGISTRY OF TOXIC EFFECTS OF CHEMICAL SUBSTANCES National Institute for Occupational Safety & Health, Cincinnati, Ohio.

SALAMAN M H and GLENDENNING O M (1957) Tumor promotion in mouse skin by sclerosing agents. *British Journal of Cancer* **11,** 434.

SAWAHATA T and NEAL R A (1983) Biotransformation of phenol to hydroquinone and catechol by rat liver microsomes. *Molecular Pharmacology* **23,** 453-460.

THOMPSON E D and GIBSON D P (1984) A method for determining the maximum tolerated dose for acute *in vivo* cytogenetic studies. *Food and Chemical Toxicology* **22,** 665-676.

THOMPSON E D and MELAMPY P J (1981) An examination of the quantitative suspension assay for mutagenesis with strains of *Salmonella typhimurium. Environmental Mutagenesis* **3,** 453-465.

TRINCHER R C and RISSING J P (1983) Contamination of potable water by phenol from a solar water tank liner — Georgia. *Morbidity and Mortality Weekly Report* **32,** 493-494.

TUNEK A, OLOFSSON T and BERLIN M (1981) Toxic effects of benzene and benzene metabolites on granulopoietic stem cells and bone marrow cellularity in mice. *Toxicology and Applied Pharmacology* **59,** 149-156.

UNITED STATES ENVIRONMENTAL PROTECTION AGENCY (1980) Ambient water quality criteria for phenol. US EPA, Criteria and Standards Division, Washington DC. EPA-440/5-80-066.

VAN DUUREN B L and GOLDSCHMIDT B M (1976) Cocarcinogenic and tumor-promoting agents in tobacco carcinogenesis. *Journal of the National Cancer Institute* **56,** 1237-1242.

VAN DUUREN B L, KATZ C and GOLDSCHMIDT B M (1973) Cocarcinogenic agents in tobacco carcinogenesis. *Journal of the National Cancer Institute* **51,** 703-705.

VERSCHUEREN K (1983) *Handbook of environmental data on organic chemicals.* Van Nostrand Reinhold Company, Second Edition.

WATER RESEARCH CENTRE (1981) Organic micropollutants in drinking water. WRc Technical Report TR 159.

WELSH WATER and NORTH WEST WATER (1984) Joint report on the pollution incident affecting the River Dee and water supplies January 1984.

WILD D, ECKHARDT K, GOCKE E and KING M T (1980) Comparative results of short-term *in vitro* and *in vivo* mutagenicity tests obtained with selected environmental chemicals. In: *Short-term Test Systems for Detecting Carcinogens* ed by K H Norpoth and R C Garner. Springer-Verlag, Berlin.

3. 2-ETHYLHEXANOL

3.1 Introduction

2-Ethylhexanol (2-ethylhexyl alcohol) is used as an intermediate in the synthesis of plasticisers and 2-ethylhexyl acrylate, and as a fragrance raw material. Of less importance are its uses as a dispersing and wetting agent, as a solvent for gums and resins, a cosolvent for nitrocellulose and in ceramics, paper coatings, rubber latex and textiles.

Much work on the hepatic effects and genetic toxicology of 2-ethylhexanol is available, primarily because it is one of the mammalian metabolites of di-(2-ethylhexyl)phthalate, a very important plasticiser.

CAS Reg No:	104-76-7
Molecular weight:	130
Boiling point:	184°C
Solubility:	1 g/l at 20°C (Verschueren 1983)
Threshold odour concentration in water:	0.27 mg/l (Verschueren 1983)

3.2 Exposure

This compound was identified in only one of 14 treated water samples examined in the WRc survey (Water Research Centre 1981). 2-Ethylhexanol has been in use since the 1950s as a fragrance. In the USA, around 25 000 lb are used for this purpose each year. The usual concentrations are 0.01% in soap, 0.001% in detergent, 0.005% in creams and lotions and 0.04% in perfume (Opdyke 1979).

3.3 Toxicokinetics

Early studies in rabbits and rats demonstrated that 2-ethylhexanol was rapidly metabolised by the liver and eliminated in the urine, primarily as a glucuronide conjugate (Kamil *et al* 1953, Knaak *et al* 1966). Albro (1975) found that of a single oral dose of 2-ethylhexanol in rats, 80–82% was excreted in the urine, 8–9% in the faeces, and 6–7% in the expired air by 28 hours. In urine, the major metabolite was 2-ethylhexanoic acid. Other minor metabolites were 2-heptanone, 4-heptanone, 2-ethyl-5-ketohexanoic acid, 2-ethyl-1,6-hexanedioic acid and 2-ethyl-5-hydroxy-hexanoic acid. About 3% of the dose was excreted unchanged. 2-Ethylhexanol appears to be a good substrate for mammalian alcohol dehydrogenase but not for yeast alcohol dehydrogenase (Albro 1975).

3.4 Health effects

A monograph on the toxicology of this compound has been published by the Research Institute for Fragrance Materials (Opdyke 1979).

3.4.1 Acute and subacute toxicity

2-Ethylhexanol is of low acute toxicity in experimental animals. Oral LD50s in the rat ranging from 3.2 to 6.4 g/kg have been documented (Opdyke 1979). LD50s, by the intraperitoneal route, are 650 mg/kg and 780 mg/kg for the rat and mouse respectively (Rowe and McCollister 1982).

Intravenous injection of 0.3–4.2 mg/kg to rabbits induced a dose-related lowering of blood pressure. This effect was not observed in rats or dogs. Both the rats and rabbits exhibited toxicity to the heart and to the smooth muscle of blood vessels (Hollenbach *et al* 1972).

Male F-344 rats fed for 3 weeks with diets containing 2% 2-ethylhexanol developed a marked proliferation of hepatic peroxisomes associated with hepatomegaly (an increase in liver weight/body weight ratio). Liver catalase activity was slightly increased, liver carnitine acetyltransferase activity (CAT, a peroxisomal enzyme) was elevated almost 15-fold, whilst serum cholesterol and triglycerides were lowered by 30% and 50% respectively (Moody *et al* 1976, Moody and Reddy 1978). A later, almost identical, study again found a 50% lowering of serum triglycerides, but only a small lowering of serum cholesterol (Moody and Reddy 1982). Lake *et al* (1975) found elevated liver weight, dilatation of the hepatic smooth endoplasmic reticulum and an increase in the number of hepatic peroxisomes and microperoxisomes in rats given seven daily oral doses of 850–1425 mg/kg of 2-ethylhexanol. Alcohol dehydrogenase and microsomal cytochrome P-450 content were also increased, and glucose-6-phosphatase activity was lowered. Rhodes *et al* (1983, 1984) found no changes in relative liver or testes weights, liver or testes pathology, number of hepatic peroxisomes, hepatic cyanide-insensitive palmitoyl-CoA oxidation or catalase activity, and plasma triglycerides and cholesterol in male rats given 130 mg/kg/day of 2-ethylhexanol by gavage for 14 days.

2-Ethylhexanol (1 mM) also induces peroxisomal proliferation in primary cultures of rat hepatocytes over 48 hours. A nine-fold increase in CAT and a doubling in 7-ethoxycoumarin *O*-deethylase activity (an indicator of microsomal mixed function oxidase activity) were found in this experiment (Gray *et al* 1982). In a further *in vitro* study, 0.2 mM 2-ethylhexanol led to a CAT activity of 151% of control, whilst 1 mM 2-ethylhexanol induced CAT activity to 583% of control. Cyanide-insensitive palmityl-CoA oxidation, thought to be a more specific peroxisomal marker than CAT, was not affected by 0.2 mM 2-ethylhexanol (Gray *et al* 1983).

2-Ethylhexanol inhibited rat liver aminopyrine *N*-demethylase and aniline hydroxylase activities *in vitro* (Seth 1982, Agarwal *et al* 1982a) while *in vivo*, elevated liver cytochrome P-450 and biphenyl-4-hydroxylase activities have been reported (Lake *et al* 1974).

Application of 2-ethylhexanol to the skin was reported to induce hepatic succinate dehydrogenase activity and lower lactate dehydrogenase activity (Schmidt *et al* 1973).

Agarwal *et al* (1982b) have also demonstrated that 2-ethylhexanol is a competitive inhibitor of mouse liver alcohol dehydrogenase activity *in vitro*. An interaction with the pharmacology of ethanol was thus proposed.

This compound has been reported to be severely irritating to the rabbit eye (Schmidt *et al* 1973, Scala and Burtis 1973) and mildly irritating to the skin of both rabbits and guinea-pigs (Opdyke 1979, Rowe and McCollister 1982, Schmidt *et al* 1973). Pathological evidence for gastrointestinal irritation has been reported in rats given near lethal oral doses of 2-ethylhexanol (Scala and Burtis 1973).

Negative results have been found in human patch tests and sensitisation tests at a concentration of 4% in petrolatum (Opdyke 1979). Mashkina (1966) reported that 2-ethylhexanol had no irritant effects in human volunteers.

3.4.2 Chronic toxicity

Evidence of slight liver and kidney damage was found in male and female rats fed 2-ethylhexanol at 2% of diet for 90 days. No effects were found in rats fed 0.01, 0.05 or 0.25%, though elevated liver weight was evident at 1.25% (Rowe and McCollister 1982).

3.4.3 Genotoxicity

2-Ethylhexanol was negative in the Ames test at 0.01–1.0 5l/plate to *Salmonella typhimurium* TA98, TA100, TA1535, TA1537 and TA1538 both with and without metabolic activation (Kirby *et al* 1983). It also proved negative in the *Bacillus subtilis* rec assay at 500 μg/disc and also in the L5178Y mouse lymphoma mutagenicity assay at concentrations of 0.013–1.0 5l/ml (Kirby *et al* 1983, Tomita *et al* 1982). However, it was reported to be weakly mutagenic in a *Salmonella typhimurium* liquid suspension assay where resistance to 8-azaguanine was the genetic marker (Seed 1982).

No significant induction of chromosome aberrations was found in Chinese hamster ovary cells treated with concentrations of 1.5–2.4 mM for 2 hours. 2-Ethylhexanol had a steep dose–response curve for toxicity (measured by cloning efficiency) with 50% survival at a concentration of 2.5 mM (Phillips *et al* 1982). This compound was also negative for induction of unscheduled DNA synthesis in primary hepatocyte cultures derived from Fischer 344 rats (Hodgson *et al* 1982).

It has been reported in the US Federal Register (1984) that this compound gave negative results in a cell transformation assay.

2-Ethylhexanol induced a dose-dependent inhibition of [^{3}H]thymidine incorporation into the replicating DNA of proliferating C57BL/6J splenic lymphoid cells. There was evidence that this was not due to suppressed cellular uptake of the tracer. However, suppression was reversed by incubation of the cells for 3 hours in the absence of the compound, suggesting that the inhibition had not been of a DNA-damaging kind (Warren *et al* 1982).

2-Ethylhexanol was not found to bind to protein, RNA or DNA of rat liver *in vitro* (Albro *et al* 1982) or to rat liver DNA *in vivo* (Albro *et al* 1983).

Oral doses of 0.02, 0.07 or 0.21 ml/kg/day (about 17, 58 and 175 mg/kg/day) of 2-ethylhexanol in corn oil were administered by gavage to Fischer 344 rats. From each experimental animal 50 bone marrow metaphase cells were examined. No significant induction of chromatid and chromosome breaks or structural rearrangements were found. Mitotic index was also unaffected (Putman *et al* 1983).

A dominant lethal study in ICR/SIM mice has also proved negative. Oral doses of 250, 500 or 1000 mg/kg in corn oil were administered to male mice on five consecutive days. After treatment each male was housed with two virgin females each week for an 8-week period. The females were killed on days 14–17 and evaluated for reproductive effects. The treatment was not found to affect fertility or the average number of dead and total implants per pregnancy (Rushbrook *et al* 1982).

3.4.4 Carcinogenicity

No carcinogenicity studies of this compound appear to have been carried out.

3.4.5 Reproductive toxicity

Incubation of 0.2 mM 2-ethylhexanol with primary cultures of mixed rat testicular cells did not result in any detectable toxic effects (Gray and Beamand 1984).

2-Ethylhexanol was administered by oral gavage to Wister rats at a dose of 0.833 or 1.67 mg/kg (1.0 or 2.0 ml/kg) on day 12 of gestation. A dose reponse in the number of foetuses showing defects was observed. These consisted of hydronephrosis, tail and limb defects (Ritter *et al* 1987).

3.5 Discussion

2-Ethylhexanol is rapidly metabolised in the liver by alcohol and aldehyde dehydrogenases and excreted primarily in the urine as the glucuronide conjugate of 2-ethylhexanoic acid. It is of low acute and subacute toxicity in rodents, the main effects at high doses being hypolipidaemia (lowering of serum triglycerides and cholesterol) and specific changes in the liver. The liver changes are characterised by hepatomegaly, an increase in the size of the smooth endoplasmic reticulum and a marked increase in the number of peroxisomes. Peroxisomal enzyme activities are often considerably elevated. As the peroxisome has recently been discovered to play a role in lipid metabolism, there may be a link between the liver changes and the lowering of serum lipids.

Compounds which are peroxisomal proliferators also tend to be able to induce liver tumours in high-dose rodent carcinogenicity bioassays. The mechanism is not thought to be one of direct genetic damage. Although there is no information available on the carcinogenicity of 2-ethylhexanol, this compound does not appear to be genotoxic.

The hazard to man of compounds which cause peroxisomal proliferation in rodents is not entirely clear. However, studies on another rat liver peroxisomal proliferator, clofibrate, did not find similar hepatic changes in monkeys or humans *in vivo*. Moreover, recent *in vitro* evidence suggests that human hepatocytes are much less sensitive to peroxisome proliferating agents than rat hepatocytes.

References

AGARWAL D K, AGARWAL S and SETH P K (1982a) Effect of di-(2-ethylhexyl)-phthalate on drug metabolism, lipid peroxidation and sulfhydryl content of rat liver. *Drug Metabolism and Disposition* **10,** 77-80.

AGARWAL D K, AGARWAL S and SETH P K (1982b) Interaction of di-(2-ethylhexyl)phthalate with the pharmacological response and metabolic aspects of ethanol in mice. *Biochemical Pharmacology* **31,** 3149-3423.

ALBRO P W (1975) The metabolism of 2-ethylhexanol in rats. *Xenobiotica* **5,** 625-636.

ALBRO P W, CORBETT J T, SCHROEDER J L, JORDAN S and MATTHEWS H B (1982) Pharmacokinetics, interactions with macromolecules and species differences in metabolism of DEHP. *Environmental Health Perspectives* **45,** 19-25.

ALBRO P W, CORBETT J T, SCHROEDER J L and JORDAN S T (1983) Incorporation of radioactivity from labeled di-(2-ethylhexyl) phthalate into DNA of rat liver *in vivo. Chemicobiological Interactions* **44,** 1-16.

GRAY T J B and BEAMAND J A (1984) Effect of some phthalate esters and other testicular toxins on primary cultures of testicular cells. *Food and Chemical Toxicology* **22,** 123-131.

GRAY T J B, BEAMAND J A, LAKE B G, FOSTER J R and GANGOLLI S D (1982) Peroxisome proliferation in cultured rat hepatocytes produced by clofibrate and phthalate ester metabolites. *Toxicology Letters* **10,** 273-279.

GRAY T J B, LAKE B G, BEAMAND J A, FOSTER J R and GANGOLLI S D

(1983) Peroxisomal effects of phthalate esters in primary cultures of rat hepatocytes. *Toxicology* **28,** 167-179.
HODGSON J R, MYHR B C, McKEON M and BRUSICK D J (1982) Evaluation of di-(2-ethylhexyl)phthalate and its major metabolites in the primary rat hepatocyte unscheduled DNA synthesis assay. *Environmental Mutagenesis* **4,** 388.
HOLLENBACH K, SCHMIDT P and STREMMEL D (1972) Tierexperimentelle untersuchungen zur blutdruckwirksamkeit von thioglykolsaureisooctylester, thioglykolsaure und 2-athylhexanol. *Zeitschrift fur gesamte Hygiene und Ihre Grenzgebiete* **18,** 418.
KAMIL I A, SMITH J N and WILLIAMS R T (1953) The formation of ester glucuronides of aliphatic acids during the metabolism of 2-ethylbutanol and 2-ethylhexanol. *Biochemical Journal* **53,** 137-140.
KIRBY P E, PIZZARELLO R F, LAWLOR T E, HAWORTH S R and HODGSON J R (1983) Evaluation of di-(2-ethylhexyl)phthalate and its major metabolites in the Ames test and L5178Y mouse lymphoma mutagenicity assay. *Environmental Mutagenesis* **5,** 657-663.
KNAAK J B, KOZBELT S J and SULLIVAN L J (1966) Metabolism of 2-ethylhexyl sulfate by the rat and rabbit. *Toxicology and Applied Pharmacology* **8,** 369-379.
LAKE B G, GANGOLLI S D, WRIGHT M G, GRASSO P and LLOYD A G (1974) Studies on the effects of the oral administration of di-(2-ethylhexyl)-phthalate on some hepatic enzymes in the rat. *Biochemical Society Transactions* **2,** 322-325.
LAKE B G, GANGOLLI S D, GRASSO P and LLOYD A G (1975) Studies on the hepatic effects of orally administered di-(2-ethylhexyl)phthalate in the rat. *Toxicology and Applied Pharmacology* **32,** 355-367.
MASHKINA O N (1966) Toxicology of 2-ethylhexanal and 2-ethylhexanol. *Mater Konf Fiziol Biokhim Farmakol Uchast Prakt Vrachei Ufa* **168.**
MOODY D E and REDDY J K (1978) Hepatic peroxisome (microbody) proliferation in rats fed plasticizers and related compounds. *Toxicology and Applied Pharmacology* **45,** 497-504.
MOODY D E and REDDY J K (1982) Serum triglyceride and cholesterol contents in male rats receiving diets containing plasticizers and analogues of the ester 2-ethylhexanol. *Toxicology Letters* **10,** 379-383.
MOODY D E, AZARNOFF D L and REDDY J K (1976) Induction of hepatic peroxisomes, peroxisome associated enzymes and hypolipidemia in rats treated with 2-ethyl hexanoic acid and 2-ethyl hexanol. *Journal of Cell Biology* **70,** 363a.
OPDYKE D L J (1979) Fragrance Raw Materials Monographs. 2-Ethyl hexanol. *Food and Cosmetics Toxicology* **17** Suppl, 775-777.
PHILLIPS B J, JAMES T E B and GANGOLLI S D (1982) Genotoxicity studies of di-(2-ethylhexyl)phthalate and its metabolites in CHO cells. *Mutation Research* **102,** 297-304.
PUTMAN D L, MOORE W A, SCHECHTMAN L M and HODGSON J R (1983) Cytogenetic evaluation of di-(2-ethylhexyl)phthalate and its major metabolites in Fischer 344 rats. *Environmental Mutagenesis* **5,** 227-231.

RITTER E J, SCOTT W J, RANDALL J L and RITTER J M (1987) Teratogenicity of di(2-ethylhexyl) phthalate, 2-ethylhexanol, 2-ethylhexanoic acid and valproic acid and potentiation by caffeine. *Teratology* **35,** 41-46.

RHODES C, ELCOMBE C R, STONARD M D, SIMPSON M G and VERNALL A (1983) The *in vivo* and *in vitro* effects of alkanols on the morphology and peroxisomal enzyme activities of rat liver. *Toxicology Letters* **18** Suppl 1, 64.

RHODES C, SOAMES T, STONARD M D, SIMPSON A J, VERNALL A J and ELCOMBE C R (1984) The absence of testicular atrophy and *in vivo* and *in vitro* effects on hepatocyte morphology and peroxisomal enzyme activities in male rats following the administration of several alkanols. *Toxicology Letters* **21,** 103-109.

ROWE V K and McCOLLISTER S B (1982) Alcohols. In: *Patty's Industrial Hygiene and Toxicology,* ed by G D Clayton and F E Clayton, 3rd Revised Edition, Vol 2C. John Wiley & Sons. pp 4620-4624.

RUSHBROOK C J, JORGENSON T A and HODGSON J R (1982) Dominant lethal study of di-(2-ethylhexyl)phthalate and its major metabolites in ICR/SIM mice. *Environmental Mutagenesis* **4,** 387.

SCALA R A and BURTIS E G (1973) Acute toxicity of a homologous series of branched-chain primary alcohols. *American Industrial Hygiene Association Journal* **34,** 493-499.

SCHMIDT P, GOHLKE R and ROTHE R (1973) Zur toxizitat einiger C8-aldehyde und-alkohole. *Zeitschrift fur Gesamte Hygiene und Ihre Grenzgebiete* **19,** 485.

SEED J L (1982) Mutagenic activity of phthalate esters in bacterial liquid suspension assays. *Environmental Health Perspectives* **45,** 111-114.

SETH P K (1982) Hepatic effects of phthalate esters. *Environmental Health Perspectives* **45,** 27-34.

TOMITA I, NAKAMURA Y, AOKI N and INUI N (1982) Mutagenic/carcinogenic potential of DEHP and MEHP. *Environmental Health Perspectives* **45,** 119-125.

UNITED STATES FEDERAL REGISTER (1984) 49, 18779-18780.

VERSCHUEREN K (1983) *Handbook of environmental data on organic pollutants.* Van Nostrand Reinhold Company, Second Edition.

WARREN J R, LALWANI N D and REDDY J K (1982) Phthalate esters as peroxisome proliferator carcinogens. *Environmental Health Perspectives* **45,** 35-40.

WATER RESEARCH CENTRE (1981) Organic micropollutants in drinking water. WRc Technical Report TR 159.

4. 2-PHENYLPHENOL

4.1 Introduction

2-Phenylphenol (*ortho*-phenylphenol, 2-hydroxybiphenyl, Dowicide 1, Preventol O extra) is produced commercially by hydrolysis of chlorobenzene with aqueous sodium hydroxide. This compound is used as a fungicide on post-harvest fruit and vegetables, in the rubber industry, in ceramic glazes, paints and polishes, metalworking fluids, textiles, glues, detergents and cosmetics.

CAS Reg No:	90-43-7
Molecular weight:	170
Boiling Point:	282°C
Solubility:	700 mg/l at 25°C (Verschueren 1983)
Threshold odour concentration in water:	0.4 mg/l (Verschueren 1983)

4.2 Exposure

In the WRc survey, this compound was detected in only one of 14 drinking water samples examined. The source of this particular sample was a groundwater (Water Research Centre 1981). 2-Phenylphenol has also been identified in groundwater samples near Melbourne, Australia (Stepan *et al* 1981) and in river water and drinking water in West Germany (Dietz and Traud 1978).

Levels of 2-phenylphenol ranging from trace to 0.2 mg/kg have been reported in fruit in the US (Johnson and Manske 1977). Much higher concentrations have been detected in fruit in Japan (Ito *et al* 1979). Food may therefore represent the major source of exposure to this compound.

4.3 Toxicokinetics

Following oral administration in mammals, most of a dose of 2-phenylphenol is conjugated with glucuronic acid and sulphate and excreted in the urine within 24 hours (Von Ernst 1965, Savides and Oehme 1980, Reitz *et al* 1983). When very high doses were given to F344 rats, around 20–30% of the dose was converted to dihydroxybiphenyl. It would appear that oxidative metabolism is important in rats at high doses of 2-phenylphenol but not at low doses (Reitz *et al* 1983).

4.4 Health effects

4.4.1 Acute and subacute toxicity

The acute toxicity of 2-phenylphenol in experimental animals is characterised by haemorrhages in the lung, liver, myocardium and gastrointestinal tract and death by respiratory failure. Oral LD50s of 2–3 g/kg, 0.9–2 g/kg and 3.5 g/kg have been reported for the rat, mouse and guinea-pig respectively (Registry of Toxic Effects of Chemical Substances).

No effects on growth rate and blood haemoglobin, total white cell count and differential white cell count were found in rats given oral doses of up to 200 mg/kg body weight/day of 2-phenylphenol in nut oil for 32 days (Macintosh 1945).

Groups of female B6C3F1 mice dosed with 0, 1, 10 or 200 mg/kg body weight/day of 2-phenylphenol by gavage for 10 days over a 2-week period gave no evidence for altered immune function or host susceptibility (Luster *et al* 1981). In an earlier study, however, some evidence for immunodepression was found in male CBA/J mice given drinking water containing either 5 or 10 mg/l of 2-phenylphenol for up to 7 weeks (La Via and La Via 1979).

No evidence for skin irritation or sensitisation was found in patch tests with 200 volunteers using a 5% solution of 2-phenylphenol in sesame oil. Both 1% and 5%

aqueous solutions of the sodium salt of 2-phenylphenol, sodium *ortho*-phenylphenate, were significantly irritant, but a 0.1% solution was not found to produce irritation or sensitisation (Hodge *et al* 1952). No evidence of skin sensitisation was found for 2-phenylphenol in the guinea-pig maximisation test. In the same study, only one of 40 animals exposed to sodium *ortho*-phenylphenate exhibited sensitisation (Andersen and Hamann 1984).

Cases of allergic contact dermatitis in man have been associated with exposure to 2-phenylphenol (Cronin 1980, Adams 1981).

4.4.2 Chronic toxicity

In a 90-day study, a group of 30 F344 rats were maintained on diets containing 2% 2-phenylphenol. Pathological changes including focal tubular collapse and focal cortical cysts were apparent in the kidney after 30 days of treatment (Reitz *et al* 1983). In earlier experiments, depression of body weight gain, but no pathological changes, was found in rats given a diet containing 2% 2-phenylphenol for 3 months (Hodge *et al* 1952). Depression of body weight gain and renal damage characterised by tubular dilation and inflammation were observed in rats maintained on diets containing 2% 2-phenylphenol for 2 years. No effects were reported at dietary levels of 0.02% and 0.2% (Hodge *et al* 1952). No pathological or haematological effects were reported in rats given 200 or 500 mg/kg body weight/day of 2-phenylphenol by stomach tube, 5 days/week for 6 months (Hodge *et al* 1952).

Pairs of dogs given oral doses of 0, 20, 200 or 500 mg/kg body weight/day of 2-phenylphenol for 1 year showed no adverse changes in body weight gain, organ weights, haematology, urinalysis or histopathology (Hodge *et al* 1952).

A group of 30 F344 rats maintained on diets containing 2.0% sodium *ortho*-phenylphenate for 90 days exhibited elevated mitosis of bladder epithelial cells after only 3 days, while hyperplasia of the bladder epithelium became apparent at 14 days. The thickness of the bladder epithelium was found to increase throughout the remainder of the 90-day treatment period (Reitz *et al* 1983). This is in contrast to B6C3F1 mice, in which no changes in the bladder were found after 13 weeks on a diet containing 2.0% sodium *ortho*-phenylphenate (Shibata *et al* 1985).

Groups of 50 male and 50 female B6C3F1 mice maintained on diets containing 0, 0.5, 1.0 and 2.0% of sodium *ortho*-phenylphenate for 96 weeks did not exhibit changes in organ weights, mortality, clinical signs, haematology or urinalysis. Some histopathological changes were reported, but these were not dose-dependent. Growth retardation was evident in males receiving the 2.0% dose level and in females receiving the 0.5, 1.0 and 2.0% dose levels. A dose-dependent increase in serum alkaline phosphatase activity was also noted in females (Hagiwara *et al* 1984).

4.4.3 Genotoxicity

Although most bacterial mutagenicity studies have given negative results for 2-phenylphenol (Cline and McMahon 1977, Shirasu *et al* 1978, Hirayama *et al* 1981, Reitz *et al* 1983, Ishidate *et al* 1984), one study has found weak direct mutagenic activity for this compound in *Salmonella typhimurium* TA1535 (Haworth *et al* 1983). There are reports that 2-phenylphenol has activity in some DNA repair assays (Nishioka and Ogasawara 1978, Hirayama *et al* 1981).

Similarly, although most studies in higher test systems have given negative results for genotoxicity (Nawai *et al* 1980, Yoshida *et al* 1980, Probst *et al* 1981, Reitz *et al* 1983, Ishidate *et al* 1984), this compound has been reported to be a weak inducer of chromosome aberrations and sister chromatid exchanges in CHO-K1 cells *in vitro* (Nawai *et al* 1984). 2-Phenylphenol was also found to be mutagenic in an ultraviolet-sensitive human cell strain where resistance to ouabain was the genetic marker (Suzuki *et al* 1985).

No evidence for covalent binding to bladder DNA was found in F344 rats given single doses of 500 mg/kg body weight of either 2-phenylphenol or its sodium salt (Reitz *et al* 1983). In a later study, however, macromolecular binding of ^{14}C-labelled 2-phenylphenol and sodium *ortho*-phenylphenate was observed in the liver, kidney and bladder of F344 rats given single doses of 50–500 mg/kg. A disproportionate increase in binding was found at the higher dose levels (Reitz *et al* 1984).

No evidence for induction of chromosome abnormalities was observed in the bone marrow of mice given single oral doses of up to 4 g/kg body weight or daily doses of up to 0.8 g/kg body weight for 5 days (Shirasu *et al* 1978). In a dominant lethal study, male C3H mice were given oral doses of 100 or 500 mg/kg body weight/day for 5 days. Each male was then mated with two virgin females each week for 6 weeks. No dominant lethal mutations were observed (Shirasu *et al* 1978, Kaneda *et al* 1978). A similar result was obtained when male mice were fed diets containing up to 4% sodium *ortho*-phenylphenate for 2 months before mating (Ogata *et al* 1980a).

4.4.4 Carcinogenicity

Both 2-phenylphenol and sodium *ortho*-phenylphenate have been tested for carcinogenicity in rodents. Studies in rats and mice have given no evidence for carcinogenicity of 2-phenylphenol. A significant increase in tumours of the urinary tract was found in rats fed sodium *ortho*-phenylphenate, but no evidence of carcinogenicity was found for this compound in mice.

In the 2-phenylphenol study, groups of 18 male and 18 female 7-day-old mice of the (C57BL/6×C3H/Anf)F1 and (C57BL/6×AKR) F1 strains were given single doses of 100 mg/kg body weight by gavage. This dose, though not subsequently adjusted for increasing body weight, was given each day till weaning at 4 weeks. From this point to the end of the study at 18 months, the animals were given a diet containing 280 mg/kg of 2-phenylphenol. No differences were apparent in the tumour incidences between the test and control animals (Innes *et al* 1969). In an earlier feeding study, no evidence for an increased tumour incidence was found in rats maintained on diets containing 2% 2-phenylphenol for 2 years (Hodge *et al* 1952).

Groups of ten male and ten female F344/Du rats were fed diets containing 0, 0.125, 0.25, 0.5, 1.0, 2.0 or 4.0% of sodium *ortho*-phenylphenate for 13 weeks (Hiraga and Fujii 1981). Tumours of the urinary bladder (some benign and some malignant) were found in male rats receiving the 1.0, 2.0 and 4.0% diets and in females receiving the 4.0% diet. In groups of male F344/Du rats fed the same dietary concentrations for 91 weeks, the incidence of transitional cell carcinomas of the urinary system (including carcinomas of the renal papilla, renal pelvis and urinary bladder) was as follows:

Dose level	0	0.125%	0.25%	0.5%	1.0%	2.0%	4.0%
Tumours/no of rats	0/20	0/20	0/20	1/21	7/21	20/21	17/20

There was no clear evidence for carcinogenicity of sodium *ortho*-phenylphenate in groups of 50 male and 50 female B6C3F1 mice maintained on diets containing 0, 0.5, 1.0 and 2.0% for 96 weeks (Hagiwara *et al* 1984).

Although F344 rats fed diets containing 2% sodium *ortho*-phenylphenate for 32 weeks developed hyperplasia and tumours in the bladder, 2-phenylphenol gave little evidence for effects on the bladder even after the rats had been pretreated with the initiating agent *N*-butyl-*N*-(4-hydroxybutyl)nitrosamine (Fukushima *et al* 1983).

There was no evidence for carcinogenicity of promoting activity of *ortho*-phenylphenol tested by application to mouse skin alone or after initiation with 7,12-dimethylbenz(*a*)anthracene (National Toxicology Program 1985).

4.4.5 Reproductive toxicity

There were no apparent teratogenic or embryotoxic effects in Sprague–Dawley rats given 0, 100, 300 or 700 mg/kg body weight/day of 2-phenylphenol by gavage on days 6–15 of gestation. Some maternal toxicity was evident at the highest dose level (John *et al* 1981). Similar results have been obtained in mice and rats by Japanese workers, though evidence of embryotoxicity has been reported at doses of 600 mg/kg and above (Kaneda *et al* 1978, Ogata *et al* 1980b).

4.5 Discussion

In mammals, 2-phenylphenol is rapidly metabolised by conjugation with glucuronic acid and sulphate, followed by excretion in the urine.

This compound appears to be of low acute toxicity and chronic toxicity, though there is insufficient information at lower dose levels. 2-Phenylphenol has given some evidence for weak genotoxic potential in the Ames test and in Chinese hamster cells and human cells *in vitro*. It was not found to be carcinogenic in rats or mice or teratogenic in rats. However, sodium *ortho*-phenylphenate has been shown to induce malignant tumours in the kidney and urinary bladder in long-term feeding studies in rats. In response to this finding, FAO/WHO (1984) have recently lowered the acceptable daily intake of 2-phenylphenol to a temporary figure of 0–20 μg/kg body weight.

In view of the relatively low toxicity of 2-phenylphenol and its infrequent occurrence in drinking water, this compound would not appear to pose a threat to the health of consumers.

References

ADAMS R M (1981) Allergic contact dermatitis due to *o*-phenylphenol. *Contact Dermatitis* **7,** 332.

ANDERSEN K E and HAMANN K (1984) The sensitizing potential of metalworking fluid biocides (phenolic and thiazole compounds) in the guinea-pig maximization test in relation to patch-test reactivity in eczema patients. *Food and Chemical Toxicology* **22,** 655-660.

CLINE J C and McMAHON R E (1977) Detection of chemical mutagens: Use of concentration gradient plates in a high capacity screen. *Research Communications in Chemical Pathology and Pharmacology* **16,** 523-533.

CRONIN E (1980) *Contact dermatitis.* Churchill Livingstone, Edinburgh p 681.

DIETZ F and TRAUD J (1978) The trace analysis of phenols, especially chlorophenols, in water by gas chromatography — methods and results. *Vom Wasser* **51,** 235-257.

FAO/WHO EXPERT GROUP ON PESTICIDES (1984) Pesticide residues in food — 1983. FAO Plant Production and Protection Paper 56, Rome.

FUKUSHIMA S, KURATA Y, SHIBATA M, IKAWA E and ITO N (1983) Promoting effect of sodium *o*-phenylphenate and *o*-phenylphenol on two-stage urinary bladder carcinogenesis in rats. *Gann* **74,** 625-632.

HAGIWARA A, SHIBATA M, HIROSE M, FUKUSHIMA S and ITO N (1984) Long-term toxicity and carcinogenicity study of sodium *o*-phenylphenate in B6C3F1 mice. *Food and Chemical Toxicology* **22,** 809-814.

HAWORTH S, LAWLOR T, MORTELMANS K, SPECK W and ZEIGER E (1983) Salmonella mutagenicity test results for 250 chemicals. *Environmental Mutagenesis* **5,** Suppl 1, 3-142.

HIRAGA K and FUJII T (1981) Induction of tumours of the urinary system in F344 rats by dietary administration of sodium *o*-phenylphenate. *Food and Cosmetics Toxicology* **19,** 303-310.

HIRAYAMA T, NOHARA M, SHINDO H and FUKUI S (1981) Mutagenicity assays of photochemical resction products of biphenyl (BP) and *o*-phenylphenol (OPP) with NOx. *Chemosphere* **10,** 223-228.

HODGE H C, MAYNARD E A, BLANCHET H J Jr, SPENCER H C and ROWE V K (1952) Toxicological studies of orthophenylphenol (Dowicide 1). *Journal of Pharmacology and Experimental Therapeutics* **104,** 202-210.

INNES J R M, ULLAND B M, VALERIO M G, PETRUCELLI L, FISHBEIN L, HART E R, PALLOTTA A J, BATES R R, FALK L, GART J J, KLEIN M, MITCHELL I and PETERS J (1969) Bioassay of pesticides and industrial chemicals for tumorigenicity in mice: A preliminary note. *Journal of the National Cancer Institute* **42,** 1101-1114.

ISHIDATE M Jr, SOFUNI T, YOSHIKAWA K, HAYASHI M, NOHMI T, SAWADA M and MATSUOKA A (1984) Primary mutagenicity screening of food additives currently used in Japan. *Food and Chemical Toxicology* **22,** 623-636.

ITO Y, TOYODA M, OGAWA S, IWAIDA M and YANAGIDA F (1979) Occurrence of orthophenylphenol during manufacture of lemon marmalade. *Journal of Food Protection* **42,** 292-293.

JOHN J A, MURRAY F J, RAS K S and SCHWETZ B A (1981) Teratological evaluation of orthophenylphenol in rats. *Fundamental and Applied Toxicology* **1,** 282-285.

JOHNSON R D and MANSKE D D (1977) Pesticide and other chemical residues in total diet samples (XI). *Pesticides Monitoring Journal* **11,** 116-131.

KANEDA M, TERAMOTO S, SHINGU A and SHIRASU Y (1978) Teratogenicity and dominant lethal studies with *o*-phenylphenol. *Journal of Pesticide Science* **3,** 365-370.

LA VIA M F and LA VIA D S (1979) Phenol derivatives are immunodepressive in mice. *Drug and Chemical Toxicology* **2,** 167-177.

LUSTER M L, DEAN J H, BOORMAN G A, ARCHER D L, LAUER L,

LAWSON L D, MOORE J A and WILSON R E (1981) The effects of orthophenylphenol, tris(2,3-dichloropropyl)phosphate and cyclophosphamide on the immune system and host susceptibility of mice following subchronic exposure. *Toxicology and Applied Pharmacology* **58,** 252-261.

MACINTOSH F C (1945) The toxicity of diphenyl and *o*-phenyl-phenol. *Analyst* **70,** 334-335.

NATIONAL TOXICOLOGY PROGRAM (1985) Toxicology and carcinogenesis studies of *ortho*-phenylphenol alone and with 7,12-dimethylbenz(*a*)anthracene in Swiss CD-1 mice. National Toxicology Program Technical Report No 301.

NAWAI S, YOSHIDA S, NAKAO T and HIRAGA K (1980) Examination of mutagens by induced sister chromatid exchange (SCE). 2 Test of two fungicides by induced SCE, *in vitro*. *Pesticide Abstracts* **13,** 289. 80-1144.

NAWAI S, YOSHIDA S, NAKAO T and HIRAGA K (1984) Induction of chromosome aberrations and sister-chromatid exchanges in CHO-K1 cells by *o*-phenylphenol. *Mutation Research* **141,** 95-99.

NISHIOKA J and OGASAWARA H (1978) Mutagenicity testing for diphenyl derivatives in bacterial systems. *Mutation Research* **54,** 248-249.

OGATA A, YOSHIDA S, NAWAI S, ANDO H, KUBO K, HIRAGA K and MASUBUCHI M (1980a) Dominant lethal tests of long term administration with sodium *ortho*-phenylphenolate (Na-OPP) in mice. *Pesticide Abstracts* **13,** 795-796. 80-2939

OGATA A, ANDO H, KUBO Y and HIRAGA K (1980b) Teratological tests of *o*-phenylphenol (OPP) and sodium *o*-phenylphenol (OPP-Na) in mice. *Pesticide Abstracts* **13,** 666. 80-2625.

PROBST G S, McMAHON R E, HILL L E, THOMPSON C Z, EPP J K and NEAL S B (1981) Chemically-induced unscheduled DNA synthesis in primary rat hepatocyte cultures: A comparison with bacterial mutagenicity using 218 compounds. *Environmental Mutagenesis* **3,** 11-32.

REGISTRY OF TOXIC EFFECTS OF CHEMICAL SUBSTANCES National Institute for Occupational Safety and Health, Cincinnati, Ohio.

REITZ R H, FOX T R, QUAST J F, HERMANN E A and WATANABE P G (1983) Molecular mechanisms involved in the toxicity of orthophenylphenol and its sodium salt. *Chemicobiological Interactions* **43,** 99-119.

REITZ R H, FOX T R, QUAST J F, HERMANN E A and WATANABE P G (1984) Biochemical factors involved in the effects of *ortho*-phenylphenol (OPP) and sodium orthophenylphenate (SOPP) on the urinary tract of male F344 rats. *Toxicology and Applied Pharmacology* **73,** 345-349.

SAVIDES M C and OEHME F W (1980) Urinary metabolism of orally administered *ortho*-phenylphenol in dogs and cats. *Toxicology* **17,** 355-363.

SHIBATA M, HAGIWARA A, TAMANO S, FUKUSHIMA S and ITO N (1985) Subchronic toxicity study of sodium *o*-phenylphenate in mice. *Toxicology Letters* **25,** 239-246.

SHIRASU Y, MORIYA M, KATO K, TEZUKA H, HENMI R, SHINGU A, KANEDA M and TERAMOTO S (1978) Mutagenicity testing on *o*-phenylphenol. *Mutation Research* **54,** 227.

STEPAN S, SMITH J F and RIHA M (1981) Movement and chemical change of organic pollutants in an aquifer. *Australian Water Resources Council Confer-*

ence Series **No.1,** 415-424.
SUZUKI H, SUZUKI N, SASAKI M and HIRAGA K (1985) Orthophenylphenol mutagenicity in a human cell strain. *Mutation Research* **156,** 123-127.
VERSCHUEREN K (1983) *Handbook of environmental data on organic chemicals.* Van Nostrand Reinhold Company, Second Edition.
VON ERNST W (1965) Conversion and elimination of 2-hydroxybiphenyl by rats. *Arzneimittel Forschung* **15,** 632-636.
WATER RESEARCH CENTRE (1981) Organic micropollutants in drinking water. WRc Technical Report TR 159.
YOSHIDA S, MASUBUCHI M and HIRAGA K (1980) Cytogenetic studies of antimicrobials on cultured cells. *Pesticide Abstracts* **13,** 665-666. 80-2624.

5. REMAINING MISCELLANEOUS OXYGENATED COMPOUNDS

5.1 Introduction

The remaining compounds of the miscellaneous oxygenated group are mostly long-chain aliphatic alcohols, though there are some chemicals of quite diverse structure.

Diacetone alcohol (4-hydroxy-4-methylpentan-2-one) is the toxic constituent of *Stipa vaseyi,* sleepy grass (Epstein *et al* 1964). It is widely used in industry, mostly as a solvent. Dihydroactinidiolide has been identified as an excretion product of some blue-green algae (Henatsch and Juttner 1983). It is also released into the aquatic environment by *Eleocharis* species, and appears to act as a growth inhibitor of other macrophytes (Stevens and Merrill 1980). Dodecanol (lauryl alcohol) is used in the manufacture of detergents and sulphuric acid esters. Hexadecanol (cetyl alcohol) is primarily used in cosmetics and perfumes. Both this compound and octadecanol (stearyl alcohol) have been used as anti-evaporating agents in ponds and lakes. Menthol is commonly employed as a peppermint flavour in confectionery, 4-(2-phenylisopropyl) phenol (cumyl phenol) is an intermediate in the manufacture of resins, insecticides and lubricants, while phthalic anhydride is used in the manufacture of phthalate esters, benzoic acids, resins and dyes.

5.2 Exposure

The remaining miscellaneous oxygenated compounds identified in UK drinking water by WRc (Water Research Centre 1981, 1982) were:

Decenol isomer
Diacetone alcohol
Dihydroactinidiolide
Dodecanol
Hexadecanol
Menthol
Methoxydihdropyran isomer
3-Methylbutan-2-ol 5-methyltetrahydropyranyl-4,3,1,1,2,3,3-pentamethylindane
Octadecanol isomers (two)
Pentadecanol isomer
Pentenol isomer

4-(2-Phenylisopropyl)phenol
4-Phenylphenol
2-Phenyl-2-propanol
Phthalic anhydride

All of these compounds occurred only infrequently in drinking water.

There is very little other information available on the presence of these compounds in water, food or air.

5.3 Toxicokinetics

For most of these compounds the major pathway of biotransformation would appear to be oxidation to the corresponding fatty acid and subsequent incorporation into intermediary metabolism. In the case of an oral dose of 2 g/kg of hexadecanol in rats, about 20% was recovered unchanged in the faeces, while a slight increase in glucuronide metabolites was found in the urine (McIsaac and Williams 1958). In another study, thoracic-duct cannulated rats were given a single dose of 0.2 mg of hexadecanol by stomach tube. About 66% of the dose was recovered from the faeces and intestinal contents, while 25.8% was collected from the lymph. Similar results were obtained after a single dose of 300 mg (Baxter *et al* 1967). Within 48 hours of an intracerebral dose of hexadecanol in rodents, almost all of the dose appeared to be incorporated into brain phospholipids (Bell *et al* 1971).

In human volunteers, most of an oral dose of 1.56 g of menthol was rapidly excreted in the urine as glucuronide conjugates (Bolund *et al* 1967).

5.4 Health effects

5.4.1 Acute and subacute toxicity

The miscellaneous oxygenated compounds appear to be of very low acute toxicity. Acute oral LD50s (g/kg) reported for the rat are as follows (Opdyke 1973, 1974, 1978, Registry of Toxic Effects of Chemical Substances):

9-Decen-1-ol	>5.0
Diacetone alcohol	4.0
1-Dodecanol	>12.8
1-Hexadecanol	6.4–12.8
Menthol	3.2
1-Octadecanol	20
Phthalic anhydride	0.8–4.0

In a very early study, rats given single doses of 1.86 g/kg of diacetone alcohol by stomach tube exhibited microscopic evidence of liver damage and lowered blood haemoglobin and erythrocyte counts (Keith 1932). Other effects of acute exposure to high doses of diacetone alcohol include lowering of blood pressure and narcosis. In groups of rats exposed to diacetone alcohol via their drinking water for 30 days, no evidence of toxicity was found at a dose level of 10 mg/kg body weight/day. At 40 mg/kg body weight/day, however, histopathological changes (unspecified) were reported (Smyth and Carpenter 1948).

Groups of ten male and ten female Wistar rats were given daily doses of 0, 200, 400 or 800 mg/kg body weight of menthol by gavage for 28 days. There were no effects on body weight gain, but absolute and relative liver weights were elevated at all dose levels in males and at the high and intermediate doses in females. Hepatocyte vacuolation was also noted in treated animals. No changes in haematology, clinical chemistry or the histopathology of a range of tissues other than the liver were reported (Thorup *et al* 1983). Menthol was reported to be cytotoxic in *in vitro* cellular systems at concentrations greater than 0.1 mM (Bernson and Pettersson 1983).

When tested in human volunteers, 9-decen-1-ol and 1-hexadecanol gave negative results for both skin irritation in patch tests and skin sensitisation (Opdyke 1974, 1978). 1-Dodecanol has also given negative results for human skin sensitisation (Opdyke 1973).

5.4.2 Chronic toxicity

None of the compounds in this group appear to have been tested for chronic toxicity in experimental animals.

5.4.3 Genotoxicity

Several members of this group have been tested for genotoxicity, and all have so far given negative results.

Dihydroactinidiolide was not found to be mutagenic in the Ames test to *Salmonella typhimurium* TA98, TA100 and TA1535, in either the presence or absence of metabolic activation, at a dose level of 100 μg/plate. It also gave negative results in the *Bacillus subtilis* rec assay at 10 mg/disk (Kinae *et al* 1981). Hexadecanol and octadecanol were found to be non-mutagenic in the Ames spot test to *Salmonella typhimurium* TA1538, TA1537, TA1535, TA100 and TA98, in either the presence or absence of metabolic activation, at a dose level of 50 μg/plate (Blevins and Taylor 1982). Phthalic anhydride was also reported to be non-mutagenic in the Ames test when tested in TA98, TA100, TA1535 and TA1537 in the presence or absence of either rat liver or hamster liver S-9 (Zeiger *et al* 1982). Menthol has given negative results for both mutagenicity in the Ames test (Andersen and Jensen 1984, Ishidate *et al* 1984) and for chromosome aberrations in a Chinese hamster cell line (Ishidate *et al* 1984). 4-Phenylphenol was also found to be negative for both mutagenicity in bacterial assays (Cline and McMahon 1977, Probst *et al* 1981) and unscheduled DNA synthesis in primary cultures of rat hepatocytes (Probst *et al* 1981).

Dobanol (a synthetic mixture comprising 41% dodecanol and 58% tridecanol) gave negative results for mutagenicity in the Ames test and *E. coli,* for mitotic gene conversion in *Saccharomyces cerevisiae,* and for chromosome damage in a rat liver cell line (Dean *et al* 1985).

5.4.4 Carcinogenicity

At 7 days of age, groups of 18 male and 18 female mice of both the (C57BL/6×C3H/Anf)F1 and (C57BL/6×AKR)F1 strains were given single doses of 464 mg/kg body weight of 4-phenylphenol by gavage. This dose, though not subsequently adjusted for changes in body weight, was then given each day for the next 4 weeks. From this time to the end of the study at 18 months, the animals were fed a diet containing 1400 mg/kg of 4-phenylphenol. There was no evidence that 4-phenylphenol was carcinogenic in this study (Innes *et al* 1969).

Phthalic anhydride has been tested in a carcinogenesis bioassay as part of the US National Toxicology Program. Groups of 50 male and 50 female F-344 rats were fed diets containing either 0, 7500 or 15 000 ppm for 102–106 weeks. A group of 50 male B6C3F1 mice were fed diets containing 0, 25 000 and 50 000 ppm for the initial 32 weeks and 0, 12 500 and 25 000 ppm for the remainder of the study. A group of 50 female mice were maintained on diets containing 0, 25 000 and 50 000 ppm for 32 weeks and 0, 6250 and 12 500 for the rest of the study. Reduced body weight gain was found in both sexes of mice, but survival was unaffected. There was no evidence for an increased tumour incidence in the treated animals (Kluwe *et al* 1982).

Neither menthol nor 1-dodecanol was found to increase the incidence of primary lung tumours in strain A mice given a range of doses by intraperitoneal injection, thrice weekly for 8 weeks and then observed until 24 weeks (Stoner *et al* 1973).

Thrice-weekly application of 1-dodecanol for 60 weeks to the skin of 30 mice previously initiated with dimethylbenzanthracene resulted in skin tumours in two of the mice. Severe skin irritation was also noted, suggesting that the possible weak tumour-promoting effect may have been due to the skin damage induced by 1-dodecanol rather than a true tumour-promotional action (Sice 1966). In an identical experiment with 1-hexadecanol, only one of 26 surviving mice developed a skin tumour (Sice 1966).

5.4.5 Reproductive toxicity

Phthalic anhydride has been reported to be teratogenic following intraperitoneal injection in CD-1 mice only at dose levels which were near lethal to the adults (Fabro *et al* 1982).

5.5 Discussion

The compounds in this group were identified only infrequently in the WRc survey. For some of them, their use would suggest that other routes of exposure may be more significant than water, but for many there is no information.

With respect to metabolism, the long-chain alcohols are probably incorporated into fatty acid biosynthesis and catabolism, but there is almost no information on the other compounds.

The acute toxic potential of these chemicals appears to be very low. However, there are no data available on chronic toxicity. Several members of the group have been tested in the Ames test and other *in vitro* assays and have given negative results. In carcinogenicity studies, 4-phenylphenol proved negative in mice while phthalic anhydride was negative in both rats and mice. Only phthalic anhydride appears to have been tested for reproductive toxicity. Evidence for teratogenicity was found only at dose levels which were near lethal to the adults.

The toxicology of this group of compounds has been poorly studied, but the limited information available would suggest that they are unlikely to present a risk to health at concentrations currently encountered in drinking water.

References

ANDERSEN P H and JENSEN N J (1984) Mutagenic investigation of peppermint oil in the *Salmonella*/mammalian-microsome test. *Mutation Research* **138,** 17-20.

BAXTER J H, STEINBERG D, MIZE C E and AVIGAN J (1967) Absorption and metabolism of uniformly ^{14}C-labeled phytol and phytanic acid by the intestine of the rat studied with thoracic duct cannulation. *Biochimica et Biophysica Acta* **137,** 277-290.

BELL O E Jr, BLANK M L and SNYDER F (1971) The incorporation of ^{18}O and ^{14}C from long-chain alcohols into the alkyl and alk-1-enyl ethers of phospholipids of developing rat brain. *Biochimica et Biophysica Acta* **231,** 579-583.

BERNSON V S M and PETTERSSON B (1983) The toxicity of menthol in short-term bioassays. *Chemicobiological Interactions* **46,** 233-246.

BLEVINS R D and TAYLOR D E (1982) Mutagenicity screening of twenty-five cosmetic ingredients with the Salmonella/microsome test. *Journal of Environmental Science and Health* [A] **17,** 217-239.

BOLUND S, FALUS F and JORGENSEN K (1967) *Scandinavian Journal of Clinical and Laboratory Investigation* **19,** 288-290.

CLINE J C and McMAHON R E (1977) Detection of chemical mutagens: use of concentration gradient plates in a high capacity screen. *Research Communications in Chemical Pathology and Pharmacology* **16,** 523-533.

DEAN B J, BROOKS T M, HODSON-WALKER G and HUTSON D H (1985) Genetic toxicology testing of 41 industrial chemicals. *Mutation Research* **153,** 57-77.

EPSTEIN W, GERBER K and KARLER R (1964) The hypnotic constituent of *Stipa vaseyi,* sleepy grass. *Experientia* **20,** 390.

FABRO S, SHULL G and BROWN N A (1982) The relative teratogenic index and teratogenic potency: proposed components of developmental toxicity risk assessment. *Teratogenesis, Carcinogenesis and Mutagenesis* **2,** 61-76.

HENATSCH J J and JUTTNER F (1983) Volatile odorous excretion products of different strains of *Synechococcus* (cyanobacteria). *Water Science and Technology* **15,** 259-266.

INNES J R M, ULLAND B M, VALERIO M G, PETRUCELLI L, FISHBEIN L, HART E R, PALLOTTA A J, BATES R R, FALK H L, GART J J, KLEIN M, MITCHELL I and PETERS J (1969) Bioassay of pesticides and industrial chemicals for tumorigenicity in mice: A preliminary note. *Journal of the National Cancer Institute* **42,** 1101-1114.

ISHIDATE M Jr, SOFUNI T, YOSHIKAWA K, HAYASHI M, NOHMI T, SAWADA M and MATSUOKA A (1984) Primary mutagenicity screening of food additives currently used in Japan. *Food and Chemical Toxicology* **22,** 623-636.

KEITH H M (1932) Effect of diacetone alcohol on the liver of the rat. *Archives of Pathology* **13,** 707-712.

KINAE N, HASHIZUME T, MAKITA T, TOMITA I, KIMURA J and KANAMORI H (1981) Studies on the toxicity of pulp and paper mill effluents. 1 Mutagenicity of the sediment samples derived from Kraft paper mills. *Water*

Research **15,** 17-24.
KLUWE W M, McCONNELL E E, HUFF J E, HASEMAN J K, DOUGLAS J F and HARTWELL W V (1982) Carcinogenicity testing of phthalate esters and related compounds by the National Toxicology Program and the National Cancer Institute. *Environmental Health Perspectives* **45,** 129-133.
McISAAC W M and WILLIAMS R T (1958) The metabolism of spermaceti. *West African Journal of Biological Chemistry* **2,** 42-44.
OPDYKE D L J (1973) Fragrance raw materials monographs: alcohol C-12. *Food and Cosmetics Toxicology* **11,** 109.
OPDYKE D L J (1974) Fragrance raw materials monographs: decylenic alcohol. *Food and Cosmetics Toxicology* **12,** 405.
OPDYKE D L J (1978) Fragrance raw materials monographs: cetyl alcohol. *Food and Cosmetics Toxicology* **16,** 683-686.
PROBST G S, McMAHON R E, HILL L E, THOMPSON C Z, EPP J K and NEAL S B (1981) Chemically-induced unscheduled DNA synthesis in primary rat hepatocyte cultures: a comparison with bacterial mutagenicity using 218 compounds. *Environmental Mutagenesis* **3,** 11-32.
REGISTRY OF TOXIC EFFECTS OF CHEMICAL SUBSTANCES National Institute for Occupational Safety and Health, Cincinnati, Ohio.
SICE J (1966) Tumor-promoting activity of *n*-alkanes 1-alkanols. *Toxicology and Applied Pharmacology* **9,** 70-74.
SMYTH H F Jr and CARPENTER C P (1948) Further experience with the range finding test in the industrial toxicology laboratory. *Journal of Industrial Hygiene and Toxicology* **30,** 63-68.
STEVENS K L and MERRILL G B (1980) Growth inhibitors from spikerush. *Journal of Agricultural and Food Chemistry* **28,** 644-646.
STONER G D, SHIMKIN M B, KNIAZEFF A J, WEISBURGER J H and GORI G B (1973) Test for carcinogenicity of food additives and chemotherapeutic agents by the pulmonary tumour response in strain A mice. *Cancer Research* **33,** 3069-3085.
THORUP I, WURTZEN G, CARSTENSEN J and OLSEN P (1983) Short term toxicity study in rats dosed with pulegone and menthol. *Toxicology Letters* **19,** 207-210.
WATER RESEARCH CENTRE (1981) Organic micropollutants in drinking water. WRc Technical Report TR 159.
WATER RESEARCH CENTRE (1982) Frequency of occurrence data for compounds identified by GC–MS in XAD-2 samples taken for mutagenic testing survey. WRc unpublished report.
ZEIGER E, HAWORTH S, SPECK W and MORTELMANS K (1982) Phthalate ester testing in the National Toxicology Program's Environmental Mutagenesis Test Development Program. *Environmental Health Perspectives* **45,** 99-101.

20

The phenyl alkanes

1. INTRODUCTION

Phenylalkanes are the mono-alkyl derivatives of benzene. They are derived from petroleum, and their principal uses are as solvents and as intermediates in the synthesis of plastics, paint, pesticides and resin coatings. Phenyldodecane is also used commercially in the manufacture of detergents.

2. EXPOSURE

2.1 Air

Although phenylalkanes have been detected in car exhaust fumes (Lonneman *et al* 1968), there is no evidence to suggest that these compounds are present at significant levels in ambient air.

2.2 Food

There appears to be no information available on the occurrence of phenylalkanes in food.

2.3 Water

The following were identified in drinking water by WRc, although all occurred only infrequently (Water Research Centre 1981).

1-Phenylhexane
2-Phenylhexane
Phenylheptane
1-Phenyloctane
2-Phenyloctane
Phenylnonane
1-Phenyldecane
2-Phenyldecane

3. TOXICOKINETICS

Phenylalkanes may be absorbed from the gastrointestinal tract, or by inhalation (Gerarde 1960b). There is insufficient evidence to assess their potential for skin penetration (Gerarde and Linden 1959). Due to the high lipid solubility of these compounds they readily accummulate in fatty tissues.

Within 72 hours of a single oral dose of phenyldodecane about 90% was metabolised, then excreted in the urine as alcohols and carboxylic acids, while 10% remained in the body tissues. Very little of the original dose was detected in the expired air. Phenyldodecane administered to rats, subcutaneously, at a dose level of 5 ml/kg had no effect on the urinary sulphate ratio, in contrast to the decrease following the administration of benzene (Gerarde 1960b).

Phenylalkanes are metabolised almost exclusively by oxidation of the aliphatic side chain. The resulting metabolites may then be excreted in the urine as glucuronide or glutathione conjugates, or they may be degraded by fatty acid β-oxidation.

4. HEALTH EFFECTS

4.1 Acute and subacute toxicity

Phenylalkanes have a low order of acute toxicity. Phenyldodecane has an oral LD50 of more than 5 ml/kg (4300 mg/kg) in the male albino rat, while Dobane, a commercial mixture of C10–C13 phenylalkanes, has an oral LD50 value of 3 ml/kg (2580 mg/kg) (Gerarde 1960a).

Aliphatic chain length influences the activity of the phenylalkanes in that acute oral toxicity decreases as the number of carbon atoms in the side chain of a phenylalkane increases. This inverse relationship is also true for skin irritation, inflammatory responses and narcotic potency (Gerarde and Linden 1959).

Inhalation and direct contact of liquid phenylalkanes with lung tissue can result in pulmonary oedema, haemorrhage and tissue necrosis. However, this is a general reaction to hydrocarbons, since their low surface tension properties enable a small volume of chemical to spread over a large surface area, causing extensive damage and membrane irritation (Gerarde 1960a).

Rats given daily subcutaneous injections of 10 ml/kg (8600 mg/kg) of an unspecified phenylalkane compound for 2 weeks showed no reduction in growth rate. The haemopoietic system also appeared to be unaffected, since the size of the white cell population remained stable and blood-forming tissue such as the spleen and thymus did not exhibit any organ enlargement.

The lack of data, particularly recent information, on phenylalkanes may be due to the apparently low industrial hazard associated with these compounds.

4.2 Chronic toxicity

Repeated contact with phenyldodecane may cause dermatitis, due to removal of natural oils from the skin (Gerarde 1960a). No recent information on the chronic toxicity of these compounds appears to be available.

4.3 Genotoxicity

Dobane was not mutagenic in the Ames test with *Salmonella typhimurium* TA98, TA100, TA1535, TA1537 or TA1538 at dose levels ranging from 125 to 4000 μg per plate, either in the presence or absence of metabolic activation. It also gave negative results for mitotic gene conversion in *Saccharomyces cerevisiae* JDI and for structural chromosome damage in a cultured rat liver cell line (Dean *et al* 1985).

No other information on the mutagenicity of phenylalkanes appears to be available.

4.4 Carcinogenicity

There is some evidence to suggest that phenylalkanes are promoting agents in mouse skin (Horton *et al* 1957). A single application of 0.6% 7,12-dimethylbenz[*a*]anthracene (DMBA) in white mineral oil upon the skin of C3H mice was followed by multiple application of a selected hydrocarbon over a period of 6 months. In this study, for a given concentration of carcinogen, long-chain hydrocarbon solvents, such as dodecane and phenyldodecane, led to a higher rate of tumour induction on mouse skin than did solutions composed of short-chain hydrocarbon solvents. These solvents, when uncontaminated with impurities, did not themselves induce tumours, although they are skin irritants.

4.5 Reproductive toxicity

No information appears to be available.

5. DISCUSSION

Phenylalkanes are released from car and motorboat exhaust and so may be detected both in the atmosphere and in water, but there are only limited data on the concentrations likely to be encountered. These compounds are readily absorbed into the body and accumulate in fatty tissues, due to their lipophilic nature. In the liver they are rapidly metabolised by oxidation of the aliphatic side chain.

Like the short-chain alkylbenzenes, the long-chain phenylalkanes appear to be of low acute and chronic toxicity. Their principal toxic effect is on the CNS, but, in contrast to the neurotoxic, convulsant properties of benzene, they are CNS depressants. They also do not share the depression in bone marrow function shown by benzene.

Dobane, a commercial mixture of phenylalkanes, displayed no genotoxic activity when tested in bacteria, yeast and in a rat liver cell line. There is some evidence that phenylalkane solvents can act as promoting agents. No information appears to be available on the reproductive toxicity of these compounds.

Although there are little recent data on phenylalkanes, from the limited information available and from evidence on the short-chain alkyl-benzenes it appears unlikely that they represent a hazard to human health at the low levels currently encountered in drinking water.

REFERENCES

DEAN B J, BROOKS T M, HODSON-WALKER G and HUTSON D H (1985) Genetic toxicology testing of 41 industrial chemicals. *Mutation Research* **153**, 57-77.

GERARDE H W (1960a) *Toxicology and biochemistry of aromatic hydrocarbons.* Elsevier Publishing Company.

GERARDE H W (1960b) The toxicology and biochemistry of the mono-cyclic aromatic hydrocarbons. *Medical Bulletin of New Jersey* **20**, 1, 74-90.

GERARDE H W and LINDEN N J (1959) Toxicological studies on hydrocarbons. III. The biochemorphology of the phenylalkanes and phenylalkenes. *AMA Archives of Industrial Health* **19**, 403-418.

HORTON A W, DENMAN D T and TROSSET R P (1957) Carcinogenesis of the skin II. The accelerating properties of aliphatic and related hydrocarbons. *Cancer Research* **17**, 758-766.

LONNEMAN W A, BELLAR T A and ALTSHULLER A P (1968) Aromatic hydrocarbons in the atmosphere of the Los Angeles basin. *Environmental Science and Technology* **2**(11), 1017-1020.

WATER RESEARCH CENTRE (1981) Organic micropollutants in drinking water. WRc Technical Report TR 159.

21

The carboxylic acids

1. INTRODUCTION

Carboxylic acids are a large group of compounds with a very wide range of industrial applications, including the manufacture of dyes, food additives, resins, plasticisers, lubricants, perfumes and soaps. Many also occur naturally in the body and in foods.

2. EXPOSURE

2.1 Air

There appears to be no information available on the occurrence of these carboxylic acids in the atmosphere.

2.2 Food

Long-chain fatty acids are present in a wide variety of foodstuffs, including meat, fruits, beverages and dairy products. They are an important and common constituent of normal diets, contributing up to 40% of the total energy requirement in a normal human diet. Lactic acid, toluic acid and long-chain fatty acids, are used extensively in the food processing industry as food additives (Food Additives and Contaminants Committee 1976).

2.3 Water

The carboxylic acids identified by WRc, with the exception of lactic, toluic and benzoic acids, were all long-chain aliphatic monocarboxylic acids (fatty acids). None were polyenoic (polyunsaturated essential fatty acids) and there was one monoenoic acid, oleic acid (Water Research Centre 1981).

The most frequently identified compounds were:

Lauric acid	6/14 samples
Myristic acid	5/14 samples
Palmitic acid	5/14 samples

The other carboxylic acids identified were:

Benzoic acid
Decanoic acid
Heptadecanoic acid
4-hydroxybenzoic acid
Isopropylbenzoic acid
Lactic acid
Nonanoic acid
Octanoic acid
Oleic acid
Pentadecanoic acid
Steric acid
Succinic acid
Tridecanoic acid
Toluic acid

A similar range of carboxylic acids have also been identified in a sample of US drinking water (Coleman *et al* 1980).

3. TOXICOKINETICS

Aliphatic carboxylic acids are readily absorbed from the intestine, although this occurs more rapidly with acids having shorter chains. Fatty acids may be used in the synthesis of phospholipids, triglycerides, cholesterol and sterol esters. Most fatty acids are metabolised by β-oxidation, resulting in formation of acetyl CoA, propionyl CoA and ketone bodies. The ketone bodies may be further metabolised or excreted unchanged in the urine (Lehninger 1975). In some cases, medium-chain fatty acids are partly oxidised by ω-oxidation, producing dicarboxylic acids which can be catabolised by β-oxidation from either end of the molecule. It is unusual for acids of more than 12 carbons to be catabolised by ω-oxidation, although it may occur in the metabolism of lauric (C-12) and palmitic (C-16) acids (Das *et al* 1968, Guest *et al* 1982), and often becomes important when the capacity for β-oxidation is either exceeded or blocked by substituents at the alpha- or beta- position of the molecule.

Experiments with human volunteers using orally administered ^{14}C-labelled fatty acids were performed by Forsgren (1969), in which each person received 10 μCi of one acid. The radiolabel recovery as exhaled CO_2 was 47%, 57% and 44% for lauric acid, decanoic acid and myristic acid, respectively.

In man and the higher primates, toluic acid is primarily excreted as the glutamine conjugate, phenylacetylglutamine (Anon 1944, Power and Sherwin 1927), although some toluic acid is excreted in an unchanged form (Power and Sherwin 1927). Phenylacetylglutamate is a normal constituent of human urine, the amounts excreted being in the order of 250–500 mg/day (Williams 1959).

Lactic acid and succinic acid are normal products of mammalian metabolism, and can thus be metabolised by incorporation into biochemical pathways.

In humans, benzoic acid is conjugated with glucuronide and excreted in the urine as hippuric acid (Bridges *et al* 1970).

4. HEALTH EFFECTS

4.1 Acute and subacute toxicity

There are acute oral LD50 data available for about half the compounds in this group. Values given for the rat range from 2.2 to 12.0 g/kg (Guest *et al* 1982, Smyth *et al* 1962, Jenner *et al* 1964, Fassett 1963, Opdyke 1979). Oro and Wretlind (1961) showed the acute intravenous LD50 of fatty acids in the mouse to range between 23 and 1725 mg/kg. Therefore it is likely that the acids identified by WRc are of low acute toxicity.

The fatty acids are slightly irritating to the skin and eyes of humans and experimental animals. This effect is more pronounced with the shorter chain acids, since they are stronger acids and have greater ability to penetrate the skin than the long-chain fatty acids (Guest *et al* 1982).

It has been shown that *ortho-*, *meta-*, and *para*-toluic acids are potential sensitisers of human skin. Three out of five human volunteers sensitised by repeated application of 50% *ortho*-toluic acid powder later reacted when challenged with 0.5% *meta*-toluic acid in petroleum. All five subjects sensitised to *ortho-* and *para*-toluic acid, by simultaneous application of both materials, also reacted later to 50% *meta*-toluic acid (Emmett and Suskind 1973).

Within minutes of a single intravenous injection in rats of 250 μl of an oleic acid suspension (oleic acid shaken in 0.1 mg/l of a solution of albumin in saline (1 : 5 v/v)) there were marked changes in the lung, including perivascular and intra-alveolar oedema, intravascular coagulation and intra-alveolar haemorrhage. After 24 hours there was extensive interstitial infiltration and vascular congestion. This lesion was characteristic of respiratory distress syndrome, in which the physiological changes include increased pulmonary and atrial pressures, decreased systemic pressures and severe hypoxemia (Dickey *et al* 1981).

Oro and Wretlind (1961) showed that intravenous injections of heptadecanoic acid into the tail vein of mice led to convulsions, collapse and hyperapnoea, at doses approaching the LD50 (36 mg/kg). Heptadecanoic acid exhibited immunosuppressive activity *in vitro* by a decrease in phytohaemagglutinin reactivity, when 0.7 μ mol and 0.1 μ mol were added to human lymphocytes and rat spleen preparations, respectively (Smith *et al* 1976).

In rats, intraperitoneal injection of 150 mg/kg/day of toluic acid for 7 days had no effect on liver mixed function oxidase, cytochrome P-450, microsomal protein content or microsomal UDP-glucuronyl transferase activity (Lake *et al* 1980).

Rats fed a dietary level of 1–2% α-toluic acid (equivalent to 500–1000 mg/kg) for 13–14 days showed an increase in liver weight, and changes in hepatocytes such as the presence of cup-shaped mitochondria and vacuoles containing amorphous dense material (Hruban *et al* 1966). The numbers of test and control animals used in these experiments were small.

4.2 Chronic toxicity

There appeared to be no effects on gross organ pathology or individual organ weights when five male rats were fed a diet containing 10% lauric acid for 18 weeks (Fitzhugh 1960). Twenty-four rats fed a diet containing 25% lauric acid triglycerides for 2 years showed no adverse pathological effects, apart from slight excess of liver cell fatty changes compared to control rats on a basic diet. The changes were no more severe, however, than those observed in control rats fed with hydrogenated vegetable oil at the same dosage.

Weekly injections of oleic acid into dogs at a dose of 90 mg/kg for 1–3 months produced pulmonary changes. The main effects observed were type 2 cell proliferation and pulmonary fibrosis (Derks and Jacobovitz-Derks 1977).

No information on the chronic toxicity of decanoic acid in man was found, but Reye's syndrome in children has been associated with high serum levels of C8–C10 carboxylic acids (Mamunes *et al* 1974). The syndrome is characterised by encephalopathy, fatty infiltration of the liver and hepatic disease.

4.3 Genotoxicity

Octanoic acid (98% purity) did not exhibit mutagenic activity in a series of *in vitro* assays with *Salmonella typhimurium* and *Saccharomyces cerevisiae*, either with or without metabolic activation (Litton Bionetics Inc 1976).

Lactic acid USP (a mixture containing 85–90% lactic acid) and calcium lactate USP at concentrations of up to 0.18% and 0.625%, respectively, did not exhibit mutagenic activity in *in vitro* assays using strains of *Saccharomyces cerevisiae* or *Salmonella typhimurium*, with or without activation by mouse, rat or monkey liver homogenates (Select Committee on GRAS substances 1980).

Oleic acid gave negative mutagenicity results in Ames tests using five strains of *Salmonella*, in either the presence or absence of rat or hamster liver S-9 (Mortelmans *et al* 1986).

Hayatsu *et al* (1981) showed that oleic acid, obtained by the ether extraction of normal human faeces, possessed antimutagenic activity against a number of compounds including pyrolysis products, benzo(*a*)pyrene, and aflatoxin B1, although the mechanism of this action is unknown. However, addition of oleic acid to the diet of rats treated with 1,2-dimethylhydrazine, a colon carcinogen, failed to protect the rats against induction of colon cancer (Nelson and Samelson 1984).

4.4 Carcinogenicity

The addition of sodium oleate (2.5% and 5.0%) in the drinking water of groups of 50 male and 50 female rats for 108 weeks did not result in any significant difference in the incidence of tumours between treated rats and controls (Hiasa *et al* 1985).

Tumours were found in female mice after repeated administration of lauric acid by subcutaneous injection. In 16 mice given a total dose of 125 mg of lauric acid in 2.5 ml of tricaprylin over 12.5 weeks there were two leukaemic lymphomas seen after the fourth and fifth months, one subcutaneous sarcoma and one pulmonary tumour after 18 months. Only five animals survived to the eighteenth month. One pulmonary tumour was observed in 29 control animals dosed with 1.0 ml of tricaprylin. Only four of the controls survived to the eighteenth month (Swern *et al* 1970). However, this study must be considered unsatisfactory due to the high mortality of the control animals.

No evidence of carcinogenicity was observed after daily topical applications of 20% and 40% lauric acid in chloroform to the skin of 60 mice for 31 weeks (Holsti 1959). Forty control animals were skin-painted with chloroform alone, and no tumours were observed after 25 weeks.

4.5 Reproductive toxicity

The English abstract of a Russian paper reports that toluic acid produced embryotoxic effects in rats. Daily oral administration of 450 mg/kg of toluic acid to pregnant rats during critical periods of embryogenesis retarded weight gain and skeletal ossification in the embryos, and reduced their liver RNA content. The number of resorbed embryos was doubled (Maganova and Zatsev 1973). Doses of 45 mg/kg/day thoughout pregnancy also retarded skeletal ossification. There was no evidence of embryotoxicity or anatomical defects at levels of 4.5 mg/kg/day (Maganova and Zatsev 1975).

Decanoic acid caused cytolysis in the eggs of amphibians after one hour's incubation (Sentien and Vannereau 1969). No data are available for the effects of decanoic acid on mammalian reproduction.

5. DISCUSSION

Most of the carboxylic acids identified by WRc in drinking water exist naturally in foods or are used as food additives. Others occur as normal metabolites in the body.

The fatty acids are readily absorbed from the gastrointestinal tract, metabolised mainly by β- or ω-oxidation and excreted via the kidneys or lungs.

The information available on carboxylic acids suggests that this group of compounds are of low acute toxicity, and few studies of the chronic toxic effects of these compounds have been performed. None of the acids tested have shown mutagenic activity, and although only limited data are available on carcinogenicity it would seem unlikely that this group of compounds would exhibit significant carcinogenic activity.

Few reproductive toxicity studies have been performed, but the existing evidence indicates that aliphatic carboxylic acids are not toxic to the reproductive system, although toluic acid has been shown to be embryotoxic to rats at high doses.

From the limited information available, the very low concentrations of fatty acids in drinking water appear unlikely to represent a hazard to human health.

6. REFERENCES

ANON (1944) Illinois Industrial Hygiene Division Laboratory Bulletin No 7, 4, and 12. *Journal of Industrial Hygiene and Toxicology* **26**, 103A (cited in Patty F A, *Industrial Hygiene and Toxicology* Vol 2, 2nd Edn, Interscience Publishers, New York).

BRIDGES J W, FRENCH M R, SMITH R L and WILLIAMS R T (1970) The fate of benzoic acid in various species. *Biochemical Journal* **118**, 47-51.

BRIGGS B B (1976) Safety studies on a series of fatty acids. *American Industrial Hygiene Association Journal* **37**, 251-253.

COLEMAN W E, MELTON R G, KOPFLER F C, BARONE K A, AURAND T A and JELLISON M G (1980) Identification of organic compounds in a mutagenic extract of a surface drinking water by a computerised gas chromatography/mass spectrometry system (GC/MS/COM). *Environmental Science and Technology* **14**, 576-588.

DAS M L, ORRENIUS S and ERNSTER L (1968) On the fatty acid and hydrocarbon hydroxylation in rat liver microsomes. *European Journal of Biochemistry* **4**, 519-523.

DERKS C M and JACOBOVITZ-DERKS D (1977) Embolic pneumopathy induced by oleic acid. *American Journal of Pathology* **87**, 143-158.

DICKEY B F, THRALL R S, McCORMICK J R and WARD P A (1981) Oleic acid induced lung injury in the rat. *American Journal of Pathology* **103**(3), 376-383.

EMMETT E A and SUSKIND R R (1973) Allergic contact sensitisation to the toluic acids. *Journal of Investigative Dermatology* **61**, 282-285.

FASSETT D W (1963) *In Industrial Hygiene and Toxicology*, 2nd edition, Vol 2 edited by D W Fassett and D D Irish. Wiley–Interscience, New York.

FITZHUGH O G (1960) Oral toxicities of lauric acid and certain lauric acid derivatives. *Toxicology and Applied Pharmacology* **2**, 59-67.

FORSGREN L (1969) Expiratory pattern of $^{14}CO_2$ in man after feeding ^{14}C-labelled fatty acids. *Arkiv for Kemi* **30**, 355-361.

GUEST D, KATZ G V and ASTILL B D (1982) Aliphatic carboxylic acids. In *Patty's Industrial Hygiene and Toxicology* edited by G D Clayton and F E Clayton, Vol 2C, 3rd Revised Edition. Wiley–Interscience, New York, pp. 4901–4988.

HAYATSU H, ARIMOTO S, TOGAWA K and MAKITA M (1981) Inhibitory effect of the ether extract of human faeces on activities of mutagens: inhibition by oleic and linoleic acids. *Mutation Research* **81**, 287-293.

HIASA Y, KONISHI N, KITAHORI Y and SHIMOYAMA T (1985) Carcinogenicity study of a commercial sodium oleate in Fischer rats. *Food and Chemical Toxicology* **23**, 610-623.

HOLSTI P (1959) Tumour promoting effects of some long chain fatty acids in experimental skin carcinogenesis in the mouse. *Acta Pathologica et Microbiologica Scandinavica* **46**, 51-58.

HRUBAN Z, SWIFT H and SLESERS A (1966) Ultrastructural alteration of hepatic microbodies. *Laboratory Investigations* **15**, 1884-1901.

JENNER P M, HAGAN E C, TAYLOR J M, COOK E L and FITZHUGH O G (1964) Food flavourings and compounds of related structure. 1. Acute oral toxicity. *Food and Cosmetics Toxicology* **2**, 327-343.

LAKE B G (1980) The effect of treatment with some phase 2 substrates on hepatic xenobiotic metabolism and the urinary excretion of metabolites of the D-glucuronic acid pathway in the rat. *Toxicology and Applied Pharmacology* **52**, 371-378.

LEHNINGER A L (1975) In *Biochemistry*, 2nd edition, Worth Publishers Inc, New York, pp. 543-559.

LITTON BIONETICS INC (1976) Mutagenic evaluation of compounds FDA 75-38 000124-07-2 caprylic acid 98%. Food and Drug Administration Report FDA/BF 76/114. National Technical Information Service Report No PB-2527872.

MAMUNES P, DEVRIES G H, MILLER C D and DAVID R B (1974) In *Proceedings on a Conference on Reye's Syndrome* p 245. Cited in Opdyke D L J. Food and Cosmetics Toxicology 1979, 735-741.

MAGANOVA N B and ZAITSEV A N (1973) A study into the embryotoxic effects of some synthetic food aromatizers. *Voprosy Pitaniya* **32**, 50-54.

MAGANOVA N B and ZAITSEV A N (1975) Embryotoxic action of some food aromatizers. *Voprosy Pitaniya* **34**, 64-68.

MORTELMANS K, HAWORTH S, LAWLOR T, SPECK W, TAINER B and ZEIGER E (1986) Salmonella mutagenicity tests: 2. Results from the testing of 270 chemicals. *Environmental Mutagenesis* **8**, suppl. 7, 1-119.

NELSON R L and SAMELSON S L (1984) Inability of the mutagen-blocking agent oleic acid to protect against colon carcinogenesis in the rat. *Mutation Research* **140**, 155-157.

NISHIKAWA Y, OKABE M, YISHIMOTO K, KURONO G and FUKUOKO F (1976) Chemical and biochemical studies on carbohydrate esters: 2. Antitumour activity of saturated fatty acids and their ester derivatives against Ehrlich Ascites Carcinoma. *Chemical and Pharmaceutical Bulletin* **24**(3), 387-393.

OPDYKE D L J (1979) Fragrance raw materials monographs: stearic acid. *Food and Cosmetics Toxicology* **17**, 383-388.

OPDYKE D L J (1979) Fragrance raw materials monographs: capric acid. *Food and Cosmetics Toxicology* **17**, 735-741.

ORO L and WRETLIND A (1961) Pharmacological effects of fatty acids, triolein and cottonseed oil. *Acta Pharmacologica et Toxicologica* **18**, 141-152.

POWER F W and SHERWIN C P (1927) The detoxication of putrefactive products by the human body. *Archives of Internal Medicine* **39**, 60-66.

SELECT COMMITTEE ON GRAS SUBSTANCES (1980) Lactic acid and calcium lactate. Report of Select Committee on GRAS substances. PB-238-713/AS. National Technical Information Service, Springfield, Virginia. (Cited in Federal Register 1980 45 32324).

SENTIEN P and VANNEREAU H (1969) *Comptes Rendus des Seances de la Societe Biologie et de ses Filiales* **163**, 1895. (Cited in Opdyke D L J 1979.)

SMITH A D, TSANG W M, WEYMAN C and BELIN J (1976) Immunosuppression by fatty acids. *Lancet* **2**, 254-255.

SMYTH H F, CARPENTER C P, WEIL C S and POZZANI U C (1954) Range-finding toxicity data. List 5. *Archives of Industrial Hygiene and Occupational Medicine* **10**, 61-68.

SWERN D, WEIDER R, McDONOUGH M, MERANZE D R and SHIMKIN M B (1970) Investigation of fatty acids and derivatives for carcinogenic activity. *Cancer Research* **30**, 1037-1046.

WATER RESEARCH CENTRE (1981) Organic micropollutants in drinking water. WRc Technical Report TR 159.

WILLIAMS A M (1959) *Detoxification mechanisms*, 2nd Edn. Chapman and Hall, London.

Index